Atlas of Sellar and Parasellar Lesions

Gabriel Zada • M. Beatriz S. Lopes
Srinivasan Mukundan Jr. • Edward R. Laws Jr.
Editors

Atlas of Sellar and Parasellar Lesions

Clinical, Radiologic, and Pathologic Correlations

Springer

Editors
Gabriel Zada
Department of Neurosurgery
University of Southern California
Los Angeles, CA
USA

Srinivasan Mukundan Jr.
Department of Radiology
Brigham and Women's Hospital
Boston, MA
USA

M. Beatriz S. Lopes
Department of Pathology
University of Virginia
Charlottesville, VA
USA

Edward R. Laws Jr.
Department of Neurosurgery
Brigham and Women's Hospital
Boston, MA
USA

ISBN 978-3-319-22854-9 ISBN 978-3-319-22855-6 (eBook)
DOI 10.1007/978-3-319-22855-6

Library of Congress Control Number: 2015953343

Springer Cham Heidelberg New York Dordrecht London

Printed on acid-free paper

Springer International Publishing AG Switzerland is part of Springer Science+Business Media (www.springer.com)

We would like to dedicate this atlas to the many gifted teachers and physicians on whose shoulders we have stood and in particular to Dr. Harvey Cushing, who laid the foundation for this work. We would also like to dedicate this atlas to our patients, who have equally taught and inspired us.

Preface

The sella turcica and parasellar area are rich and intricate anatomic regions of the intracranial cavity. They form a unique spatial confluence of numerous key anatomic and physiologic systems. The normal anatomic organization and functional integrity of the important structures contained within this small space may be easily distorted by any number of diverse pathological processes arising in and around this region. For this reason, patients presenting with diseases of the sellar and parasellar region may seek the expertise of numerous medical practitioners, including family practitioners, neurologists, ophthalmologists, otolaryngologists, endocrinologists, and neurosurgeons, among many others. In addition, optimization of treatment for patients with pituitary disease and other lesions of the sellar and parasellar region is best provided by a multidisciplinary team comprised of these very specialties, with the assistance of neuroradiologists, radiation oncologists, neuro-oncologists, neuropathologists, and others. The spectrum of disease arising in the sellar region ranges from functional pituitary adenomas causing hormonal excess syndromes such as acromegaly or Cushing's disease, to a variety of cystic lesions, to metastatic or other malignant tumors, infections, inflammatory diseases, and vascular lesions, among many others. The assortment of entities presenting in this small yet immensely critical region is as diverse as anywhere else in the human body.

After treating many patients with sellar lesions, one begins to develop a sense for both the typical features and uniqueness of each patient and his or her disease, with regard to the clinical presentation, anatomic features, imaging characteristics, and pathology. Fortunately, patterns in the clinical presentation and underlying disease processes do emerge and can be used to understand the disease process and to optimally treat patients. An understanding of the endocrinologic, visual, and neurologic features of processes occurring in this region is paramount to diagnosing sellar and parasellar lesions and managing these patients. Similarly, a thorough understanding of the anatomic relationships among the pituitary gland, infundibulum, optic chiasm and nerves, internal carotid arteries, cranial nerves, hypothalamus, and third ventricle is mandatory. Our collective ability to effectively manage the variety of sellar and parasellar pathology has evolved tremendously over the past three decades, resulting from the development of many technological advances, including improved imaging modalities, radioimmunoassay techniques, hormone replacement therapy, the operative microscope and microsurgical technique, endoscopic neurosurgery, and radiosurgery.

Most cases in this atlas have been collected over the senior author's experience of over three decades of treating patients with sellar and parasellar disease. Traversing the sphenoid sinus more than 5000 times in order to treat patients with a wide spectrum of sellar and parasellar lesions has led to a deep appreciation for the amazing catalogue of findings possible in this region. It is our hope that the cases, images, and clinical and operative "pearls" in this atlas will convey a sense of marvel for the intricacy of this region of the body and will impart the benefit of our experience in precisely accessing this region surgically, improving the lives of patients with the many types of pathologic processes occurring here.

Los Angeles, CA, USA — Gabriel Zada, MD, MS
Charlottesville, VA, USA — M. Beatriz S. Lopes, MD, PhD
Boston, MA, USA — Srinivasan Mukundan Jr., PhD, MD
Boston, MA, USA — Edward Laws Jr., MD

Acknowledgments

This work could not have been accomplished without the same kind of multidisciplinary approach that we utilize clinically. With the assistance of so many experts from a variety of perspectives and roles, we have been successful. Those involved include our office and medical assistants, our nurses, nurse practitioners and physician assistants, our residents and fellows, and so many of our medical and surgical colleagues.

Particular mention goes to Dr. Raymond Huang, who was essential in creating the imaging segments; Dr. Kyle Hurth who helped with selected pathology images; Dr. Eric Ojerholm who collated and organized the case material; and Lee Klein from Springer who masterfully coordinated the production of this atlas.

Contents

Contributors

Paolo Cappabianca, MD Division of Neurosurgery, Department of Neurosciences, Reproductive and Odontostomatological Sciences, Universita' degli Studi di Napoli Federico II, Naples, Italy

John D. Carmichael, MD Division of Endocrinology and Diabetes, Department of Medicine, University of Southern California Pituitary Center, Los Angeles, CA, USA

Luigi Maria Cavallo, MD, PhD Division of Neurosurgery, Department of Neurosciences, Reproductive and Odontostomatological Sciences, Universita' degli Studi di Napoli Federico II, Naples, Italy

Ching-Jen Chen, MD Department of Neurosurgery, University of Virginia Health System, Charlottesville, VA, USA

Dale Ding, MD Department of Neurosurgery, University of Virginia, Charlottesville, VA, USA

Ian F. Dunn, MD Department of Neurosurgery, Brigham and Women's Hospital, Boston, MA, USA

Raymond Y. Huang, MD, PhD Department of Radiology, Brigham and Women's Hospital, Boston, MA, USA

Edward Laws Jr , MD Department of Neurosurgery, Brigham and Women's Hospital, Boston, MA, USA

M. Beatriz S. Lopes, MD, PhD Department of Pathology (Neuropathology), University of Virginia School of Medicine, Charlottesville, VA, USA

Joshua W. Lucas, MD Department of Neurosurgery, Keck School of Medicine, University of Southern California, Los Angeles, CA, USA

Srinivasan Mukundan Jr , PhD, MD Department of Radiology, Brigham and Women's Hospital, Boston, MA, USA

Miriam Padilla, MD Division of Endocrinology and Diabetes, Department of Medicine, University of Southern California Pituitary Center, Los Angeles, CA, USA

Jason Sheehan, MD, PhD Department of Neurosurgery, University of Virginia, Charlottesville, VA, USA

Domenico Solari, MD, PhD Division of Neurosurgery, Department of Neurosciences, Reproductive and Odontostomatological Sciences, Universita' degli Studi di Napoli Federico II, Naples, Italy

Teresa Somma, MD Division of Neurosurgery, Department of Neurosciences, Reproductive and Odontostomatological Sciences, Universita' degli Studi di Napoli Federico II, Naples, Italy

Robert M. Starke, MD Department of Neurosurgery, University of Virginia, Charlottesville, VA, USA

Alessandro Villa, MD Division of Neurosurgery, Department of Neurosciences, Reproductive and Odontostomatological Sciences, Universita' degli Studi di Napoli Federico II, Naples, Italy

Gabriel Zada, MD, MS Department of Neurological Surgery, Keck School of Medicine, University of Southern California, Los Angeles, CA, USA

Part I

Basic Principles

Anatomy of the Sellar and Parasellar Region

1

Luigi Maria Cavallo, Domenico Solari, Alessandro Villa, Teresa Somma, and Paolo Cappabianca

1.1 Introduction

The skull base is one of the most complex anatomical regions, incorporating many different anatomical structures. The pathology of the skull base may involve a variety of lesions, neoplastic and otherwise, whose management can be difficult. In the past, this area has been accessed by many extensive and often aesthetically disfiguring transcranial and/or transfacial approaches, including the anterior, anterolateral, and posterolateral routes.

The transsphenoidal route facilitates access to the skull base via the nose. Because of its versatility, it can be considered the least traumatic route to the sella. The transsphenoidal route provides excellent visualization of the pituitary gland and related pathology, and it offers lower morbidity and mortality than open approaches to this region [1–3]. The wider, panoramic view offered by the endoscope has propelled the development of a variety of modifications of the transsphenoidal approach targeted to the entire skull base [4–8]. Direct exposure of the suprasellar, retrosellar, and retroclival spaces can now be gained using these approaches. With the evolution of technical procedures in such critical areas reached through narrow corridors, perfect understanding and knowledge of the surgical anatomy is fundamental.

L.M. Cavallo, MD, PhD (✉) • D. Solari, MD, PhD • A. Villa, MD
T. Somma, MD • P. Cappabianca, MD
Division of Neurosurgery, Department of Neurosciences, Reproductive and Odontostomatological Sciences, Universita' degli Studi di Napoli Federico II, Naples, Italy
e-mail: lcavallo@unina.it; d.solari.md@gmail.com; alessandrovilla83@gmail.com; teresa.somma85@gmail.com; paolo.cappabianca@unina.it

1.2 Endoscopic Anatomy of the Sphenoid Sinus

The anatomy of the sphenoid sinus cavity and skull base as seen from the endoscopic endonasal point of view can be divided into four areas, according to the different surgical approaches:

- The sellar area
- The suprasellar area, explored through the transtuberculum-transplanum approach
- The parasellar area (for lesions of the cavernous sinus and Meckel's cave)
- The clival area

1.2.1 Basic Concepts

The endoscopic endonasal procedure is usually performed using a rigid 0° endoscope, 18 cm in length and 4 mm in diameter (Karl Storz Endoscopy, Tuttlingen, Germany), as the sole visualizing tool; angled scopes can be used to further explore the suprasellar area. A high-definition (HD) camera, connected to a widescreen HD monitor, guarantees excellent image quality. Dedicated surgical instruments with different angled tips are needed to permit movements in all the visible corners of the surgical field [9]. To increase the working space and the maneuverability of the instruments (above all in extended approaches), it may be advisable to perform a middle turbinectomy on one side, a middle turbinate lateral luxation in the other nostril, and removal of the posterior portion of the nasal septum. A wider anterior sphenoidotomy is recommended, especially in the lateral and superior directions, where bony spurs are flattened to create adequate space for the endoscope during the deeper steps of the procedure [5].

G. Zada et al. (eds.), *Atlas of Sellar and Parasellar Lesions: Clinical, Radiologic, and Pathologic Correlations*,
DOI 10.1007/978-3-319-22855-6_1

1.2.2 Head Positioning

The head is not placed in a neutral position. According to the target area of interest, it can be extended approximately 10–15° for anterior approaches, or it may be slightly flexed for approaches to the clivus, to facilitate the mobility of the endoscope and prevent surgical instruments from being restricted by the thorax. The surgeon works from the patient's right side.

1.3 Standard Endoscopic Endonasal Approach to the Sellar Region

The endoscope is usually introduced through one nostril, sliding along the floor of the nasal cavity following the inferior turbinate; the choana is identified, limited medially by the vomer (which is often a reliable midline marker) and superiorly by the floor of the sphenoid sinus [10, 11].

Thereafter, the middle turbinate is compressed laterally to enlarge the space between the middle turbinate and the nasal septum, and the endoscope is angled upward along the roof of the choana approximately 1.5 cm, until the sphenoid ostium is identified.

It is not always mandatory to visualize the sphenoid ostium once the choana is identified; access to the sphenoid cavity can also be achieved by ascending along the spheno-ethmoidal recess for approximately 1–1.5 cm.

Thereafter, the nasal septum is detached from the sphenoid rostrum, and the anterior wall of the sphenoid sinus is enlarged circumferentially, taking care to not extend too aggressively in an inferolateral direction, where the sphenopalatine artery or its major branches lie [12].

Septa inside the sphenoid sinus should be identified and resected or carefully drilled down so that the posterior and lateral walls of the sphenoid sinus are visible, with the sellar floor at the center, the planum sphenoidale above, and the clival indentation below (Fig. 1.1). The pituitary gland is situated within the hypophyseal fossa, a fibro-osseous compartment near the center of the cranial base. This fossa is limited laterally and superiorly by reflections of dura mater and anteriorly, posteriorly, and inferiorly by the sella turcica, a depression in the body of the sphenoid bone. The sellar floor lies at the center on the posterior sphenoid sinus wall and continues above to the planum sphenoidale and below to the clivus. The optic nerve prominences, above, are formed by the bony covering of the optic nerves; the carotid prominences, below, cover the internal carotid arteries, with the opticocarotid recess in between [11, 13]. The lateral opticocarotid recess is created by the pneumatization of the optic strut of the anterior clinoid process. Although it is rarely visible in the cavity of the sphenoid sinus, it is important to define the position of the medial opticocarotid recess, representing a key point in entering the suprasellar area [14].

Once the sellar dura is opened, the anterior lobe of the pituitary gland comes into view. Its inferior surface usually conforms to the shape of the sellar floor, but its lateral and superior margins vary in shape because these walls are composed of soft tissue rather than bone. Posteriorly, the neurohypophysis (posterior pituitary gland) can be observed and is often softer, gelatinous, and more densely adherent to the posterior sellar wall, the dorsum sellae. Above, the diaphragma sellae covers the pituitary gland, except for a small central opening through which the pituitary stalk (infundibulum) passes. Folds of dura mater, which constitute the lateral walls of the hypophyseal fossa, also comprise the medial wall of the cavernous sinuses; the internal carotid artery (ICA) coursing through the cavernous sinus can be appreciated at this level [11, 13].

The pituitary gland derives its blood supply from two major groups of arteries. The superior hypophyseal artery primarily supplies the anterior lobe, the pituitary stalk, and the inferior surface of the optic nerve and chiasm, whereas the inferior hypophyseal artery is primarily related to the pars nervosa. The superior hypophyseal artery can arise from the supraclinoid portion of the ICA or from the posterior communicating artery, whereas the inferior hypophyseal artery arises from the meningohypophyseal trunk, a branch of the cavernous segment of the ICA.

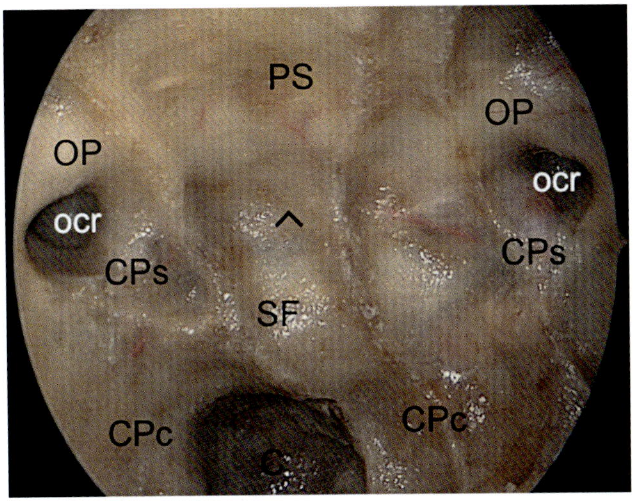

Fig. 1.1 Anatomical picture showing the posterior wall of the sphenoid sinus; all the anatomical landmarks are visible, but they may vary according to the degree of pneumatization of the sphenoid sinus. ^ tuberculum sellae as seen from the endoscopic endonasal view (recently called the "suprasellar notch"), *C* clival indentation, *CPc* paraclival segment of the carotid protuberance, *CPs* parasellar segment of the carotid protuberance, *ocr* lateral optocarotid recess, *OP* optic protuberance, *PS* planum sphenoidale, *SF* sellar floor

1.4 Extended Endoscopic Transsphenoidal Approaches

1.4.1 Suprasellar Area

The sphenoid sinus represents a window of access to the midline skull base via the endonasal corridor; when the sinus is well pneumatized, all main bony landmarks can be identified. The sellar floor occupies a central position, with the planum sphenoidale above and the clival indentation below; on both sides, lateral to the sellar floor, are the two bony prominences of the intracavernous internal carotid arteries, and the optic nerves can be identified slightly superiorly. Between these two protuberances, depending on the degree of pneumatization of the sphenoid sinus, the projection of the optic strut of the anterior clinoid process creates the lateral opticocarotid recess [7, 13–15].

Immediately above, the tuberculum sellae can be seen as an indentation represented by the angle formed by the convergence of the planum sphenoidale with the sellar floor. Recently, we renamed this structure as the "suprasellar notch" [16]. Anteriorly lies the planum sphenoidale, which is limited on both sides by the optic nerve protuberances, diverging toward the orbits.

The removal of the upper half of the sella, the tuberculum sellae, and the posterior portion of the planum sphenoidale offers the possibility of exploring and operating in the suprasellar region (Fig. 1.2). The entire suprasellar region can be divided into four intradural areas: the suprachiasmatic region, the subchiasmatic region, the retrosellar region, and the ventricular region [15].

In the suprachiasmatic region, the chiasmatic and the lamina terminalis cisterns are accessible. The anterior margin of the optic chiasm and the medial portion of the optic nerves, the anterior cerebral arteries, the anterior communicating artery, and the recurrent arteries of Heubner can be identified, together with the gyri recti of the frontal lobes [17].

In the subchiasmatic space, the pituitary stalk is encountered below the optic chiasm, with the superior hypophyseal arteries and their perforating branches supplying the inferior surface of the optic chiasm and the optic nerves (Fig. 1.3). The superior aspect of the pituitary gland and the dorsum sellae are also visible.

The retrosellar area, explored by passing with the endoscope between the pituitary stalk and the ICA above the dorsum sellae, includes the upper third of the basilar artery, the pons, the superior cerebellar arteries, the oculomotor nerves, the posterior cerebral arteries, the mammillary bodies, and the floor of the third ventricle [18, 19].

The third ventricle can be opened at the level of the tuber cinereum and the endoscope can be advanced into the ventricular cavity, obtaining a panoramic view of the ventricular area, including the thalami and the massa intermedia, the foramina of Monro and anterior commissure anteriorly, the choroid plexus of the third ventricle, the pineal and the suprapineal recesses, the posterior commissure, the habenular commissure, the habenular trigone, and the cerebral aqueduct posteriorly.

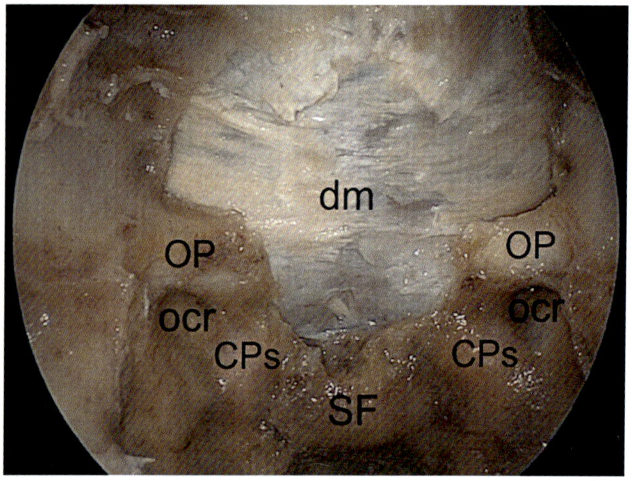

Fig. 1.2 The pattern of bony removal of the planum sphenoidale resembles a chef's hat, limited in its posterior part by the medial border of the lateral optocarotid recess (ocr) and by the bony prominence of the optic nerve. *CPc* paraclival segment of the carotid protuberance, *CPs* parasellar segment of the carotid protuberance, *dm* dura mater of the planum sphenoidale, *OP* optic protuberance, *SF* sellar floor

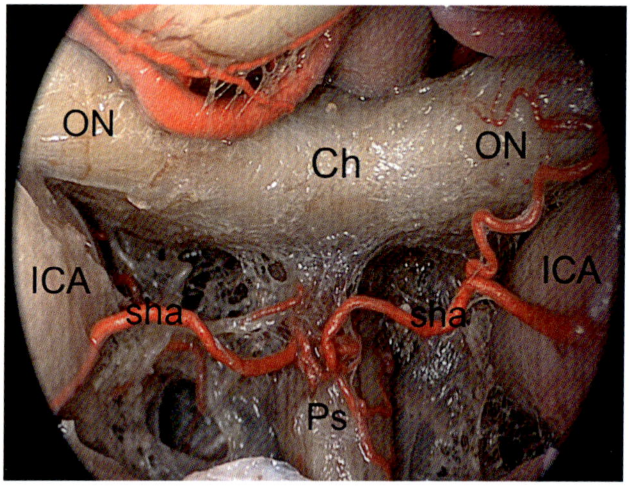

Fig. 1.3 Intradural exploration of the suprasellar area after removal of the tuberculum sellae and planum sphenoidale. *Ch* chiasm, *ICA* internal carotid artery, *ON* optic nerve, *Ps* pituitary stalk, *sha* superior hypophyseal artery

1.4.2 The Parasellar Area

The parasellar area is accessible through the lateral wall of the sphenoid sinus. The cavernous sinus apex and the trigeminal maxillary and mandibular nerve protuberances usually lie on its bony surface (Fig. 1.4). Once bone has been removed, the medial cavernous sinus wall (composed of fibrous trabecular tissue) is visualized, enclosing the C-shaped segment of the intracavernous internal carotid artery [20–23] (Fig. 1.5).

Displacing the ICA superolaterally, it is possible to visualize the meningohypophyseal trunk; the inferolateral trunk lies lateral to the carotid artery (Fig. 1.6). As seen from the endoscopic endonasal standpoint, the oculomotor nerve partially covers the trochlear nerve, whereas the V1 branch of the trigeminal nerve can be partially hidden by the sixth nerve. The oculomotor and trochlear nerves are parallel structures, coursing in a slight caudocranial direction and crossing the C-shaped ICA segment toward the superior orbital fissure. The sixth cranial nerve runs inferiorly after crossing the lower paraclival tract of the carotid artery; it usually receives sympathetic fibers from the ICA adventitia. All these nerves, together with the ophthalmic nerve, course in a slightly lateral and superior direction toward the superior orbital fissure, while the maxillary nerve runs inferiorly to reach the foramen rotundum [24] (Fig. 1.7). The oculomotor nerve, the trochlear nerve, and first two divisions of the trigeminal nerve are embedded in the lateral wall of the cavernous sinus, lying between the endothelial lining and the dura mater, whereas the abducens nerve is contained within the sinus itself. The cavernous sinus also envelops a portion of the ICA and the sympathetic nerve plexus encircling it. The intracavernous segment of the ICA extends forward, adjacent to the superolateral surface of the body of the sphenoid bone, in a groove called the carotid sulcus.

The oculomotor and abducens nerves create a triangular area whose base is represented by the lateral loop of the ICA: the outer surface of this area contains the fourth cranial nerve and a portion of V1. The abducens nerve and V2 enclose a quadrangular area, laterally limited by the bony surface of the lateral wall of the sphenoid sinus, extending from the superior orbital fissure to the foramen rotundum and medially by the ICA. Finally, an inferior quadrangular area can be identified, which is limited superiorly by V2 and inferiorly by the Vidian nerve; its anterior margin is represented by the bony surface of the lateral wall of the sphenoid sinus from the foramen rotundum to the pterygoid canal, and its posterior margin is the intrapetrous segment and the caudal portion of the ICA. This quadrangular area can be used to enter Meckel's cave [20].

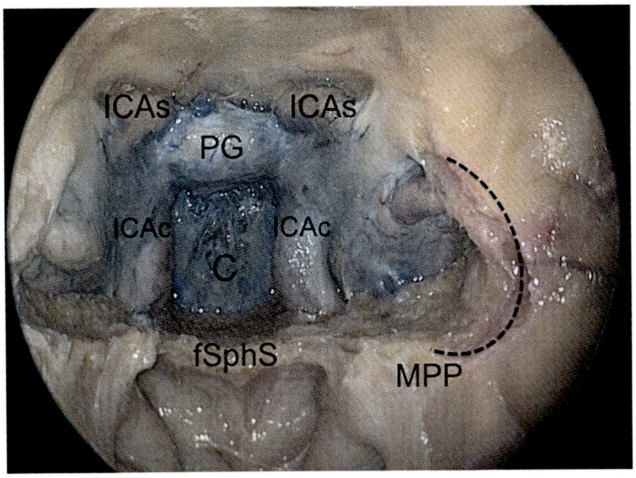

Fig. 1.4 Endoscopic view after bony removal of the sella, clivus (*C*), and the intracavernous internal carotid arteries. The medial pterygoid process has been drilled away, thus allowing a wide exposure of the lateral recess of the sphenoid sinus. The *dotted line* represents the lateral recess of the sphenoid sinus after drilling of the medial pterygoid process. *ICAc* paraclival segment of the internal carotid artery, *ICAs* parasellar segment of the internal carotid artery, *fSphS* floor of the sphenoid sinus, *MPP* medial pterygoid plate, *PG* pituitary gland

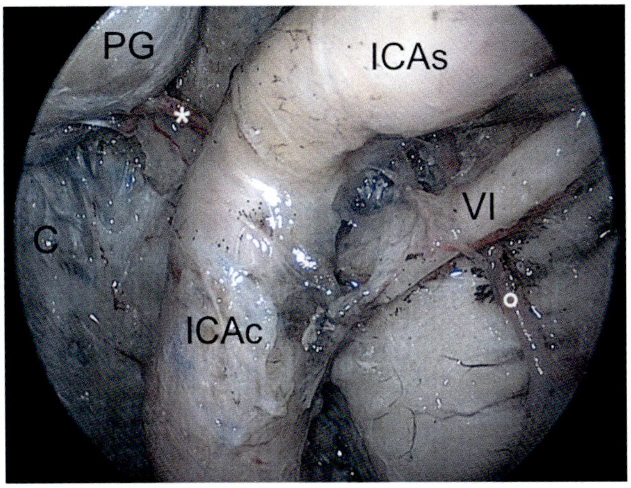

Fig. 1.6 Endoscopic close-up view of the branches of the left intracavernous internal carotid artery, including the inferior hypophyseal artery (*white asterisk*) and the inferolateral trunk (*white circle*). *C* clivus, *ICAc* paraclival segment of the internal carotid artery, *ICAs* parasellar segment of the internal carotid artery, *PG* pituitary gland, *VI* abducens nerve

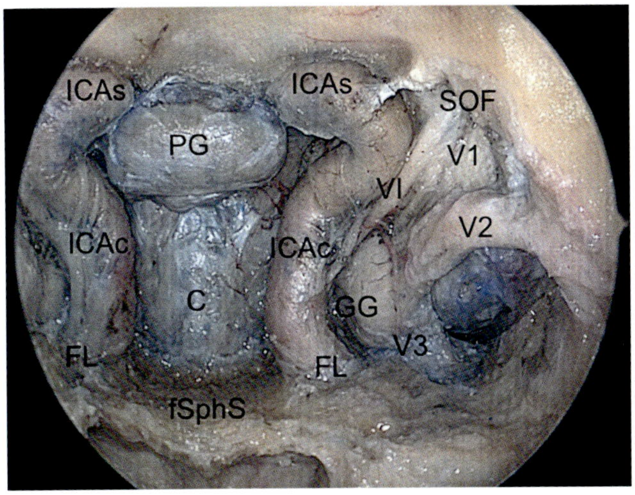

Fig. 1.5 Endoscopic view after bony removal of the lateral recess of the sphenoid sinus. *C* clivus, *ICAc* paraclival segment of the internal carotid artery, *ICAs* parasellar segment of the internal carotid artery, *FL* foramen lacerum, *fSphS* floor of the sphenoid sinus, *GG* Gasserian ganglion, *PG* pituitary gland, *SOF* superior orbital fissure, *V1* first branch of trigeminal nerve, *V2* second branch of trigeminal nerve, *V3* third branch of trigeminal nerve, *VI* abducens nerve

1.4.3 The Clival Area

From an endonasal perspective, the clivus represents the anterior gateway to the posterior cranial fossa: two corridors can be pursued, the sphenoidal (upper clivus) and the rhinopharyngeal (lower clivus) [13, 25].

The vomer and the inferior wall of the sphenoid sinus need to be removed completely in an anteroposterior direction to allow the exposure of both the sphenoidal and rhinopharyngeal parts of the clivus (Figs. 1.6 and 1.7). The Vidian nerves, which represent the lateral limits of this exposure, can be identified lateral to the vomer-sphenoid junction [26]. These nerves, after crossing the intrapetrous carotid artery from above, reach the pterygopalatine fossa at a level inferior to that of the intrapetrous ICA. Extending posteriorly with bony removal and staying medial to these nerves, one can limit the risk of ICA injury. The lateral limit of clival bone removal is represented by the paraclival course of the intracavernous internal carotid arteries, whose bony protuberances are often clearly visible (Fig. 1.7).

Removing clival bone to the carotid protuberances, the retroclival dura harboring the basilar plexus is visualized; in the middle third of the clival area, it is possible to recognize the sixth cranial nerve entering the cavernous sinus posterior to the paraclival intracavernous carotid artery in close contact to the dorsal meningeal artery, which provides the arterial blood supply to the dura of the clival region [24] (Fig. 1.8).

Upon dural opening—performed below the vertebrobasilar junction in order to spare the sixth cranial nerve origin at the brainstem—the basilar artery and its branches, as well as the upper cranial nerves, are seen along their courses. The intradural compartment can be divided into three major regions:

- The upper third, whose main neurovascular structures are the oculomotor nerves and the posterior cerebral and superior cerebellar arteries
- The middle third, whose main landmark is represented by the sixth cranial nerves
- The lower third, including the vertebrobasilar junction, the vertebral arteries, and the ninth to twelfth cranial nerves

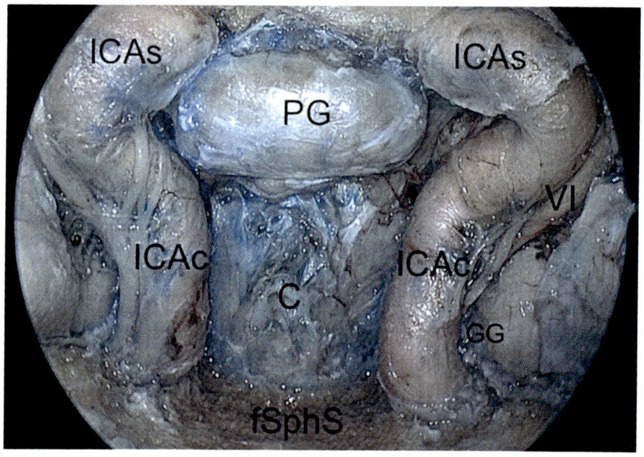

Fig. 1.7 Endoscopic view of the sellar and clival areas, enclosed between the internal carotid arteries. *C* clivus, *fSphS* floor of the sphenoid sinus, *GG* Gasserian ganglion, *ICAc* paraclival segment of the internal carotid artery, *ICAs* parasellar segment of the internal carotid artery, *PG* pituitary gland, *VI* abducens nerve

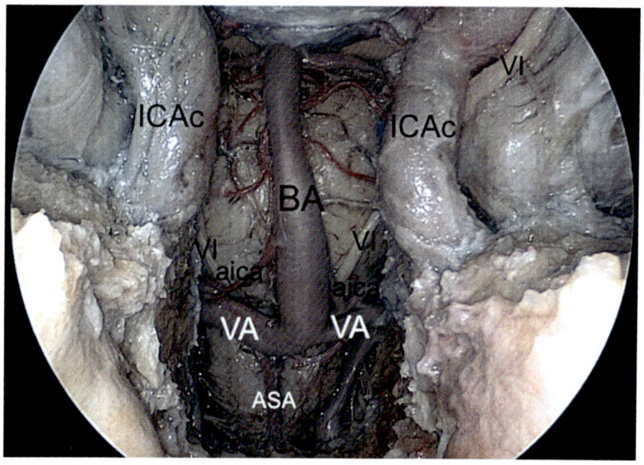

Fig. 1.8 Intradural exploration of the retroclival area after the transclival approach is extended inferiorly to C1. *AICA* anterior inferior cerebellar artery, *ASA* anterior spinal artery, *BA* basilar artery, *ICAc* paraclival segment of the internal carotid artery, *VA* vertebral artery, *VI* abducens nerve

References

1. Laws ER, Jane Jr JA. Pituitary tumors–long-term outcomes and expectations. Clin Neurosurg. 2001;48:306–19.
2. Laws ER Jr. Transsphenoidal surgery. In: Apuzzo MLJ, editor. Brain surgery: complications avoidance and management, vol. 1. New York: Churchill Livingstone; 1993. p. 357–62.
3. Weiss MH. The transnasal transsphenoidal approach. In: Apuzzo MLJ, editor. Surgery of the third ventricle. Baltimore: Williams & Wilkins; 1987. p. 476–94.
4. de Divitiis E, Cappabianca P, Cavallo LM. Endoscopic transsphenoidal approach: adaptability of the procedure to different sellar lesions. Neurosurgery. 2002;51:699–705; discussion 705–7.
5. Kassam AB, Snyderman C, Carrau RL. An evolving paradigm to the ventral skull base. Skull Base. 2004;14 Suppl 1:23.
6. Frank G, Pasquini E, Mazzatenta D. Extended transsphenoidal approach. J Neurosurg. 2001;95:917–8.
7. Cappabianca P, Cavallo LM, Esposito F, de Divitiis O, Messina A, de Divitiis E. Extended endoscopic endonasal approach to the midline skull base: the evolving role of transsphenoidal surgery. In: Pickard JD, Akalan N, Di Rocco C, et al., editors. Advances and technical standards in neurosurgery. New York: Springer; 2008. p. 152–99.
8. Laufer I, Anand VK, Schwartz TH. Endoscopic, endonasal extended transsphenoidal, transplanum transtuberculum approach for resection of suprasellar lesions. J Neurosurg. 2007;106:400–6.
9. Cappabianca P, Alfieri A, Thermes S, Buonamassa S, de Divitiis E. Instruments for endoscopic endonasal transsphenoidal surgery. Neurosurgery. 1999;45:392–5; discussion 395–6.
10. Tschabitscher M, Galzio RJ. Endoscopic anatomy along the transnasal approach to the pituitary gland and the surrounding structures. In: de Divitiis E, Cappabianca P, editors. Endoscopic endonasal transsphenoidal surgery. New York: Springer; 2003. p. 21–39.
11. Rhoton Jr AL. The sellar region. Neurosurgery. 2002;51:S335–74.
12. Cavallo LM, Solari D, Esposito F, Cappabianca P. Endoscopic endonasal approach for pituitary adenomas. Acta Neurochir (Wien). 2012;154:2251–6.
13. Cavallo LM, Messina A, Cappabianca P, Esposito F, de Divitiis E, Gardner P, Tschabitscher M. Endoscopic endonasal surgery of the midline skull base: anatomical study and clinical considerations. Neurosurg Focus. 2005;19, E2.
14. Kassam A, Snyderman CH, Mintz A, Gardner P, Carrau RL. Expanded endonasal approach: the rostrocaudal axis. Part I. Crista galli to the sella turcica. Neurosurg Focus. 2005;19(E3):1–12.
15. Cavallo LM, de Divitiis O, Aydin S, Messina A, Esposito F, Iaconetta G, et al. Extended endoscopic endonasal transsphenoidal approach to the suprasellar area: anatomic considerations–part 1. Neurosurgery. 2007;61(3 Suppl):24–33.
16. de Notaris M, Solari D, Cavallo LM, D'Enza AI, Ensenat J, Berenguer J, et al. The "suprasellar notch," or the tuberculum sellae as seen from below: definition, features, and clinical implications from an endoscopic endonasal perspective. J Neurosurg. 2012;116: 622–9.
17. Rhoton Jr AL. The supratentorial arteries. Neurosurgery. 2002;51: S53–120.
18. Silva D, Attia M, Kandasamy J, Alimi M, Anand VK, Schwartz TH. Endoscopic endonasal transsphenoidal "above and below" approach to the retroinfundibular area and interpeduncular cistern-cadaveric study and case illustrations. World Neurosurg. 2014;81:374–84.
19. Kassam AB, Prevedello DM, Thomas A, Gardner P, Mintz A, Snyderman C, Carrau R. Endoscopic endonasal pituitary transposition for a transdorsum sellae approach to the interpeduncular cistern. Neurosurgery. 2008;62:57–72; discussion 72–4.
20. Cavallo LM, Cappabianca P, Galzio R, Iaconetta G, de Divitiis E, Tschabitscher M. Endoscopic transnasal approach to the cavernous sinus versus transcranial route: anatomic study. Neurosurgery. 2005;56(2 Suppl):379–89.
21. Frank G, Pasquini E. Endoscopic endonasal cavernous sinus surgery, with special reference to pituitary adenomas. Front Horm Res. 2006;34:64–82.
22. Kassam AB, Prevedello DM, Carrau RL, Snyderman CH, Gardner P, Osawa S, et al. The front door to Meckel's cave: an anteromedial corridor via expanded endoscopic endonasal approach–technical considerations and clinical series. Neurosurgery. 2009;64(3 Suppl):71–82; discussion 82–3.
23. Rhoton Jr AL. The cavernous sinus, the cavernous venous plexus, and the carotid collar. Neurosurgery. 2002;51(4 Suppl):S375–410.
24. Prevedello DM, Ditzel Filho LF, Solari D, Carrau RL, Kassam AB. Expanded endonasal approaches to middle cranial fossa and posterior fossa tumors. Neurosurg Clin N Am. 2010;21:621–35.
25. Kassam A, Snyderman CH, Mintz A, Gardner P, Carrau RL. Expanded endonasal approach: the rostrocaudal axis. Part II. Posterior clinoids to the foramen magnum. Neurosurg Focus. 2005;19, E4.
26. Kassam AB, Vescan AD, Carrau RL, Prevedello DM, Gardner P, Mintz AH, et al. Expanded endonasal approach: vidian canal as a landmark to the petrous internal carotid artery. J Neurosurg. 2008;108:177–83.

Imaging of the Sellar Region

2

Raymond Y. Huang and Srinivasan Mukundan Jr.

Imaging of the sellar and parasellar regions is clinically indicated in patients with symptoms or signs of endocrinopathy or visual field deficiency. However, a greater proportion of sellar and parasellar pathologies are often discovered incidentally as cross-sectional imaging of the brain is increasingly performed during diagnostic evaluation of unrelated neurologic problems or during staging of systemic malignancy. The latest improvements in high-resolution magnetic resonance imaging (MRI) and computed tomography (CT) techniques have greatly increased our ability to detect small sellar lesions and delineate the extent of disease prior to surgical resection. Understanding both the advantages and limitations of these imaging techniques is essential for optimizing imaging protocol and improving diagnostic accuracy.

2.1 Imaging Strategies

2.1.1 Computed Tomography (CT)

Modern CT equipment is capable of multiplanar reformation, allowing precise assessment of the bony anatomy of the sella for surgical planning. Similar to the traditional role of lateral projection of head radiographs, the shape and size of sellae are readily visualized on CT using sagittal-plane reformatted images. Moreover, with proper windowing, the pituitary gland and stalk can often be distinctly visualized apart from the cerebrospinal fluid (Fig. 2.1). While intrapituitary lesions, specifically small pituitary adenomas or cysts, are often not detectable on CT because of its less than optimal soft-tissue contrast, CT can be a useful screening test to exclude the presence of large sellar lesions, especially those that extend out of the sella causing visual field symptoms, particularly if MRI is contraindicated.

In evaluating sellar lesions, CT has an advantage over MRI because of its superior capability in visualizing bony detail and calcifications. For example, pituitary adenomas often grow slowly, allowing time for bone remodeling that is evident by demonstration of smooth cortical margins (Fig. 2.2). In contrast, an aggressive process such as a malignancy or infection can permeate or erode the bone, resulting in indistinct cortical margins. CT is also sensitive to the presence of soft-tissue calcifications that are uniquely found in a subset of sellar pathology, including vascular aneurysm, germ cell neoplasm, and craniopharyngioma. Finally, CT angiography can be helpful in confirming the presence of aneurysms that may mimic pituitary pathology and can demonstrate the spatial relationship between sellar lesions and adjacent intracranial arteries during preoperative planning.

R.Y. Huang, MD, PhD • S. Mukundan Jr., MD, PhD (✉)
Department of Radiology, Brigham and Women's Hospital, Boston, MA, USA
e-mail: ryhuang@partners.org; smukundan@partners.org

G. Zada et al. (eds.), *Atlas of Sellar and Parasellar Lesions: Clinical, Radiologic, and Pathologic Correlations*, DOI 10.1007/978-3-319-22855-6_2

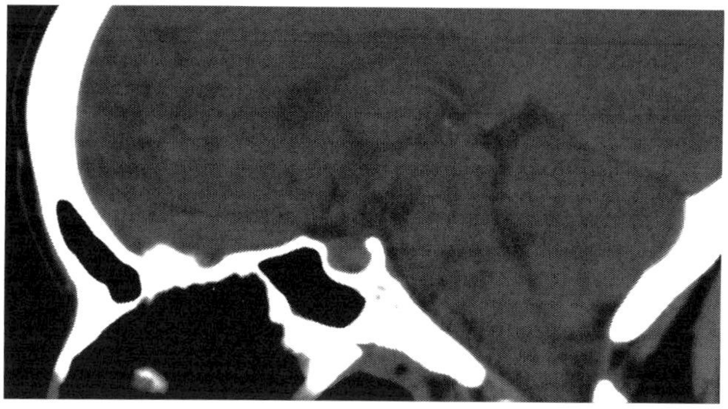

Fig. 2.1 CT image in sagittal-plane reformation shows the shape and size of the sella, with the pituitary gland and stalk clearly visualized

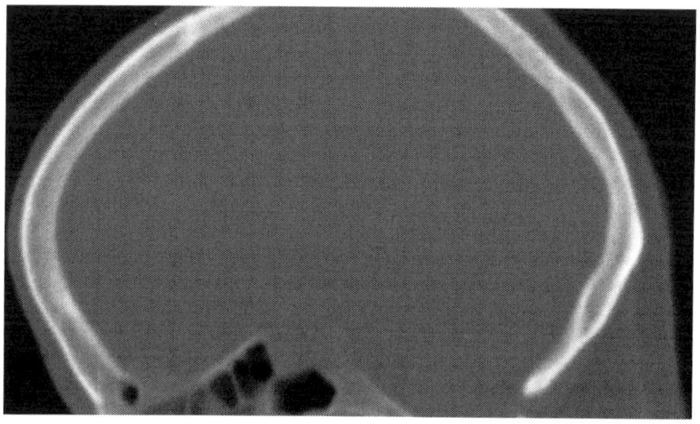

Fig. 2.2 Sagittal-plane CT image in bone window shows smooth expansion of the sella caused by a pituitary macroadenoma

2.1.1.1 Magnetic Resonance Imaging (MRI)

Because of its exquisite soft-tissue contrast and lack of ionizing radiation, MRI is the imaging modality of choice for evaluation of sellar and parasellar pathology. Because the dimensions of the sella turcica are approximately $10 \times 10 \times 10$ mm for normal adults, an inter-slice thickness of smaller or equal to 3 mm (without gap) is needed to generate at least 3 slices through the content of the sella (Fig. 2.3). When the sella is imaged in coronal and sagittal planes at 3-mm inter-slice thickness, lesions larger than 3 mm should be detectable on both planes. The multiplanar capability of MRI not only allows initial diagnosis of sellar pathology but also facilitates preoperative planning and posttreatment surveillance for recurrence.

Although noncontrast-enhanced MRI can detect and characterize sellar pathology larger than the normal gland, small adenomas often exhibit image contrast nearly identical to the surrounding pituitary gland unless the lesions contain fluid or proteinaceous or hemorrhagic material. The standard pituitary protocol used in our institution includes sagittal and coronal T1-weighted spin-echo sequences through the sella using a small field of view (20×25 cm), thin slices (3 mm), and a high-resolution matrix (256×512), performed both before and following intravenous gadolinium administration. The protocol also includes 0.5-mm volumetric 3D T2-weighted steady-state free precession (T2 SSFP) sequence (e.g., FIESTA, CISS, etc.) in the sagittal plane through the sella, whole-brain axial fluid-attenuated inversion recovery (FLAIR), diffusion-weighted imaging (DWI), and postgadolinium volumetric 3D T1-weighted sequence (e.g., MPRAGE or SPGR). The whole-brain 3D volumetric postgadolinium sequence provides lesion coregistration to surgical guidance software and also allows confirmation of small lesions (equal to or smaller than 3 mm) occasionally observed only on one of the two 3-mm spin-echo imaging planes. In our experience, this protocol could identify a majority of sellar/parasellar pathology, greatly reducing the need to perform repeated evaluations for small adenomas using dynamic gadolinium-enhanced MRI.

For detection of small pituitary adenomas that are not apparent on delayed contrast-enhanced MRI, dynamic contrast MRI can be performed to increase lesion-to-gland contrast based on different contrast wash-in and wash-out properties between adenomas and pituitary tissues. Immediately following an intravenous bolus injection of gadolinium (0.05 mmol/kg), six sequential sets of three images are acquired every 10 s using a three-dimensional Fourier transformation gradient echo or fast turbo spin-echo sequence. For a normal pituitary gland, the stalk and posterior part of the gland enhance first because of their direct arterial supply, followed by the anterior part of the gland that receives blood from the hypophyseal-portal system. The entire gland enhances homogeneously between 30 and 60 s. The maximal difference in the degree of enhancement between the normal pituitary tissue and adenomas often occurs during 30–60 s after the contrast administration, with the majority of adenomas appearing relatively hypoenhancing relative to the avidly enhancing pituitary gland. After 60 s, the contrast medium within the pituitary gland begins to wash out, but the adenomas often continue to take up contrast; peak enhancement occurs up to 200 s [1]. As a result, the imaging contrast between the adenoma and the pituitary tissue reduces after reaching maximum enhancement and can become reversed, with adenomas appearing more hyperintense compared with the pituitary gland on delayed imaging [2]. Some adenomas may enhance very early following contrast administration, possibly secondary to direct arterial supply, and dynamic contrast MRI can identify these adenomas as hyperintense lesions during the earliest time points [3].

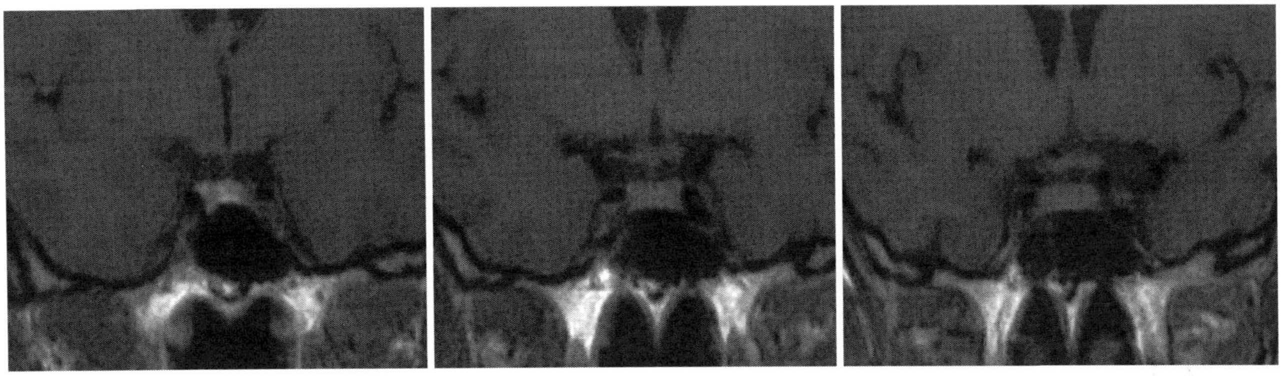

Fig. 2.3 Three consecutive coronal-plane T1-weighted images through the sella demonstrate a normal sized pituitary gland. The image on the left shows T1 shortening within the posterior pituitary

2.2 Normal Sellar Anatomy on Imaging

Sagittal T1-weighted imaging through the midline plane provides a good overall survey of the shape of the sella and its content as well as the surrounding structures (Fig. 2.4). On coronal planes through the sella, paired cavernous sinuses are located lateral to the sella (Fig. 2.5).

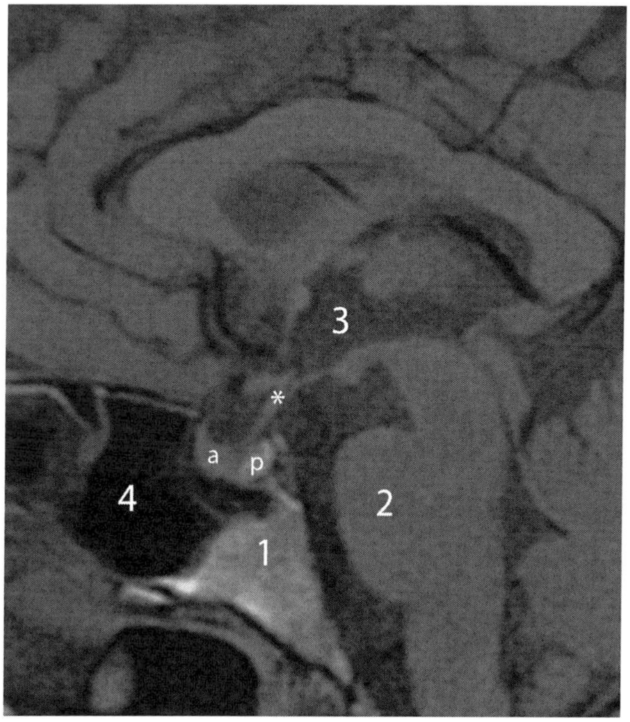

Fig. 2.4 Sagittal T1-weighted image without contrast. *Asterisk* indicates pituitary stalk. Key: *1* clivus, *2* Pons, *3* third ventricle, *4* sphenoid sinus, *a* anterior pituitary gland, *b* posterior pituitary gland

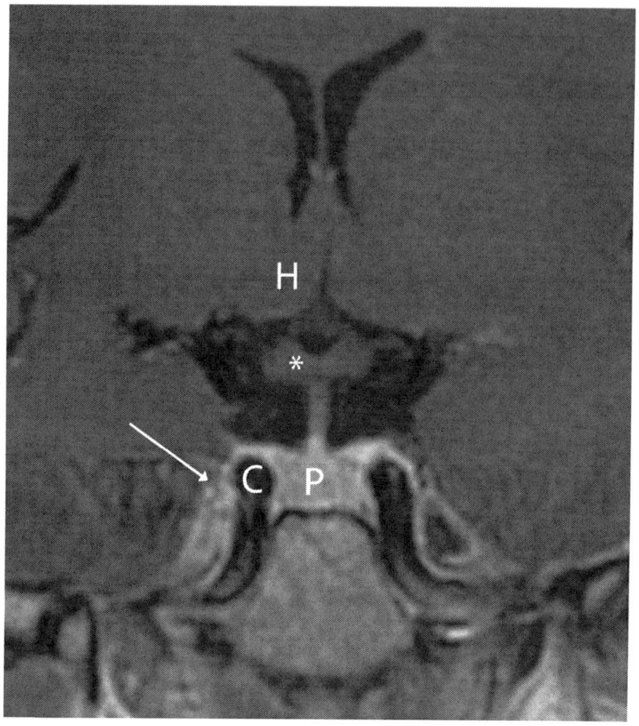

Fig. 2.5 Coronal T1-weighted image without contrast. *Asterisk* indicates optic chiasm. Key: *C* cavernous sinus (*arrow*), *H* hypothalamus, *P* pituitary gland

2.2.1 Pituitary Gland

The two anatomically and functionally distinct lobes of the pituitary gland—the anterior lobe (adenohypophysis) and the posterior lobe (neurohypophysis)—can often be distinguished on noncontrast sagittal T1-weighted images, since the posterior lobe is usually more hyperintense (posterior pituitary bright spot) than the anterior lobe (Fig. 2.6). The posterior pituitary hyperintensity is thought to result from the T1-shortening effect of the neurosecretory vesicles in the posterior pituitary lobe [4]. Absence of this T1-hyperintense spot in the posterior sella can be a sign of congenital/developmental abnormality as well as pathologic interruption of hypothalamic secretion, which often clinically accompanies diabetes insipidus. There is normal variation in the size of the pituitary bright spot, with the long axis ranging from 0.4 to 4.4 mm [5]. The size of the spot is also age-dependent, resulting in a visibility rate decline of approximately 1 % per year [6]. It is important to distinguish the posterior pituitary from bone marrow within the nearby dorsum sella that can also appear hyperintense on T1-weighted imaging.

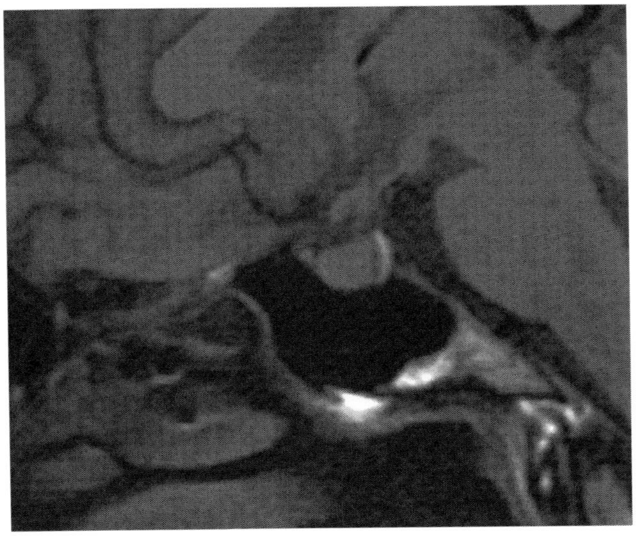

Fig. 2.6 Sagittal T1-weighted image without contrast shows posterior pituitary T1 shortening

2.2.1.1 Normal Gland Size

The size and shape of the pituitary glands are variable and can be influenced by age and sex. The height of the gland can be as much as 9 mm, and the superior margin of the gland may appear convex in normal female patients, particularly at a younger age [7]. The pituitary height in normal female subjects, on average, is greater than that in normal male subjects [8]. If stratified by age groups, the sex-related differences were significant only in the 10- to 19-, 20- to 29-, and 50- to 59-year-old age groups. The pituitary height peaked in the 20–29 age group and tended to decline with age. A practical rule of determining normal gland height can be summarized as 6 mm for children, 8 mm in men and postmenopausal women, 10 mm in women of reproductive age, and 12 mm for women in late pregnancy or postpartum women [9].

2.2.1.2 Pituitary Stalk

On midline sagittal plane, the pituitary stalk extends from the infundibular recess of the third ventricle anteriorly and inferiorly to the pituitary gland. The stalk normally enhances homogeneously immediately following contrast administration. The superior segment of the stalk can appear thicker than the caudal/anterior segment, but the transition should be smooth (Fig. 2.7). This should be differentiated from the nodular thickening of the stalk in pathologic conditions. On high-resolution MRI at 3 T, the normal pituitary stalk in adults has an anteroposterior diameter of 2.32 plus or minus 0.39 mm near the insertion and 3.35 plus or minus 0.44 mm at the level of the optic chiasm [10]. Thickening of the pituitary stalk by more than 4 mm, with or without gland involvement, can be seen in a wide variety of inflammatory and neoplastic processes. With high-resolution T2-weighted SSFP imaging, the superior portion of the stalk can appear hollow (Fig. 2.8). Deviation of the stalk from the sagittal midline plane can result from the mass effect of an underlying pituitary lesion in the opposite direction of the stalk deviation (Fig. 2.9). With suprasellar extension of an intrasellar mass, the pituitary stalk can be superiorly displaced (Fig. 2.10). Other common causes of stalk deviation include previous surgery or the presence of an arachnoid cyst. In the postoperative setting, the stalk can be markedly thinned and may not be completely visualized using standard MRI sequences. Interruption of the pituitary stalk can occur, often in the setting of congenital growth hormone insufficiency, and is usually associated with an ectopic posterior pituitary bright spot as well as a hypoplastic anterior gland [11].

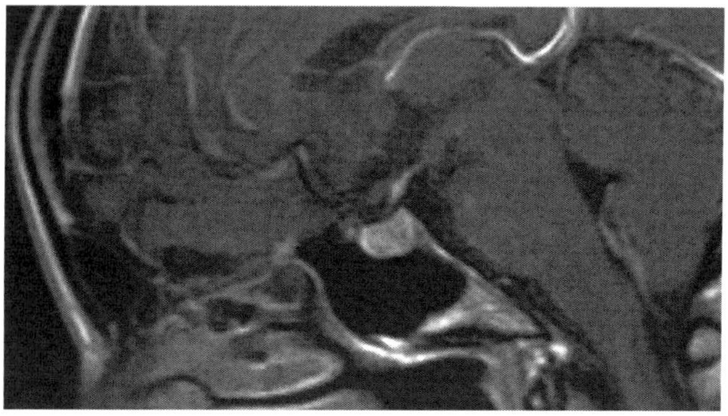

Fig. 2.7 Sagittal T1-weighted image with intravenous contrast demonstrates the appearance of the normal pituitary stalk. The cranial part of the stalk often appears thicker than the caudal component

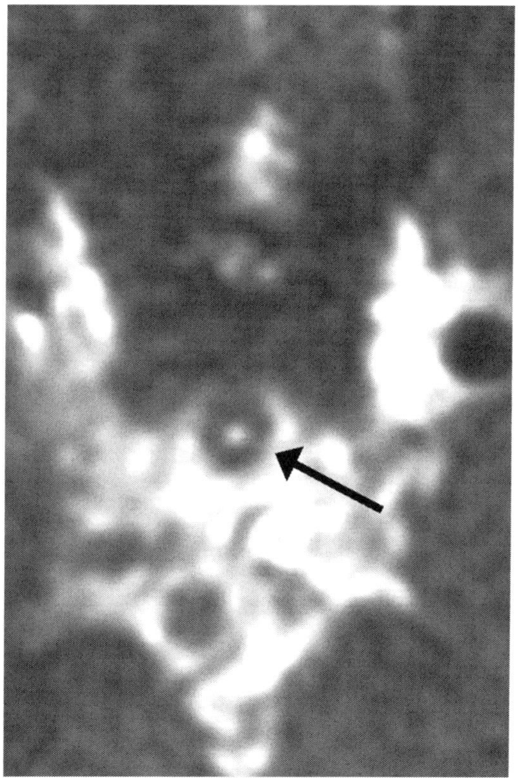

Fig. 2.8 Axial 3D FIESTA image through the cranial insertion of the stalk shows a hollow center with the CSF signal within the stalk. *Arrow* indicates hollow pituitary stalk

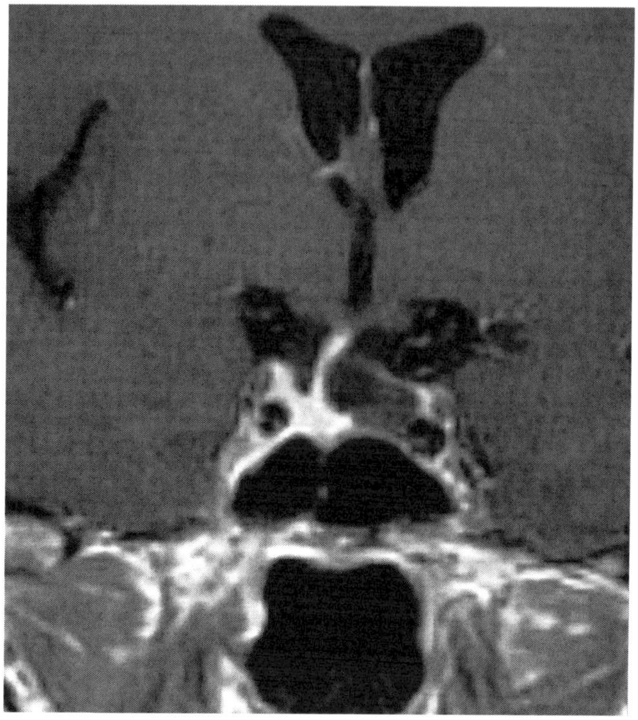

Fig. 2.9 Coronal T1-weighted image with intravenous contrast reveals a hypoenhancing mass in the left sella, displacing the stalk to the right

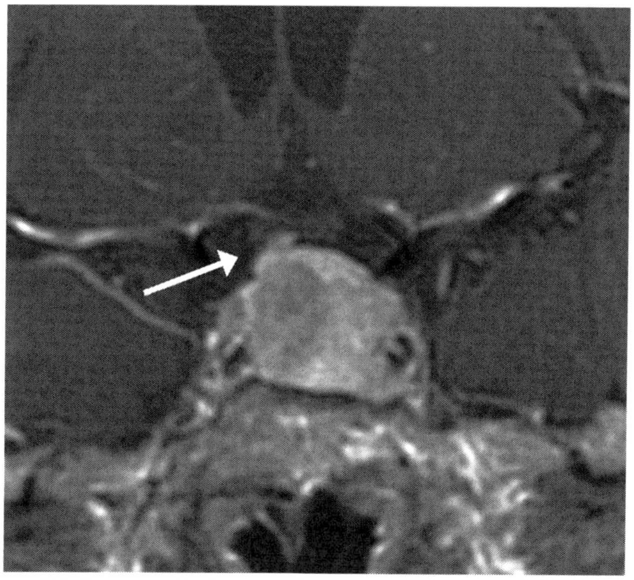

Fig. 2.10 Coronal T1-weighted image with intravenous contrast shows a large heterogeneously enhancing mass extending from the sella to the suprasellar cistern, displacing the stalk (*arrow*) superiorly

2.2.1.3 Optic Nerves, Chiasm, and Tracts

Delineating the relationship between a sellar lesion and the suprasellar optic apparatus is important in evaluating sellar anatomy as part of preoperative planning. For lesions involving the suprasellar cistern, the optic chiasm is often displaced by direct mass effect, and this finding is often associated with clinical findings of visual field cut. With significant mass effect, the optic chiasm can be markedly compressed and not readily identified, although coronal high-resolution pregadolinium T1-weighted imaging and T2-weighted SSFP imaging may allow tracing of the prechiasmatic nerve to the optic chiasm (Fig. 2.11 **a** and **b**). Occasionally, a parasellar mass can extend into the optic canal, and precise delineation of the extent of disease in this setting can greatly impact the surgical approach. Because of its obliquity from standard planes of imaging, the optic canal can be better assessed using oblique-plane high-resolution MRI by making the plane of imaging parallel and perpendicular to the segment of optic nerve within the optic canal (Fig. 2.12).

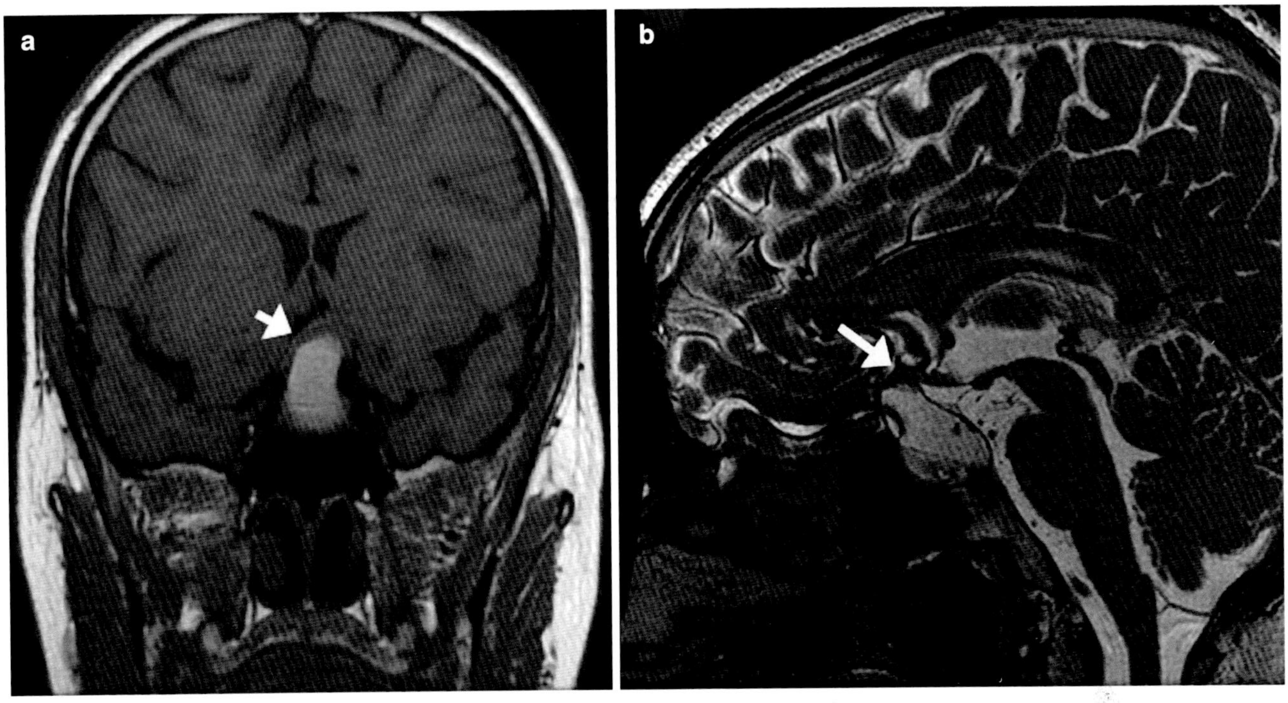

Fig. 2.11 (**a**) Coronal T1-weighted image without contrast shows superiorly displaced optic chiasm indicated by a *white arrow*. (**b**) Sagittal FIESTA image shows superiorly displaced optic chiasm indicated by a *white arrow*

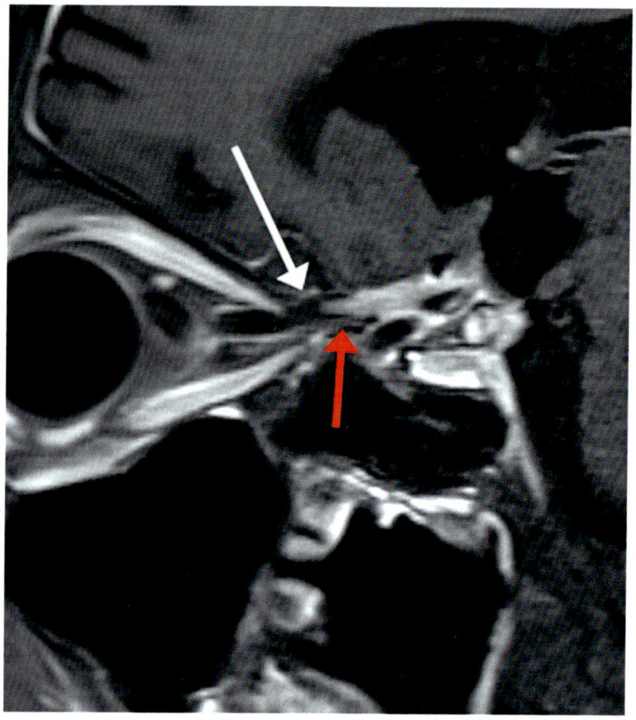

Fig. 2.12 Oblique sagittal-plane T1-weighted image with fat saturation demonstrates the extent of involvement within the optical canal. The *red arrow* indicates the most distal (peripheral) component of enhancement within the optic canal. The *white arrow* indicates the remaining intraorbital segment of the optic nerve

2.2.1.4 Cavernous Sinuses

Cavernous sinuses provide the lateral boundaries of the sella and are best characterized on coronal-plane images. While the size of cavernous sinuses can vary, they are usually symmetric when compared side-to-side. Other than normal variation, significant asymmetry in the size of cavernous sinuses can be seen in vascular abnormalities, including cavernous sinus thrombosis and cavernous-carotid fistula and neoplasms. The cavernous internal carotid arteries (ICAs) usually occupy greater than half of the volume of the cavernous sinuses. Depending on imaging sequence and contrast timing, the arterial flow within the ICAs may appear hyper-, hypo-, or isointense to the remaining part of the cavernous sinuses that is predominantly made up of venous flow unless arterialized by fistula connection(s). In some patients the course of the ICA can be highly tortuous and on occasion significantly medialized to encroach on the sellar or presellar space. Similarly, medially directed ICA aneurysms can also extend into the sella, mimicking intrasellar or suprasellar pathology. Identification of the vascular anatomy around the sella and exclusion of vascular imitators are a critical part of preoperative imaging.

2.2.1.5 Sphenoid Sinuses

The pattern of sphenoid pneumatization is highly variable. It is important to recognize the potential variations in order to avoid mistakes of interpreting them as pathologies. For example, partial or arrested pneumatization can mimic mass lesions owing to its asymmetric sclerosis on CT, but it can be readily recognized by means of location, nonexpansile appearance, and the presence of a hyperintense marrow signal on T1-weighted imaging [12]. For preoperative assessment, depending on the relationship of the sphenoid sinuses to the sella, the configuration of the sella can be categorized into three types: conchal, presellar, and sellar/postsellar (Fig. 2.13) [13]. This has a direct implication with respect to the endoscopic transsphenoidal approach; the sellar/postsellar configuration has a wide window allowing direct access to most parts of sella, whereas the conchal configuration requires significant drilling of bone to gain access to the posterior part of the sella [14]. The pattern of intersphenoid septum (or septae) also varies significantly at the points of insertion, including at the sellar floor, the carotid canal, and the optic canal [15, 16]. These variations are best evaluated on coronal CT images.

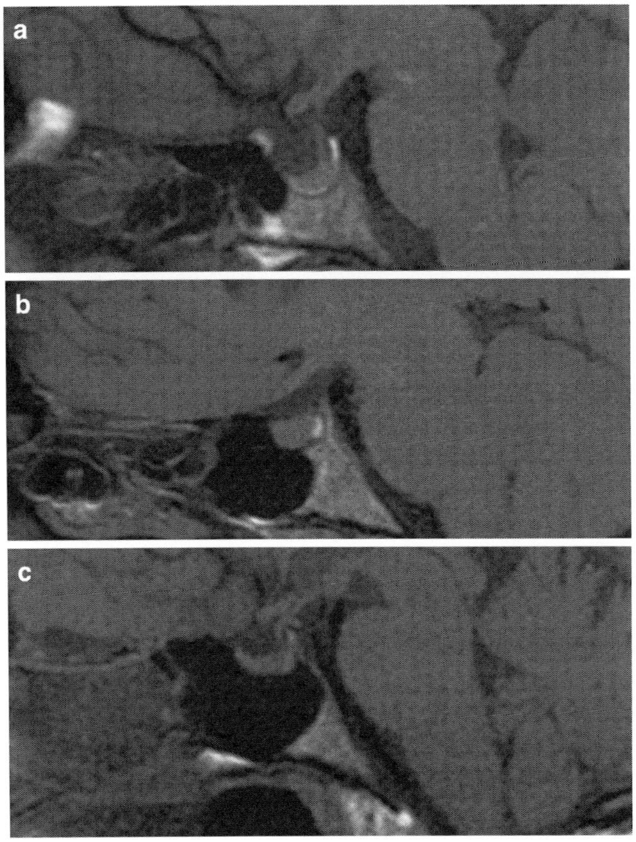

Fig. 2.13 Classification of sellar configuration based on the pneumatization pattern of the sphenoid sinuses. (**a**) Conchal; (**b**) presellar; (**c**) sellar/postsellar

2.3 Preoperative Assessment of Lesion Consistency

Knowledge of pituitary adenoma consistency can be helpful as part of preoperative evaluation. While most pituitary adenomas have a soft consistency and are easily removed, approximately 10 % of adenomas may be fibrous and not readily removed using transsphenoidal endoscopic technique [17]. Because of its short acquisition time and high sensitivity to intracranial pathology, diffusion-weighted imaging (DWI) is included in our standard sellar imaging protocol. Another study has shown that lesions with hard consistency often demonstrate high mean apparent diffusion coefficient (ADC) values, and the ADC values correlate with the percentage of collagen content [18]. More recently, FIESTA sequence has also been used as an imaging predictor of tumor consistency by categorizing adenomas based on different imaging textures: homogeneous or solid versus mosaic type containing intratumoral hyperintense dots [19].

2.4 Postoperative Imaging

The postoperative appearance of sellae largely depends on the time of imaging since surgery. The immediate postoperative MRI often reveals highly heterogeneous content within the sella, consisting of air, debris, blood, packing material, and pituitary gland tissue and possible residual tumor (Figs. 2.14 and 2.15). Unless a significant amount of residual tumor is present, distinguishing residual tumor from other tissue types is often not possible on early postoperative MRI. Serial imaging remains much more reliable in assessing residual tumor, since fat-packing material, fluid collections, and blood products typically get resorbed over time, whereas residual tumors demonstrate progressive growth.

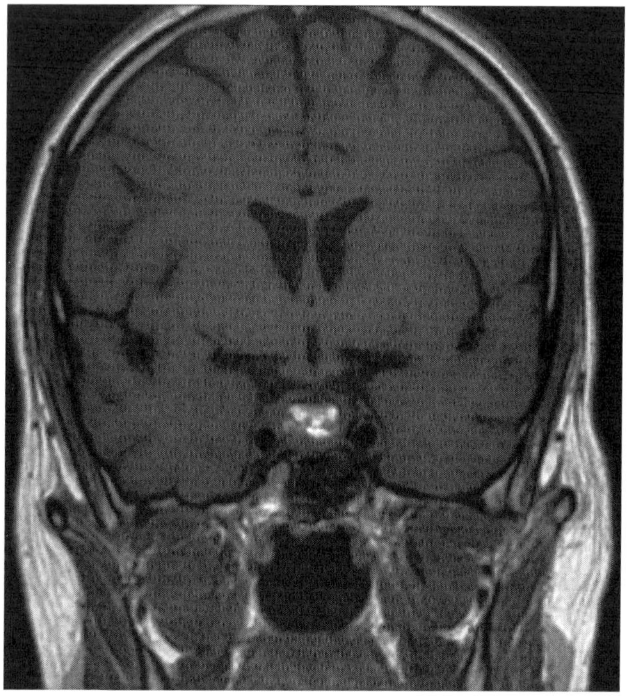

Fig. 2.14 Coronal T1-weighted image without contrast. Postoperative appearance of the sella following transsphenoidal approach resection of a sellar tumor, with fat-packing material in place manifested as lobular-shape of T1 shortening

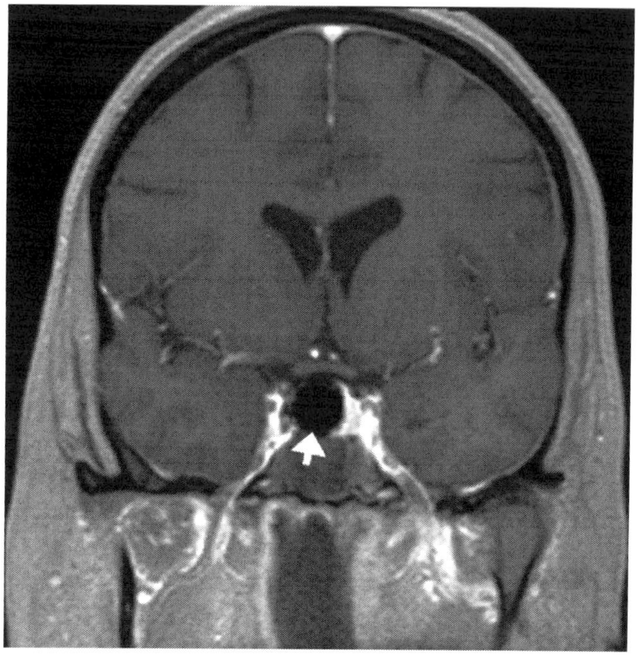

Fig. 2.15 Coronal T1-weighted image with intravenous contrast. Postoperative appearance of the sella following a transsphenoidal approach resection of a sellar tumor, with Gelfoam packing material in place (*arrow*) manifested as homogeneous T1 hypointensity

Acknowledgment ARRS/ASNR Scholar Award (Dr. Woang)

References

1. Sakamoto Y, Takahashi M, Korogi Y, Bussaka H, Ushio Y. Normal and abnormal pituitary glands: gadopentetate dimeglumine-enhanced MR imaging. Radiology. 1991;178:441–5.
2. Dwyer AJ, Frank JA, Doppman JL, Oldfield EH, Hickey AM, Cutler GB, et al. Pituitary adenomas in patients with Cushing disease: initial experience with Gd-DTPA-enhanced MR imaging. Radiology. 1987;163:421–6.
3. Yuh WT, Fisher DJ, Nguyen HD, Tali ET, Gao F, Simonson TM, Schlechte JA. Sequential MR enhancement pattern in normal pituitary gland and in pituitary adenoma. AJNR Am J Neuroradiol. 1994;15:101–8.
4. Mark LP, Haughton VM, Hendrix LE, Daniels DL, Williams AL, Czervionke LF, Asleson RJ. High-intensity signals within the posterior pituitary fossa: a study with fat-suppression MR techniques. AJNR Am J Neuroradiol. 1991;12:529–32.
5. Côté M, Salzman KL, Sorour M, Couldwell WT. Normal dimensions of the posterior pituitary bright spot on magnetic resonance imaging. J Neurosurg. 2014;120:357–62.
6. Brooks BS, el Gammal T, Allison JD, Hoffman WH. Frequency and variation of the posterior pituitary bright signal on MR images. AJNR Am J Neuroradiol. 1989;10:943–8.
7. Wolpert SM, Molitch ME, Goldman JA, Wood JB. Size, shape, and appearance of the normal female pituitary gland. Am J Roentgenol. 1984;143:377–81.
8. Tsunoda A, Okuda O, Sato K. MR height of the pituitary gland as a function of age and sex: especially physiological hypertrophy in adolescence and in climacterium. AJNR Am J Neuroradiol. 1997;18:551–4.
9. Elster AD. Imaging of the sella: anatomy and pathology. Semin Ultrasound CT MR. 1993;14:182–94.
10. Satogami N, Miki Y, Koyama T, Kataoka M, Togashi K. Normal pituitary stalk: high-resolution MR imaging at 3T. AJNR Am J Neuroradiol. 2010;31:355–9.
11. Kyriacou V, Mavridou C, Bintoudi A, Tzikos F, Kotziamani N, Tsitouridis I. Pituitary stalk interruption syndrome: the role of MRI and review of the literature. Neuroradiol J. 2010;23:607–12.
12. Welker KM, DeLone DR, Lane JI, Gilbertson JR. Arrested pneumatization of the skull base: imaging characteristics. Am J Roentgenol. 2008;190:1691–6.
13. Hamberger CA, Hammer G, Noren G, Sjogren B. Transantrosphenoidal hypophysectomy. Arch Otolaryngol. 1961;74: 2–8.
14. Zada G, Du R, Laws Jr ER. Defining the "edge of the envelope": patient selection in treating complex sellar-based neoplasms via transsphenoidal versus open craniotomy. J Neurosurg. 2011;114: 286–300.
15. Hamid O, El Fiky L, Hassan O, Kotb A, El Fiky S. Anatomic variations of the sphenoid sinus and their impact on trans-sphenoid pituitary surgery. Skull Base. 2008;18:9–15.
16. Sirikci A, Bayazit YA, Bayram M, Mumbuç S, Güngör K, Kanlikama M. Variations of sphenoid and related structures. Eur Radiol. 2000;10:844–8.
17. Naganuma H, Satoh E, Nukui H. Technical considerations of transsphenoidal removal of fibrous pituitary adenomas and evaluation of collagen content and subtype in the adenomas. Neurol Med Chir. 2002;42:202–12; discussion 213.
18. Pierallini A, Caramia F, Falcone C, Tinelli E, Paonessa A, Ciddio AB, et al. Pituitary macroadenomas: preoperative evaluation of consistency with diffusion-weighted MR imaging–initial experience. Radiology. 2006;239:223–31.
19. Yamamoto J, Kakeda S, Shimajiri S, Takahashi M, Watanabe K, Kai Y, et al. Tumor consistency of pituitary macroadenomas: predictive analysis on the basis of imaging features with contrast-enhanced 3D FIESTA at 3T. AJNR Am J Neuroradiol. 2014;35: 297–303.

Pituitary Physiology and Endocrinology

3

Miriam Padilla and John Carmichael

The hypothalamic-pituitary unit plays a vital role in several crucial bodily functions. The hypothalamus integrates stimuli from a wide array of sources to control behavioral, metabolic, and autonomic processes. Homeostatic mechanisms governed by the hypothalamus include water metabolism, appetite control, temperature regulation, sleep-wake cycles, and autonomic functions. It also plays a role in memory, behavior, and emotions. Importantly, the hypothalamus regulates the production and secretion of pituitary hormones. Through this function, it serves a critical role in the integration of neural and hormonal activity.

The pituitary gland, under control from peripheral hormonal feedback, intrapituitary paracrine action, and hypothalamic signaling, has a profound role in the endocrine and metabolic function of the body. The hypothalamus governs pituitary function through the release of adenohypophysiotropic hormones:

- Thyrotropin-releasing hormone (TRH)
- Gonadotropin-releasing hormone (GnRH)
- Dopamine
- Corticotropin-releasing hormone (CRH)
- Growth hormone-releasing hormone (GHRH)
- Somatostatin (somatotropin release-inhibiting factor, or SRIF)

These hypothalamic factors are secreted by neurosecretory cells within various nuclei of the hypothalamus and are released into the primary plexus of the hypophyseal portal circulation. There, they make contact with the median eminence and are then swept down the pituitary stalk vasculature to the anterior pituitary gland.

In response to the hypothalamic factors, the anterior pituitary, in turn, releases other hormones in exquisitely controlled pulsatile fashion:

- Thyroid-stimulating hormone (TSH)
- Adrenocorticotropin hormone (ACTH)
- Prolactin (PRL)
- Growth hormone (GH)
- Follicle-stimulating hormone (FSH)
- Luteinizing hormone (LH)

The hormones from the anterior pituitary are released from five hormone-producing cell types: thyrotrophs, lactotrophs, corticotrophs, somatotrophs, and gonadotrophs. The anterior lobe of the pituitary is only one part of the pituitary gland, but it constitutes the majority of the pituitary mass.

The pituitary also includes a vestigial intermediate lobe and a posterior lobe. The posterior pituitary gland stores and releases antidiuretic hormone (ADH), also known as vasopressin, and oxytocin. The cells of origin of the neurons secreting vasopressin and oxytocin are located in the paraventricular nuclei and the supraoptic nuclei of the hypothalamus. A broad overview of the hypothalamic-pituitary axes can be found in Table 3.1.

M. Padilla, MD
Division of Endocrinology and Diabetes, Department of Medicine, Los Angeles County/University of Southern California Medical Center, Los Angeles, CA, USA
e-mail: miriampadilla@gmail.com

J. Carmichael, MD (✉)
Division of Endocrinology and Diabetes, Department of Medicine, University of Southern California Pituitary Center, Los Angeles, CA, USA
e-mail: john.carmichael@med.usc.edu

G. Zada et al. (eds.), *Atlas of Sellar and Parasellar Lesions: Clinical, Radiologic, and Pathologic Correlations*,
DOI 10.1007/978-3-319-22855-6_3

Table 3.1 Hypothalamic-pituitary axis

Hypothalamic hormone	Main pituitary hormone	Target organs	Target hormones
CRH	Increases ACTH	Adrenal gland	Increases cortisol, DHEA, aldosterone, 17-hydroxyprogesterone
GHRH	Increases GH	Liver	Increases IGF-1
Somatostatin	Inhibits GH		
GnRH	Increases LH/FSH	Ovaries, testes	Increases progesterone, estradiol, testosterone
TRH	Increases TSH	Thyroid, bone	Increases T3, T4
Serotonin and opiates	Increase prolactin	Mammary gland	Increases PTHrP
Dopamine	Inhibits prolactin		
	Oxytocin	Uterus, mammary gland, ovary, testes, hippocampus, amygdala	Increases prolactin, LH, FSH, oxytocin, ANP Inhibits GH, TSH, ADH
	ADH	Kidneys, CNS	Increases ACTH secretion

ACTH adrenocorticotropin hormone, *ADH* antidiuretic hormone, *ANP* atrial natriuretic peptide, *CNS* central nervous system, *CRH* corticotropin-releasing hormone, *DHEA* dehydroepiandrosterone, *FSH* follicle-stimulating hormone, *GH* growth hormone, *GHRH* growth hormone-releasing hormone, *GnRH* gonadotropin-releasing hormone, *IGF* insulin-like growth factor, *LH* luteinizing hormone, *PTHrP* parathyroid hormone-related peptide, *T3* triiodothyronine, *T4* prohormone thyroxine, *TRH* thyrotropin-releasing hormone, *TSH* thyroid-stimulating hormone

3.1 Anterior Pituitary

The cells of the anterior lobe constitute 80 % of the pituitary gland by weight. The hypothalamic neurons that produce SRIF, GHRH, CRH, TRH, and GnRH send their axons through the median eminence to release these hormones into the hypophyseal portal circulation, which surrounds the pituitary stalk and penetrates the anterior lobe of the pituitary. These hypothalamic neurohormones stimulate and modulate the anterior pituitary cells to secrete GH, ACTH, TSH, LH, and FSH. Four glycoproteins—LH, FSH, TSH, and human chorionic gonadotropin (hCG)—share structural homology, having evolved from a common ancestral gene [1]. They all share an alpha subunit, whereas the beta subunit of each hormone is unique. SRIF is produced in the hypothalamus and works in concert with GHRH to modulate GH secretion from the pituitary. Approximately 50 % of cells of the anterior pituitary are somatotrophs that produce GH [2]. These cells are predominantly located in the lateral wings of the anterior lobe, but they can also be scattered in the median wedge. Prolactin-secreting lactotrophs account for 15 % of the cells in the anterior pituitary. Lactotrophs are randomly distributed throughout the lobe, but most are in the posteromedial and posterolateral portions [2]. Corticotrophs comprise 15 % of anterior pituitary cells; they mostly cluster in the central mucoid wedge but are also scattered in the lateral wings [2]. Thyrotroph cells comprise approximately 5 % of functional anterior pituitary cells and are situated predominantly in the anteromedial areas of the gland [1]. Finally, gonadotrophs, which produce LH and FSH, represent 5–15 % of the human anterior pituitary cell population [3].

3.1.1 Luteinizing Hormone and Follicle-Stimulating Hormone

The gonadotropins LH and FSH are produced by gonadotroph cells of the anterior pituitary in response to pulsatile secretion of GnRH from the hypothalamus [3]. GnRH is a 10-amino acid peptide that is released in synchronized pulses from hypothalamic nerve endings into the hypophyseal portal system every 30–120 min [4]. GnRH half-life is about 2–4 min [5]. The gonadotropins regulate gonadal steroid production and secretion and are responsible for germ cell development and the secretion of peripheral sex hormones. Although LH and FSH are co-secreted by the gonadotroph cells, their secretion is governed separately and their serum levels are not always concordant. The regulation of LH and FSH secretion is complex and corresponds to developmental age- and gender-specific feedback mechanisms. Several factors feed back to the hypothalamus, ultimately converging their signaling to the GnRH neurons, which integrate these stimuli to drive gonadotropin secretion.

Feedback inhibition of the gonadal axis is sexually dimorphic, but in general it is mediated by sex steroids and gonadal peptides that are secreted in response to LH and FSH secretion. In men, LH secretion is mediated by testosterone and by estradiol after aromatization of testosterone, at the level of the pituitary and hypothalamus [6, 7]. FSH secretion in men is controlled by both steroid hormones and inhibin B, a peptide secreted by germ cells in response to gonadotropins, through direct GnRH inhibition [8]. In men, LH induces intratesticular testosterone synthesis in the Leydig cells, and FSH mediates spermatogenesis in concert with testosterone.

In women, the feedback mechanisms responsible for the menstrual cycle and ovulation vary according to the phases of the menstrual cycle. In the early follicular phase, estradiol, progesterone, and inhibin A levels are low, leading to increased GnRH pulsation and a consequent small rise in FSH [9]. As the follicular phase progresses, increasing levels of estradiol feed back to the pituitary and hypothalamus to suppress FSH and LH secretion [10]. Mid-cycle, peripheral suppression of gonadotropins shifts to a transient positive feedback effect resulting in the LH surge [11]. The LH surge causes ovulation and leads to increased progesterone and inhibin A secretion with increased feedback inhibition to the gonadotrophs [12]. As the luteal phase progresses, peripheral progesterone and estradiol levels fall, resulting in the onset of menses and the release of FSH inhibition, allowing the cycle to begin again.

Other principal factors in gonadotropin feedback include stimulation of GnRH development and action by kisspeptin, via interaction with the orphan G protein-coupled receptor 54 (GPR54), and leptin, a product of adipose tissue that has stimulatory effects on GnRH pulsation [13, 14]. With the onset of menopause, gonadotropins rise in response to the decreased peripheral production of sex steroids.

Several pathophysiologic and physiologic factors can influence gonadotropic function or lead to gonadotropin deficiency. Deficiencies can be either congenital or acquired and can vary in severity from mild to complete gonadal dysfunction. Central congenital causes include a variety of genetic mutations involved in migration or function of GnRH neurons and the development and function of the gonadotroph cells. Functional causes are numerous; they include excessive exercise, stress, malnutrition, obesity, chronic illness, depression, and medications including opiates and antidepressants. Tumors, infiltrative diseases of the pituitary and hypothalamus, trauma, and malignancies also can lead to hypogonadotropic hypogonadism.

3.1.2 Thyroid-Stimulating Hormone

TSH is a glycoprotein hormone comprising a heterodimer of noncovalently linked alpha and beta subunits [1]. TRH induces TSH alpha and beta subunit gene transcription [1]. TRH is derived from pro-TRH by prohormone convertases. Once it is released from the paraventricular nucleus of the hypothalamus to the median eminence, it reaches the pituitary and stimulates the synthesis and release of TSH [15]. TSH binds to the TSH receptor, a seven-transmembrane glycosylated G protein-coupled receptor, resulting in thyroid follicular growth and thyroid hormone secretion from the thyroid gland [16]. TRH has a half-life of 2–6 min, and TSH can be seen as quickly as 30 min after administration of TRH [17]. Daily TSH production is about 100–400 mIU, with a half-life of 30–50 min [17]. TSH secretion is pulsatile, with pulses occurring every 2–3 h. Peak TSH secretion occurs between 11 PM and 5 AM [1]. TSH stimulates the thyroid to secrete the prohormone thyroxine (T4) and, to a lesser extent, the hormone triiodothyronine (T3) [18]. Most T3 is generated by peripheral conversion of T4 by intracellular iodothyronine deiodinases [18]. In normal conditions, production of T3 and T4 exerts a negative feedback control on the level of the hypothalamus and the pituitary [19]. T3 inhibits TRH gene transcription, as well as inhibiting TSH synthesis and release [2].

Several biological phenomena can affect TSH secretion. TSH production rises with age, but this phenomenon can be confounded by many situations that inhibit TSH secretion in the elderly, such as decreased exercise, reduced caloric intake, exposure to glucocorticoids, traumatic brain injury, and psychiatric depression [20]. Pharmacologic doses of glucocorticoids can inhibit basal TSH secretion and abolish the circadian TSH rhythm [21]. Furthermore, in severe and prolonged nutritional restriction, as in anorexia nervosa, increased cortisol secretion may contribute to the suppression of TSH release [21]. In humans, food deprivation results in several neuroendocrine responses [22]:

- Increasing ACTH and cortisol
- Decreasing thyroid hormone concentrations, thereby slowing metabolic rate
- Increasing GH concentration, thereby mobilizing energy stores
- Decreasing insulin growth factor 1 concentration, thereby slowing energy-demanding growth-related processes
- Decreasing reproductive hormone concentrations, thereby reducing fertility and preventing pregnancy

Leptin, discovered as a factor produced by adipose tissue, induces satiety and is an indicator of the body's nutritional status [17]. Leptin is a 167-amino acid peptide that is produced predominantly in the adipose tissue but is also expressed in the placenta, ovaries, mammary, epithelium, bone marrow, and lymphoid tissues [22]. Leptin replacement during fasting prevents the starvation-induced changes in the hypothalamic-pituitary-thyroid axis [22]. Several studies have shown that leptin is involved in regulating the release of TRH from the paraventricular nucleus, as low levels of circulating leptin are accompanied by a decrease in TRH mRNA [23]. Fasting and infection upregulate type II deiodinase expression, resulting in a local increase of T3, which may explain a reactive decrease in TSH observed during fasting or inflammatory diseases [2]. In contrast, chronic fatigue syndrome, morbid obesity, and diabetes type 2 may increase TSH secretion [20].

3.1.3 Prolactin

Prolactin (PRL) is a 199-amino acid polypeptide that circulates in blood in various sizes, including 23-kd monomeric prolactin, 48- to 56-kd dimeric prolactin ("big prolactin"), and polymeric complexes larger than 100 kd, referred to as "big, big prolactin" [1]. The monomeric form is the most bioactive form. PRL secretion differs from the secretion of other anterior pituitary hormones in that it is not regulated by negative feedback from peripheral hormones. PRL is regulated by tonic inhibition from dopaminergic neurons from the hypothalamus. Dopamine is secreted into the portal system and inhibits PRL through binding to type 2 dopamine (D2) receptors on the lactotroph cell surface. Normal daily PRL production ranges from 200 to 500 µg/day per square meter of body surface area [24]. It is secreted in 4–14 secretory pulses over 24 h, each lasting 67–76 min [25, 26]. The half-life of PRL ranges from 26 to 47 min. The highest levels occur during sleep, and the lowest levels occur between 10 AM and noon [24]. Levels are higher in women than in men, are higher during ovulation, and fall with age in both men and women [20]. After menopause, PRL secretion during nighttime falls by 40 % [20].

Lactotroph cells of the anterior pituitary are the main source for circulating PRL, but other sources of production include lymphocytes, skin fibroblasts, brain, breast, decidua, prostate, and adipose tissue cells [27]. The main function of PRL in humans is to stimulate milk production, but it is also involved in mammary development, melanin synthesis, and parental behavior [1]. During pregnancy, increasing estrogen secretion stimulates the growth and proliferation of the lactotrophs; as a result, PRL secretion increases [27]. The size of the pituitary doubles during pregnancy, owing to hyperplasia and hypertrophy of lactotrophs [27]. The absolute number of lactotrophs does not change during pregnancy, however, and the lactotroph hyperplasia resolves within several months after delivery [1]. During pregnancy, PRL, together with estradiol, progesterone, placental lactogen, insulin, and cortisol, cause mammary gland growth and development [27]. Prolactin prepares the mammary gland for postpartum lactation, but the high estrogen concentration during pregnancy inhibits the lactation effect in the mammary gland while the woman is still pregnant [27]. Then, as estrogen levels fall after delivery, the initiation of lactation can occur [27]. After delivery, suckling is essential for the continued secretion of PRL; if the woman does not breast-feed, PRL levels can return to normal within 7 days [1]. Suckling stimulates neurons of the hypothalamus to secrete opioids, which in turn decrease dopamine secretion in the hypothalamus and relieve the lactotroph cells from dopaminergic inhibition [27]. During lactation, mobilization of bone is critical to ensuring availability of large amounts of calcium exported into milk [28]. PRL helps this to occur by indirectly allowing for the secretion of parathyroid hormone-related peptide (PTHrP). PRL causes dilatation of the mammary gland alveoli, which in turn synthesize serotonin in the mammary epithelial cells [28]. Serotonin then controls the expression of PTHrP in the mammary glands [28]. PTHrP is secreted in large quantities from lactating mammary glands, causing bone resorption [28]. Elevated PRL during and immediately after pregnancy also inhibits ovulation by suppressing LH and FSH secretion [27]. Similarly, feedback to the hypothalamus from pathologic hyperprolactinemia of any etiology can inhibit GnRH-mediated LH and FSH secretion, thereby inducing a hypogonadotropic hypogonadism [29].

Beyond elevations seen during pregnancy, PRL production is stimulated by many other factors, including psychological and physical stress, breast stimulation, hypoglycemia, estrogen, use of dopamine-2-receptor antagonist medications, sexual activity, hyperthermia, sleep, food intake, opiates, and exercise [1]. Some hormones that stimulate secretion include TRH, oxytocin, ghrelin, vasoactive intestinal polypeptide (VIP), epidermal growth factor, serotonin, angiotensin II, estradiol, oxytocin, galanin, and GHRH at high doses [27]. Estrogen increases PRL secretion mainly by reducing expression of lactotroph dopamine receptors [2]. In rats, a short feedback loop for PRL has been described, with PRL increasing tyrosine hydroxylase activity in the tuberoinfundibular neurons [1]. Other than dopamine, growth factor B1, noradrenaline, gamma-aminobutyric acid (GABA), serotonin, histamine, somatostatin, chromogranin, orexin-A, cortistatin, nitrogen oxide, and endothelin-1 also inhibit prolactin secretion [27].

Abnormal elevations of PRL secretion can arise from prolactinomas (benign pituitary adenomas derived from lactotroph cells) or can be due to non-prolactinoma tumors located in the sellar and parasellar regions through the so-called stalk effect, in which PRL is secreted from nontumor cells when dopaminergic inhibition is interrupted. Drugs, inflammation (hypophysitis), neurogenic chest wall stimulation, and reduced PRL clearance are other causes of hyperprolactinemia. PRL deficiency is rare and can be due to trauma or inflammatory or genetic causes.

3.1.4 Growth Hormone

Somatotroph cells from the anterior pituitary secrete GH, a hormone principally responsible for linear growth during development, but with many other metabolic functions. GH circulates primarily as a 22-kD, 191-amino acid, single-chain peptide bound to GH binding protein. GH secretion is normally episodic and exhibits a diurnal rhythm with approximately two thirds of the total daily GH secretion occurring at night, triggered by the onset of slow-wave sleep [1]. Normal GH secretion is characterized by secretory episodes separated by troughs of minimal basal secretion during which GH is undetectable [1].

GH secretion is regulated by hypothalamic secretion of growth hormone-releasing hormone (GHRH) and somatostatin (SRIF) [30]. Several hypothalamic factors influence SRIF and GHRH secretion; the secretion of these hormones in concert determines the pulsation frequency and amplitude of GH secretion [31]. The somatotroph cell responds to signaling from GHRH, SRIF, and growth hormone secretagogues to secrete GH. SRIF, a cyclopeptide consisting of 14–28 amino acids, is expressed in many tissues throughout the body, including the central nervous system, hypothalamus, gastrointestinal tract, and the pancreas [32, 33].

Once in circulation, GH binds to GH receptors to stimulate production and secretion of insulin-like growth factors (IGFs), of which IGF-1 is the principal target growth factor [31]. IGF-1 circulates bound to IGF-binding proteins and participates in feedback inhibition of GH secretion via inhibition at the level of the pituitary and stimulation of SRIF release [34].

GH concentration is high in fetal circulation, falls during early childhood, and then rises again at the onset of puberty [1]. Daily production of GH in the prepubertal state is 200–600 μg, which then rises to 1000–1800 μg at the pubertal peak [31]. Secretion of GH then proceeds to decline progressively throughout adulthood [35]. Adiposity that accompanies the aging process accounts for a significant component of the decline in GH output with increasing age [36]. Basal and stimulated GH levels can be reduced in patients with obesity, especially visceral adiposity [37]. Aged adults secrete less GH than do young individuals during fasting, exercise, or sleep, in response to nearly all secretagogues [20].

IGF-1 is produced mainly in the liver in response to GH and is a mediator of GH effects on protein anabolism [1]. IGF-1 strongly stimulates protein synthesis and inhibits protein breakdown [38]. This action is especially relevant in situations of starvation, in which GH and IGF-1 secretion both limit catabolism of protein and instead encourage the mobilization of fat stores [39]. GH has been shown to promote fat metabolism by enhancing lipolysis and fatty acid oxidation [38]. In this situation, elevation of free fatty acids (FFAs) then acts as a negative feedback to suppress further GH secretion [40].

Ghrelin, which is produced in the gastric mucosal neuroendocrine cells and in the hypothalamus, binds to the GH secretagogue receptor (a receptor that was discovered before the endogenous ligand ghrelin) to induce GH release [41, 42]. Ghrelin concentrations have been shown to be decreased in situations where GHRH expression is muted, such as in cases of glucocorticoid excess, hyperthyroidism, and food deprivation [23]. Ghrelin specifically is involved in encouraging appetite and increased food intake [43]. Once ghrelin levels rise in anticipation of food intake, GH is produced, which then exerts some insulin-like effects, stimulating amino acid uptake and protein synthesis [44]. However, in opposition to insulin, GH suppresses glucose oxidation and utilization while enhancing hepatic glucose production [38]. It has long been known that there is a relationship between glucose metabolism and GH secretion [45]. This relationship has been capitalized upon to develop testing for GH deficiency with insulin-induced hypoglycemia and testing for acromegaly with suppression of GH with glucose administration [45, 46].

Several other peripheral factors, hormones, and clinical settings influence GH secretion. Testosterone stimulates GH secretion centrally, whereas estrogen influences GH secretion indirectly [1]. Oral estrogen not only increases growth hormone binding protein but also stimulates GH secretion by inhibiting IGF-1 production, thus decreasing IGF-1 feedback inhibition [1]. Dopamine and interleukin-1 beta (IL-1B) can stimulate SRIF release [47]. Beta-blockers like propranolol can decrease hypothalamic SRIF secretion [47]. Certain medications with alpha-adrenergic effects, such as clonidine and L-dopa, have demonstrated increased GH secretion [1]. Norepinephrine also works via the alpha-adrenergic pathways to increase GH secretion, whereas beta-adrenergic pathways in turn decrease GH release [1]. When patients are left with GH deficiency, they may have increased visceral adiposity, abnormal lipid profiles, premature atherosclerosis, decreased muscle mass, osteoporosis, and decreased quality of life [48]. Conversely, the GH excess found in acromegaly exerts profound metabolic and growth abnormalities, including soft tissue and bony growth, hypertension, diabetes, cardiac disease, sleep abnormalities, and shortened survival [49].

3.1.5 Adrenocorticotropin Hormone

The corticotroph cells of the pituitary play an essential role in maintaining metabolic homeostasis and reacting in response to stress stimuli through secretion of ACTH, which regulates serum levels of glucocorticoids in the body. The corticotroph cell is under hypothalamic control, and secretion of ACTH is mediated through a negative feedback loop involving peripheral glucocorticoids.

Corticotroph cells produce ACTH through the processing of the pre-prohormone proopiomelanocortin (POMC). Products of this precursor include ACTH and beta-lipotropin, which is cleaved to form alpha-lipotropin and beta-endorphin [1]. ACTH can be cleaved to form a melanocyte-stimulating hormone (alpha-MSH) [1].

CRH acts on corticotropin-releasing factor receptor 1 (CRFR1) receptors on the anterior pituitary corticotrophs to stimulate the release of ACTH [50]. Vasopressin acts synergistically with CRH to augment the release of ACTH in humans [50]. ACTH is then secreted by corticotroph cells [1]. ACTH then enters the blood stream and acts via melanocortin type 2 receptors (MC2R) in the adrenal gland cortex to stimulate the synthesis and release of adrenal glucocorticoids, androgenic steroids such as dehydroepiandrosterone (DHEA), and, to a small degree, mineralocorticoids [50]. ACTH signals via adenyl cyclase to regulate cytochrome P450 enzyme transcription, which then controls the synthesis and secretion of cortisol, aldosterone, 17-hydroxyprogesterone, and adrenal androgens [51]. Secretory cortisol pulses follow ACTH pulses within 5–10 min [1]. Once cortisol levels increase, a prominent negative feedback system then acts to inhibit further CRH production and release from the hypothalamus [50]. By this negative feedback, both basal and stimulated ACTH secretions are blunted in response to glucocorticoids [52]. Although cortisol rapidly inhibits hypothalamic CRH and pituitary ACTH secretion in a long feedback loop, chronic exposure to glucocorticoids can suppress the hypothalamic-pituitary-adrenal (HPA) axis for a longer period that depends on the duration, potency, and dose of the steroid. Feedback is also mediated in a short feedback loop whereby ACTH inhibits CRH secretion as well as an ultrashort loop of ACTH suppression of the corticotroph itself [1].

ACTH and cortisol follow a 24-h circadian rhythm that is driven by CRH [53]. Human ACTH and cortisol begin rising between 1 and 4 AM, peak during early morning, have a lower peak in the early afternoon, then fall during the rest of the day, and reach a nadir about midnight [2]. The ACTH circadian rhythm is influenced by visual cues—specifically, the light and dark cycle [54]—but the normal HPA axis can be disrupted by conditions including mania, depression, dementia, chronic fatigue syndrome, alcoholism, visceral adiposity, diabetes mellitus, polycystic ovary syndrome (PCOS), acute illness, systemic disease, or multiorgan failure [55].

In response to stress, there is stimulation of the parvocellular neurons of the hypothalamic paraventricular nucleus (PVN) and consequent release of CRH and vasopressin (ADH). CRH, which has a half-life of 4 min, then stimulates the pituitary to release ACTH, which peaks 30 min after the release of CRH [56]. The result is stimulation of glucocorticoid secretion by the adrenal cortex, which is essential for stress adaptation [56]. Stimulants of CRH release include endogenous and exogenous stress, such as the stress of hypoglycemia [1]. Other stressors that stimulate CRH and ACTH release include pain, infection, inflammation, hemorrhage, hypovolemia, trauma, and psychological stress [1]. In situations of inflammation, IL-6, tumor necrosis factor (TNF) alpha, and IL-1 normally increase CRH release, resulting in increasing glucocorticoid levels, which then limit inflammation by inhibiting lymphocyte proliferation and production of immunoglobulins and cytokines [2]. Exercise stimulates ACTH release and glucocorticoid production, especially during intense anaerobic exercise [57]. The stimulation of CRH by exercise is important because CRH increases heart rate and venous return to the heart, increases mesenteric and aortic blood flow, and at the same time reduces food intake [5]. CRH is able to have such widespread effects on the body because CRH receptors have been found not only in the anterior pituitary gland but also in the retina, heart, skeletal muscle, vasculature, adrenal gland, and gastrointestinal tissue [5]. These widely distributed receptors allow for CRH effects to vary from reducing gastric acid secretion to protecting cardiac myocytes from lethal ischemic injury [50].

ACTH excess may result from corticotroph-derived pituitary adenomas. It causes excess cortisol secretion. When this cortisol excess is caused by a pituitary tumor, it is called Cushing's disease, whereas the general term Cushing's syndrome is used for all other forms. The syndrome consists of myriad symptoms and comorbidities, including central weight gain, muscle atrophy, fatty tissue dysplasia, hypertension, diabetes mellitus, and osteoporosis, among others.

ACTH deficiency can be due to congenital or acquired causes, including genetic deletions, inflammatory and infiltrative diseases of the hypothalamus and pituitary, trauma, and compression from local tumors or other masses. The effects of adrenal insufficiency that arise from ACTH deficiency can be fatal if not adequately treated; manifestations include cardiovascular collapse, metabolic derangements, acute abdominal pain, nausea, and vomiting, all culminating in adrenal crisis if not recognized early in the course of illness.

3.2 Posterior Pituitary

Oxytocin and vasopressin are nine-amino acid-long peptides that differ from each other at only two amino acid positions [58]. Oxytocin and vasopressin neuron bodies, located in the hypothalamus, send axons through the pituitary stalk to terminate in the posterior pituitary, where they release oxytocin and vasopressin.

3.2.1 Vasopressin (ADH)

Vasopressin, also known as antidiuretic hormone (ADH), is synthesized in the nerve cell bodies of the supraoptic and paraventricular nuclei [59]. The hormone is packaged into secretory granules and transported down long axons that terminate in the pituitary stalk and posterior pituitary [59]. ADH is secreted from the neurohypophysis in response to reductions in plasma volume and increases in the plasma osmolality [60]. Blood volume status is monitored by baroreceptors present in the left atrium and large pulmonary veins, while serum osmolality changes are detected by peripheral and hypothalamic osmoreceptors [59]. ADH acts to promote water conservation through the V2 receptors of the distal tubules and collecting ducts of the kidneys by increasing their water permeability through the aquaporin-II water channels [61]. This allows water to be reabsorbed from the urine. A lack of ADH causes central diabetes insipidus, whereas an inability of the kidney to respond normally to ADH causes nephrogenic diabetes insipidus. ADH is also involved in increasing arterial blood pressure and in regulating CRH secretion [60]. In addition to the usual control of ADH secretion and production through baroreceptor and osmoreceptor pathways, other stimuli for ADH release include nausea, vomiting, nicotine, hypoglycemia, hypoxia, barbiturates, beta-adrenergic drugs, morphine, tricyclic antidepressants, cholinergic drugs, and pain [59]. Inhibitors of ADH release include ethanol, alpha-adrenergic drugs, atropine, chlorpromazine, alpha blockers, and glucocorticoids [59].

3.2.2 Oxytocin

Oxytocin is involved in a wide variety of physiological functions such as sexual activity, penile erection, ejaculation, pregnancy, uterus contraction, milk ejection, and maternal behavior [62]. Oxytocin is produced in the supraoptic and paraventricular nuclei of the hypothalamus and is mainly released from the neurohypophysis [62].

Some of the social behaviors influenced by oxytocin include social memory, attachment, sexual activity, maternal behavior, aggression, pair bonding, and trust [60]. Oxytocin abnormalities have been implicated in the development of autism spectrum disorders as well as in obsessive-compulsive disorders. Some of the nonsocial behaviors that involve oxytocin include brain development, learning and memory, feeding, respiration, cardiovascular activity, digestion, energy balance, thermoregulation, immune regulation, pain perception, lactation, and parturition [60]. Plasma oxytocin levels increase during sexual arousal in both women and men and are significantly higher than prior baseline levels during orgasm/ejaculation [60].

In women, oxytocin fluctuates throughout the menstrual cycle. During labor, oxytocin can elicit uterine smooth muscle contraction to facilitate parturition and postpartum recovery of the uterus [60]. Oxytocin as a medication is used to induce or augment maternal labor, especially for those who are after term [62]. Shortly before delivery, maternal oxytocin crossing the placenta reaches the fetal brain and induces a switch in the action of GABA from excitatory to inhibitory fetal neurons [60]. This action increases the resistance of fetal neurons to hypoxia insults during labor [60]. Following parturition, oxytocin becomes an essential tool for the development of mother-child attachment [60]. Suckling stimulates a bolus release of oxytocin, which (along with prolactin) causes ejection of the milk from the mammary glands [60].

Conclusion

The hypothalamic-pituitary axis is critical in maintaining body endocrine homeostasis. Through the production and secretion of the anterior pituitary hormones PRL, ACTH, TSH, LH, FSH, and GH—each governed by hypothalamic hypophysiotropic neuropeptides—the pituitary serves to regulate serum levels of several important hormones responsible for metabolism, growth, reproduction, and lactation. The posterior pituitary hormones oxytocin and vasopressin (ADH) are vital to labor, delivery, breastfeeding, and water homeostasis.

References

1. Melmed S, Kleinberg DL, Ho K. Pituitary physiology and diagnostic evaluation. In: Melmed S, Polonsky KS, Larsen PR, Kronenberg HM, editors. Williams textbook of endocrinology. 12th ed. Philadelphia: Saunders; 2011. p. 175–228.
2. Ben-Shlomo A, Melmed S. Regulation of anterior pituitary function. In: Melmed S, editor. The pituitary. 3rd ed. Waltham: Academic; 2011. p. 21–45.
3. Thackray VG, Mellon PL, Coss D. Hormones in synergy: regulation of the pituitary gonadotropin genes. Mol Cell Endocrinol. 2010;314:192–203.
4. Vadakkadath Meethal S, Atwood CS. The role of hypothalamic-pituitary-gonadal hormones in the normal structure and functioning of the brain. Cell Mol Life Sci. 2005;62:257–70.
5. Quintanar JL, Guzman-Soto I. Hypothalamic neurohormones and immune responses. Front Integr Neurosci. 2013;7:56.
6. Matsumoto AM, Bremner WJ. Modulation of pulsatile gonadotropin secretion by testosterone in man. J Clin Endocrinol Metab. 1984;58:609–14.
7. Hayes FJ, Seminara SB, Decruz S, Boepple PA, Crowley Jr WF. Aromatase inhibition in the human male reveals a hypothalamic site of estrogen feedback. J Clin Endocrinol Metab. 2000;85:3027–35.
8. O'Connor AE, De Kretser DM. Inhibins in normal male physiology. Semin Reprod Med. 2004;22:177–85.
9. Hall JE, Schoenfeld DA, Martin KA, Crowley Jr WF. Hypothalamic gonadotropin-releasing hormone secretion and follicle-stimulating hormone dynamics during the luteal-follicular transition. J Clin Endocrinol Metab. 1992;74:600–7.
10. Sherman BM, Korenman SG. Hormonal characteristics of the human menstrual cycle throughout reproductive life. J Clin Invest. 1975;55:699–706.
11. Adams JM, Taylor AE, Schoenfeld DA, Crowley Jr WF, Hall JE. The midcycle gonadotropin surge in normal women occurs in the face of an unchanging gonadotropin-releasing hormone pulse frequency. J Clin Endocrinol Metab. 1994;79:858–64.
12. Stocco C, Telleria C, Gibori G. The molecular control of corpus luteum formation, function, and regression. Endocr Rev. 2007;28:117–49.
13. Gutierrez-Pascual E, Martinez-Fuentes AJ, Pinilla L, Tena-Sempere M, Malagon MM, Castano JP. Direct pituitary effects of kisspeptin: activation of gonadotrophs and somatotrophs and stimulation of luteinising hormone and growth hormone secretion. J Neuroendocrinol. 2007;19:521–30.
14. Moschos S, Chan JL, Mantzoros CS. Leptin and reproduction: a review. Fertil Steril. 2002;77:433–44.
15. Costa-e-Sousa RH, Hollenberg AN. Minireview: the neural regulation of the hypothalamic-pituitary-thyroid axis. Endocrinology. 2012;153:4128–35.
16. Colaianni G, Cuscito C, Colucci S. FSH and TSH in the regulation of bone mass: the pituitary/immune/bone axis. Clin Dev Immunol. 2013;2013:382698.
17. Moura EG, Moura CC. Regulation of thyrotropin synthesis and secretion. Arq Bras Endocrinol Metabol. 2004;48:40–52.
18. Mebis L, van den Berghe G. The hypothalamus-pituitary-thyroid axis in critical illness. Neth J Med. 2009;67:332–40.
19. Mebis L, Debaveye Y, Visser TJ, Van den Berghe G. Changes within the thyroid axis during the course of critical illness. Endocrinol Metab Clin North Am. 2006;35:807–21.
20. Veldhuis JD. Changes in pituitary function with ageing and implications for patient care. Nat Rev Endocrinol. 2013;9:205–15.
21. Fisher DA. Physiological variations in thyroid hormones: physiological and pathophysiological considerations. Clin Chem. 1996;42:135–9.
22. Mantzoros CS, Magkos F, Brinkoetter M, Sienkiewicz E, Dardeno TA, Kim SY, et al. Leptin in human physiology and pathophysiology. Am J Physiol Endocrinol Metab. 2011;301:E567–84.
23. Guillemin R. Hypothalamic hormones a.k.a. hypothalamic releasing factors. J Endocrinol. 2005;184:11–28.
24. Cooper DS, Ridgway EC, Kliman B, Kjellberg RN, Maloof F. Metabolic clearance and production rates of prolactin in man. J Clin Invest. 1979;64:1669–80.
25. Veldhuis JD, Johnson ML. Operating characteristics of the hypothalamo-pituitary-gonadal axis in men: circadian, ultradian, and pulsatile release of prolactin and its temporal coupling with luteinizing hormone. J Clin Endocrinol Metab. 1988;67:116–23.
26. Greenspan SL, Klibanski A, Rowe JW, Elahi D. Age alters pulsatile prolactin release: influence of dopaminergic inhibition. Am J Physiol. 1990;258:E799–804.
27. Ignacak A, Kasztelnik M, Sliwa T, Korbut RA, Rajda K, Guzik TJ. Prolactin–not only lactotrophin. A "new" view of the "old" hormone. J Physiol Pharmacol. 2012;63:435–43.
28. Horseman ND, Gregerson KA. Prolactin actions. J Mol Endocrinol. 2014;52:R95–106.
29. Serri O, Chik CL, Ur E, Ezzat S. Diagnosis and management of hyperprolactinemia. CMAJ. 2003;169:575–81.
30. Corpas E, Harman SM, Blackman MR. Human growth hormone and human aging. Endocr Rev. 1993;14:20–39.
31. Giustina A, Veldhuis JD. Pathophysiology of the neuroregulation of growth hormone secretion in experimental animals and the human. Endocr Rev. 1998;19:717–97.
32. Reichlin S. Somatostatin. N Engl J Med. 1983;309:1495–501.
33. Reichlin S. Somatostatin (second of two parts). N Engl J Med. 1983;309:1556–63.
34. Jones JI, Clemmons DR. Insulin-like growth factors and their binding proteins: biological actions. Endocr Rev. 1995;16:3–34.
35. Zadik Z, Chalew SA, McCarter Jr RJ, Meistas M, Kowarski AA. The influence of age on the 24-hour integrated concentration of growth hormone in normal individuals. J Clin Endocrinol Metab. 1985;60:513–6.
36. Vahl N, Jorgenson JO, Jurik AG, Christiansen JS. Abdominal adiposity and physical fitness are major determinants of the age

associated decline in stimulated GH secretion in healthy adults. J Clin Endocrinol Metab. 1996;81:2209–15.
37. Rasmussen MH, Frystyk J, Andersen T, Breum L, Christiansen JS, Hilsted J. The impact of obesity, fat distribution, and energy restriction on insulin-like growth factor-1 (IGF-1), IGF-binding protein-3, insulin, and growth hormone. Metabolism. 1994;43:315–9.
38. Takahashi Y. Essential roles of growth hormone (GH) and insulin-like growth factor-I (IGF-I) in the liver. Endocr J. 2012;59: 955–62.
39. Brick DJ, Gerweck AV, Meenaghan E, Lawson EA, Misra M, Fazeli P, et al. Determinants of IGF1 and GH across the weight spectrum: from anorexia nervosa to obesity. Eur J Endocrinol. 2010;163:185–91.
40. Casanueva FF, Villanueva L, Dieguez C, Diaz Y, Cabranes JA, Szoke B, et al. Free fatty acids block growth hormone (GH) releasing hormone-stimulated GH secretion in man directly at the pituitary. J Clin Endocrinol Metab. 1987;65:634–42.
41. Howard AD, Feighner SD, Cully DF, Arena JP, Liberator PA, Rosenblum CI, et al. A receptor in pituitary and hypothalamus that functions in growth hormone release. Science. 1996;273:974–7.
42. Kojima M, Hosoda H, Date Y, Nakazato M, Matsuo H, Kangawa K. Ghrelin is a growth-hormone-releasing acylated peptide from stomach. Nature. 1999;402:656–60.
43. Smith RG, Jiang H, Sun Y. Developments in ghrelin biology and potential clinical relevance. Trends Endocrinol Metab. 2005;16: 436–42.
44. Moller N, Jorgenson JO, Abildgard N, Orskov L, Schmitz O, Christiansen JS. Effects of growth hormone on glucose metabolism. Horm Res. 1991;36 Suppl 1:32–5.
45. Roth J, Glick SM, Yalow RS, Berson SA. The influence of blood glucose on the plasma concentration of growth hormone. Diabetes. 1964;13:355–61.
46. Earll JM, Sparks LL, Forsham PH. Glucose suppression of serum growth hormone in the diagnosis of acromegaly. JAMA. 1967;201: 628–30.
47. Buonomo FC, Baile CA. The neurophysiological regulation of growth hormone secretion. Domest Anim Endocrinol. 1990;7: 435–50.
48. de Boer H, Blok GJ, Van der Veen EA. Clinical aspects of growth hormone deficiency in adults. Endocr Rev. 1995;16:63–86.
49. Melmed S. Acromegaly pathogenesis and treatment. J Clin Invest. 2009;119:3189–202.
50. Bale TL, Vale WW. CRF and CRF receptors: role in stress responsivity and other behaviors. Annu Rev Pharmacol Toxicol. 2004;44: 525–57.
51. Keeney DS, Waterman MR. Regulation of steroid hydroxylase gene expression: importance to physiology and disease. Pharmacol Ther. 1993;58:301–17.
52. Keller-Wood ME, Dallman MF. Corticosteroid inhibition of ACTH secretion. Endocr Rev. 1984;5:1–24.
53. Buckley TM, Schatzberg AF. On the interactions of the hypothalamic-pituitary-adrenal (HPA) axis and sleep: normal HPA axis activity and circadian rhythm, exemplary sleep disorders. J Clin Endocrinol Metab. 2005;90:3106–14.
54. Gomez MT, Magiakou MA, Mastorakos G, Chrousos GP. The pituitary corticotroph is not the rate limiting step in the postoperative recovery of the hypothalamic-pituitary-adrenal axis in patients with Cushing syndrome. J Clin Endocrinol Metab. 1993;77:173–7.
55. Veldhuis JD, Sharma A, Roelfsema F. Age-dependent and gender-dependent regulation of hypothalamic-adrenocorticotropic-adrenal axis. Endocrinol Metab Clin North Am. 2013;42:201–25.
56. Aguilera G. HPA axis responsiveness to stress: implications for healthy aging. Exp Gerontol. 2011;46:90–5.
57. Kanaley JA, Weltman JY, Pieper KS, Weltman A, Hartman ML. Cortisol and growth hormone responses to exercise at different times of day. J Clin Endocrinol Metab. 2001;86:2881–9.
58. Donaldson ZR, Young LJ. Oxytocin, vasopressin, and the neurogenetics of sociality. Science. 2008;322:900–4.
59. Braunstein G. The hypothalamus. In: Melmed S, editor. The pituitary. 3rd ed. Waltham: Academic; 2011. p. 303–37.
60. Yang HP, Wang L, Han L, Wang SC. Nonsocial functions of hypothalamic oxytocin. ISRN Neurosci. 2013;2013:179272.
61. Agre P, King LS, Yasui M, Guggino WB, Ottersen OP, Fujiyoshi Y, et al. Aquaporin water channels–from atomic structure to clinical medicine. J Physiol. 2002;542:3–16.
62. Viero C, Shibuya I, Kitamura N, Verkhratsky A, Fujihara H, Katoh A, et al. REVIEW: oxytocin: crossing the bridge between basic science and pharmacotherapy. CNS Neurosci Ther. 2010;16: e138–56.

4 Pathology and Molecular Biology of the Pituitary Region

M. Beatriz S. Lopes

4.1 Introduction

Tumors of the pituitary gland and sellar region represent approximately 10–15 % of all brain tumors [1]. Numerous types of tumors may involve the sellar region, reflecting its complex anatomy. Table 4.1 lists the most frequent tumors arising in the pituitary and sellar region. By far the most common of these are pituitary adenomas, benign epithelial tumors derived from cells of the adenohypophysis. In fact, pituitary adenomas represent the third most common primary intracranial tumor in neurosurgical practice, outnumbered only by gliomas and meningiomas [1]. Pituitary adenomas predominantly affect women between the third and sixth decades, but no age group is spared [1]. Adenomas are uncommon in the pediatric population, and most tumors of childhood are clinically functioning adenomas that are thought to be more aggressive [2]. Rates for pituitary tumors in the United States are slightly higher among African Americans than Caucasians [1]. Incidental adenomas can be found in nearly 10 % of autopsied patients [3].

Table 4.1 Tumors and tumor-like conditions of the pituitary gland and sellar region

Tumor origin	Specific entity
Neuroendocrine tumors	Pituitary adenoma
	Atypical adenoma
	Pituitary carcinoma
Non-neuroendocrine tumors	Pituicytoma
	Granular cell tumor
	Spindle cell oncocytoma
	Gangliocytoma
Tumors of non-pituitary origin	Craniopharyngioma
	Meningioma
	Chordoma
	Langerhans cell histiocytosis
	Germ cell tumors
	Metastases
Cystic lesions	Rathke's cleft cyst
	Arachnoid cyst
	Epidermoid/dermoid cyst
Inflammatory lesions	Lymphocytic hypophysitis
	Granulomatous hypophysitis
	Sarcoidosis

M.B.S. Lopes, MD, PhD
Department of Pathology (Neuropathology), University of Virginia School of Medicine, 1215 Lee Street, Room 3060–HEP, Charlottesville, VA 22908, USA
e-mail: msl2e@virginia.edu

G. Zada et al. (eds.), *Atlas of Sellar and Parasellar Lesions: Clinical, Radiologic, and Pathologic Correlations*, DOI 10.1007/978-3-319-22855-6_4

4.2 Pituitary Adenomas

4.2.1 Classification

Pituitary adenomas are classified clinically into two main groups: clinically functioning adenomas and clinically nonfunctioning adenomas, according to whether an endocrine syndrome is present. Most adenomas are functioning tumors, which may produce prolactin (PRL), growth hormone (GH), adrenocorticotropic hormone (ACTH), or thyroid-stimulating hormone (TSH) [4]. However, about a third of all pituitary adenomas are unassociated with either clinical or biochemical evidence of hormone excess [5]. This group includes gonadotroph adenomas, which produce follicle-stimulating hormone (FSH) and luteinizing hormone (LH), the less differentiated null-cell adenomas, and the silent adenomas. These clinically nonfunctioning adenomas commonly present with symptoms related to local mass effect, such as headaches, neurologic deficits in the cranial nerves (including visual field disturbances), and mild hyperprolactinemia due to pituitary stalk compression (the so-called stalk effect).

According to tumor size and gross anatomic features, adenomas are divided into microadenomas (tumors < 1 cm in diameter) and macroadenomas (tumors ≥ 1 cm in diameter). Giant adenomas (tumors > 4 cm) are rare. Macroadenomas show an increased tendency toward suprasellar extension, gross invasion, and recurrence.

A number of attempts to histologically classify pituitary adenomas have been made over the years. The recommended World Health Organization (WHO) classification from 2004 [6], which is used by most laboratories, incorporates the clinical and radiological presentation of the tumor with its morphologic features, immunohistochemical profile, and ultrastructural appearance (Table 4.2). Pituitary adenomas are classified according to the hormone content of the tumor cells as assessed by immunohistochemical stains. The immunohistochemical classification provides significant information for clinical practice [4], but immunohistochemistry alone does not discriminate between a number of specific subtypes of tumors that have prognostic clinical significance. In these instances, analysis of the ultrastructure of adenomas is necessary [4].

The WHO classification employs updated lineage studies that result in new and appropriate clustering of a variety of tumor subtypes. This classification not only has changed our understanding of the pathogenesis of these tumors but also opens new avenues of pharmacological treatment, which may result in increasing levels of hormonal control. A few highlights of the WHO classification include the continuing evidence that morphological features, including ultrastructure, may correlate with aggressive tumor behavior, as seen in the sparsely granulated GH adenoma, the mammosomatotroph cell adenoma, the acidophilic stem cell adenoma, and the silent adenoma subtype III.

Table 4.2 Morphofunctional classification of pituitary adenomas

Clinical presentation	Adenoma subtyping
PRL-secreting adenomas	Sparsely granulated lactotroph adenoma
	Densely granulated lactotroph adenoma
	Acidophilic stem cell adenoma
GH-secreting adenomas	Densely granulated somatotroph adenoma
	Sparsely granulated somatotroph adenoma
GH- and PRL-secreting adenomas	Mixed somatotroph-lactotroph adenoma
	Mammosomatotroph-cell adenoma
ACTH-secreting adenomas	Corticotroph adenoma
TSH-secreting adenomas	Thyrotroph adenoma
Gonadotropin-secreting adenomas	Gonadotroph adenoma
Nonfunctioning adenomas	Null-cell adenoma
	Oncocytoma
Silent adenomas	Silent corticotroph adenomas (subtypes I and II)
	Silent adenoma subtype III

ACTH adrenocorticotropic hormone, *GH* growth hormone, *PRL* prolactin, *TSH* thyroid-stimulating hormone

4.2.2 Grading

Perhaps the most controversial aspect of the WHO classification is the introduction of a grading system for pituitary endocrine tumors. These tumors are now categorized as typical pituitary adenoma (ICD code 8272/0), atypical pituitary adenoma (8272/1), and pituitary carcinoma (8272/3).

Most pituitary adenomas are typical, with bland histologic features, infrequent mitotic figures, and a Ki-67 proliferative index less than 3 %. The designation of atypical adenoma is reserved for tumors that show "atypical morphologic features suggestive of aggressive behavior such as invasive growth" [7]. Other features also seen in these tumors include elevated mitotic index, a Ki-67 labeling index greater than 3 %, and extensive nuclear staining for the p53 protein by immunohistochemistry [7]. Close follow-up of patients with atypical adenomas is recommended.

Pituitary carcinomas are very rare, comprising less than 1 % of all pituitary neoplasms [7–9]. By definition, pituitary carcinomas are characterized by demonstration of either craniospinal dissemination or systemic metastases [7]. The majority of cases are endocrinologically functioning tumors; the most common are PRL-secreting tumors, followed by ACTH-secreting tumors [8, 9]. Nonfunctioning carcinomas (about 15–20 % of cases) include gonadotroph, silent corticotroph, and rarely null-cell carcinomas [8, 9].

There are no morphologic criteria to distinguish locally aggressive or even markedly atypical adenomas from carcinomas when the tumor is confined to the sella turcica. Standard morphologic features associated with malignancy, including hypercellularity, nuclear and cellular pleomorphism, increased mitotic activity, necrosis, and dural or bony invasion, are commonly present but are not necessarily diagnostic of carcinoma. Ki-67 labeling indices are quite variable and show considerable overlap with ordinary pituitary adenomas, but they are often higher in metastatic deposits. Additionally, unlike pituitary adenomas, carcinomas appear to show overexpression of the p53 protein by immunohistochemistry [8].

4.2.3 Invasiveness and Proliferative Potential of Pituitary Adenomas

Pituitary adenomas either grow expansively or invade adjacent structures. In the first case, the tumors are usually small, well demarcated, and restricted to the sella turcica. Invasive adenomas usually have a more rapid growth rate, spreading into neighboring tissues such as the sphenoid sinus, the cavernous sinus, and, in some cases, the brain [10].

The mechanisms of progression of pituitary adenomas to more aggressive, invasive tumors are not yet totally understood. A proliferative continuum from benign adenoma to invasive adenoma and carcinoma has not been demonstrated in the great majority of tumors. The propensity of pituitary adenomas to infiltrate locally and invade adjacent structures appears to be independent of histologic features of the tumors. Invasive adenomas do not necessarily show histologic features of tumor aggressiveness, including pleomorphism, nuclear atypia, and mitotic activity, as seen in atypical adenomas. Although both clinically functioning and nonfunctioning adenomas may present as invasive tumors, gross invasion appears to be more frequent in functioning tumors [10]. On the other hand, there is an apparent relationship between invasiveness and tumor size: macroadenomas have a higher frequency of invasion than microadenomas [10].

Studies of proliferative potential of pituitary adenomas have been applied as an adjuvant tool for distinguishing aggressive pituitary adenomas from the most common benign tumors [11]. These studies have revealed that the majority of adenomas show a low growth fraction, with most Ki-67 indices being less than 3 %. The mean growth fractions among invasive adenomas and pituitary carcinomas are significantly higher than those of noninvasive adenomas [11]. Although these data may suggest that a significant correlation exists between Ki-67 labeling index and pituitary tumor invasiveness, a significant correlation between the proliferative index and tumor recurrence has not yet been demonstrated [12].

4.2.4 Molecular Genetics of Pituitary Adenomas

The mechanisms involved in human pituitary tumorigenesis and tumor progression are still not well understood. Pituitary adenomas appear to develop through a multistep and multicausal process in which endocrine factors, hereditary genetic disposition, and specific somatic mutations may serve as contributory factors. An extended review of the mechanisms of pituitary tumorigenesis is beyond the scope of this chapter.

Pituitary adenomas arise mostly in a sporadic manner; only a minority is part of hereditary or familial syndromes [13]. The large majority of pituitary adenomas are monoclonal expansions, as demonstrated by X-chromosomal inactivation analysis [14]. The development of pituitary adenomas is associated with some hereditary conditions:

- Multiple endocrine neoplasia type 1 (MEN-1), linked to somatic mutations of the *MEN-1* gene
- Carney complex, linked to mutations of the tumor suppressor gene *PRKAR1A*
- McCune-Albright syndrome, linked to activating mutation of the *gsp* oncogene (see below).

A few other rare familial syndromes are also associated with pituitary adenomas:

- Pituitary adenoma predisposition (PAP), which is associated with a germline mutation of the *AIP* (aryl hydrocarbon receptor-interacting protein) gene
- Isolated familial somatotrophinomas (IFS), which is associated with a loss of heterozygosity at the 11q13 locus but is not associated with the *MEN-1* gene
- Familial isolated pituitary adenomas (FIPA), in which there is no characterization of a single genetic alteration. Mutations of the *AIP* gene have been described in about 15 % of families with this syndrome, however [15].

The primary genetic defect remains unknown for the majority of sporadic adenomas. A number of oncogenes and tumor suppressor genes have been recognized as potential participants in tumorigenesis of pituitary adenomas. The most commonly found genetic alteration in sporadic tumors is activating mutation of the *gsp* gene, an oncogene mostly identified in GH cell adenomas [16–18]. The *gsp* mutation has been identified in about 40 % of GH-secreting adenomas [17–19], but it is rare in other pituitary tumor subtypes, occurring in only 10 % of clinically nonfunctioning pituitary adenomas and in 5 % of corticotroph adenomas [19].

Other oncogenes and tumor suppressor genes that have been shown to be linked to pituitary tumorigenesis include the oncogene *PTTG* (pituitary tumor-transforming gene), the proto-oncogene *H-ras*, and the tumor suppressor genes *RB* and *TP53*. However, it seems that these genes are not directly associated with pituitary adenoma tumorigenesis but may play a role during the progression and malignant transformation of these tumors [20]; details can be found in several outstanding reviews.

4.2.5 Conclusions

One of the most important prognostic features of pituitary adenomas remains their hormonal profile and pathological subtype classification. The recognition of specific subtypes of adenomas that have a higher propensity for aggressive clinical behavior (*e.g.*, the sparsely granulated growth hormone adenoma, the densely granulated lactotroph adenoma, the silent type III adenoma, and the silent corticotroph adenoma) in a systematic grading designation may assist in clinical management and understanding of the epidemiology of these tumors.

Nevertheless, a number of areas with regard to the classification of pituitary tumors remain controversial. Among these is the phenomenon of the invasion of tissues surrounding the tumor, including the brain, the cavernous sinuses, and the skull base, and the correlation of invasion with recurrence and worse clinical outcomes.

4.3 Tumors of the Sellar Region of Non-neuroendocrine Origin

4.3.1 Overview

Although much less frequent than the main tumors of the sellar region—the pituitary adenomas—pituicytomas, granular cell tumors, and spindle cell oncocytomas are important entities in the differential diagnosis of sellar masses. All three tumors are low-grade, non-neuroendocrine neoplasms of the sella that can clinically mimic nonfunctioning pituitary adenomas.

The term "pituicytoma" has been used to describe a number of tumors in the region of the sella turcica, including pilocytic astrocytomas and granular cell tumors. In 2000, Brat and colleagues [21] formally defined "pituicytoma" as a distinctive low-grade glial neoplasm that arises from pituicytes—the specialized glia of the neurohypophysis and the pituitary stalk, with a sustentacular function in the posterior pituitary.

Granular cell tumors of the pituitary, unlike those elsewhere in the gastrointestinal tract and skin, which are thought to be of Schwann cell origin, are considered to be unique neoplasms of the neurohypophysis and pituitary stalk and have also been suggested to derive from pituicytes [22].

Spindle cell oncocytomas were described in 2002 by Roncaroli and colleagues [23] as non-neuroendocrine neoplasms arising in the adenohypophysis and characterized by mitochondrion-rich, spindle to epithelioid cells. The cellular origin of spindle cell oncocytomas remains uncertain; Roncaroli et al. [23] proposed a folliculostellate cell origin based on similarities of their ultrastructural and immunohistochemical features. However, recent data on the shared immunoreactivity for the thyroid transcription factor-1 (TTF-1) of pituicytomas, granular cell tumors, and spindle cell oncocytomas may suggest more similarity in origin than was originally suspected [24, 25].

4.3.2 A Common Origin for the Non-neuroendocrine Tumors of the Pituitary Gland

Pituicytes are embryologically derived from the floor of the diencephalon. Recent data have revealed that the floor of the diencephalon is an area under the influence of TTF-1, a transcription factor known to be critical for the development of lungs and thyroid, and now discovered to play a role in the induction of the infundibular anlage during development of the posterior pituitary and infundibulum [25]. Similar to normal, nontumorous pituicytes, these three tumors—pituicytomas, granular cell tumors, and spindle cell oncocytomas—show diffuse nuclear expression for TTF-1 [24, 25]. On the other hand, folliculostellate cells, the sustentacular cells of the adenohypophysis, are negative for TTF-1 [25].

Furthermore, the ultrastructural morphology of these tumors shows similarities with the described variants of normal pituicytes, another indication of a possible common pituicyte lineage [24]. Pituicytes have five distinct ultrastructural variants: light (or major), dark, granular, ependymal, and oncocytic [26]. The current hypothesis is that these non-neuroendocrine pituitary tumors would originate from specific variants of pituicytes: pituicytomas from the light/major variant, granular cell tumors from the granular variant, and spindle cell oncocytomas from the oncocytic variant [24].

4.3.3 Conclusion

Pituicytomas, granular cell tumors, and spindle cell oncocytomas may be a challenge to diagnose because their clinical presentation resembles that of the much more common pituitary adenomas and their morphological and immunohistochemical features also overlap. Diffuse TTF-1 expression in these three tumors provides a diagnostic marker to distinguish these lesions from other entities including adenomas, schwannomas, and meningiomas.

References

1. Ostrom QT, Gittleman H, Liao P, Rouse C, Chen Y, Dowling J, et al. CBTRUS statistical report: primary brain and central nervous system tumors diagnosed in the United States in 2007–2011. Neuro Oncol. 2014;16 Suppl 4:iv1–63.
2. Jagannathan J, Dumont AS, Jane Jr JA. Diagnosis and management of pediatric sellar lesions. In: Laws Jr ER, Sheehan JP, editors. Pituitary surgery – a modern approach. Basel: Karger; 2006. p. 83–104.
3. Ezzat S, Asa SL, Couldwell WT, Barr CE, Dodge WE, Vance ML, et al. The prevalence of pituitary adenomas: a systematic review. Cancer. 2004;101:613–9.
4. Horvath E, Kovacs K. The adenohypophysis. In: Kovacs K, Asa SL, editors. Functional endocrine pathology. Boston: Blackwell Scientific; 1991. p. 245–81.
5. Greenman Y, Stern N. Non-functioning pituitary adenomas. Best Pract Res Clin Endocrinol Metab. 2009;23:625–38.
6. DeLellis RA, Lloyd RV, Heitz PU, Eng C, editors. Pathology and genetics of tumours of endocrine organs, World Health Organization classification of tumours, vol. 8. 3rd ed. Lyon: IARC Press; 2004.
7. Lloyd RV, Kovacs K, Young Jr WF, Farell WE, Asa SL, Trouillas J, et al. Pituitary tumours: introduction. In: DeLellis RA, Lloyd RV, Heitz PU, Eng C, editors. Pathology and genetics of tumours of endocrine organs, World Health Organization classification of tumours, vol. 8. 3rd ed. Lyon: IARC Press; 2004. p. 10–3.
8. Scheithauer BW, Kovacs K, Horvath E, Roncaroli F, Ezzat S, Asa SL, et al. Pituitary carcinoma. In: DeLellis RA, Lloyd RV, Heitz PU, Eng C, editors. Pathology and genetics of tumours of endocrine organs, World Health Organization classification of tumours, vol. 8. 3rd ed. Lyon: IARC Press; 2004. p. 36–9.
9. Lopes MB, Scheithauer BW, Schiff D. Pituitary carcinoma: diagnosis and treatment. Endocrine. 2005;28:115–21.
10. Meij BP, Lopes MB, Ellegala DB, Alden TD, Laws Jr ER. The long-term significance of microscopic dural invasion in 354 patients with pituitary adenomas treated with transsphenoidal surgery. J Neurosurg. 2002;96:195–208.
11. Salehi F, Agur A, Scheithauer BW, Kovacs K, Lloyd RV, Cusimano M. Ki-67 in pituitary neoplasms: a review–part I. Neurosurgery. 2009;65:429–37.
12. Prevedello DM, Jagannathan J, Jane Jr JA, Lopes MB, Laws Jr ER. Relevance of high Ki-67 in pituitary adenomas. Case report and review of the literature. Neurosurg Focus. 2005;19(5), E11.
13. Daly AF, Tichomirowa MA, Beckers A. Genetic, molecular and clinical features of familial isolated pituitary adenomas. Horm Res. 2009;71 Suppl 2:116–22.
14. Clayton RN, Farrell WE. Pituitary tumour clonality revisited. Front Horm Res. 2004;32:186–204.
15. Vierimaa O, Georgitsi M, Lehtonen R, Vahteristo P, Kokko A, Raitila A, et al. Pituitary adenoma predisposition caused by germline mutations in the AIP gene. Science. 2006;312:1228–30.
16. Vallar L, Spada A, Giannattasio G. Altered Gs and adenylate cyclase activity in human GH-secreting pituitary adenomas. Nature. 1987;330:566–8.
17. Landis CA, Masters SB, Spada A, Pace AM, Bourne HR, Vallar L. GTPase inhibiting mutations activate the alpha-chain of Gs and stimulate adenylyl cyclase in human pituitary tumors. Nature. 1989;340:692–6.
18. Landis CA, Harsh G, Lyons J, Davis RL, McCormick F, Bourne HR. Clinical characteristics of acromegalic patients whose pituitary tumors contain mutant Gs protein. J Clin Endocrinol Metab. 1990;71:1416–20.
19. Lania A, Mantovani G, Spada A. Genetics of pituitary tumors: focus on G-protein mutations. Exp Biol Med. 2003;228:1004–17.
20. Asa SL, Ezzat S. The pathogenesis of pituitary tumors. Annu Rev Pathol. 2009;4:97–126.
21. Brat DJ, Scheithauer BW, Staugaitis SM, Holtzman RN, Morgello S, Burger PC. Pituicytoma: a distinctive low-grade glioma of the neurohypophysis. Am J Surg Pathol. 2000;24:362–8.
22. Lopes MB, Scheithauer BW, Saeger W. Granular cell tumor. In: DeLellis RA, Lloyd RV, Heitz PU, Eng C, editors. World Health Organization classification of tumours, Pathology and genetics of tumours of endocrine organs, vol. 8. 3rd ed. Lyon: IARC Press; 2004. p. 44–5.
23. Roncaroli F, Scheithauer BW, Cenacchi G, Horvath E, Kovacs K, Lloyd RV, et al. 'Spindle cell oncocytoma' of the adenohypophysis: a tumor of folliculostellate cells? Am J Surg Pathol. 2002;26:1048–55.
24. Mete O, Lopes MB, Asa SL. Spindle cell oncocytomas and granular cell tumors of the pituitary are variants of pituicytoma. Am J Surg Pathol. 2013;37:1694–9.
25. Lee EB, Tihan T, Scheithauer BW, Zhang PJ, Gonatas NK. Thyroid transcription factor 1 expression in sellar tumors: a histogenetic marker? J Neuropathol Exp Neurol. 2009;68:482–8.
26. Takei Y, Seyama S, Pearl GS, Tindall GT. Ultrastructural study of the human neurohypophysis. II. Cellular elements of neural parenchyma, the pituicytes. Cell Tissue Res. 1980;205:273–87.

The Direct Endoscopic Endonasal Transsphenoidal Approach to the Pituitary Gland

5

Gabriel Zada, Joshua W. Lucas, and Edward R. Laws Jr.

Over the past two decades, the endoscopic endonasal transsphenoidal approach to the pituitary gland and sellar region for the treatment of pituitary pathology has evolved rapidly. Integration of the endoscope into pituitary surgery affords the surgeon superior panoramic visualization and illumination compared with the traditional microscopic approach. Additionally, the endoscopic approach facilitates two-handed surgical microdissection and the ability to look around anatomic surgical corners using angled lenses, which in turn may promote maximal tumor resection and preservation of the normal pituitary gland. This chapter focuses on key anatomic landmarks and operative strategies pertaining to the direct endoscopic endonasal approach to the sella. Continued experience and familiarity with the endoscopic transsphenoidal approach, combined with technologic advancements and improved instrumentation, are likely to contribute to improved surgical outcomes in the future.

The transsphenoidal approach to the pituitary gland and sellar region has undergone extensive evolution over the past century. It was not until the 1990s, however, that the first descriptions of routine, fully endoscopic approaches to the pituitary region were reported as a result of collaboration between neurosurgeons and rhinologists experienced in endoscopic sinus surgery [1]. Over the past two decades, routine use of the endoscope has become commonplace in providing access to the pituitary region and has expanded our ability to surgically access the entire midline skull base. The use of the endoscope for transsphenoidal surgery offers numerous advantages, including panoramic visualization, the ability to use angled lenses to look around anatomic "corners," improved illumination, and improved instrument mobility. The endonasal endoscopic transsphenoidal approach to the sellar region consists of four major stages: the nasal, sphenoid, sellar, and reconstruction stages. This chapter provides a brief overview of surgical techniques and operative pearls utilized during these four stages of an endoscopic endonasal transsphenoidal pituitary operation.

G. Zada, MD, MS (✉)
Department of Neurological Surgery, Keck School of Medicine, University of Southern California, 1200 N State Street, #3300, Los Angeles, CA 90033, USA
e-mail: gzada@usc.edu

J.W. Lucas, MD
Department of Neurosurgery, Keck School of Medicine, University of Southern California, Los Angeles, CA USA
e-mail: joshuawlucas@gmail.com

E.R. Laws Jr., MD
Department of Neurosurgery, Brigham and Women's Hospital, 15 Francis Street, Boston, MA 02115, USA
e-mail: elaws@partners.org

G. Zada et al. (eds.), *Atlas of Sellar and Parasellar Lesions: Clinical, Radiologic, and Pathologic Correlations*,
DOI 10.1007/978-3-319-22855-6_5

5.1 A Brief History of Endoscopic Transsphenoidal Surgery

The first documented transsphenoidal approach for resection of a pituitary lesion dates back to 1906 by Schloffer [2]. By 1914, Dr. Harvey Cushing had refined his sublabial transseptal technique, which reduced the degree of nasal trauma associated with earlier external rhinotomy incisions. In the 1960s, integration of the operative microscope into pituitary surgery by Hardy revitalized the transsphenoidal procedure by providing the magnification and illumination that made more precise tumor resection possible, especially for pituitary microadenomas [2].

Surgical endoscopy first emerged in the fields of otolaryngology, gastroenterology, and urology and was originally used primarily for visualization purposes [3]. Endoscopic procedures, however, quickly became possible with the advent of specially designed endoscopic surgical instruments and the electrocautery. Walter Dandy was among the greatest pioneers of early neuroendoscopy, performing endoscopic intraventricular operations as early as 1920 and contributing greatly to the development of improved endoscopic instrumentation [3]. The use of the endoscope in conjunction with the microsurgical approach to the sella was first proposed in 1963, even though the procedure was later abandoned because of inadequate visualization [4]. In 1977, the use of angled (70- to 120-degree) endoscopes to visualize parasellar regions following microsurgical tumor resection was reported [5]. In the 1990s, teams of neurosurgeons and otolaryngologists began to develop "pure" endoscopic techniques for removal of sellar lesions. In 1996, Jho and Carrau described their technique of a pure endoscopic approach in detail, and in 1997 they published their report of endoscopic removal of pituitary adenomas in 44 patients [1, 6]. Another team helped subsequently to pioneer the pure endoscopic approach and introduced the concept of functional endoscopic pituitary surgery (FEPS) in 1998 [7]. The endoscopic approach to the sella continued to be refined during the early twenty-first century, and with technologic advancements, including neuro-navigation and micro-Doppler ultrasonography, endonasal endoscopy has now expanded to include extended approaches to adjacent regions of the skull base. Current endoscopic endonasal approaches to the skull base can now provide access to a wide arc of pathology along the midline skull base, spanning from the frontal sinuses to the foramen magnum and upper cervical spine (Fig. 5.1).

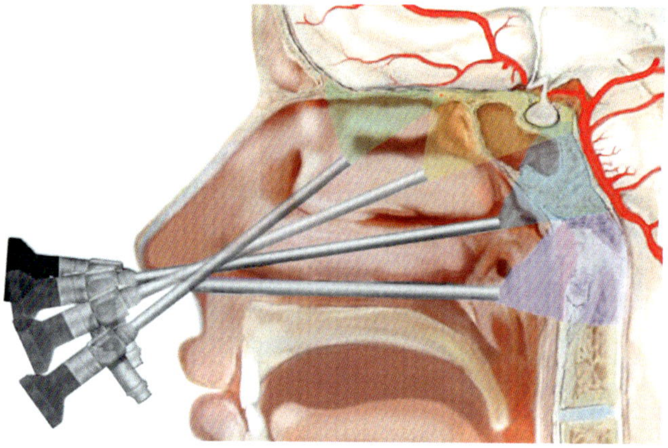

Fig. 5.1 Extended endoscopic approaches allow access from the anterior skull base anteriorly to the foramen magnum and upper cervical spine inferiorly (Courtesy of Dr. Luigi Cavallo)

5.2 Comparison of Endoscopic and Microsurgical Approaches for Pituitary Lesions

Despite early skepticism regarding the application of endoscopic techniques to the resection of sellar lesions, numerous studies have shown equivalent rates of tumor excision and incidence of complications with endoscopic pituitary approaches compared with microsurgical approaches [8–10]. In addition to similar effectiveness rates, endoscopic techniques may offer some distinct technical advantages over microsurgical techniques. Well-recognized drawbacks of the microsurgical approach include a narrower surgical field that is limited by the width of the nasal speculum, reduced illumination near the surgical target, and limited ability to visualize specific anatomic landmarks such as the carotid protuberances that define the limits of the sella [2, 11]. Pure endoscopic techniques allow improved panoramic visualization and illumination, obviating the need for a nasal speculum. From this widened surgical field, modified endoscopic transsphenoidal procedures have been developed to access lesions arising or extending outside of the sella, including the cavernous sinus, suprasellar, planum sphenoidale/olfactory groove, and retroclival lesions in which prior exposure via a microsurgical transsphenoidal approach was accompanied by formidable challenges. Improved instrument mobility and two-handed surgical dissection facilitated by endoscopic approaches are other major benefits of this technique.

Potential disadvantages associated with the endoscopic technique include a loss of binocular three-dimensional vision, a steep initial learning curve, and potential injury to the nasal mucosa that is not under direct visualization upon insertion or withdrawal of instruments from the surgical field. Endoscopic techniques are, by necessity, limited by the projection of a three-dimensional image onto a two-dimensional screen, whereas three-dimensional visualization is readily available with the operating microscope. This shortcoming can be partially corrected for by the use of large high-resolution (HD) video monitors and the reliance on tactile or haptic feedback to help gauge surgical depth. Also, the use of a two-surgeon, three-handed technique that allows dynamic movement of the endoscope and comparison between that movement and the motion of the surgical instruments can partially help offset the loss of depth perception. Newer three-dimensional visualization systems are rapidly improving and may one day all but obviate this shortcoming associated with endoscopic surgery [12].

5.3 Equipment and Surgical Instrumentation

The continued development and refinement of endoscopic equipment and surgical instrumentation have greatly contributed to the advancement of endoscopic surgery as a viable procedure for transsphenoidal approaches to the sella. Basic components of the endoscopic setup include the rigid-lens endoscope, a high-definition camera, a fiberoptic cable and light source, a large high-definition video monitor, and a video recording system. The most commonly used endoscope is 4 mm in diameter with a length of 18 or 30 cm (Fig. 5.2). Variations in lens angulation are available for specific steps of the operation, including a 0-degree scope, a 30-degree scope, and a 45-degree scope. Larger-angle scopes ranging between 70 and 120 degrees are available but are rarely required for a majority of endoscopic skull base operations.

In general, endoscopic instruments are long, rotating tools with a single straight shaft equipped with angled tips. The angled tips on the working ends of many surgical instruments permit a wider range of motion than standard instruments. Compared to the microsurgical technique, in which bayoneted instruments are typically employed to avoid interference with the light source, the use of straight-shaft instruments is preferred with endoscopy. The endoscope may be introduced into the nostrils along with a sheath, which is connected to an irrigation system that allows cleaning of the lens without repeated removal and reentry of the telescope. An endoscope holder may be used during the sellar phase of the procedure to stabilize the view of the surgical field, but its use limits the dynamic movement that helps to compensate for loss of depth perception. The use of neuro-navigation systems, although not required, can be helpful in patients with recurrent lesions or abnormal sellar or paranasal sinus anatomy and for extended endonasal approaches.

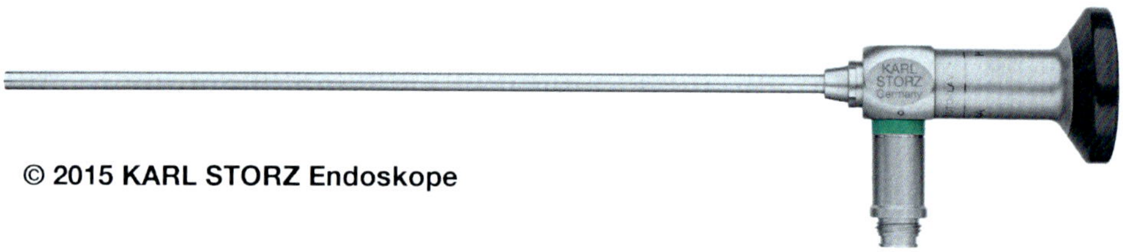

Fig. 5.2 A modern glass-rod lens endoscope used for endoscopic transsphenoidal neurosurgery (Courtesy of Karl Storz, Inc.)

5.4 Preoperative Assessment of Neuroimaging

Preoperative imaging is imperative for assessing the relevant anatomy that will be encountered during the surgical approach. Magnetic resonance imaging (MRI) of the head with and without gadolinium contrast and computed tomography (CT) imaging of the head will show the degree of pneumatization of the sphenoid sinuses and the anatomy of the sphenoid septations. Identification of the target lesion, normal pituitary gland, stalk, optic chiasm and optic nerves, and the course of the internal carotid arteries should also be assessed, often relying on sagittal and coronal images as the most useful planes to assess relevant neuroanatomic relationships.

The anatomy of the sella turcica, sphenoid sinus, and adjacent anterior and central skull base structures is highly variable. Preoperative imaging, specifically midsagittal MR images with contrast, must be assessed to identify the morphology of the sellar floor and the configuration of sphenoid sinus septations (Fig. 5.3). The sellar angle, defined as the angle between lines drawn tangential to the sellar floor originating at the tuberculum sellae point and the sellar-clival point, can be used to classify the different sellar floor morphologies (Fig. 5.4) [13]. Prominent sellar floors (sellar angle <90 degrees) and curved sellar floors (sellar angle between 90 and 150 degrees) can usually be easily identified during surgery using identifiable anatomic landmarks. On the other hand, flat sellar floors (sellar angle >150 degrees) or conchal (no sellar floor) sphenoid phenotypes occur in 11 % and 1 % of patients, respectively, and are more difficult to identify intraoperatively. Neuro-navigation systems are recommended in patients with these anatomic subtypes (Figs. 5.5 and 5.6) [13]. Additionally, neuro-navigation systems are recommended for patients who exhibit complex sphenoid sinus configurations (29 % of patients) consisting of two asymmetric septa, three or more septa, or horizontal septa and patients who have undergone previous transsphenoidal surgery [13].

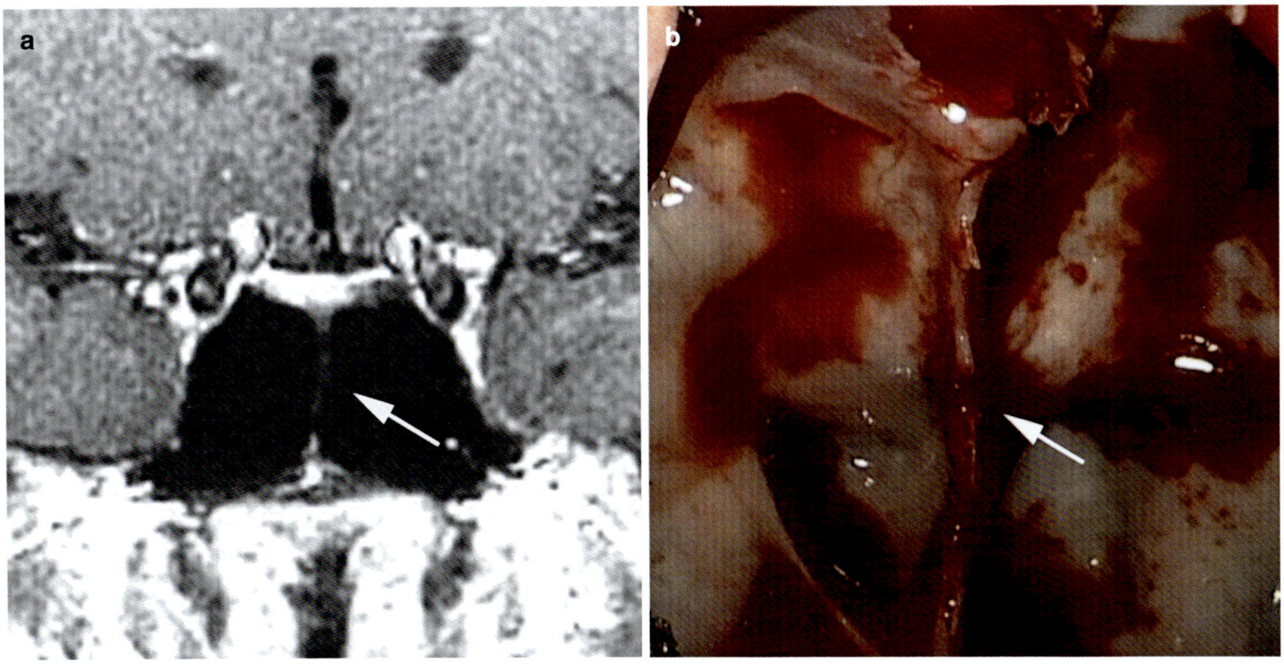

Fig. 5.3 Correlation of coronal MR imaging and intraoperative endoscopic views of vertical sphenoid septations in patients with simple sphenoid sinus morphology. The presence of one midline septum (**a**, **b**, *white arrows*) can be used to identify the anatomic midline. The presence of two symmetric septa (**c**, **d**, *white arrows*) can be used to approximate the lateral boundaries of the sella (From Zada et al. [13]; with permission)

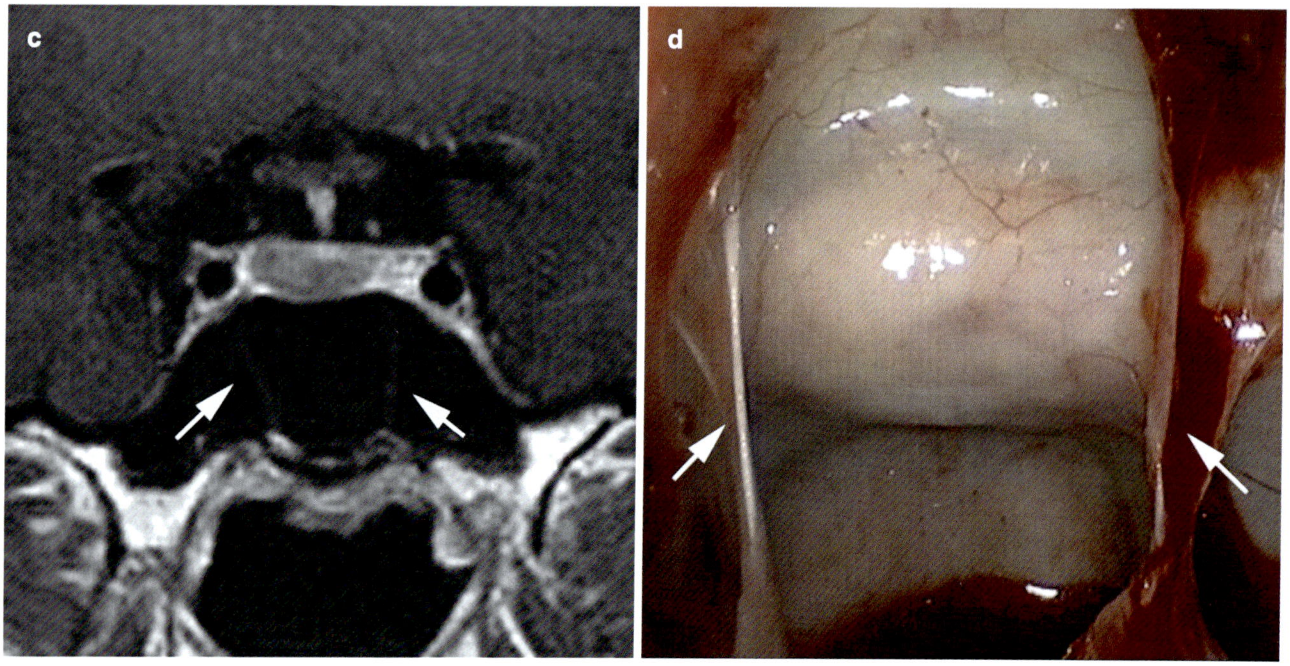

Fig. 5.3 (continued)

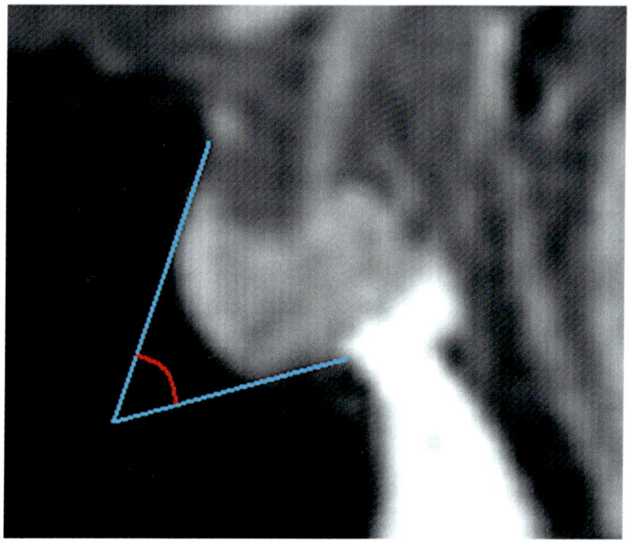

Fig. 5.4 The sellar angle, defined as the angle formed from lines drawn tangentially to the sella originating at the tuberculum sellae and the sellar-clival junction (From Zada et al. [13]; with permission)

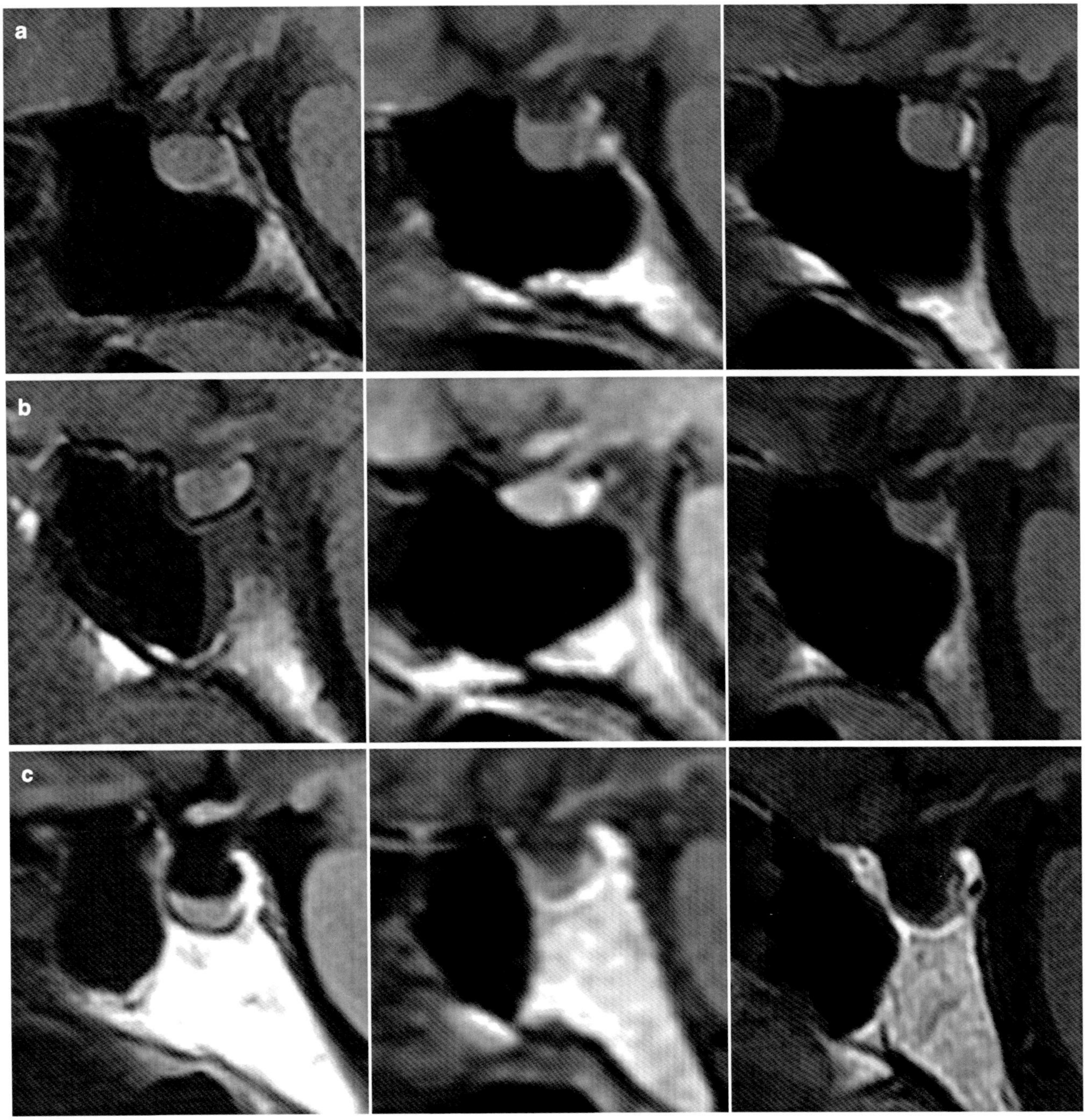

Fig. 5.5 Variations in sellar phenotypes on MRI. (**a**) Prominent sellar floor. (**b**) Curved sellar floor. (**c**) Flat sellar floor or conchal sphenoid phenotype (From Zada et al. [13]; with permission)

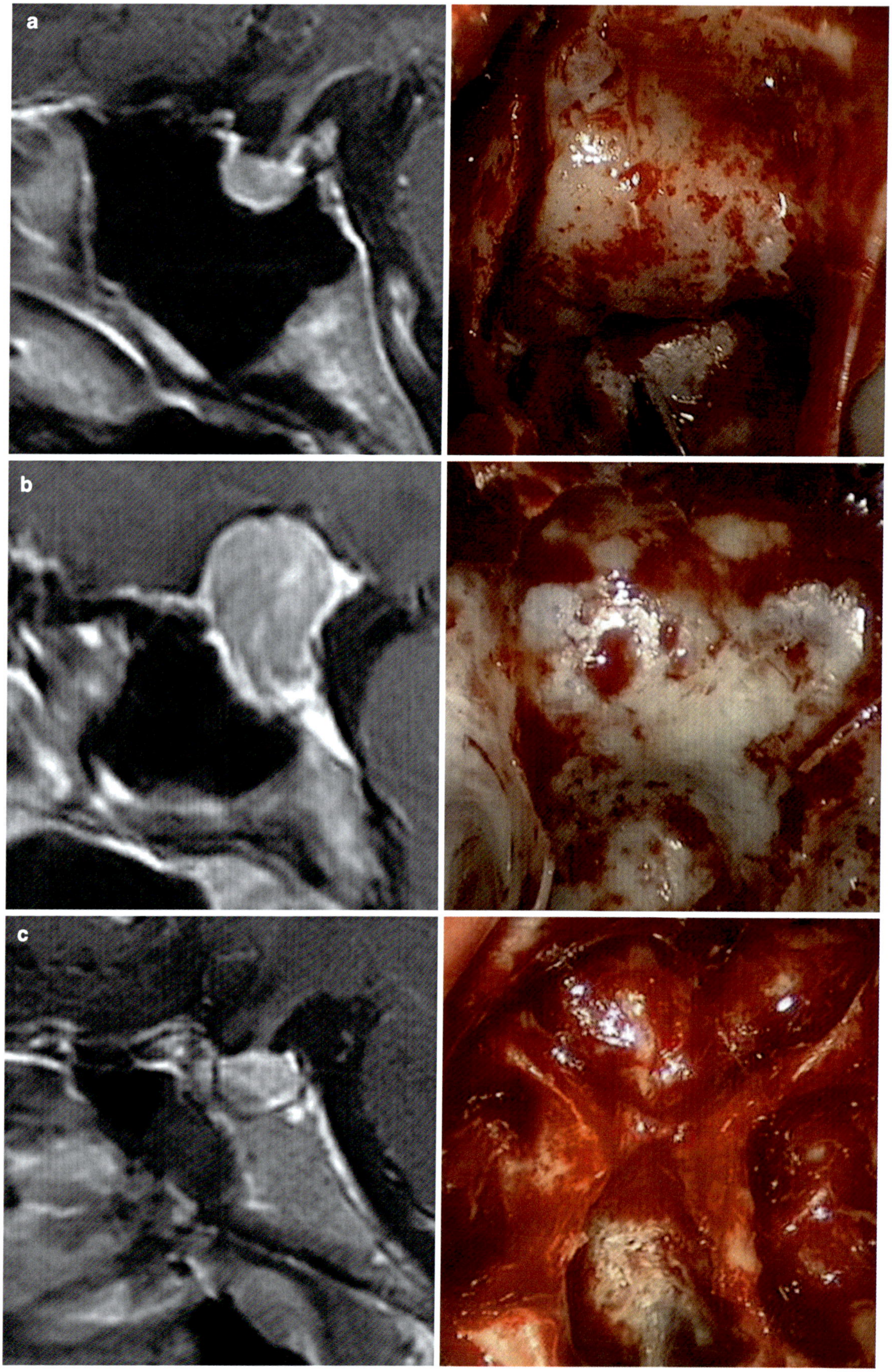

Fig. 5.6 Sagittal MRI and corresponding intraoperative endoscopic images of the sellar floor. (**a**) Prominent sella phenotype that is easily identifiable intraoperatively. (**b**) Curved sella phenotype. (**c**) Flat sella phenotype that is very difficult to differentiate from the clivus, making neuro-navigation extremely important (From Zada et al. [13]; with permission)

5.5 Surgical Technique

The endoscopic transsphenoidal approach to pituitary pathology has been continuously refined since it was first described [2, 22]. Although many variations to the procedure exist, the following represents the authors' preferred surgical technique utilized for this approach [14].

5.5.1 Preparation and Positioning

The video monitor is positioned behind the patient's head and in the direct line of sight of the surgeon who, in most cases, stands on the patient's right side. The anesthesiologist is positioned on the patient's left side. The head of the bed is turned approximately 120 degrees away from the anesthesiologist, and the patient is placed in a semirecumbent position with the thorax elevated to 15 degrees in order to optimize venous outflow. The head is positioned with a slight degree of rotation, approximately 10 degrees toward the surgeon, with the midline of the patient's head parallel to the lateral walls of the operating room and the bridge of the patient's nose parallel to the floor. The degree of flexion/extension of the patient's head is dependent on the location of the lesion. Lesions located primarily in the clivus or sphenoid sinus often require slight flexion of the head in order to permit working space for the endoscope. Lesions located more anteriorly, such as those based in the planum sphenoidale, require the head to be in a neutral or slightly hyperextended position. As with any operation, all endoscopic equipment and instrumentation should be checked prior to the operation to ensure proper function. The surgeon must also communicate with the anesthesia team to discuss administration of appropriate medications, especially with regard to hormone replacement and antibiotics. Routine use of an intraoperative checklist prior to commencement of the surgery may help ensure that all necessary laboratory and equipment components of the operation are functional [15].

Following intubation, the endotracheal and orogastric tubes are positioned at the left side of the patient's mouth and taped downward so as to keep the upper lip free. All lines and monitoring devices are preferentially positioned on the patient's left side. These maneuvers free the patient's right side for the surgeon. The nasal cavity is then prepared by administration of a nasal decongestant (e.g., oxymetazoline), followed by intranasal cleansing with an aqueous antiseptic such as chloroxylenol USP 3 % (Techni-Care Solution) or iodine solution. Finally, the nasal region is prepped externally and draped. The abdomen or lateral thigh is also prepared under sterile conditions in the event that autologous fat and/or fascial graft harvesting is required during the reconstruction phase.

5.5.1.1 Nasal Stage

The nasal stage of the operation begins with the surgeon using a short (18-cm) 0-degree endoscope. Upon introduction of the endoscope, the floor of the nasal cavity, inferior turbinate (laterally), nasal septum (medially), and the choana (posteriorly) should be identified (Fig. 5.7). The surgeon should assess for anatomic variations, including a deviated septum or septal perforation, septal spurs, polyps, or synechiae. Once the choana is identified, maneuvering the endoscope superiorly allows identification of the middle turbinate, which arises from the ethmoid region superiorly. A blunt instrument such as a Freer dissector is used to gently displace the middle turbinate laterally while attempting to preserve the integrity of the overlying mucosa and minimize bleeding. Subsequent packing with lidocaine/epinephrine pledgets placed between the middle turbinate and nasal septum helps to maintain the developed working space between the middle turbinate and nasal septum and to promote hemostasis. Following sufficient lateral displacement of the middle turbinate, the endoscope is advanced and angled slightly superiorly in order to identify the superior turbinate posteriorly. In rare cases, resection of the middle turbinate helps to widen the surgical corridor; this maneuver is typically reserved for extended skull base operations or patients with acromegaly and enlarged turbinates.

The next landmark that should be identified and posterior the sphenoid ostium, which is usually located just medial to the inferior aspect of the superior turbinate, approximately 1.5 cm superior to the superior edge of the choana. The sphenoid ostium is occasionally concealed by mucosa or a thin layer of bone, in which case attempting to first identify the ostium on the opposite side may be of benefit. Use of neuronavigation may also be helpful in confirming the trajectory into the sphenoid sinus, after which a small dissector instrument can be used to probe gently for the ostium and enter the sinus. If a pedicled nasoseptal flap is being prepared, this should be performed at this point. Once the ostium is identified, its mucosal edges are coagulated using mild monopolar cautery, which can be extended down the medial and inferior surfaces of the sphenoid rostrum (Fig. 5.7). Avoidance of inferolateral cauterization and dissection helps to prevent arterial bleeding from septal branches of the sphenopalatine artery.

Local anesthesia (lidocaine 1 % with epinephrine 1:100,000) is then injected medially into the posterior nasal septum using a spinal needle with the tip bent to 20 degrees. An anterior sphenoidotomy is initialized using a mushroom (Stammberger) punch to widen the aperture of the sphenoid ostium and begin to remove the sphenoid rostrum in a direction inferior and medial to the ostium. This maneuver is almost always performed on both sides of the nasal cavity, although the approach may be entirely from one side, depending on the size and location of the target lesion and the requirement for using instruments through both nostrils.

A Cottle elevator is used to create a vertical incision in the posterior nasal septum immediately overlying the keel of the sphenoid rostrum (the vomer and perpendicular plate of the ethmoid) at its junction with the cartilaginous septum. The Cottle elevator or a suction instrument (i.e., suction Freer) is used to develop the nasal mucosal flap along a subperiosteal plane on both sides of the vomer, creating two mucosal flaps and exposing the entire bony sphenoid rostrum. Once adequate exposure of the bony keel is achieved, it can be removed using a stout pituitary or Smith-Ferris rongeur (Fig. 5.8). The remaining superior and inferior-most aspects of the bony keel of the vomer serve as useful midline markers during the remainder of the operation (Fig. 5.9). Soft tissue from the posterior septum and elevated superior mucosal flaps are typically preserved for future development of a “rescue” flap. A backbiter instrument may be utilized to extend the posterior septectomy more anteriorly as required to improve communication between both sides of the nasal cavity, improve visualization and instrument mobility, and minimize the likelihood of instrument collisions. The lateral and superior soft tissue and bony overhang of the sphenoid rostrum and sinus may be resected using a Kerrison rongeur, a micro-débrider, or Blakesley forceps in order to provide adequate room to dock the endoscope superolaterally at the ten o’clock position. The bony rostrum is typically removed down to the level of the floor of the sphenoid sinus using a Kerrison rongeur or high-speed drill in order to maximize workspace for the endoscope and two instruments (Fig. 5.10).

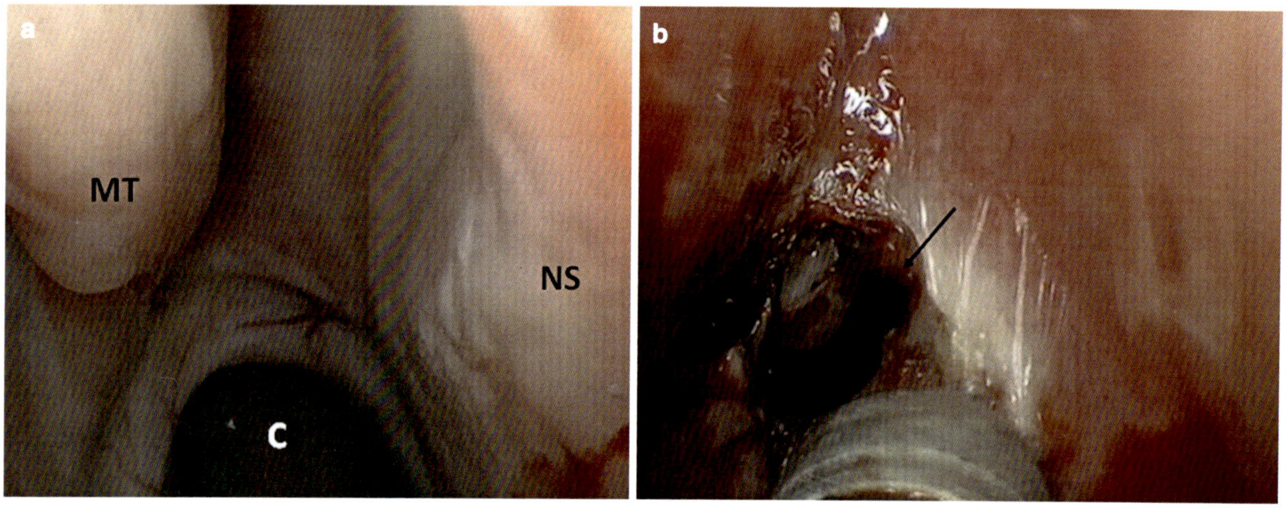

Fig. 5.7 The nasal stage. (**a**) Upon entering the nares, the choana (*C*) is immediately visualized, with the middle turbinate (*MT*) identified laterally and the nasal septum (*NS*) medially. (**b**) The sphenoid ostium (*black arrow*) is identified and coagulated in preparation for gaining access to the sphenoid sinus

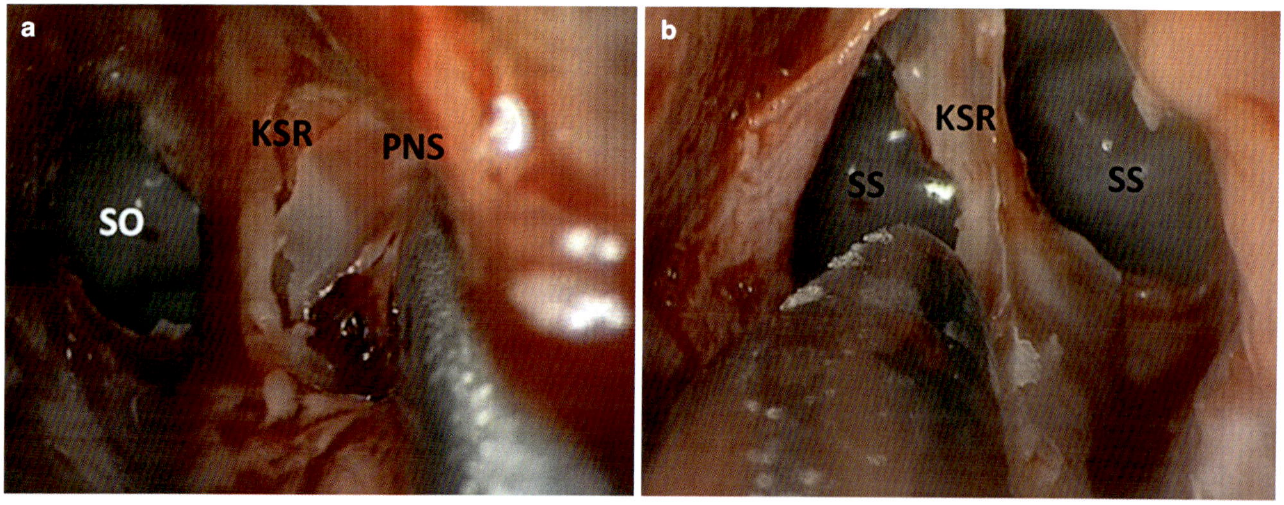

Fig. 5.8 The nasal stage. (**a**) A posterior septectomy is performed through the posterior nasal septum (*PNS*) after enlarging the sphenoid ostium (*SO*). The keel of the sphenoid rostrum (*KSR*) is identified. (**b**) Removal of the posterior nasal septum allows bimanual access to the sphenoid sinus (*SS*)

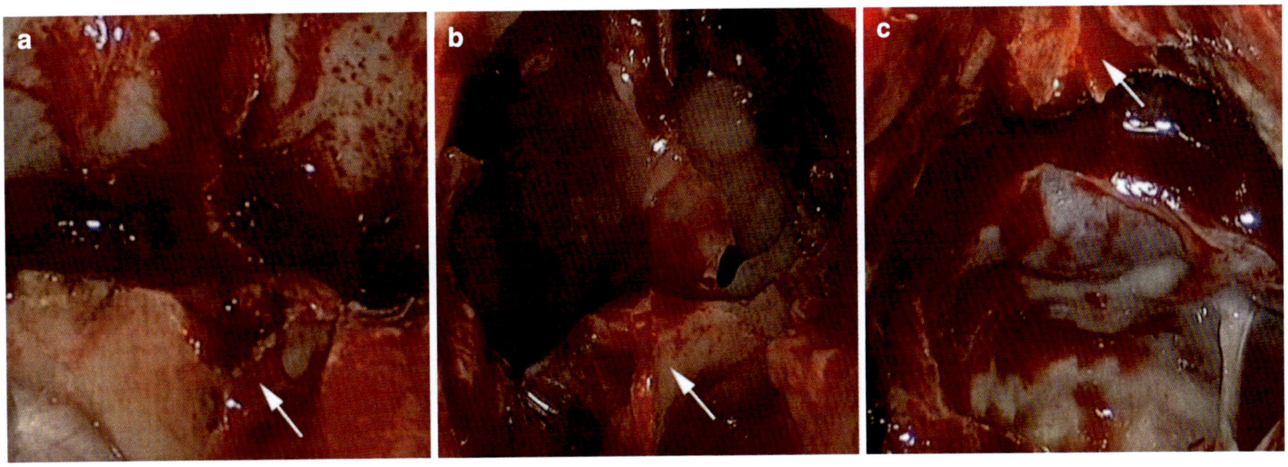

Fig. 5.9 The nasal stage. Intraoperative endoscopic images of relatively constant midline markers that can often be used even in the presence of complex sphenoid sinus configurations. These markers include the base of the vomer (**a**, **b**, *white arrows*) and the superior rostrum of the sphenoid (**c**, *white arrow*) (From Zada et al. [13]; with permission)

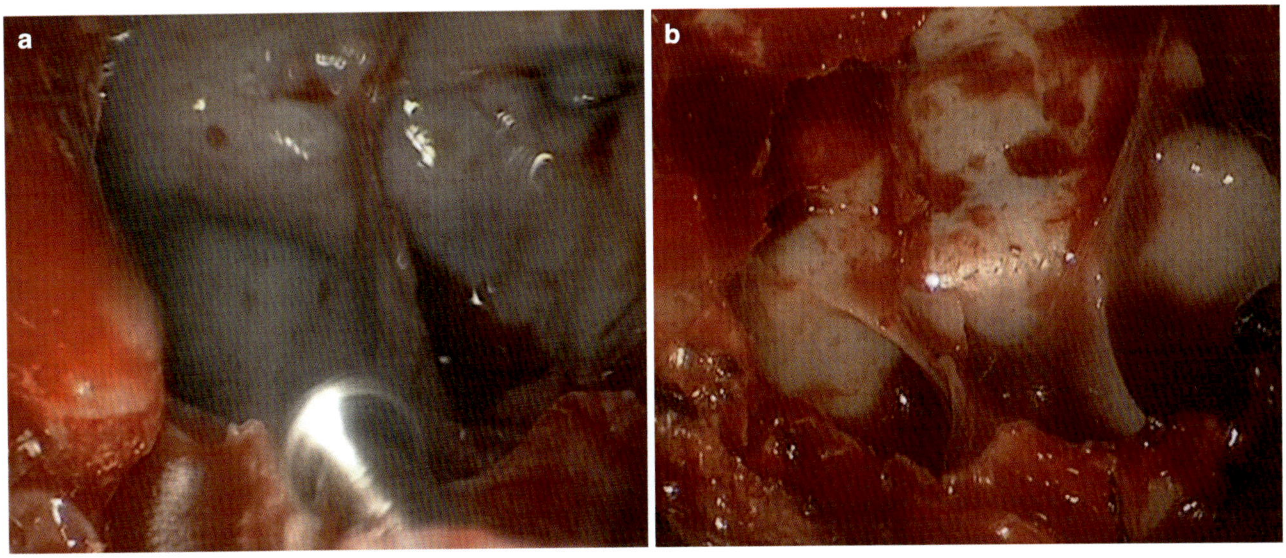

Fig. 5.10 The nasal stage. (**a**) The bony rostrum is removed to the level of the floor of the sphenoid sinus using a high-speed drill. (**b**) The endoscope and instruments are subsequently advanced through the aperture into the sphenoid sinus

5.5.1.2 Sphenoid Stage

Upon entering the sphenoid sinus, the initial goal is to identify key anatomic landmarks and correlate them with pertinent neuroimaging findings. The surgeon must always study the anatomy of the sphenoid sinus on preoperative imaging, including the morphology and curvature of the sellar floor, the location and course of the carotid arteries, and the configuration of sphenoid septations. Septations within the sphenoid sinus should be correlated with MR and CT imaging and often lead directly to the carotid arteries laterally and posteriorly. Careful removal of these septations is performed using a pituitary forceps, Kerrison rongeur, or high-speed drill. A dehiscent bony covering of the internal carotid artery may be identified in up to 10 % of the population. The sphenoid mucosa can be stripped and removed as needed using suction and a small-cup forceps.

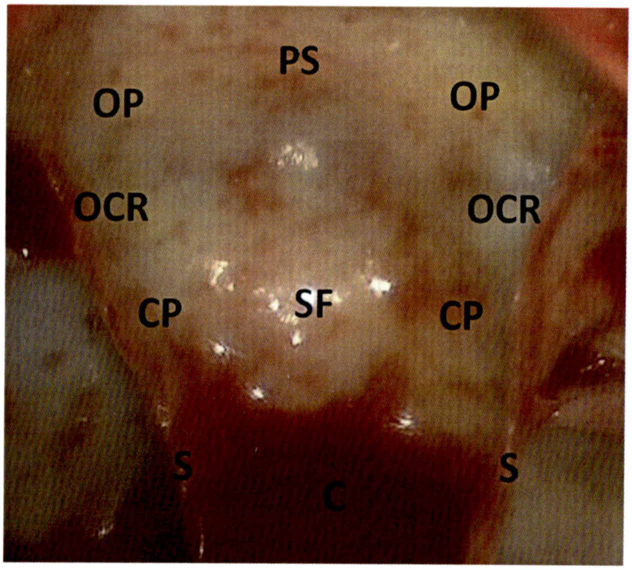

Fig. 5.11 The sphenoid stage. Anatomic landmarks surrounding the sellar floor (*SF*) are identified. Paired sphenoid septa (*S*) can be used as lateral guidelines for dissection if confirmed on preoperative MRI. *C* clivus, *CP* carotid protuberance, *PS* planum sphenoidale, *OCR* opticocarotid recess, *OP* optic protuberance

Once the posterior wall of the sphenoid sinus is visible, the surgeon should identify the sellar floor, the tuberculum sphenoidale and planum sphenoidale located superiorly, and the clivus located inferiorly (Fig. 5.11). Lateral to the sellar floor, the bony prominences of the cavernous carotid arteries and optic nerves can be identified, with the opticocarotid recesses between them. The floor of the sella turcica is prominent and thus easily recognizable in the majority of patients, but a flat, less prominent variety is seen in approximately 10 % of patients [13]. Although neuro-navigation is not required for the procedure, it can be extremely beneficial to confirm the identification of key anatomic landmarks in patients with flat sellar subtypes and presellar or conchal sphenoid sinuses as well as in patients who have undergone prior transsphenoidal surgery. Finally, thorough saline irrigation of the sinus using a large bulb syringe is performed to remove blood and bone fragments in preparation for the sellar stage.

5.5.1.3 Sellar Stage

For the sellar phase, the operation is converted to a two-surgeon, "four-handed" technique so that bimanual microdissection can be safely performed. Alternatively, the endoscope is fixed with an endoscope holder to permit a single surgeon to work with both hands. The floor of the sella, when expanded and thinned by an intrasellar lesion, can usually be fractured open using a pituitary rongeur or blunt microdissector (Fig. 5.12). In some cases, a thicker sellar floor precludes this maneuver, requiring the use of an osteotome, drill, or ultrasonic bony curette. A wide sellar exposure is then performed using a 2-mm Kerrison rongeur, typically spanning from one cavernous sinus to the other (Fig. 5.13). In addition to identifying the cavernous sinuses laterally, the anterior intercavernous sinus is frequently identified in the rostral aspect of the exposure. A micro-Doppler probe and neuro-navigation are routinely used to check for the location of the internal carotid arteries and to confirm the site of the planned dural opening. The dura is incised using a retractable micro-blade, ensuring penetration of both dural layers (Fig. 5.14). The dural opening is typically performed in a cruciate or X-shaped fashion; in cases where a dural specimen is desired for pathologic examination, a rectangular dural "window" can be resected for analysis. Following dural opening, a blunt nerve hook or microdissector is used to develop a circumferential subdural, extraglandular, or extracapsular plane.

Following adequate exposure of the pituitary gland and target lesion, the intrasellar pathology may be addressed using two-handed microdissection techniques. The surgeon should maintain constant awareness of the normal anterior and posterior pituitary glands in an effort to identify and preserve them. For microadenomas and small intrasellar macroadenomas, microdissectors may be used to develop an extracapsular plane around the tumor pseudocapsule prior to delivering it. For larger tumors, angled curettes and small-cup forceps can be used to fragment and deliver the tumor, first working inferiorly along the sellar floor, then laterally to the cavernous sinus on each side, and finally in a superior direction (Fig. 5.15a, b). Removing the superior portion of a macroadenoma before the lateral and inferior portions can cause early prolapse of the diaphragma sella and arachnoid into the surgical field, obscuring visualization and increasing the risk of an early cerebrospinal fluid leak. Care should be taken to remove as much tumor as possible for pathology and/or tissue banking (Fig. 5.15c). Once a sufficient specimen has been collected, curettes and suction can be used to remove the remainder of the tumor (Fig. 5.15d). The arachnoid may descend into the field of view at this point and should be manipulated carefully and protected with a cotton pledget, thereby avoiding direct suction on it. Venous cavernous sinus bleeding may be encountered following tumor removal and can be controlled using temporary gelatin foam packing and/or an injectable gelatin hemostatic matrix followed by gentle pressure with a cottonoid. A 30- or 45-degree endoscope can be inserted to look laterally and superiorly into the cavernous sinuses in order to assess for residual tumor. In cases of macroadenomas with extensive suprasellar extension, the tumor will often descend spontaneously given enough time and gentle curettage. In patients with tumors that have a firmer consistency, a brief Valsalva maneuver can be performed to assist delivery of the tumor. Intrasellar and cavernous sinus hemostasis can typically be achieved using temporary packing with a gelatin sponge, followed by lining the tumor cavity with oxidized cellulose (Surgicel).

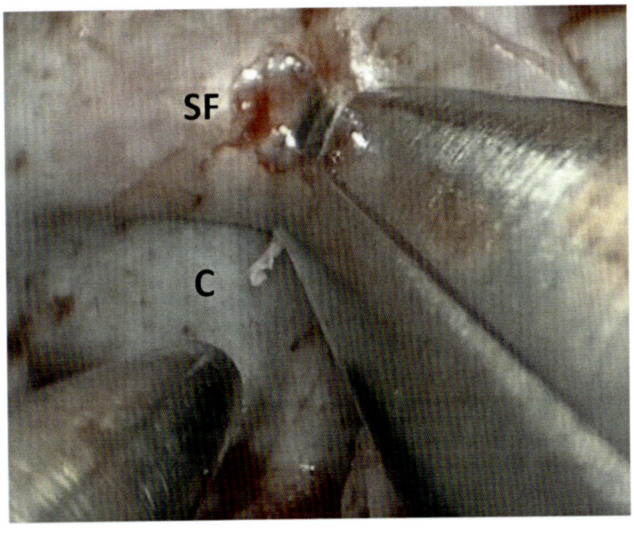

Fig. 5.12 The sellar stage. When sufficiently thinned by an intrasellar lesion, the sellar floor (*SF*) can be easily fractured with a pituitary forceps and then removed with a Kerrison rongeur. The clivus (*C*) aids in localizing the sellar floor

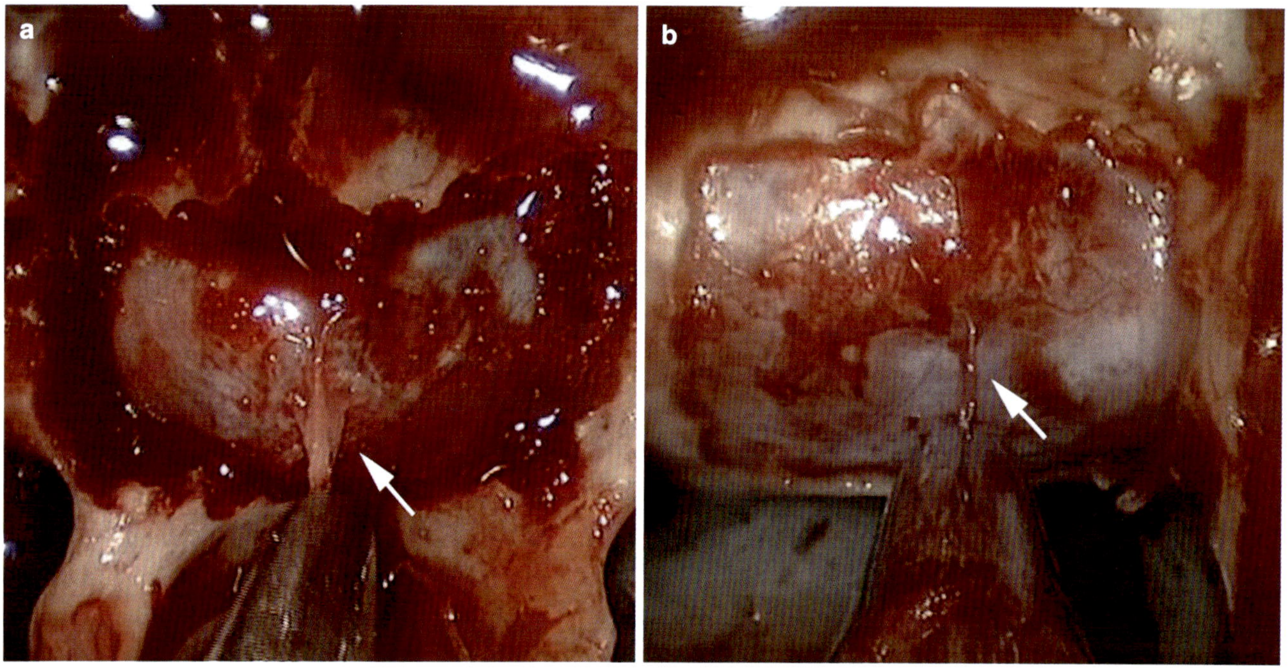

Fig. 5.13 The sellar stage. Intraoperative endoscopic images following removal of the bony sellar floor. A midline dural filum (**a**, **b**, *white arrows*) can be identified in approximately 50 % of patients (From Zada et al. [13]; with permission)

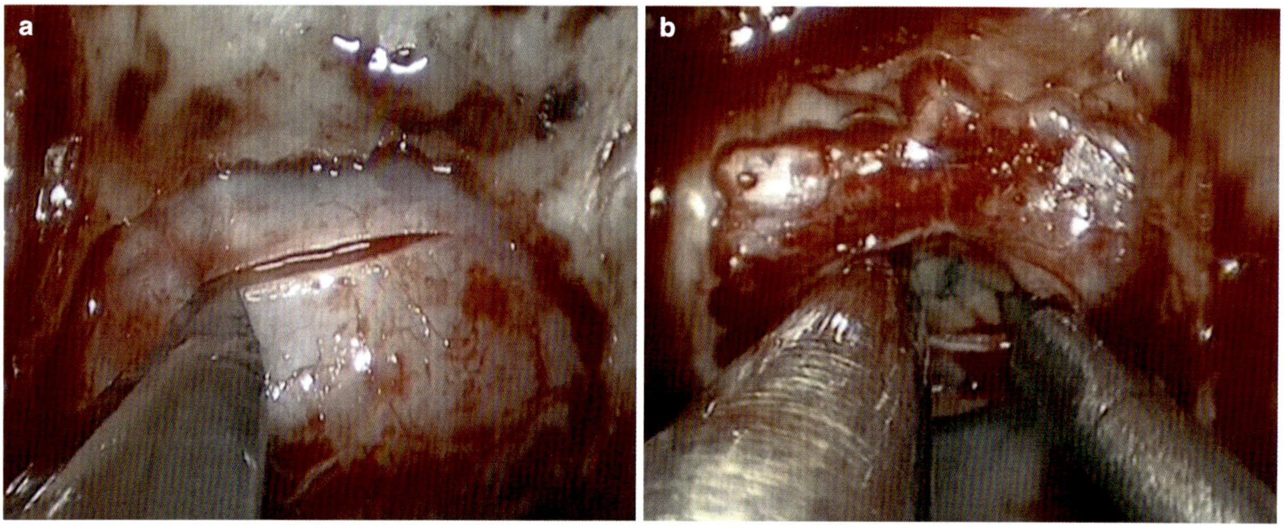

Fig. 15.14 The sellar stage. Various methods of dural opening. (**a**) A horizontal superior incision is made to create a "dural window" in order to send a dural specimen to pathology to inspect for evidence of dural invasion. (**b**) An X-shaped incision is used to maximize exposure to the gland and tumor

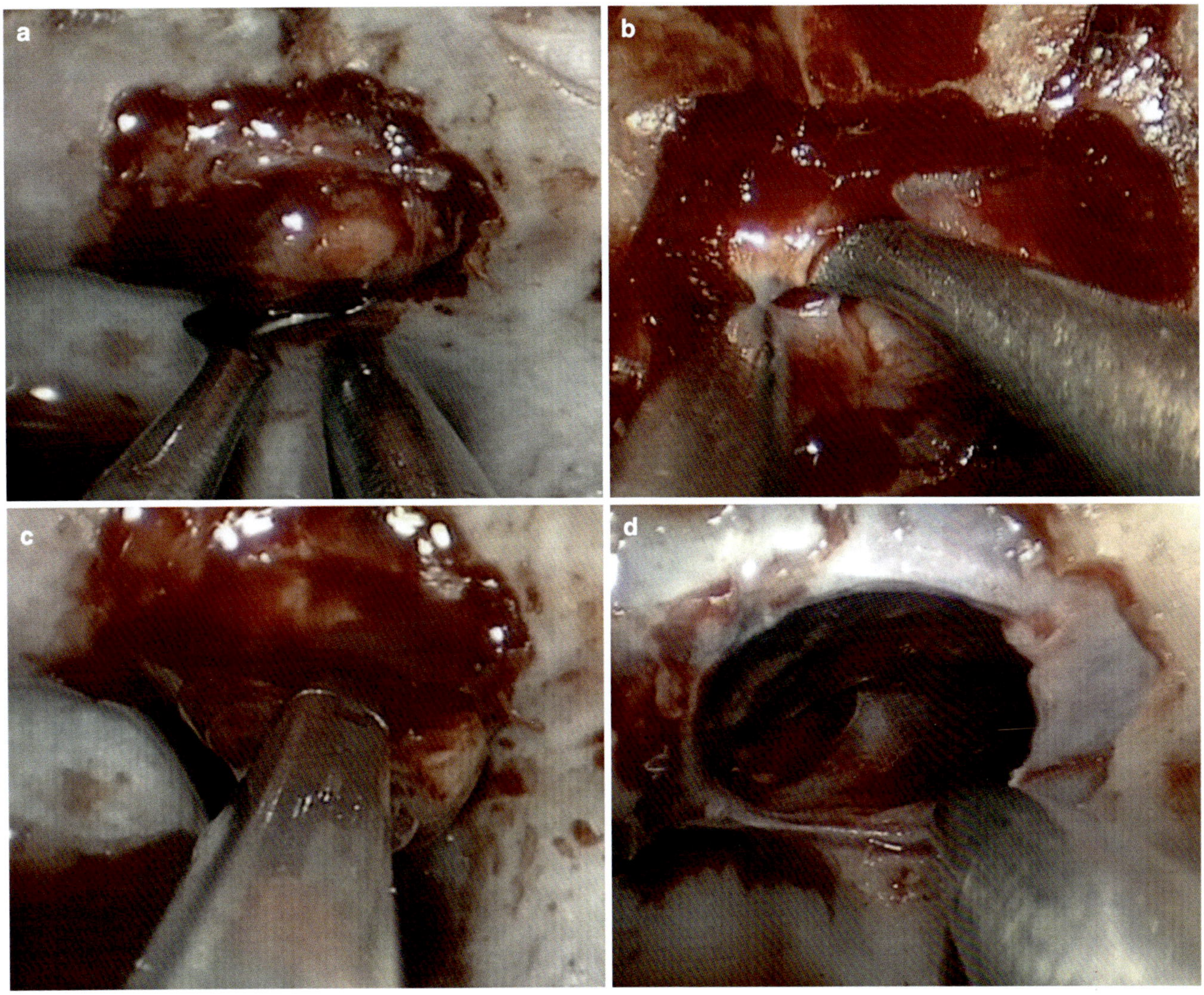

Fig. 5.15 The sellar stage. (**a**, **b**) An extracapsular plane is created by first dissecting inferiorly and then laterally to aid with tumor delivery. (**c**) Small-cup forceps are then used to remove the lesion. (**d**) The sella is subsequently examined for residual tumor prior to closure

5.5.1.4 Reconstruction and Closure

Once tumor resection is completed and hemostasis is achieved, the goal of reconstructing the skull base defect and repairing any possible cerebrospinal fluid fistula begins. Multiple methods of achieving reconstruction exist, including conventional repairs with autologous or artificial grafts, formation and rotation of a vascularized pedicled nasoseptal flap, and multilayered closure techniques using dural and bony substitutes.

The first goal of reconstruction is to assess for a cerebrospinal fluid leak, if not already evident. A Valsalva maneuver can be helpful in identifying a subtle or weeping leak. In simpler cases where no intraoperative leak is identified, the tumor cavity is lined with cellulose (Surgicel), and the sella can be packed with gelatin sponge. Insertion of a rigid buttress is avoided if no intraoperative cerebrospinal leak is observed. If an intraoperative leak is identified, an abdominal fat graft is typically harvested, although for smaller "weeping" cerebrospinal fluid leaks an allograft or dural substitute in combination with fibrin glue may be sufficient [16]. A two-layered fascial closure using a fascial apposition method is also an excellent way of achieving a durable sellar floor repair while avoiding the use of a rigid buttress [17]. In extended transsphenoidal cases, fascia lata from the thigh may be harvested for a multilayer reconstruction, and a pedicled nasoseptal flap may be developed ahead of time if a large cerebrospinal fluid leak is anticipated. Following packing of the sella using any combination of gelatin foam, fat, or fascia lata, an absorbable plate may be tailored for larger sellar defects and inserted as an epidural inlay underneath the lateral edges of the bony sellar face to provide buttressing of the underlying grafts (Fig. 5.16).

Gentle irrigation and hemostasis is then carried out. Sphenoid sinus and nasal hemostasis is typically achieved using cautery and absorbable cellulose and/or a gelatin sponge. The mucosal margins surrounding the sphenoid rostrum are inspected for any bleeding and appropriately cauterized, preferably with a bipolar cautery. The nasal septum is also inspected for any bleeding. The middle turbinates are medialized in order to reapproximate their natural position. Nasal packing is not routinely used but may be placed if bleeding persists. The choanae and oropharynx are carefully suctioned.

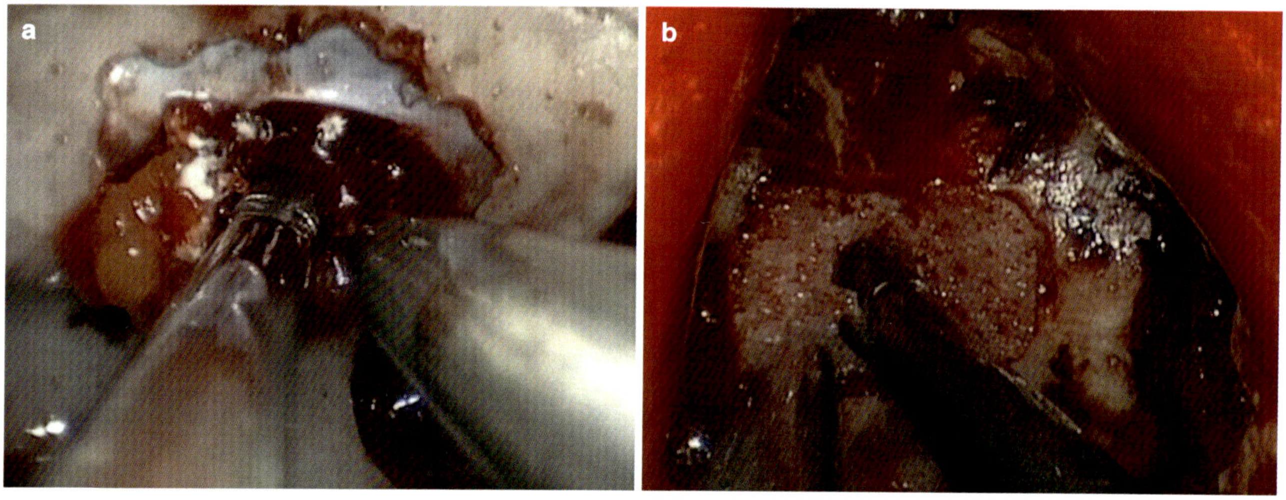

Fig. 5.16 The reconstruction stage. The sella is packed (**a**), and an epidural inlay is placed to aid in buttressing the absorbable graft (**b**)

5.6 Complications

Despite the minimally invasive nature of transsphenoidal approaches to the sella turcica, complications may arise. Complications encountered within the nasal cavity during the approach include anosmia, nasal septal perforation, crusting, saddlenose deformity, orbital fracture, cribriform plate injury with subsequent cerebrospinal fluid leak, and epistaxis. Complications arising within the sphenoid sinus may include sinusitis, mucocele formation, and optic nerve or carotid artery injury from fracture of the sphenoid body. Potential complications associated with tumor resection and the sellar phase include cerebrospinal fluid leak, hypopituitarism, diabetes insipidus, meningitis, postoperative hematoma, carotid artery or other vascular injury, optic nerve injury, ophthalmoplegia, subarachnoid hemorrhage, vasospasm, and tension pneumocephalus, among others.

For both microscopic and endoscopic transsphenoidal surgery, the most common nonendocrine complications include cerebrospinal fluid leak, meningitis, and sinusitis [18–20]. Recent studies have shown endoscopic techniques to be associated with similar or reduced rates of complications as compared to microsurgical techniques [20–22]. In 1997 Ciric and colleagues published a widely renowned analysis describing the observed rates of complications from microscopic transsphenoidal surgery [18]. In 2002, Cappabianca and coworkers published a large series of pure endoscopic techniques that analyzed the complication rates observed in these procedures and compared them to the complication rates of microsurgical procedures observed in Ciric's study [23]. They found an overall decreased incidence of complications with the endoscopic technique. A recent systematic review analyzed nine studies with 821 total patients treated with endoscopic transsphenoidal surgery [22]. The study found pooled complication rates equal to or less than complication rates for microsurgical techniques reported in the literature.

5.7 Postoperative Care and Follow-Up

Following endoscopic transsphenoidal pituitary procedures, patients must be observed very closely for evidence of visual dysfunction, epistaxis, neurologic deterioration, and hormonal deficits, including diabetes insipidus. A majority of patients are discharged home on postoperative day two or three. In most patients, serum sodium levels and urine output are followed every 6–8 h for the first 48 h. Patients with any evidence of new hypocortisolemia must receive adequate replacement treatment. Patients with functional pituitary adenomas typically undergo basic nonstimulation hormonal testing (e.g., serum prolactin, cortisol, or growth hormone) on postoperative days one and two. If nasal packing is utilized (in a minority of cases), it is typically removed on postoperative day one. Following discharge, patients usually are followed up in clinic 1 week after the operation, with a routine serum sodium level obtained on postoperative day seven to rule out occult hyponatremia [24]. Routine early postoperative imaging is not performed in a majority of patients. Most patients undergo standard MRI 3 months following the operation.

Conclusions

Despite its relatively short existence in the realm of transsphenoidal resection of pituitary lesions, the endoscopic approach has been extensively refined and is quickly becoming the preferred technique over microsurgical transsphenoidal approaches. Integration of the endoscope into pituitary surgery affords the surgeon superior panoramic visualization and illumination as well as improved surgical freedom and mobility compared to the traditional microscopic approach. The future of endoscopy for the resection of pituitary lesions will likely be based on continued miniaturization of the endoscope camera and optical technology, innovation in design of surgical instrumentation, application of three-dimensional cameras and viewing systems to compensate for the loss of depth perception, and the introduction of robotics. Combined with increasing surgical experience and comfort using the endoscopic technique, these advances will likely contribute to improved surgical outcomes in the future.

References

1. Jho HD, Carrau RL. Endoscopy assisted transsphenoidal surgery for pituitary adenoma. Technical note. Acta Neurochir. 1996;138:1416–25.
2. Jane Jr JA, Han J, Prevedello DM, Jagannathan J, Dumont AS, Laws Jr ER. Perspectives on endoscopic transsphenoidal surgery. Neurosurg Focus. 2005;19:E2.
3. Zada G, Liu C, Apuzzo ML. "Through the looking glass:" optical physics, issues, and the evolution of neuroendoscopy. World Neurosurg. 2012;77:92–102.
4. Guiot G, Rougerie J, Fourestier M. Intracranial endoscopic explorations [in French]. Presse Med. 1963;71:1225–8.
5. Apuzzo ML, Heifetz MD, Weiss MH, Kurze T. Neurosurgical endoscopy using the side-viewing telescope. J Neurosurg. 1977;46:398–400.
6. Carrau RL, Jho HD, Ko Y. Transnasal-transsphenoidal endoscopic surgery of the pituitary gland. Laryngoscope. 1966;106:914–8.
7. Cappabianca P, Alfieri A, de Divitiis E. Endoscopic endonasal transsphenoidal approach to the sella: towards functional endoscopic pituitary surgery (FEPS). Minim Invasive Neurosurg. 1998;41:66–73.
8. Dallapiazza R, Bond AE, Grober Y, Louis RG, Payne SC, Oldfield EH, Jane Jr JA. Retrospective analysis of a concurrent series of microscopic versus endoscopic transsphenoidal surgeries for Knosp Grades 0–2 nonfunctioning pituitary macroadenomas at a single institution. J Neurosurg. 2014;121:511–7.

9. Goudakos JK, Markou KD, Georgalas C. Endoscopic versus microscopic trans-sphenoidal pituitary surgery: a systematic review and meta-analysis. Clin Otolaryngol. 2011;36:212–20.
10. Dehdashti AR, Ganna A, Karabatsou K, Gentili F. Pure endoscopic endonasal approach for pituitary adenomas: early surgical results in 200 patients and comparison with previous microsurgical series. Neurosurgery. 2008;62:1006–15; discussion 1015–7.
11. Cappabianca P, Cavallo LM, de Divitiis O, Solari D, Esposito F, Colao A. Endoscopic pituitary surgery. Pituitary. 2008;11:385–90.
12. Tabaee A, Anand VK, Fraser JF, Brown SM, Singh A, Schwartz TH. Three-dimensional endoscopic pituitary surgery. Neurosurgery. 2009;64 Suppl 2:288–93; discussion 294–5.
13. Zada G, Agarwalla PK, Mukundan Jr S, Dunn I, Golby AJ, Laws Jr ER. The neurosurgical anatomy of the sphenoid sinus and sellar floor in endoscopic transsphenoidal surgery. J Neurosurg. 2011;114: 1319–30.
14. Lucas JW, Zada G. Endoscopic surgery for pituitary tumors. Neurosurg Clin N Am. 2012;23:555–69.
15. Christian E, Harris B, Wrobel B, Zada G Endoscopic endonasal transsphenoidal surgery: implementation of an operative and perioperative checklist. Neurosurg Focus. 2014(4):E1
16. Esposito F, Dusick JR, Fatemi N, Kelly DF. Graded repair of cranial base defects and cerebrospinal fluid leaks in transsphenoidal surgery. Neurosurgery. 2007;60 Suppl 2:295–303; discussion 303–94.
17. Couldwell WT, Kan P, Weiss MH. Simple closure following transsphenoidal surgery. Technical note. Neurosurg Focus. 2006;20:E11.
18. Ciric I, Ragin A, Baumgartner C, Pierce D. Complications of transsphenoidal surgery: results of a national survey, review of the literature, and personal experience. Neurosurgery. 1977;40:225–36; discussion 236–7.
19. Zada G, Kelly DF, Cohan P, Wang C, Swerdloff R. Endonasal transsphenoidal approach for pituitary adenomas and other sellar lesions: an assessment of efficacy, safety, and patient impressions. J Neurosurg. 2003;98:350–8.
20. Berker M, Hazer DB, Yucel T, Gurlek A, Cila A, Aldur M, Onerci M. Complications of endoscopic surgery of the pituitary adenomas: analysis of 570 patients and review of the literature. Pituitary. 2012;15:288–300.
21. Cappabianca P, Cavallo LM, de Divitiis E. Endoscopic endonasal transsphenoidal surgery. Neurosurgery. 2004;55:933–40; discussion 940–1.
22. Tabaee A, Anand VK, Barron Y, Hiltzik DH, Brown SM, Kacker A, et al. Endoscopic pituitary surgery: a systematic review and meta-analysis. J Neurosurg. 2009;111:545–54.
23. Cappabianca P, Cavallo LM, Esposito F, Valente V, De Divitiis E. Sellar repair in endoscopic endonasal transsphenoidal surgery: results of 170 cases. Neurosurgery. 2002;51:1365–71; discussion 1371–2.
24. Zada G, Liu CY, Fishback D, Singer PA, Weiss MH. Recognition and management of delayed hyponatremia following transsphenoidal pituitary surgery. J Neurosurg. 2007;106:66–71.

Transcranial and Skull Base Surgical Approaches to the Sellar and Parasellar Region

6

Ian F. Dunn

The surgeon approaching tumors in the sellar region must contend with a highly congested neurovascular anatomy surrounding the pituitary gland and stalk. In particular, the optic chiasm and nerves, carotid artery and branches, and upper cranial nerves merit meticulous attention. Although the transsphenoidal approach is used to resect the vast majority of sellar lesions and an increasing number of lesions with extrasellar extension, facility with open transcranial approaches is still necessary for safe resection of lesions with particular anatomical characteristics for which endonasal approaches are ill-advised.

The subfrontal and pterional approaches are the most common surgical approaches used to access lesions in the sella. The subfrontal approach provides direct anterior access to the sella, but the pterional corridor permits anterolateral access, superior vascular control, enhanced superior access, and routes to cavernous sinus and posterior fossa extension. Further refinements of the subfrontal and pterional approaches include the supraorbital and cranio-orbitozygomatic approaches, respectively; these approaches enhance exposure and minimize brain retraction. More recently, the keyhole craniotomy via an eyebrow or eyelid-crease incision has gained popularity in the transcranial management of small parasellar lesions.

6.1 Indications for a Transcranial Approach

The most common tumors in the neurosurgeon's practice in the sellar and parasellar region are pituitary adenomas, meningiomas, and craniopharyngiomas. The surgeon should at least consider using a transcranial rather than (or in addition to) a transsphenoidal approach if a lesion in this region features one or more of these characteristics [1]:

- Suprasellar or retrosellar extension
- Lateral cavernous sinus extension
- Posterior fossa extension
- Firm consistency
- Brain invasion
- Prior radiation
- Encasement of the optic apparatus or large cerebral vessels

Clear insinuation of a tumor in this region into the optic canals, in most hands, continues to be a strong indication for a transcranial surgical approach.

I.F. Dunn, MD
Department of Neurosurgery, Brigham and Women's Hospital, Boston, MA, USA
e-mail: idunn@partners.org

G. Zada et al. (eds.), *Atlas of Sellar and Parasellar Lesions: Clinical, Radiologic, and Pathologic Correlations*, DOI 10.1007/978-3-319-22855-6_6

6.2 The Range of Approaches

Selection of one approach over the others depends on the precise geometry and growth trajectory of the tumor, the need for vascular control, and the surgeon's preference and experience. One may consider approaches to this region in a modular fashion, which mimics their evolution: The base unit, the frontal craniotomy, may be performed via eyebrow incision or may be extended bilaterally for bifrontal access. To this approach may be added a superior orbital rim osteotomy in one piece, yielding a supraorbital approach. One or both orbital rims may be removed, but usually one is sufficient. The frontal craniotomy may be extended temporally to confer a pterional approach [2]. To the pterional approach, a superior and lateral orbital rim removal and zygomatic osteotomy may be added, yielding the cranio-orbitozygomatic exposure (Fig. 6.1) [3, 4]. The various approaches occupy a spectrum of access to the region and versatility; the pterional approach is more flexible than the bifrontal approach, with skull base modifications of each (as reviewed later) providing additional exposure and minimizing brain retraction.

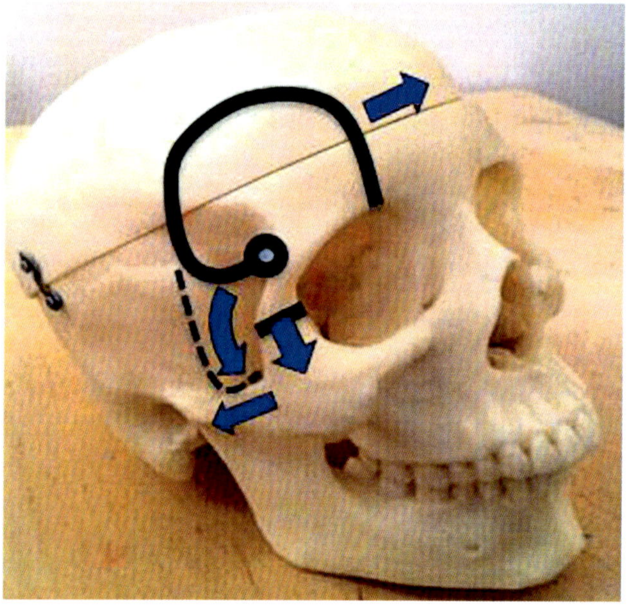

Fig. 6.1 A supraorbital flap (*dark black*), based on the true keyhole, may be modified by involving more of the lateral orbit, extending medially (bifrontal) or extending temporally with or without a zygomatic osteotomy

6.3 Frontal Approaches

The unifrontal or bifrontal approach is the oldest cranial approach employed for lesions of the sellar region [5]; its main advantage is its "straight-shot" trajectory beneath the frontal lobe to the optic chiasm and sella. A lumbar drain facilitates brain relaxation. A three-fourths bicoronal incision or a full bicoronal incision, sparing the temporalis, is fashioned behind the hairline for a unilateral or a bilateral subfrontal approach, respectively. Excessive extension of the head results in an overly oblique orientation of the planum and tuberculum away from the surgeon. A pericranial flap from one temporal line to the other, based anteriorly on the supraorbital vessels and extending under the posterior aspect of the incision, should be raised during the opening in anticipation of frontal sinus entry or violation of the ethmoid or sphenoid sinuses, which would merit repair with a vascularized graft. A bifrontal craniotomy follows, which should be taken as low as possible to decrease the distance to the anterior fossa floor and minimize brain retraction.

The dura is opened low and transversely—across a ligated sagittal sinus, if bilateral—and is reflected inferiorly. The olfactory tracts are identified and separated from the frontal lobe to prevent avulsion. The optic nerves and chiasm are readily seen with gentle frontal lobe retraction. Ventricular extension of the lesion may be reached through the lamina terminalis; limitations include a prefixed optic chiasm and lateral/cavernous sinus or substantial superior extension. Additional extradural dissection after frontal craniotomy may add to the exposure in select cases; the planum and tuberculum may be drilled for more inferior exposure beneath a prefixed chiasm, and the optic canals can be opened for greater maneuverability around the optic apparatus. Any parasellar or frontal sinus should be exenterated, obliterated, and covered with a large pericranial graft.

The surgeon may also consider the subfrontal "keyhole" approach [6], through either an eyebrow or eyelid incision. This approach has been used to access the sellar and parasellar regions. The incision most commonly is placed in the eyebrow with a slight lateral extension, being sure to stay lateral to the supraorbital nerve. The craniotomy, intended to be situated lateral to the frontal sinus, is small, and the main advantage is cosmetic.

6.4 Supraorbital Approach

The supraorbital approach, like the bifrontal approach, provides access to pathology of the planum, tuberculum, clinoid, and sella with minimal or no extension lateral to the carotid. The main conceptual advantage is that removal of the superior and lateral orbital rims reduces the amount of frontal lobe retraction required and may facilitate removal of more superiorly projecting midline tumors through enhanced visualization.

We perform the supraorbital approach based on the approach originally described by Jane et al. [7]. A spinal drain is optional. The scalp incision is begun 1 cm anterior to the tragus and is continued in curvilinear fashion behind the hairline to the level of the superior temporal line on the opposite side. The superficial temporal artery is behind the incision, and the facial nerve branches are in front of it. A large pericranial flap based on the supraorbital and frontal vessels, beginning well behind the skin incision and extending from one superior temporal line to the other, is raised and reflected over the scalp flap anteriorly and dissected off the superior and lateral orbital walls. The supraorbital nerve is freed from its notch or freed from its foramen with a high-speed drill.

Only the superior aspect of the temporalis muscle needs to be mobilized. To do this, a subfascial dissection of the temporalis fascia is carried out by incising both layers of the fascia to expose the temporalis muscle, beginning at the keyhole and proceeding behind the course of the facial nerve to approximately the level of the sylvian fissure. The fascial layers are reflected forward, and the temporalis muscle, dissected free from its overlying fascia, is released from its insertion at the superior temporal line and along the superior and lateral orbit and reflected inferiorly. The junction of the zygomatic, sphenoidal, and frontal bones is thus exposed.

The bone flap is usually a unilateral supraorbital bone flap (Fig. 6.2a), although large tumors may be approached with a bifrontal supraorbital flap, with a one-piece intent for cosmetic purposes. The unilateral flap begins with placement of a burr hole at the anatomical keyhole about 1 cm behind the frontozygomatic suture. When drilled correctly, the superior half exposes frontal lobe dura and the lower half exposes the periorbita, with the orbital roof in the center of the burr hole separating the frontal lobe and orbit. An additional cut is made in the lateral orbital rim anywhere above the zygoma while the lateral periorbita is protected and continued to the orbital half of the keyhole. Finally, the flap is completed with a superior orbital roof osteotomy, done by placing a chisel straddling the lateral aspect of the superior orbit exposed in the keyhole and completing the osteotomy, with cottonoids protecting the frontal dura and the periorbita. It is important to angle the chisel superiorly, to ensure that the medial end of the osteotomy is well away from the orbital apex. It is also critical to complete the osteotomy rather than to "crack" the bone flap off manually, which may lead to unintended angles of roof compromise through the optic canal.

If the frontal sinus is entered during the exposure, the sinus is exenterated and its posterior wall is removed. A small piece of fat or temporalis muscle is used to pack the sinus and obliterate the frontonasal duct.

This approach provides excellent access to the optic nerves and chiasm and to pathology in the sellar region in or in front of the sella and medial to the carotids. Both optic canals can be accessed and opened from this vantage point.

The pituitary stalk is distinct in its color and vascular arborization. Tuberculum sellae meningiomas usually displace the stalk posteriorly; rarely, they will engulf the stalk, requiring careful microdissection. Hypophyseal branches off the carotid are spared.

The involved dura of the tuberculum and planum is resected and any hyperostotic bone is drilled with a high-speed diamond burr. Paranasal sinus entry is handled by exenterating the sinus mucosa and packing the spaces with fat. A piece of free pericranium or fascia lata is then placed intradurally and secured to the native dura over the resected dura. After dural closure, the pericranial flap is turned over the orbit and frontal bone and is spread over any defect in the anterior fossa floor.

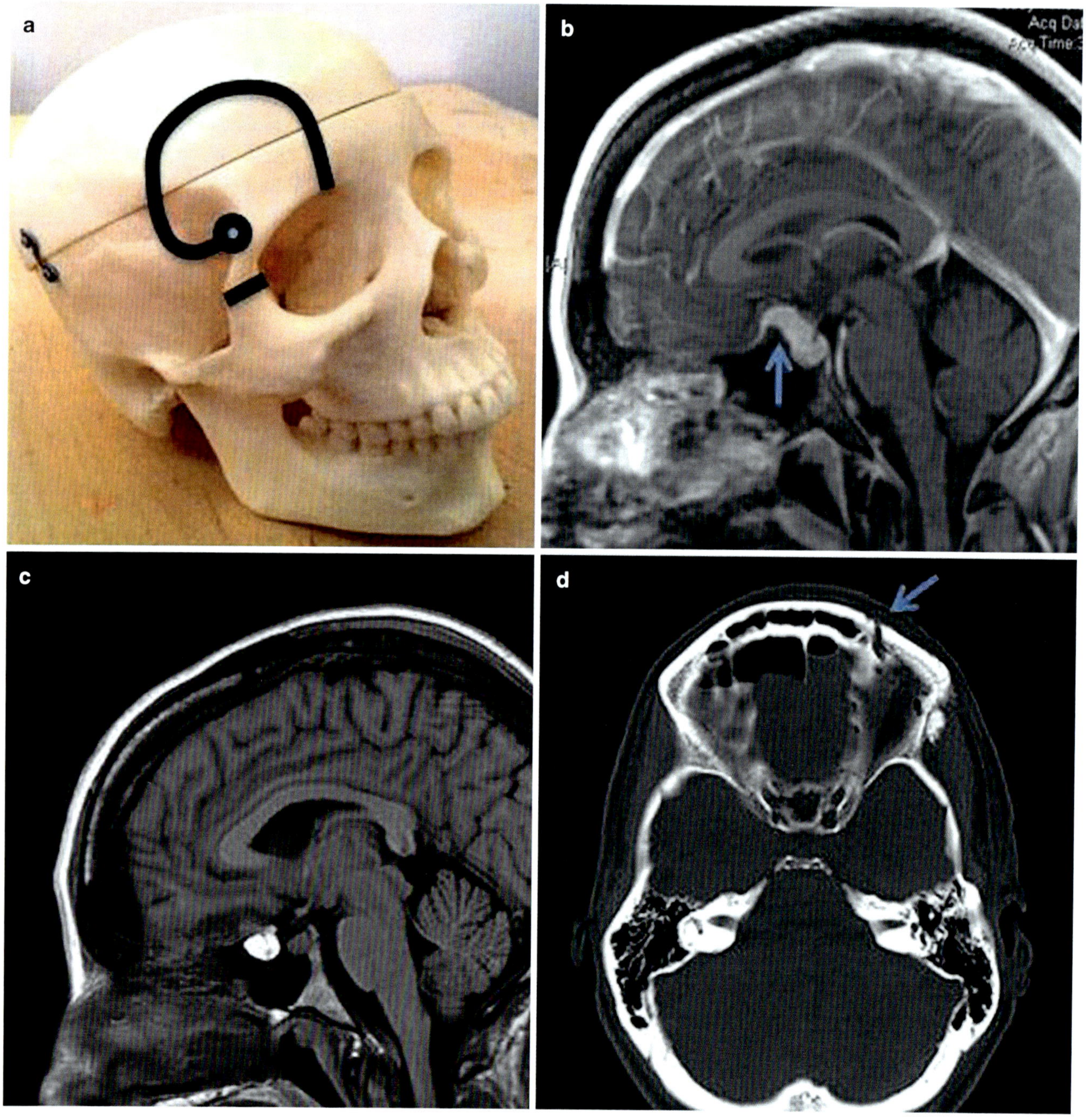

Fig. 6.2 (**a**) Supraorbital bone flap. (**b**) Sagittal T1 contrast MRI showing a tuberculum sella meningioma with significant hyperostosis (*blue arrow*). (**c**) Postoperative T1 MRI showing fat in the roof of the sphenoid sinus after involved bone is drilled away. (**d**) Postoperative CT scan showing the superior orbital osteotomy just lateral to the frontal sinus (*arrow*)

6.4.1 Application to Parasellar Tumors: Tuberculum Sellae Meningiomas

Tuberculum sellae meningiomas, originating in front of the sella and arising from the tuberculum, chiasmatic sulcus, and limbus sphenoidale, accounted for 5–10 % of meningiomas in Cushing's and Eisenhardt's series [8]. These tumors often invade the floor of the anterior fossa and cause hyperostosis, commonly in front of the sella (Fig. 6.2b). As they enlarge, they displace the optic nerves laterally and the chiasm superiorly; they also impinge on the pituitary stalk posteriorly, as well as the basilar artery, and they can extend to the interpeduncular space. They frequently insinuate into one or both optic canals. The blood supply is typically inferiorly from the posterior ethmoidal arteries. Meticulous attention must be paid to the anterior cerebral artery (ACA) complex, which (depending on the tumor's size) may be encased or displaced superiorly. Careful attention also must be paid to small, medial lenticulostriates.

6.4.2 Specific Surgical Principles

The main principles of the supraorbital approach as it pertains to tuberculum sellae tumors are the low frontobasal exposure, which facilitates access to the tumor without undue frontal retraction, and access to both optic canals (Fig. 6.2c, d). Once the dura is opened, the ipsilateral olfactory tract is quickly encountered and should be dissected off from the frontal lobe in order to prevent its avulsion. A drop of fibrin glue applied to the olfactory tract may further decrease the risk of damage to the tract. When the tumor is encountered, its basal posterior ethmoidal arterial feeders are coagulated to devascularize the tumor; central debulking then may be undertaken by ultrasonic aspiration or other means. The optic chiasm is usually displaced superiorly, and the optic nerves, superiorly and laterally. Should the nerves be engulfed in tumor, dissection should begin at the chiasm and proceed proximally. The arterial supply to the optic chiasm and nerves is preserved. All associated dura is resected, and any hyperostotic bone at the tuberculum and planum is drilled away with a high-speed diamond bit.

Decompressing the visual apparatus is not complete until the optic canals are unroofed. In a recent series, 67 % of tuberculum sellae tumors were associated with tumor extension into one optic canal (40 %) or both canals (60 %) [9]. Moreover, tumor left inside the optic canal may be the source of recurrence or of diminished visual improvement after surgery [10]. One or both optic canals are exposed and unroofed with a high-speed drill under constant irrigation, to avoid thermal injury to the optic nerve. The falciform ligament and optic sheath are opened sharply. Optic nerve decompression should proceed as far anterior toward the globe as is needed to ensure that all optic extension of the tumor has been extirpated. Even if the clinical presentation suggests extension of the tumor into only one optic canal, the surgeon should be prepared to decompress both canals on the basis of intraoperative findings. Even the slightest suggestion of canalicular extension should prompt at least the opening of the falciform ligament.

6.5 Pterional Approach

The pterional or frontotemporal approach, popularized by Yasargil and Fox [11], has the additional benefit of providing a lateral corridor to sellar lesions, access to cavernous sinus extension, and more superior access than afforded by an anteriorly directed frontal or supraorbital approach. Importantly, it allows for a greater degree of vascular control, given the excellent access it provides to the parasellar vasculature. Lesions that extend to the cavernous sinus should be approached with, at minimum, a pterional approach.

The placement of a lumbar drain is optional; it is less important than in frontal approaches because of the access the pterional approach affords to the sylvian cisterns. The head is turned 30° away and extended, bringing the lateral aspect of the malar eminence to an uppermost position. This position also usually places the ipsilateral optic nerve perpendicular to the floor.

The scalp incision extends from the zygomatic root within 1 cm of the tragus, arcing behind the hairline to the midline and staying above the temporalis fascia, sparing the superficial temporal artery. To minimize obstruction in the desired line of sight, we reflect the temporalis inferiorly after a subfascial dissection and detachment from its temporal line insertion. We turn a standard pterional bone flap, which spans the sylvian fissure but often includes a generous frontal extension, with the craniotomy extending to just above the supraorbital rim. The sphenoid ridge is generously drilled from lateral to medial aspects to expose the superior orbital fissure and the posterior aspect of the orbit, such that the anterior and middle fossa floors are flush with each other.

Once the pterional flap is turned, the anterior clinoid process may be removed for access to the subclinoid carotid in order to enlarge the opticocarotid window for improved intrasellar access [12]. Sectioning the dural ring permits mobilization of the carotid. Anterior clinoid removal also allows opening of the oculomotor trigone for superior entry to the cavernous sinus. The pterional approach also allows lateral cavernous sinus access. Once the anterior clinoid is removed, the temporal dura propria may be dissected from the lateral wall of the cavernous sinus extradurally, exposing the divisions of the trigeminal nerve and the superior orbital fissure. In this fashion, tumor extensions from the sella into the cavernous sinus may be approached extradurally through such corridors as Parkinson's triangle [13] between the trochlear and first division of the trigeminal nerve.

The dura is then opened in a C-shaped fashion, spanning the sylvian fissure and reflected anteriorly. Attention is then turned to achieving adequate brain relaxation. The arachnoid over the optic nerve is opened to allow the frontal lobe to be elevated, and the sylvian fissure is then widely split. This step is performed with patience, gradually withdrawing sufficient CSF to optimize brain relaxation and minimize retraction pressures. Wide sylvian fissure opening permits the development of the working corridor between the frontal and temporal lobes and easy access to the carotid for vascular control.

Several operative corridors are available. In most instances, obvious tumor is encountered behind the tuberculum and between the optic nerves. The opticocarotid window, which may be expanded by lateral reflection of the carotid artery after anterior clinoid removal, is a standard corridor for removal of sellar lesions. Extension to the third ventricle may be accessed through the lamina terminalis. Cavernous sinus extension may be accessed superiorly through the oculomotor window once the clinoid is removed or laterally following separation of the temporal dura from the lateral wall of the sinus.

In general, pituitary tumors are internally debulked once their capsules are opened, and the capsule is only removed where safe. Great care should be exercised in dealing with portions of the tumor or capsule attached to the optic apparatus, as dissection may damage these structures or their microvasculature, which may be shared by the tumor capsule.

6.6 Cranio-Orbitozygomatic Approach

The cranio-orbitozygomatic (COZ) approach adds a superior and lateral orbital osteotomy and zygomatic osteotomy to the standard pterional approach, rendering it ideal for accessing tumors that may engulf or displace structures superiorly and laterally in the parasellar region. The skin incision is similar to the incision for the supraorbital or pterional approach. A subfascial dissection of the temporalis fascia is performed to preserve the frontal branches of the facial nerve. The zygomatic arch and superior and lateral orbital margins are exposed by subperiosteal dissection, after which the zygoma is divided at either end and displaced inferiorly on its masseteric pedicle (Fig. 6.3a). The temporalis muscle is then elevated in subperiosteal fashion, beginning low on the temporal squama and proceeding superiorly to detach the muscle at the superior temporal line. The entire temporalis muscle is then reflected inferiorly with the freed zygoma.

The cranio-orbital flap is raised as described for the supraorbital approach, except that the lateral orbital osteotomy is taken down to the malar eminence, and the inferior aspect of the frontal craniotomy is taken to the floor of the temporal fossa. With the orbit now exposed, electromyographic electrodes may be directly placed into the superior oblique, superior rectus, and lateral rectus muscles to monitor cranial nerves III, IV, and VI.

If the tumor engulfs the carotid, proximal control may be obtained either in the neck or in the petrous segment, to which the COZ approach provides access through exposure of Glasscock's triangle. Proximal control may be obtained by sufficient exposure for placement of a temporary clip on the petrous carotid artery, if necessary. Alternatively, a Fogarty catheter may be inserted into the carotid canal. Should vascular control be required, the catheter balloon can be inflated to occlude the carotid artery in the carotid canal [14].

Medial exposure of the cavernous sinus and exposure of the paraclinoid carotid artery are obtained by drilling out the remainder of the orbital roof, the superior orbital fissure, the anterior clinoid process, and the optic strut. The anterior clinoid process is cored out with the drill and then disarticulated by drilling out the optic strut. The clinoid is subperiosteally dissected and resected. The superior orbital fissure is opened by drilling along the lesser sphenoid wing. This procedure exposes the subclinoid portion of the carotid artery, which is both extradural and extracavernous, and provides distal control of the carotid artery.

Entrance into the cavernous sinus has been described in relationship to the intervals between the neurovascular structures of the cavernous sinus. These intervals have been annotated as 10 triangles distributed among the parasellar, middle fossa, and paraclival locations [15]. The actual approach taken must be individualized for each patient; it depends on the anatomy of the lesion in relationship to the cavernous sinus structures. In general, there are two approaches for entry into the cavernous sinus: a superior approach and a lateral approach. The superior approach is particularly suited to those lesions adjacent to the anterior loop of the carotid artery and those that are superior and/or medial to the cavernous carotid artery. The lateral approach lends itself well to exposing lesions that are lateral and/or inferior to the carotid artery, as well as those that are posteriorly located within the cavernous sinus. These approaches often are combined for lesions widely involving the sinus.

Reconstruction after the COZ approach begins by directing attention toward prevention of CSF leaks by searching for and obliterating any feature of the dissection that may result in a CSF leak. Any entrance into the paranasal sinuses or the eustachian tube should be obliterated with fat and fascia. Any tenuous or incomplete dural closures should be reinforced with tissue—preferably autologous—such as fascia, muscle, or fat. Fibrin glue can be used for further reinforcement. The thick pericranial flap can be brought down under the frontal lobe, over the orbit, and over any sinus entries in the middle fossa or petrous apex. The orbital roof is reconstructed to prevent late enophthalmos. If the frontal sinus has been entered, the mucosa should be exenterated and the cavity packed with fat or tissue to prevent mucocele formation and CSF leakage. The cranio-orbital flap is secured in place with titanium miniplates. Bony defects can be obliterated with titanium plates or mesh, or with any of a number of cranioplastic materials, such as hydroxyapatite cement. The temporalis muscle is sutured to the superior temporal line. The zygoma is plated into position with titanium miniplates.

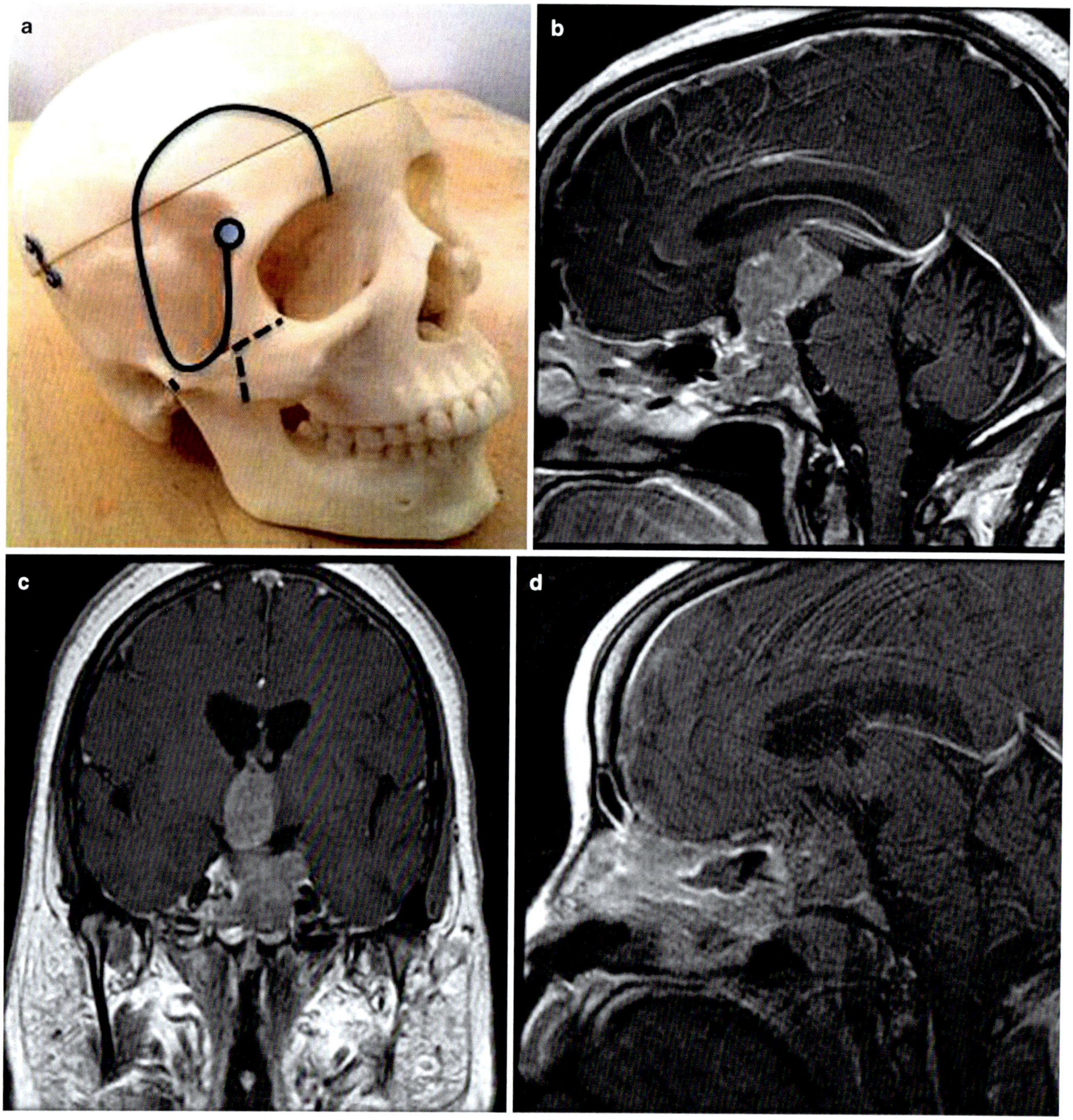

Fig. 6.3 (**a**) Cranio-orbitozygomatic (COZ) flap, with a lateral orbital cut and zygomatic cuts (*dashed lines*). (**b**) Preoperative T1 contrast MRI showing a sellar mass with significant suprasellar and retrosellar extension to the level of the internal cerebral veins. (**c**) Preoperative coronal MRI showing the superior extent of the mass in the third ventricle. (**d**) Postoperative sagittal MRI

6.6.1 Applications to Parasellar Tumors: Pituitary Macroadenomas (Superior and Lateral Projections)

The increasing flexibility of—and experience with—extended endonasal approaches has dramatically diminished the application of transcranial approaches to pituitary tumors, but conventional open cranial microsurgical approaches continue to play a role in the management of pituitary adenomas, though their indications are rarer. A number of preoperative radiographic features may favor transcranial surgery [1, 16]:

- An overly small sella
- Tumor above and lateral to the supraclinoid carotid
- Encasement of subarachnoid arteries
- Presence of tumor predominantly in the cavernous sinus
- A very narrow diaphragma sellae and a large supradiaphragmatic component
- T2 changes in the brain
- History of prior radiation in cases of vascular encasement
- Significant retrosellar or posterior fossa extension

In addition, the discovery of an overly vascular or fibrous tumor during transsphenoidal surgery for a tumor with a significant suprasellar extent may prompt consideration of a second transcranial approach. If postoperative apoplexy occurs when residual tumor has been left in the suprasellar space, transcranial surgery should be strongly considered [16].

Patients with documented fibrous tumors with significant suprasellar and retrosellar extension with residual tumor after incomplete transsphenoidal resection are candidates for a transcranial approach. Another common indication is the presence of substantial tumor burden in the cavernous sinus lateral to the carotid artery, where progressive growth or symptoms mandate treatment and radiation is deferred. Technical advances in microsurgery have established the cavernous sinus as an approachable space whose contents may be navigated successfully. Core principles of these approaches include maximal bone removal for exposure, the avoidance of brain retraction, precise knowledge of cranial nerve anatomy, and control of the carotid artery in its petrous, cavernous, and/or clinoid segments.

6.6.2 Specific Surgical Principles

The COZ approach affords wide exposure of the entire cavernous sinus and the proximal and distal carotid artery, with minimal cerebral retraction. In cases of fibrous tumor with significant superior extension (with or without posterior fossa extension), the pterional component of the COZ permits a wide splitting of the sylvian fissure while the superior and lateral orbital osteotomy component minimizes frontal lobe retraction during access to the superiorly projecting tumor. Sellar components of tumor also may be accessed easily. The patient in Fig. 6.3, with a dopamine-refractory prolactinoma, had undergone multiple transsphenoidal attempts at removal, followed by radiation. Long-term dopamine agonist use had rendered the tumor extremely fibrous. In this patient, the COZ approach permitted sylvian fissure access, vascular control, a superolateral trajectory, and sellar access. Figure 6.4 shows a lesion with a substantial frontal and posterior fossa component and encasement of the arteries of the circle of Willis. This patient underwent four transsphenoidal operations, radiation therapy, and temozolomide chemotherapy, mandating a transcranial approach in which vascular control and the middle fossa corridor to the posterior fossa component allowed safe microsurgical resection.

Significant progressively enlarging or symptomatic lateral cavernous sinus tumor burden left during transsphenoidal surgery continues to be an indication for transcranial surgery, as in Fig. 6.5. The surgical principles germane to removing the right lateral cavernous sinus component are superior and lateral access to the cavernous sinus, the ability to obtain vascular control, visualization of the optic apparatus, and clinoid removal (achieved using the COZ approach). Monitoring the abducens and oculomotor nerve functions by placing needles in the appropriate orbital musculature may confer an additional degree of safety.

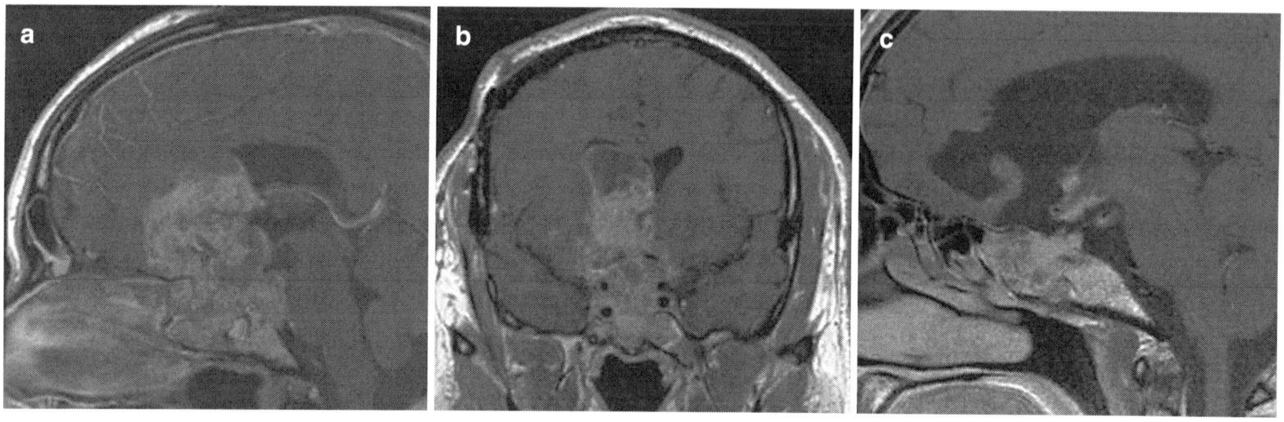

Fig. 6.4 (**a**) Preoperative sagittal MRI showing a macroadenoma with A2 encasement and posterior fossa extension. (**b**) Preoperative coronal MRI showing the superior and lateral extent and encasement of bilateral A1. (**c**) Postoperative sagittal MRI

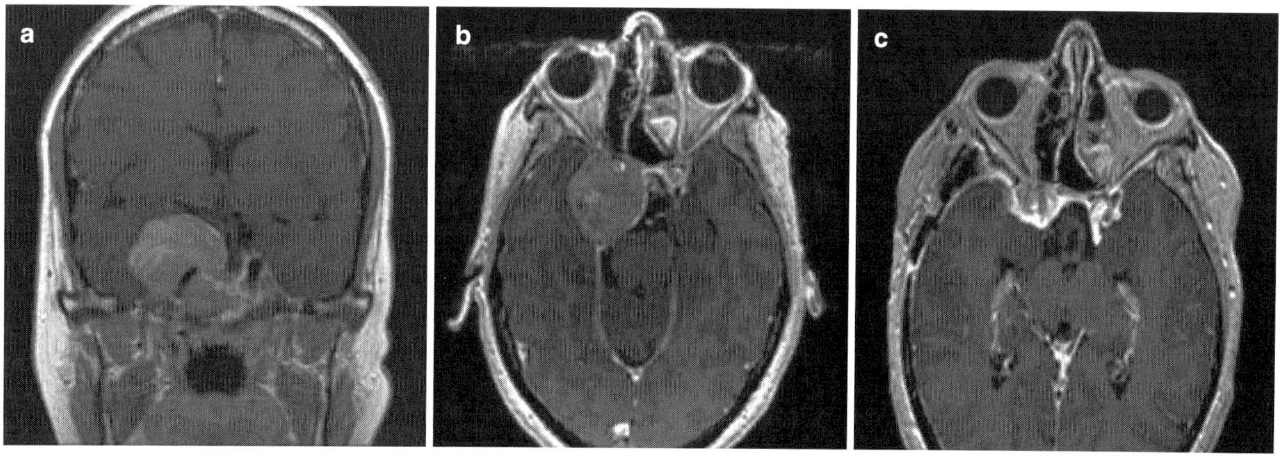

Fig. 6.5 Preoperative coronal (**a**) and axial (**b**) MRIs showing extensive lateral cavernous sinus tumor burden. (**c**) Postoperative axial MRI

Conclusion

The evolution and refinement of transsphenoidal surgery have dramatically reduced the use of transcranial approaches to sellar and parasellar pathology, but transcranial approaches remain vital means of approaching tumors in this area for which an endonasal solution is ill-advised. Frontal or pterional craniotomies, with the addition of superior orbital, lateral orbital, and/or zygomatic osteotomies, are the primary approaches to the region. The selection of the best approach for each case is driven by anatomical characteristics (Table 6.1) and surgeon preference.

Table 6.1 Considerations in selecting a transcranial surgical approach

Subfrontal/supraorbital approach	Pterional/cranio-orbitozygomatic (COZ) approach
Excellent frontobasal exposure	Excellent anterior and middle fossa exposure
Minimizes frontal lobe retraction	Minimizes frontal and temporal lobe retraction
Excellent for sellar, suprasellar, or tuberculum pathology	Excellent for clinoidal or suprasellar and all parasellar pathology
Use if pathology is medial to carotid or optic apparatus	Strongly consider if pathology extends lateral to carotid or optic apparatus or if superior extension merits lateral exposure
	Preferable for vascular control

References

1. Zada G, Du R, Laws Jr ER. Defining the "edge of the envelope": patient selection in treating complex sellar-based neoplasms via transsphenoidal versus open craniotomy. J Neurosurg. 2011;114:286–300.
2. Cawley CM, Zipfel GJ, Day AL. Surgical treatment of paraclinoid and ophthalmic aneurysms. Neurosurg Clin N Am. 1998;9:765–83.
3. Al-Mefty O. Supraorbital-pterional approach to skull base lesions. Neurosurgery. 1987;21:474–7.
4. Al-Mefty O, Fox JL. Superolateral orbital exposure and reconstruction. Surg Neurol. 1985;23:609–13.
5. Landolt AM. History of pituitary surgery from the technical aspect. Neurosurg Clin N Am. 2001;12:37–44, vii–viii.
6. Reisch R, Perneczky A. Ten-year experience with the supraorbital subfrontal approach through an eyebrow skin incision. Neurosurgery. 2005;57:242–55.
7. Jane JA, Park TS, Pobereskin LH, Winn HR, Butler AB. The supraorbital approach: technical note. Neurosurgery. 1982;11:537–42.
8. Cushing H, Eisenhardt L. Suprasellar meningiomas. In: Meningiomas: their classification, regional behavior, life history, and surgical end results. Baltimore: Charles C. Thomas; 1938. p. 224–49.
9. Mahmoud M, Nader R, Al-Mefty O. Optic canal involvement in tuberculum sellae meningiomas: influence on approach, recurrence, and visual recovery. Neurosurgery. 2010;67(3 Suppl Operative):ons108–18; discussion ons118–9.
10. Schick U, Hassler W. Surgical management of tuberculum sellae meningiomas: involvement of the optic canal and visual outcome. J Neurol Neurosurg Psychiatry. 2005;76:977–83.
11. Yasargil MG, Fox JL. The microsurgical approach to intracranial aneurysms. Surg Neurol. 1975;3:7–14.
12. Youssef AS, Agazzi S, van Loveren HR. Transcranial surgery for pituitary adenomas. Neurosurgery. 2005;57:168–75.
13. Dolenc VV. Transcranial epidural approach to pituitary tumors extending beyond the sella. Neurosurgery. 1997;41:542–50; discussion 551–2.
14. Wascher TM, Spetzler RF, Zabramski JM. Improved transdural exposure and temporary occlusion of the petrous internal carotid artery for cavernous sinus surgery. Technical note. J Neurosurg. 1993;78:834–7.
15. Borba LAB, Al-Mefty O. Normal anatomy of the cavernous sinus. In: Eisenberg MB, Al-Mefty O, editors. The cavernous sinus: a comprehensive text. Philadelphia: Lippincott Williams & Wilkins; 2000. p. 21–33.
16. Pratheesh R, Rajaratnam S, Prabhu K, Mani SE, Chacko G, Chacko AG. The current role of transcranial surgery in the management of pituitary adenomas. Pituitary. 2013;16:419–34.

Radiosurgery of the Sellar and Parasellar Region

7

Robert M. Starke, Ching-Jen Chen, Dale Ding, and Jason Sheehan

7.1 Introduction

Tumors of the sellar and parasellar regions have posed tremendous challenges to neurosurgeons over the past century. Conventional microsurgical techniques alone are often insufficient in providing definitive treatment. Attempts at complete resection are often hindered by tumor proximity to critical vascular, neuronal, and hormonal structures. Treatment combinations including surgery, radiosurgery, radiation therapy, and medical management are often utilized to improve remission rates. Since Dr. Harvey Cushing used the "radium bomb" to treat intracranial tumors in 1923, ionizing radiation has been used as a primary or adjuvant treatment for sellar and parasellar tumors by both neurosurgeons and radiation oncologists [1, 2].

In recent years, radiosurgery has become the method of choice in delivering ionizing radiation to tumors located in the sellar and parasellar regions. Radiosurgery is characterized by its ability to deliver focused, high-dose radiation in a single session to target tumors, even as its steep radiation dose falloff at the tumor margins limits the exposure of adjacent normal tissue to significant doses of radiation. Radiosurgery delivery devices include proton beam units, linear accelerator (LINAC)–based systems, and Gamma Knife (Elekta AB, Stockholm, Sweden).

Proton beam radiosurgery takes advantage of the Bragg phenomenon, in which the peak energy deposition of an accelerated proton occurs immediately before it comes to rest, so that the surrounding tissues are relatively spared of radiation doses [3]. Currently, only a few centers in the world offer this treatment; most deliver protons in a fractionated fashion rather than using them for radiosurgery. The number of proton centers is expected to increase over the next decade, however, as these units become more compact and cost-effective.

In LINAC-based systems (CyberKnife, TrueBeam Stx, Novalis TX, Trilogy, and Axesse), photons are produced from the collision of an accelerated electron with a high z target. The photon beams are delivered in multiple, noncoplanar arcs that intersect at the target lesion, producing submillimeter target accuracy [4]. Most use a stereotactic frame to restrict patient motion during treatment, although a few systems (CyberKnife and Novalis TX) have moved toward frameless, image-guided techniques.

In Gamma Knife radiosurgery (GKRS), a dose plan conforming to the contours of the target lesion is constructed using multiple isocenters. In the Gamma Knife Perfexion system, gamma ray beams produced by the radioactive decay of cobalt 60 converge on each isocenter, which comprises eight sectors of beams, with up to 192 simultaneous beams per sector. Beam diameters vary from 0 to 16 mm. The number and locations of isocenters are dictated by the size, shape, and location of the lesion. GKRS also achieves submillimeter target accuracy. At approximately 50 % isodose line, the cobalt-based system can achieve the steepest radiation dose falloff at the tumor margins, compared with an 80–90 % isodose line for the LINAC-based systems. Patient immobilization during treatment is generally achieved using rigid frame fixation to the skull.

Patients must be assessed individually to determine their candidacy for stereotactic radiosurgery. Characteristics such as lesion volume, lesion shape, and proximity to vital structures influence treatment decisions. If the lesion is more than 30 mm in diameter, or if it abuts extremely radiation-sensitive structures such as the optic system, treatment using multisession radiosurgery (e.g., the Gamma Knife Extend™ system) may be favored. This chapter reviews the recent radiosurgical experience in the treatment of major sellar and parasellar lesions.

R.M. Starke, MD • C.-J. Chen, MD • D. Ding, MD
J. Sheehan, MD, PhD (✉)
Department of Neurosurgery, University of Virginia, Charlottesville, VA, USA
e-mail: RMS6BX@virginia.edu; dmd7q@hscmail.mcc.virginia.edu; jsheehan@virginia.edu; cc5hx@virginia.edu

G. Zada et al. (eds.), *Atlas of Sellar and Parasellar Lesions: Clinical, Radiologic, and Pathologic Correlations*,
DOI 10.1007/978-3-319-22855-6_7

7.2 Nonfunctioning Pituitary Adenomas

Microsurgical resection of nonfunctioning pituitary macroadenomas achieves tumor control rates that vary from 50 to 80 % [5–7]. Literature has demonstrated that radiosurgery is an effective treatment for patients with tumor recurrence or progression following surgery. The goal of radiosurgery is the prevention of tumor growth, with or without tumor volume reduction. In a recent study, Wilson et al. [8] observed a 100 % tumor control rate following LINAC radiosurgery for nonfunctioning adenomas (NFAs) in 51 patients, using a mean margin dose of 14 Gy. Starke et al. [9] also found a comparable control rate of 90 % in a population of 140 patients following GKRS, using an average margin dose of 18 Gy. Recent series in radiosurgery for NFAs suggest a mean tumor control rate of 96 % (range, 83–100 %), with tumor reduction in an average of 57 % of patients (range, 26–91 %) [5, 7–26]. An average margin dose of 16 Gy (range, 12–20 Gy) was reported in these series. Table 7.1 summarizes radiosurgical results from recent studies for nonfunctioning adenomas.

Although the rates of neurologic deficits (mean, 1.8 %; range, 0–6.7 %) and endocrine deficits (mean, 11.3 %; range, 0–39 %) are relatively low, vision decline and hypopituitarism are the most frequently reported complications. Large tumor volume has been observed to be associated with an increased incidence of neurologic deficits and delayed hypopituitarism following radiosurgery [9, 11, 12]. In contrast, improvement in visual function with or without tumor volume reduction has been observed in other series [10, 15]. Current evidence suggests that radiosurgery is a safe and effective treatment for recurrent or residual disease in patients with NFAs, but continued long-term follow-up remains essential, as growth or reduction of these slow-growing tumors may not be immediately apparent [11, 16].

Table 7.1 Comparison of radiosurgical results for nonfunctioning pituitary adenomas

Study	Year	Patients	Prior surgical resection, %	Radiosurgery	F/U, *mo*	Maximal dose, *Gy*	Margin dose, *Gy*	Tumor volume change, %			Tumor control, %	Neurologic deficit, %	New hormone deficit, %
								Decreased	Unchanged	Increased			
Wilson et al. [8]	2012	51	–	LINAC	37.2	–	14	91.1	8.9	0	100	6.7	0
El-Shehaby et al. [10]	2012	21	90.5	GKRS	44	–	12	52	43	5	95	0	14.3
Starke et al. [9]	2012	140	90.7	GKRS	60	38.6	18	–	–	10	90	0	30.3
Gopalan et al. [11]	2011	48	97.9	GKRS	95	41.3	18.4	75	8	17	83	6.3	39
Park et al. [12]	2011	125	88	GKRS	62	27.9	13	52.8	36.8	10.4	89.6	2.4	24
Hayashi et al. [13]	2010	43	–	GKRS	36	–	18.2	–	–	–	100	0	0
Hoybye and Rahn [5]	2009	23	100	GKRS	78	50	20	78.3	17.4	4.3	100	4.3	0
Pollock et al. [14]	2008	62	95.2	GKRS	64	34.5	16	60	37	3	97	1.6	27
Liscak et al. [15]	2007	79	85	GKRS	60	40	20	88.6	11.4	0	100	0	2.5
Mingione et al. [16]	2006	90	91.1	GKRS	44.9	41.5	18.5	65.5	26.7	7.8	92.2	0	19.7
Voges et al. [17]	2006	37	–	LINAC	56.6	–	13.4	40.5	59.5	0	100	–	–
Picozzi et al. [18]	2005	51	100	GKRS	40.6	–	16.5	–	–	3.9	96.1	–	–
Iwai et al. [19]	2005	28	100	GKRS	36.4	–	12.3	–	–	–	93	0	7
Losa et al. [20]	2004	52	100	GKRS	41.1	33.2	16.6	38.5	57.7	3.8	96.2	0	9.6
Muacevic et al. [21]	2004	51	100	GKRS	21.7	–	16.5	–	–	–	95	0	3.9
Petrovich et al. [22]	2003	56	–	GKRS	34	30[a]	15[a]	–	–	0	100	–	–
Muramatsu et al. [23]	2003	8	100	LINAC	30	–	15[a]	–	–	0	100	–	–
Sheehan et al. [7]	2002	42	–	GKRS	31.2	32	16.2	42.9	54.8	2.4	97.6	4.8	0
Wowra and Stummer [24].	2002	30	96.7	GKRS	57.7	28.9	16	–	–	–	93	0	10
Izawa et al. [25]	2000	23	69.6	GKRS	30.1	–	19.5	26.1	–	–	95.6	4.3	4.3
Shin et al. [26]	2000	3	–	GKRS	18.7	–	16	33.3	66.7	0	100	0	0

Mean or median values used
F/U follow-up, *GKRS* Gamma Knife radiosurgery, *LINAC* linear accelerator–based radiosurgery, *mo* months
[a]Includes dose for other adenomas

7.3 Cushing's Disease

Hypersecretion of adrenocorticotropic hormone (ACTH) is responsible for 80 % of endogenous Cushing's syndrome, and pituitary adenomas are often the source of the hormone overproduction [27]. Microsurgical and endoscopic resection are the primary treatments for Cushing's disease, but a surgical cure remains a challenge when there is tumor invasion of surrounding structures or difficult tumor delineation on imaging. Radiosurgery serves as an invaluable adjunctive treatment following resection in these circumstances. Although the updated 2008 guidelines from the Endocrine Society recommend the use of postoperative morning serum cortisol levels in establishing biochemical remission [27], there remains significant variability in the literature regarding its definition. Most studies define endocrine remission using normal serum cortisol or normal 24-h urinary-free cortisol (UFC). In a large study of 90 patients at the University of Virginia who were treated with GKRS, we have observed a biochemical remission rate of 54.4 % defined by 24-h UFC and a tumor control rate of 95.5 % [28, 29]. Table 7.2 shows a summary of radiosurgical results for Cushing's disease from recent studies. These studies demonstrate a mean tumor control rate of 93 % (range, 77–100 %) and a biochemical remission rate of 54 % (range, 16.7–100 %), with a mean margin dose of 23.5 Gy (range, 15–35 Gy) [13, 22, 25, 26, 28–46].

In most series, rates of new neurologic deficits following radiosurgery are low, with an average of 2.8 % (range, 0–15.4 %), but the incidence of new endocrine deficit is higher, at a mean of 23 % (range, 0–68.8 %). These complication rates are both higher than what has been observed in radiosurgery for NFA; this difference could represent radiation damage to the normal pituitary and nerves secondary to the higher margin doses delivered to ACTH-secreting adenomas. Despite biochemical remission and hormone reduction offered by radiosurgery, late recurrence rates of up to 20 % have been reported, so long-term follow-up is very important for these patients [28, 40].

Table 7.2 Comparison of radiosurgical results for Cushing's disease

Study	Year	Patients	Radiosurgery	F/U, *mo*	Maximal dose, *Gy*	Margin dose, *Gy*	Biochemical remission rate, %	Tumor control, %	Neurologic deficit, %	New hormone deficit, %
Grant et al. [45]	2013	15	GKRS	40.2	–	35	73	100	–	40
Wein et al. [46]	2012	17	LINAC	23	31.9	17.8	59	–	0	11.8
Sheehan et al. [29]	2011	82	GKRS	31	–	24[a]	54	–	–	22
Hayashi et al. [13]	2011	13	GKRS	36	–	25.2[a]	38	77	15.4	0
Castinetti et al. [42]	2009	18	GKRS	95.5	–	28.5	50	100	–	–
Wan et al. [43]	2009	68	GKRS	67.3	–	23	27.9	86.8	–	1.5
Kobayashi et al. [44]	2009	30	GKRS	64.1	–	28.7	35	–	–	–
Pollock et al. [39]	2008	8	GKRS	73	40	20	87	100	–	–
Tinnel et al. [40]	2008	12	GKRS	37	30	25	50	–	0	50
Petit et al. [41]	2008	33	PSR	58.5	–	20	52	94	0	43.8
Kong et al. [37]	2007	7	GKRS	25.4	–	25.1[a]	100	–	0	–
Castinetti et al. [38]	2007	40	GKRS	54.7	–	29.5	42.5	–	5	15
Jagannathan et al. [28]	2007	90	GKRS	36/41.3[b]	49	23	54.4	95.5	5.6	22.2
Voges et al. [17]	2006	17	LINAC	58.7	33.7[a]	15.3[a]	52.9	88.2	–	–
Devin et al. [36]	2004	35	LINAC	42	33.7	14.7	49	91	0	40
Wong et al. [34]	2003	5	LINAC	38	16–20	14.8–19.2	80	–	0	20
Petrovich et al. [22]	2003	4	GKRS	34	30[a]	15[a]	50	–	–	–
Choi et al. [35]	2003	9	GKRS	42.5	54.1[a]	28.5[a]	55.6	85.7	0	0
Kobayashi et al. [32]	2002	20	GKRS	64.1	49.4[a]	28.7[a]	35	100	–	–
Pollock et al. [33]	2002	9	GKRS	36/42.4[b]	40[a]	20[a]	78	100	11.1	–
Hoybye et al. [31]	2001	18	GKRS	202	71.4	–	44	–	0	68.8
Izawa et al. [25]	2000	12	GKRS	26.4	–	24.2[a]	16.7	83	0	0
Sheehan et al. [30]	2000	43	GKRS	44	47	20	63	100	2.3	16.3
Shin et al. [26]	2000	6	GKRS	88.2	–	32.3	50	100	–	16.7

Mean or median values used

F/U follow-up, *GKRS* Gamma Knife radiosurgery, *LINAC* linear accelerator–based radiosurgery, *mo* months, *PSR* proton stereotactic radiosurgery

[a]Includes dose for other adenomas

[b]Imaging follow-up/endocrine follow-up

7.4 Nelson's Syndrome

Adrenalectomy is the ultimate treatment for patients with Cushing's disease refractory to conventional surgical, radiosurgical, and medical managements. Although definitive treatment for hypercortisolemia can be offered by adrenalectomy, up to 23 % of patients subsequently develop Nelson's syndrome, which can lead to rapid growth of the adenoma and parasellar invasion [47]. Relatively few studies in the literature have evaluated the role of radiosurgery in the treatment of Nelson's syndrome. In the largest series thus far, Mauermann et al. [48] observed a 90.9 % rate of tumor control and a 20 % rate of ACTH normalization in a population of 23 patients treated with GKRS. In a recent study of 22 patients treated with GKRS, Sheehan et al. [29] found the same hormone normalization rate of 20 %. Table 7.3 shows a summary of radiosurgical results for Nelson's syndrome from recent studies. These studies show an average tumor control rate of 95 % (range, 82–100 %) and a hormone normalization rate of 30 % (range, 0–100 %), using a mean margin dose of 22 Gy (range, 12–28.7 Gy) [17, 32, 41, 48–51]. Despite the low hormone normalization rates reported in the series, studies have demonstrated significant reduction in ACTH following radiosurgery [48, 50, 51].

Common adverse effects of radiosurgery for Nelson's syndrome include visual and hormonal deficits; recent series show the incidence of neurologic deficits to be 2.7 % (range, 0–9.1 %) and the incidence of hormonal deficits to be 32.6 % (range, 0–50 %). Current literature demonstrates that radiosurgery is effective in controlling tumor progression and reducing ACTH levels, but hormone normalization may be difficult to achieve with radiosurgery alone.

Table 7.3 Comparison of radiosurgical results for Nelson's syndrome

Study	Year	Patients	Radiosurgery	F/U, *mo*	Maximal dose, *Gy*	Margin dose, *Gy*	Hormone normalization, %	Tumor volume change, %			Tumor control, %	Neurologic deficit, %	New hormone deficit, %
								Decreased	Unchanged	Increased			
Sheehan et al. [29]	2011	22	GKRS	31	–	24[a]	20	–	–	–	–	–	28
Vik-Mo et al. [51]	2009	10	GKRS	84	53.4	26.2	10	90	10	0	100	0	40
Petit et al. [41]	2008	5	PSR	109	–	20	100	–	–	0	100	0	50
Mauermann et al. [48]	2007	23	GKRS	20/50[b]	50	25	20	54.5	36.4	9.1	90.9	4.5	50
Voges et al. [17]	2006	9	LINAC	63.1	57.4	20	22.2	44.4	44.4	11.2	88.8	–	–
Kobayashi et al. [32]	2002	6	GKRS	64.1	49.4[a]	28.7[a]	33.3	–	–	0	100	–	–
Pollock and Young [50]	2002	11	GKRS	37	40	20	36.3	54.5	27.3	18.2	82	9.1	27.3
Wolffenbuttel et al. [49]	1998	1	GKRS	33	40	12	0	100	0	0	100	0	0

Mean or median values used
F/U follow-up, *GKRS* Gamma Knife radiosurgery, *LINAC* linear accelerator–based radiosurgery, *mo* months, *PSR* proton stereotactic radiosurgery
[a]Includes dose for other adenomas
[b]Imaging follow-up/endocrine follow-up

7.5 Acromegaly

Although surgical resection remains the first-line treatment in most cases of acromegaly, endocrine cure by surgery alone is unlikely, particularly for patients with tumor involvement of the dura and cavernous sinus [52]. Because complete surgical resection may not always be feasible, radiosurgery provides a viable alternative or adjunct treatment for those who cannot tolerate first-line management or who have residual disease following surgery. Radiosurgery following surgical resections achieves almost total tumor control; in contrast, the average biochemical remission rate is only 48 % (range, 17–100 %) across recent series, using a mean margin dose of 23 Gy (range, 15–35 Gy) [13, 17, 22, 23, 25, 26, 29, 33, 35, 39, 40, 42, 43, 45, 53–70]. Precise criteria for biochemical remission following radiosurgery vary across case series. The most recent 2010 guidelines for remission have not been extensively validated following treatment with radiosurgery [71], and most studies define remission using a random serum growth hormone (GH) level less than 2 ng/mL, a GH level less than 1 ng/mL following an oral glucose tolerance test, or normal insulin-like growth factor-1 level adjusted for age and sex [72, 73]. In the largest study thus far, Sheehan et al. [29] reported a biochemical remission rate of 53 % in 130 patients treated with GKRS. More recently, in a smaller cohort of patients treated with GKRS, Franzin et al. [74] observed a more favorable remission rate of 60.7 %. Table 7.4 shows a summary of recent radiosurgical results for acromegaly.

Several studies have found decreased biochemical remission rates and delayed remission in patients treated with hormone-suppressing medications such as octreotide at the time of radiosurgery [29, 33, 62, 75]. The mechanism involved remains unclear; it is believed that suppression of the tumor cell cycle by medication leads to decreased cell susceptibility to the effects of ionizing radiation [73]. The reported rate of neurologic deficits following radiosurgery is 1.6 % (range, 0–11.1 %), and the rate of endocrine deficits is 16.7 % (range, 0–40 %). Current literature supports maximum safe surgical resection followed by radiosurgery for the management of patients presenting with acromegaly.

Table 7.4 Comparison of radiosurgical results for acromegaly

Study	Year	Patients	Radiosurgery	F/U, *mo*	Maximal dose, *Gy*	Margin dose, *Gy*	Biochemical remission, %	Neurologic deficit, %	New hormone deficit, %
Grant et al. [45]	2013	13	GKRS	40.2	–	35[a]	61	–	31
Erdur et al. [70]	2012	22	GKRS	60	47.2	23.8	54.5	0	28.6
Franzin et al. [74]	2012	112	GKRS	71	–	22.5	60.7	0	7.8
Liu et al. [69]	2012	40	GKRS	72	–	21	47.5	0	40
Sheehan et al. [29]	2011	130	GKRS	31	–	24[a]	53	–	34
Poon et al. [68]	2010	40	GKRS	73.8	–	20–35	69.2	0	11.4
Hayashi et al. [13]	2010	25	GKRS	36	–	25.2[a]	40	0	0
Iwai et al. [67]	2010	26	GKRS	84	40	20	38.5	0	8
Ronchi et al. [66]	2009	35	GKRS	114	40	20	42.9	0	50
Castinetti et al. [42]	2009	43	GKRS	99.7	–	25.7	41.9	5.3	21
Wan et al. [43]	2009	103	GKRS	67.3	–	21.4	36.9	–	1.9
Jagannathan et al. [65]	2008	95	GKRS	57	47	22	53	4.2	34
Losa et al. [64]	2008	83	GKRS	69	42	21.5	60.2	0	8.5
Pollock et al. [39]	2008	27	GKRS	46.9	45	20	67	–	–
Tinnel et al. [40]	2008	9	GKRS	35	–	25	44.4	11	22
Petit et al. [63]	2007	22	PSR	75.6	–	20	59.1	0	38
Pollock et al. [62]	2007	46	GKRS	63	43.5	20	50	2.2	33
Vik-Mo et al. [61]	2007	61	GKRS	66	53.4	26.5	17	3.3	13.1
Jezkova et al. [60]	2006	96	GKRS	53.7	63	32	50	0	27.1
Voges et al. [17]	2006	64	LINAC	37.2	33.7[a]	15.3[a]	37.5	–	–
Castinetti et al. [59]	2005	82	GKRS	49.5	–	25.7	17	1.2	17.1
Gutt et al. [58]	2005	44	GKRS	22.8	36	18	41	0	–
Kobayashi et al. [57]	2005	67	GKRS	63.3	35.3	18.9	4.8	11.1	14.6
Attanasio et al. [56]	2003	30	GKRS	46	40	20	23	0	6.7
Choi et al. [35]	2003	12	GKRS	42.5	54.1[a]	28.5[a]	50	0	0
Muramatsu et al. [23]	2003	4	LINAC	30	–	15[a]	50	–	–
Petrovich et al. [22]	2003	5	GKRS	34	30[a]	15[a]	100	–	–
Pollock et al. [33]	2002	26	GKRS	36/42.4[b]	40[a]	20[a]	42	0	–
Fukuoka et al. [55]	2001	9	GKRS	42	41	20	50	0	0
Ikeda et al. [54]	2001	17	GKRS	59.1	–	25	82	0	0
Izawa et al. [25]	2000	29	GKRS	26.4	–	24.2[a]	41.4	0	0
Shin et al. [26]	2000	6	GKRS	42.7	–	34.4	66.7	–	0
Zhang et al. [53]	2000	68	GKRS	>12	–	31.3	40	2.9	4.4

Mean or median values used

F/U follow-up, *GKRS* Gamma Knife radiosurgery, *LINAC* linear accelerator–based radiosurgery, *mo* months

[a]Includes dose for other adenomas

[b]Imaging follow-up/endocrine follow-up

7.6 Prolactinomas

Prolactinomas are the most common hormone-secreting pituitary adenomas. Unlike acromegaly or Cushing's disease, the mainstay therapy for patients with prolactinomas remains medical management using dopamine agonists such as bromocriptine or cabergoline. Although most patients can be managed using medical therapy alone, a small subset of patients is refractory or intolerant to the medications. These refractory prolactinomas may harbor biological atypia not seen in other prolactinomas. In this challenging cohort, surgical resection and radiosurgery are viable treatment alternatives. Despite reports in the literature of excellent tumor control rates that approach 100 % following radiosurgery, rates of biochemical remission without the antisecretory medications remain poor, at a mean of 37 % (range, 15.4–100 %) [17, 22, 25, 29, 35, 39, 40, 42–45, 50, 75–81]. Peripheral radiation doses used in these series ranged from 15 to 35 Gy, and most series define biochemical remission using normal serum prolactin levels. Wan et al. [43] observed a remission rate of only 23.3 % in the largest study, yet comprising 176 patients who underwent GKRS for prolactinomas. Although radiosurgery leads to serum prolactin reduction in most cases, hormone normalization rates following radiosurgery for prolactinomas appear to be lower than those for Cushing's disease and acromegaly. However, as with acromegaly, reports have suggested improved remission rates in patients who did not have concurrent treatment with dopamine agonists at the time of radiosurgery [29, 75, 80, 81]. Table 7.5 summarizes recent studies of radiosurgical results for prolactinomas. In these series, the mean rate of neurologic deficit following radiosurgery has been reported to be 3.1 % (range, 0–11 %), and the mean rate of endocrine deficit has been 13.7 % (range, 0–38 %). Despite the relatively low remission rates, radiosurgery remains a safe adjunctive treatment for prolactinomas refractory to surgical resection and medical management.

Table 7.5 Comparison of radiosurgical results for prolactinomas

Study	Year	Patients	Radiosurgery	F/U, *mo*	Maximal dose, *Gy*	Margin dose, *Gy*	Biochemical remission, %	Neurologic deficit, %	New hormone deficit, %
Grant et al. [45]	2013	2	GKRS	40.2	–	35[a]	100	–	0
Liu et al. [76]	2013	22	GKRS	37.5/36[b]	–	15	27.3	0	4.5
Sheehan et al. [29]	2011	32	GKRS	31	–	24[a]	26	–	38
Tanaka et al. [77]	2010	22	GKRS	60	50	25	18	4.5	38
Kobayashi et al. [44]	2009	23	GKRS	37.4	–	18.4	43.5	0	0
Castinetti et al. [42]	2009	15	GKRS	86.2	–	25.5	46.6	–	–
Jezkova et al. [78]	2009	35	GKRS	75.5	70	34	37.1	0	14.3
Wan et al. [43]	2009	176	GKRS	67.3	–	22.4	23.3	–	1.7
Pollock et al. [39]	2008	11	GKRS	48	50	25	18	–	–
Tinnel et al. [40]	2008	2	GKRS	19.5	–	30	50	11	22
Ma et al. [79]	2007	51	GKRS	37	50.41	26.1	40	–	17.6
Pouratian et al. [80]	2006	23	GKRS	52/58[b]	42.2	18.6	26	7	28
Voges et al. [17]	2006	13	LINAC	56	33.7[a]	15.3[a]	15.4	–	–
Choi et al. [35]	2003	21	GKRS	42.5	54.1[a]	28.5[a]	23.8	0	0
Petrovich et al. [22]	2003	12	GKRS	34	30[a]	15[a]	83.3	–	–
Pollock et al. [33]	2002	7	GKRS	36/42.4[b]	40[a]	20[a]	29	0	–
Izawa et al. [25]	2000	15	GKRS	26.4	–	24.2[a]	20	6.7	0
Landolt and Lomax [75]	2000	20	GKRS	28.6	–	25.2	25	5	–
Pan et al. [81]	2000	128	GKRS	33.2	44.6	31.2	52	0	–

Mean or median values used
F/U follow-up, *GKRS* Gamma Knife radiosurgery, *LINAC* linear accelerator–based radiosurgery, *mo* months
[a]Includes dose for other adenomas
[b]Imaging follow-up/endocrine follow-up

7.7 Meningiomas

Surgical resection of meningiomas in the parasellar location is not without risks of morbidity and mortality, despite improvements in microsurgical techniques and the often-benign histologic appearance of these tumors [82–91]. Tumor involvement of vascular and neuronal structures such as the internal carotid arteries and cranial nerves in the cavernous sinus renders complete resection difficult, and any resection that is short of complete tumor removal is complicated by high recurrence rates [92]. The goal of treatment has shifted from absolute tumor resection to aggressive surgical resection with functional preservation. Hence, radiosurgery has become an important adjuvant treatment; in many cases, it is the primary treatment of these tumors. In a retrospective study that compared the results of primary radiosurgery to surgical resection for intracranial meningiomas, Pollock et al. [93] found that radiosurgery is associated with significantly lower rates of tumor progression or recurrence (2 % *vs.* 12 %). Furthermore, Simpson grade I resections did not offer significant benefit for the rate of progression-free survival (PFS), and resections of grades II and III–IV had significantly lower PFS rates than radiosurgery alone at 3 and 7 years. In a recent study by Williams et al. [94], radiosurgery for 138 patients with parasellar meningiomas produced PFS rates of 95 %, 86 %, and 69 % at 5, 7, and 10 years, respectively. In an earlier study, Hasegawa et al. [95] found comparable PFS rates of 87 % at 5 years and 73 % at 10 years. Overall local tumor control rates following radiosurgery for parasellar meningiomas ranged from 71 to 100 %, and similar rates of 71 to 98 % have been reported at 10-year follow-up [93–117]. Radiation-induced cranial nerve injury is the most common complication following radiosurgery for parasellar meningiomas; its incidence has been reported to range from 0 to 12 %, compared with 18 to 41 % after surgical resection [82–91, 93, 95–118]. Table 7.6 shows a summary of radiosurgical results for parasellar meningiomas from recent large studies. Intracavernous portions of parasellar meningiomas are best treated with radiosurgery, given its high tumor control rates and low complication rates. Microsurgical resection can be attempted on extracavernous portions of the tumors (Fig. 7.1).

Table 7.6 Comparison of radiosurgical results for parasellar meningiomas

Study	Year	Patients	Radiosurgery	F/U, *mo*	Tumor control rates, %	CN deficits, %	Complications, %
Williams et al. [94]	2011	138	GKRS	84	95 and 71 (5 and 10 y)	10	10
Takanashi et al. [117]	2009	38	GKRS	52	95.5	0	0
Kimball et al. [102]	2009	49	LINAC	50	100 and 98 (5 and 10 y)	2	2
Hasegawa et al. [95]	2007	115	GKRS	62	94 and 92 (5 and 10 y)	–	12
Pollock et al. [113]	2005	49	GKRS	58	100	12	14
Metellus et al. [109]	2005	36	GKRS	63.6	94.4	0	2.8
Selch et al. [118]	2004	45	LINAC	36	97.4 (3 y)	0	2.2
Kuo et al. [103]	2004	57	GKRS	15.2	100	1.8	1.8
Iwai et al. [101]	2003	43	GKRS	49	92 (5 y)	0	0
Spiegelmann et al. [116]	2002	42	LINAC	38	97.5 and 97.5 (3 and 7 y)	7.1	14
Lee et al. [105]	2002	159	GKRS	35	93 and 93 (5 and 10 y)	5	6.9
Nicolato et al. [110]	2002	122	GKRS	48.9	96.5 (5 y)	1	1
Chen et al. [97]	2001	35	GKRS	30	100	0	0
Shin et al. [115]	2001	40	GKRS	42	86.4 and 82.3 (3 and 10 y)	2.5	2.5
Roche et al. [114]	2000	80	GKRS	30.5	93 (5 y)	3	3.8
Liscak et al. [106]	1999	53	GKRS	19	100	–	–
Chang et al.	1997	55	LINAC	48	98 (2 y)	2	4

Mean or median values used

CN cranial nerve, *F/U* follow-up, *GKRS* Gamma Knife radiosurgery, *LINAC* linear accelerator–based radiosurgery, *mo* months, *y* years

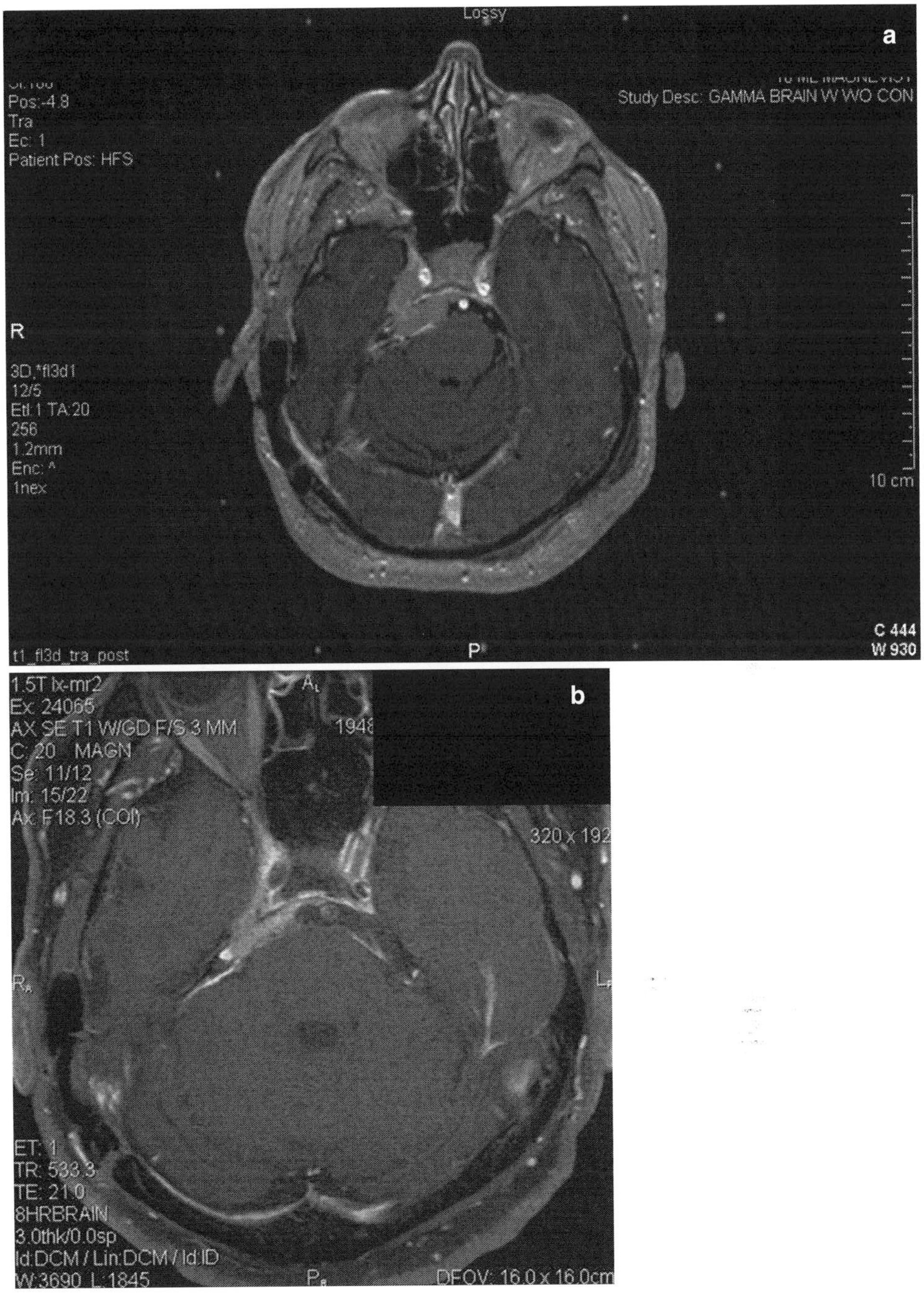

Fig. 7.1 The patient had a right parasellar meningioma treated with Gamma Knife radiosurgery. (**a**) His stereotactic radiosurgery MRI depicts the tumor, which was treated with 15 Gy to the 50 % isodose line. (**b**) On follow-up 2 years later, the tumor demonstrates marked regression in size

7.8 Lymphocytic Hypophysitis

Optimal treatment for lymphocytic hypophysitis remains controversial; the treatments that have been used with variable results include high-dose steroid therapy, methotrexate, transsphenoidal surgery, and radiotherapy [119–127]. The current standard therapies are corticosteroids and surgical resection, but long-term use of corticosteroids is associated with adverse effects, and suprasellar extension or adherence to surrounding dura often leads to incomplete surgical resection and recurrence. Limited data have been published with regard to the use of radiation in the treatment of lymphocytic hypophysitis. Selch et al. [127] reported two cases successfully treated using stereotactic radiotherapy with 24 Gy given in 12 fractions. Ray et al. [128] reported the only case in literature treated with radiosurgery [128]. The patient did not respond to surgical and medical interventions and was therefore treated using single-session GKRS with a prescription dose of 15 Gy to the 50 % isodose line in a treatment volume of 3.5 cm^3. Reduction in lesion size was seen on imaging more than 12 months following radiosurgery, and the patient did not experience recurrence of symptoms. No complications were associated with the radiosurgical treatment. Future studies may show radiosurgery to be a viable treatment option for patients with lymphocytic hypophysitis resistant to surgical and medical interventions.

7.9 Craniopharyngiomas

Recent studies have suggested that radiosurgery is a valuable treatment option for patients with residual or progressive craniopharyngioma [129–142]. Target localization with the use of stereotaxis and dose planning has allowed for the precise delivery of the radiation dose in a single fraction with steep dose falloff at tumor margins. In the largest series, involving 98 patients treated with GKRS, Kobayashi et al. [132] reported a local tumor control rate of 79.6 % with mean follow-up of 65.5 months for mean tumor size of 3.5 cm^3 at a mean margin dose of 11.5 Gy. PFS rates of 60.8 % and 53.8 % with respective actuarial 5-year and 10-year survival rates of 94.1 % and 91 % were observed in the study, and the rate of complications was low, at 6.1 %. In a more recent study, Niranjan et al. found a similar local tumor control rate of 76 % with a low complication rate of 2.2 % [143].

Table 7.7 shows a summary of radiosurgical results for craniopharyngiomas from recent studies. Local tumor control rates following radiosurgery for craniopharyngiomas ranged from 36 to 100 %, with a mean of 76 %. Overall complication rates ranged from 0 to 19 %, with a mean of 3.7 %. Visual field deficits and worsening endocrine function are the most commonly described complications, but their rates are considerably less than for surgical resection, which has reported rates of visual deficits up to 41 % and reported rates of endocrine dysfunction up to 100 % [144, 145]. Higher tumor control rates have been observed for single-type tumors, either solid or cystic, compared with mixed-type tumors. Solid tumors have an average tumor control rate of 90 % (range, 57–100 %), and the control rate for cystic tumors is 89 % (range, 74–100 %), whereas the average rate for mixed-type tumors is 62 % (range, 21–86 %) [129–133, 135, 136, 138–140, 143]. Despite current controversy regarding the optimal treatment modality for craniopharyngiomas, maximal safe surgical resection followed by radiosurgery is recommended [130, 132, 143, 146]. Current literature suggests that radiosurgery is both an effective and safe adjuvant treatment following subtotal resection.

Table 7.7 Comparison of radiosurgical results for craniopharyngiomas

Study	Year	Patients/ tumors	Age, *y*	Prior tumor resection, %	Pre-radiosurgery treatment, %			Radiosurgery	F/U, *mo*	Margin dose, Gy	Tumor size, *cm3*	Local tumor control rate, %				Complications, %
					Intracavitary isotope	Bleomycin	RT					Solid	Cyst	Mix	Total	
Xu et al. [130]	2011	37	33.2	76	27	3	5	GKRS	50	14.5	3.24	–	–	67.5[b]	67.5[b]	–
Niranjan et al. [143]	2010	46	23.5	93	24	0	4	GKRS	62.2	13	1	81.8	80	75[a]	76[a]	2.2
Yomo et al. [140]	2009	18	38.4	85	0	0	20	GKRS	26.8	11.6	1.8	100	100	66.7	94	0
Kobayashi et al. [132]	2005	98	38 < 15, 62 > 15	100	0	3	13	GKRS	65.5	11.5	3.5	93	79	61	79.6	6.1
Albright et al. [138]	2005	5	13	0	0	0	0	GKRS	29	–	6.5	–	–	80[b]	80[b]	0
Barua et al. [134]	2003	7	–	100	–	–	–	GKRS	50.4	14.2	–	–	–	–	100	–
Amendola et al. [137]	2003	14	11.5	86	8	0	7.1	GKRS	39.2	14	3.7	–	–	–	86	0
Ulfarsson et al. [129]	2002	21/22	11 < 15, 10 > 15	56	19	0	0	GKRS	90	5	7.8	57	100	21	36	19
Chiou et al. [135]	2001	10/12	14.5	50	30	0	10	GKRS	63	16.4	1.74	100	–	37.5	58	10
Chung et al. [131]	2000	31	32	74	6.5	0	6.5	GKRS	36	12.2	8.94	100	100	75	87.2	3.2
Yu et al. [139]	2000	46	39	61	72	0	–	GKRS	16	8–18	13.5	90	–	86	89	0
Mokry et al. [133]	1999	23	31.4	39	0	43	–	GKRS	24	7.8–9.7	7	–	74	–	74	0
Prasad et al. [136]	1995	9	38.1	67	44	0	–	GKRS	–	12.9	10	100	–	50	62.5	0

Mean or median values used
F/U follow-up, *GKRS* Gamma Knife radiosurgery, *mo* months, *RT* radiotherapy, *y* years
[a]Includes treatment for solid-only portions
[b]All treated for solid portions only

Conclusions

Tumor involvement of critical structures in the sellar and parasellar regions often prohibits complete surgical resection, leading to residual disease and recurrence. Radiosurgery serves as an effective and low-risk adjunctive treatment following maximum safe surgical resection and in some cases may be used as primary treatment. Current literature clearly demonstrates that radiosurgery offers exceptional tumor control rates for NFAs. Despite moderate to low biochemical remission rates for hormone-secreting adenomas, radiosurgery provides excellent tumor control rates and significant hormone reductions. High tumor control rates are also observed for craniopharyngiomas and parasellar meningiomas treated with radiosurgery. Complications following radiosurgery are relatively uncommon, and neurologic preservation or even improvement is typically achieved following radiosurgery.

References

1. Schulder M, Loeffler JS, Howes AE, Alexander 3rd E, Black PM. Historical vignette: the radium bomb: Harvey Cushing and the interstitial irradiation of gliomas. J Neurosurg. 1996;84:530–2.
2. Seymour ZA, Cohen-Gadol AA. Cushing's lost cases of "radium bomb" brachytherapy for gliomas. J Neurosurg. 2010;113:141–8.
3. Chen CC, Chapman P, Petit J, Loeffler J. Proton radiosurgery in neurosurgery. Neurosurg Focus. 2007;23(6):E5.
4. Friedman WA, Foote KD. Linear accelerator radiosurgery in the management of brain tumours. Ann Med. 2000;32:64–80.
5. Hoybye C, Rahn T. Adjuvant gamma knife radiosurgery in nonfunctioning pituitary adenomas; low risk of long-term complications in selected patients. Pituitary. 2009;12:211–6.
6. Laws ER, Sheehan JP, Sheehan JM, Jagnathan J, Jane Jr JA, Oskoulan R. Stereotactic radiosurgery for pituitary adenomas: a review of the literature. J Neurooncol. 2004;69:257–72.
7. Sheehan JP, Kondziolka D, Flickinger J, Lunsford LD. Radiosurgery for residual or recurrent nonfunctioning pituitary adenoma. J Neurosurg. 2002;97:408–14.
8. Wilson PJ, De-Loyde KJ, Williams JR, Smee RI. A single centre's experience of stereotactic radiosurgery and radiotherapy for nonfunctioning pituitary adenomas with the Linear Accelerator (Linac). J Clin Neurosci. 2012;19:370–4.
9. Starke RM, et al. Gamma Knife surgery for patients with nonfunctioning pituitary macroadenomas: predictors of tumor control, neurological deficits, and hypopituitarism. J Neurosurg. 2012;117(1):129–35.
10. El-Shehaby AM, Reda WA, Tawadros SR, Abdel Karim KM. Low-dose Gamma Knife surgery for nonfunctioning pituitary adenomas. J Neurosurg. 2012;117(Suppl):84–8.
11. Gopalan R, Schlesinger D, Vance ML, Laws E, Sheehan J. Long-term outcomes after Gamma Knife radiosurgery for patients with a nonfunctioning pituitary adenoma. Neurosurgery. 2011;69:284–93.
12. Park KJ, Kano H, Parry PV, Niranian A, Flickinger JC, Lunsford LD, et al. Long-term outcomes after gamma knife stereotactic radiosurgery for nonfunctional pituitary adenomas. Neurosurgery. 2011;69:1188–99.
13. Hayashi M, Chernov M, Tamura N, Nagai M, Yomo S, Ochiai T, et al. Gamma Knife robotic microradiosurgery of pituitary adenomas invading the cavernous sinus: treatment concept and results in 89 cases. J Neurooncol. 2010;98:185–94.
14. Pollock BE, Cochran J, Natt N, Brown PD, Erickson D, Link MJ, et al. Gamma knife radiosurgery for patients with nonfunctioning pituitary adenomas: results from a 15-year experience. Int J Radiat Oncol Biol Phys. 2008;70:1325–9.
15. Liscak R, Vladyka V, Marek J, Simonova G, Vymazal J. Gamma knife radiosurgery for endocrine-inactive pituitary adenomas. Acta Neurochir (Wien). 2007;149:999–1006; discussion 1006.
16. Mingione V, Yen CP, Vance ML, Steiner M, Sheehan J, Laws ER, et al. Gamma surgery in the treatment of nonsecretory pituitary macroadenoma. J Neurosurg. 2006;104:876–83.
17. Voges J, Kocher M, Runge M, Poggenborg J, Lehrke R, Lenartz D, et al. Linear accelerator radiosurgery for pituitary macroadenomas: a 7-year follow-up study. Cancer. 2006;107:1355–64.
18. Picozzi P, Losa M, Mortini P, Valle MA, Franzin A, Attuati L, et al. Radiosurgery and the prevention of regrowth of incompletely removed nonfunctioning pituitary adenomas. J Neurosurg. 2005;102(Suppl):71–4.
19. Iwai Y, Yamanaka K, Yoshioka K, Yoshimura M, Honda Y, Matsusaka Y, et al. The usefulness of adjuvant therapy using gamma knife radiosurgery for the recurrent or residual nonfunctioning pituitary adenomas. No Shinkei Geka. 2005;33:777–83.
20. Losa M, Valle M, Mortini P, Franzin A, da Passano CF, Cenzato M, et al. Gamma knife surgery for treatment of residual nonfunctioning pituitary adenomas after surgical debulking. J Neurosurg. 2004;100:438–44.
21. Muacevic A, Uhl E, Wowra B. Gamma knife radiosurgery for nonfunctioning pituitary adenomas. Acta Neurochir Suppl. 2004;91:51–4.
22. Petrovich Z, Jozsef G, Yu C, Apuzzo ML. Radiotherapy and stereotactic radiosurgery for pituitary tumors. Neurosurg Clin N Am. 2003;14:147–66.
23. Muramatsu J, Yoshida M, Shioura H, Kawamura Y, Ito H, Takeuchi H, et al. Clinical results of LINAC-based stereotactic radiosurgery for pituitary adenoma. Nippon Igaku Hoshasen Gakkai Zasshi. 2003;63:225–30.
24. Wowra B, Stummer W. Efficacy of gamma knife radiosurgery for nonfunctioning pituitary adenomas: a quantitative follow up with magnetic resonance imaging-based volumetric analysis. J Neurosurg. 2002;97:429–32.
25. Izawa M, Hayashi M, Nakaya K, Satoh H, Ochiai T, Hori T, et al. Gamma knife radiosurgery for pituitary adenomas. J Neurosurg. 2000;93 Suppl 3:19–22.
26. Shin M, Kurita H, Sasaki T, Tago M, Morita A, Ueki K, et al. Stereotactic radiosurgery for pituitary adenoma invading the cavernous sinus. J Neurosurg. 2000;93 Suppl 3:2–5.
27. Biller BM, Grossman AB, Stewart PM, Melmed S, Bertagna X, Bertherat J, et al. Treatment of adrenocorticotropin-dependent Cushing's syndrome: a consensus statement. J Clin Endocrinol Metab. 2008;93:2454–62.
28. Jagannathan J, Sheehan JP, Pouratian N, Laws ER, Steiner L, Vance ML. Gamma Knife surgery for Cushing's disease. J Neurosurg. 2007;106:980–7.
29. Sheehan JP, Pouratian N, Steiner L, Laws ER, Vance ML. Gamma Knife surgery for pituitary adenomas: factors related to radiological and endocrine outcomes. J Neurosurg. 2011;114:303–9.
30. Sheehan JM, Vance ML, Sheehan JP, Ellegala DB, Laws Jr ER. Radiosurgery for Cushing's disease after failed transsphenoidal surgery. J Neurosurg. 2000;93:738–42.
31. Hoybye C, Grenback E, Rahn T, Degerblad M, Thoren M, Hulting AL. Adrenocorticotropic hormone-producing pituitary tumors: 12- to 22-year follow-up after treatment with stereotactic radiosurgery. Neurosurgery. 2001;49:284–91; discussion 291–2.

32. Kobayashi T, Kida Y, Mori Y. Gamma knife radiosurgery in the treatment of Cushing disease: long-term results. J Neurosurg. 2002;97(5 Suppl):422–8.
33. Pollock BE, Nippoldt TB, Stafford SL, Foote RL, Abboud CF. Results of stereotactic radiosurgery in patients with hormone-producing pituitary adenomas: factors associated with endocrine normalization. J Neurosurg. 2002;97:525–30.
34. Wong GK, Leung CH, Chiu KW, Ma R, Cockram CS, Lam MJ, et al. LINAC radiosurgery in recurrent Cushing's disease after transsphenoidal surgery: a series of 5 cases. Minim Invasive Neurosurg. 2003;46:327–30.
35. Choi JY, Chang JH, Chang JW, Ha Y, Park YG, Chung SS. Radiological and hormonal responses of functioning pituitary adenomas after gamma knife radiosurgery. Yonsei Med J. 2003;44:602–7.
36. Devin JK, Allen GS, Cmelak AJ, Duggan DM, Blevins LS. The efficacy of linear accelerator radiosurgery in the management of patients with Cushing's disease. Stereotact Funct Neurosurg. 2004;82:254–62.
37. Kong DS, Lee JI, Limdo H, Kim KW, Shin HJ, Nam DH, et al. The efficacy of fractionated radiotherapy and stereotactic radiosurgery for pituitary adenomas: long-term results of 125 consecutive patients treated in a single institution. Cancer. 2007;110:854–60.
38. Castinetti F, Nagai M, Dufour H, Kuhn JM, Morange I, Jaquet P, et al. Gamma knife radiosurgery is a successful adjunctive treatment in Cushing's disease. Eur J Endocrinol. 2007;156:91–8.
39. Pollock BE, Brown PD, Nippoldt TB, Young Jr WF. Pituitary tumor type affects the chance of biochemical remission after radiosurgery of hormone-secreting pituitary adenomas. Neurosurgery. 2008;62:1271–6; discussion 1276–8.
40. Tinnel BA, Henderson MA, Witt TC, Fakiris AJ, Worth RM, Des Rosiers PM, et al. Endocrine response after gamma knife-based stereotactic radiosurgery for secretory pituitary adenoma. Stereotact Funct Neurosurg. 2008;86(5):292–6.
41. Petit JH, Biller BM, Yock TI, Swearingen B, Coen JJ, Chapman P, et al. Proton stereotactic radiotherapy for persistent adrenocorticotropin-producing adenomas. J Clin Endocrinol Metab. 2008;93:393–9.
42. Castinetti F, Nagai M, Morange I, Dufour H, Caron P, Chanson P, et al. Long-term results of stereotactic radiosurgery in secretory pituitary adenomas. J Clin Endocrinol Metab. 2009;94:3400–7.
43. Wan H, Chihiro O, Yuan S. MASEP gamma knife radiosurgery for secretory pituitary adenomas: experience in 347 consecutive cases. J Exp Clin Cancer Res. 2009;28:36.
44. Kobayashi T. Long-term results of stereotactic gamma knife radiosurgery for pituitary adenomas. Specific strategies for different types of adenoma. Prog Neurol Surg. 2009;22:77–95.
45. Grant RA, Whicker M, Lleva R, Knisely JP, Inzucchi SE, Chiang VL. Efficacy and safety of higher dose stereotactic radiosurgery for functional pituitary adenomas: a preliminary report. World Neurosurg. 2013. doi:10.1016/j.wneu.2013.01.127.
46. Wein L, Dally M, Bach LA. Stereotactic radiosurgery for treatment of Cushing disease: an Australian experience. Intern Med J. 2012;42:1153–6.
47. Nagesser SK, van Seters AP, Klevit J, Hermans J, Krans HM, van de Velde CJ. Long-term results of total adrenalectomy for Cushing's disease. World J Surg. 2000;24:108–13.
48. Mauermann WJ, Sheehan JP, Chernavvsky DR, Laws ER, Steiner L, Vance ML. Gamma Knife surgery for adrenocorticotropic hormone-producing pituitary adenomas after bilateral adrenalectomy. J Neurosurg. 2007;106:988–93.
49. Wolffenbuttel BH, Kitz K, Beuls EM. Beneficial gamma-knife radiosurgery in a patient with Nelson's syndrome. Clin Neurol Neurosurg. 1998;100:60–3.
50. Pollock BE, Young Jr WF. Stereotactic radiosurgery for patients with ACTH-producing pituitary adenomas after prior adrenalectomy. Int J Radiat Oncol Biol Phys. 2002;54:839–41.
51. Vik-Mo EO, Øksnes M, Pedersen PH, Wentzel-Larsen T, Redahl E, Thorsen F, et al. Gamma knife stereotactic radiosurgery of Nelson syndrome. Eur J Endocrinol. 2009;160:143–8.
52. Jane Jr JA, Starke RM, Elzoghby MA, Reames DL, Payne SC, Thorner MO, et al. Endoscopic transsphenoidal surgery for acromegaly: remission using modern criteria, complications, and predictors of outcome. J Clin Endocrinol Metab. 2011;96: 2732–40.
53. Zhang N, Pan L, Wang EM, Dai Z, Wang BJ, Cai PW. Radiosurgery for growth hormone-producing pituitary adenomas. J Neurosurg. 2000;93 Suppl 3:6–9.
54. Ikeda H, Jokura H, Yoshimoto T. Transsphenoidal surgery and adjuvant gamma knife treatment for growth hormone-secreting pituitary adenoma. J Neurosurg. 2001;95:285–91.
55. Fukuoka S, Ito T, Takanashi M, Hojo A, Nakamura H. Gamma knife radiosurgery for growth hormone-secreting pituitary adenomas invading the cavernous sinus. Stereotact Funct Neurosurg. 2001;76:213–7.
56. Attanasio R, Epaminonda P, Motti E, Giugni E, Ventrella L, Cozzi R, et al. Gamma-knife radiosurgery in acromegaly: a 4-year follow-up study. J Clin Endocrinol Metab. 2003;88:3105–12.
57. Kobayashi T, Mori Y, Uchiyama Y, Kida Y, Fujitani S. Long-term results of gamma knife surgery for growth hormone-producing pituitary adenoma: is the disease difficult to cure? J Neurosurg. 2005;102(Suppl):119–23.
58. Gutt B, Wowra B, Alexandrov R, Uhl E, Schaaf L, Stalla GK, et al. Gamma-knife surgery is effective in normalising plasma insulin-like growth factor I in patients with acromegaly. Exp Clin Endocrinol Diabetes. 2005;113:219–24.
59. Castinetti F, Taieb D, Kuhn JM, Chanson P, Tamura M, Jaquet P, et al. Outcome of gamma knife radiosurgery in 82 patients with acromegaly: correlation with initial hypersecretion. J Clin Endocrinol Metab. 2005;90:4483–8.
60. Jezkova J, Marek J, Hana V, Krsek M, Weiss V, Vladyka V, et al. Gamma knife radiosurgery for acromegaly – long-term experience. Clin Endocrinol. 2006;64:588–95.
61. Vik-Mo EO, Oksnes M, Pedersen PH, Wentzel-Larsen T, Rødahl E, Thorsen F, et al. Gamma knife stereotactic radiosurgery for acromegaly. Eur J Endocrinol. 2007;157:255–63.
62. Pollock BE, Jacob JT, Brown PD, Nippoldt TB. Radiosurgery of growth hormone-producing pituitary adenomas: factors associated with biochemical remission. J Neurosurg. 2007;106:833–8.
63. Petit JH, Biller BM, Coen JJ, Swearingen B, Ancukiewicz M, Bussiere M, et al. Proton stereotactic radiosurgery in management of persistent acromegaly. Endocr Pract. 2007;13:726–34.
64. Losa M, Gioia L, Picozzi P, Franzin A, Valle M, Giovanelli M, et al. The role of stereotactic radiotherapy in patients with growth hormone-secreting pituitary adenoma. J Clin Endocrinol Metab. 2008;93:2546–52.
65. Jagannathan J, Sheehan JP, Pouratian N, Laws Jr ER, Steiner L, Vance ML. Gamma knife radiosurgery for acromegaly: outcomes after failed transsphenoidal surgery. Neurosurgery. 2008;62:1262–9; discussion 1269–70.
66. Ronchi CL, Attanasio R, Verrua E, Cozzi R, Ferrante E, Loli P, et al. Efficacy and tolerability of gamma knife radiosurgery in acromegaly: a 10-year follow-up study. Clin Endocrinol (Oxf). 2009;71:846–52.
67. Iwai Y, Yamanaka K, Yoshimura M, Kawasaki I, Yamagami K, Yoshioka K. Gamma knife radiosurgery for growth hormone-producing adenomas. J Clin Neurosci. 2010;17:299–304.
68. Poon TL, Leung SC, Poon CY, Yu CP. Predictors of outcome following Gamma Knife surgery for acromegaly. J Neurosurg. 2010;113(Suppl):149–52.
69. Liu X, Kano H, Kondziolka D, Park KJ, Iyer A, Niranjan A, et al. Gamma knife radiosurgery for clinically persistent acromegaly. J Neurooncol. 2012;109:71–9.

70. Erdur FM, Kilic T, Peker S, Celik O, Kadioglu P. Gamma knife radiosurgery in patients with acromegaly. J Clin Neurosci. 2011;18:1616–20.
71. Giustina A, Chanson P, Bronstein MD, Klibanski A, Lamberts S, Casanueva FF, et al. A consensus on criteria for cure of acromegaly. J Clin Endocrinol Metab. 2010;95:3141–8.
72. Stapleton CJ, Liu CY, Weiss MH. The role of stereotactic radiosurgery in the multimodal management of growth hormone-secreting pituitary adenomas. Neurosurg Focus. 2010;29(4):E11.
73. Rolston JD, Blevins Jr LS. Gamma knife radiosurgery for acromegaly. Int J Endocrinol Print. 2012;2012:821579.
74. Franzin A, Spatola G, Losa M, Picozzi P, Mortini P. Results of gamma knife radiosurgery in acromegaly. Int J Endocrinol Print. 2012;2012:342034.
75. Landolt AM, Lomax N. Gamma knife radiosurgery for prolactinomas. J Neurosurg. 2000;93 Suppl 3:14–8.
76. Liu X, Kano H, Kondziolka D, Park KJ, Iyer A, Shin S, et al. Gamma knife stereotactic radiosurgery for drug resistant or intolerant invasive prolactinomas. Pituitary. 2013;16:68–75.
77. Tanaka S, Link MJ, Brown PD, Stafford SL, Young Jr WF, Pollock BE. Gamma knife radiosurgery for patients with prolactin-secreting pituitary adenomas. World Neurosurg. 2010;74:147–52.
78. Jezkova J, Hana V, Krsek M, Weiss V, Vladyka V, Liscak R, et al. Use of the Leksell gamma knife in the treatment of prolactinoma patients. Clin Endocrinol (Oxf). 2009;70:732–41.
79. Ma ZM, Qui B, Hou YH, Liu YS. Gamma knife treatment for pituitary prolactinomas. Zhong Nan Da Xue Xue Bao Yi Xue Ban. 2006;31:714–6.
80. Pouratian N, Sheehan J, Jagannathan J, Laws Jr ER, Steiner L, Vance ML. Gamma knife radiosurgery for medically and surgically refractory prolactinomas. Neurosurgery. 2006;59:255–66.
81. Pan L, Zhang N, Wang EM, Wang BJ, Dai JZ, Cai PW. Gamma knife radiosurgery as a primary treatment for prolactinomas. J Neurosurg. 2000;93 Suppl 3:10–3.
82. Cusimano MD, Sekhar LN, Sen CN, Pomonis S, Wright DC, Biglan AW, et al. The results of surgery for benign tumors of the cavernous sinus. Neurosurgery. 1995;37:1–9; discussion 9–10.
83. De Jesus O, Sekhar LN, Parikh HK, Wright DC, Wagner DP. Long-term follow-up of patients with meningiomas involving the cavernous sinus: recurrence, progression, and quality of life. Neurosurgery. 1996;39:915–9; discussion 919–20.
84. DeMonte F, Smith HK, al-Mefty O. Outcome of aggressive removal of cavernous sinus meningiomas. J Neurosurg. 1994;81:245–51.
85. Kim DK, Grieve J, Archer DJ, Uttley D. Meningiomas in the region of the cavernous sinus: a review of 21 patients. Br J Neurosurg. 1996;10:439–44.
86. Klink DF, Sampath P, Miller NR, Brem H, Long DM. Long-term visual outcome after nonradical microsurgery in patients with parasellar and cavernous sinus meningiomas. Neurosurgery. 2000;47: 24–31; discussion 31–2.
87. Knosp E, Perneczky A, Koos WT, Fries G, Matula C. Meningiomas of the space of the cavernous sinus. Neurosurgery. 1996;38:434–42; discussion 442–4.
88. Landeiro JA, Ribeiro CH, Lapenta MA, Flores MS, Lopes CA, Marins J. Meningiomas of the cavernous sinus: the surgical resectability and complications. Arq Neuropsiquiatr. 2001;59:746–53.
89. O'Sullivan MG, van Loveren HR, Tew Jr JM. The surgical resectability of meningiomas of the cavernous sinus. Neurosurgery. 1997;40:238–44; discussion 245–7.
90. Sekhar LN, Patel S, Cusimano M, Wright DC, Sen CN, Bank WO. Surgical treatment of meningiomas involving the cavernous sinus: evolving ideas based on a ten year experience. Acta Neurochir Suppl. 1996;65:58–62.
91. Sindou M, Wydh E, Jouanneau E, Nebbal M, Liutaud T. Long-term follow-up of meningiomas of the cavernous sinus after surgical treatment alone. J Neurosurg. 2007;107:937–44.
92. Simpson D. The recurrence of intracranial meningiomas after surgical treatment. J Neurol Neurosurg Psychiatry. 1957;20: 22–39.
93. Pollock BE, Stafford SL, Utter A, Giannini C, Schreiner SA. Stereotactic radiosurgery provides equivalent tumor control to Simpson Grade 1 resection for patients with small- to medium-size meningiomas. Int J Radiat Oncol Biol Phys. 2003;55: 1000–5.
94. Williams BJ, Yen CP, Starke RM, Basina B, Nguyen J, Rainey J, et al. Gamma Knife surgery for parasellar meningiomas: long-term results including complications, predictive factors, and progression-free survival. J Neurosurg. 2011;114:1571–7.
95. Hasegawa T, Kida Y, Yoshimoto M, Koike J, Iizuka H, Ishii D. Long-term outcomes of Gamma Knife surgery for cavernous sinus meningioma. J Neurosurg. 2007;107:745–51.
96. Chang SD, Adler Jr JR, Martin DP. LINAC radiosurgery for cavernous sinus meningiomas. Stereotact Funct Neurosurg. 1998;71:43–50.
97. Chen JC, Giannotta SL, Yu C, Petrovich Z, Levy ML, Apuzzo ML. Radiosurgical management of benign cavernous sinus tumors: dose profiles and acute complications. Neurosurgery. 2001;48:1022–30; discussion 1030–2.
98. Chang SD, Doty JR, Martin DP, Hancock SL, Adler JR. Treatment of cavernous sinus tumors with linear accelerator radiosurgery. Skull Base Surg. 1999;9:195–200.
99. Duma CM, Lunsford LD, Kondziolka D, Harsh 4th GR, Flickinger JC. Stereotactic radiosurgery of cavernous sinus meningiomas as an addition or alternative to microsurgery. Neurosurgery. 1993;32:699–704; discussion 704–5.
100. Friedman WA, Murad GJ, Bradshaw P, Amdur RJ, Mendenhall WM, Foote KD, et al. Linear accelerator surgery for meningiomas. J Neurosurg. 2005;103:206–9.
101. Iwai Y, Yamanaka K, Ishiguro T. Gamma knife radiosurgery for the treatment of cavernous sinus meningiomas. Neurosurgery. 2003;52:517–24; discussion 523–4.
102. Kimball MM, Friedman WA, Foote KD, Bova FJ, Chi YY. Linear accelerator radiosurgery for cavernous sinus meningiomas. Stereotact Funct Neurosurg. 2009;87:120–7.
103. Kuo JS, Chen JC, Yu C, Zelman V, Giannotta SL, Petrovich Z, et al. Gamma knife radiosurgery for benign cavernous sinus tumors: quantitative analysis of treatment outcomes. Neurosurgery. 2004;54:1385–93; discussion 1393–4.
104. Kurita H, Sasaki T, Kawamoto S, Taniguchi M, Terahara A, Tago M, et al. Role of radiosurgery in the management of cavernous sinus meningiomas. Acta Neurol Scand. 1997;96:297–304.
105. Lee JY, Niranjan A, McInerney J, Kondziolka D, Flickinger JC, Lunsford LD. Stereotactic radiosurgery providing long-term tumor control of cavernous sinus meningiomas. J Neurosurg. 2002;97:65–72.
106. Liscak R, Simonova G, Vymazal J, Janouskova L, Vladyka V. Gamma knife radiosurgery of meningiomas in the cavernous sinus region. Acta Neurochir (Wien). 1999;141:473–80.
107. Malik I, Rowe JG, Walton L, Radatz MW, Kemeny AA. The use of stereotactic radiosurgery in the management of meningiomas. Br J Neurosurg. 2005;19:13–20.
108. Maruyama K, Shin M, Kurita H, Kawahara N, Morita A, Kirino T. Proposed treatment strategy for cavernous sinus meningiomas: a prospective study. Neurosurgery. 2004;55:1068–75.
109. Metellus P, Regis J, Muracciole X, Fuentes S, Dufour H, Nanni I, et al. Evaluation of fractionated radiotherapy and gamma knife radiosurgery in cavernous sinus meningiomas: treatment strategy. Neurosurgery. 2005;57:873–86.
110. Nicolato A, Foroni R, Alessandrini F, Bricolo A, Gerosa M. Radiosurgical treatment of cavernous sinus meningiomas: experience with 122 treated patients. Neurosurgery. 2002;51: 1153–9; discussion 1159–61.

111. Nicolato A, Foroni R, Alessandrini F, Maluta S, Bricolo A, Gerosa M. The role of Gamma Knife radiosurgery in the management of cavernous sinus meningiomas. Int J Radiat Oncol Biol Phys. 2002;53:992–1000.
112. Pendl G, Schrottner O, Eustacchio S, Ganz JC, Feichtinger K. Cavernous sinus meningiomas – what is the strategy: upfront or adjuvant gamma knife surgery? Stereotact Funct Neurosurg. 1998;70 Suppl 1:33–40.
113. Pollock BE, Stafford SL. Results of stereotactic radiosurgery for patients with imaging defined cavernous sinus meningiomas. Int J Radiat Oncol Biol Phys. 2005;62:1427–31.
114. Roche PH, Regis J, Dufour H, Fournier HD, Delsanti C, Pellet W, et al. Gamma knife radiosurgery in the management of cavernous sinus meningiomas. J Neurosurg. 2000;93 Suppl 3:68–73.
115. Shin M, Kurita H, Sasaki T, Kawamoto S, Tago M, Kawahara N, et al. Analysis of treatment outcome after stereotactic radiosurgery for cavernous sinus meningiomas. J Neurosurg. 2001;95: 435–9.
116. Spiegelmann R, Nissim O, Menhel J, Alezra D, Pfeffer MR. Linear accelerator radiosurgery for meningiomas in and around the cavernous sinus. Neurosurgery. 2002;51:1373–9; discussion 1379–80.
117. Takanashi M, Fukuoka S, Hojyo A, Sasaki T, Nakagawara J, Nakamura H. Gamma knife radiosurgery for skull-base meningiomas. Prog Neurol Surg. 2009;22:96–111.
118. Selch MT, Ahn E, Laskari A, Lee SP, Agazaryan N, Solberg TD, et al. Stereotactic radiotherapy for treatment of cavernous sinus meningiomas. Int J Radiat Oncol Biol Phys. 2004;59:101–11.
119. Hashimoto K, Asaba K, Tamura K, Takao T, Nakamura T. A case of lymphocytic infundibuloneurohypophysitis associated with systemic lupus erythematosus. Endocr J. 2002;49:605–10.
120. Nishioka H, Ito H, Fukushima C. Recurrent lymphocytic hypophysitis: case report. Neurosurgery. 1997;41:684–6; discussion 686–7.
121. Tubridy N, Saunders D, Thom M, Asa SL, Powell M, Plant GT, et al. Infundibulohypophysitis in a man presenting with diabetes insipidus and cavernous sinus involvement. J Neurol Neurosurg Psychiatry. 2001;71:798–801.
122. Yamagami K, Yoshioka K, Sakai H, Fukumoto M, Yamakita T, Hosoi M, et al. Treatment of lymphocytic hypophysitis by high-dose methylprednisolone pulse therapy. Intern Med. 2003;42: 168–73.
123. Thodou E, Asa SL, Kontogeorgos G, Kovacs K, Horvath E, Ezzat S. Clinical case seminar: lymphocytic hypophysitis: clinicopathological findings. J Clin Endocrinol Metab. 1995;80:2302–11.
124. Buxton N, Robertson I. Lymphocytic and granulocytic hypophysitis: a single centre experience. Br J Neurosurg. 2001;15:242–5; discussion 245–6.
125. Holck S, Laursen H. Prolactinoma coexistent with granulomatous hypophysitis. Acta Neuropathol. 1983;61:253–7.
126. Su SB, Zhang DJ, Yue SY, Zhang JN. Primary granulomatous hypophysitis: a case report and literature review. Endocr J. 2011;58:467–73.
127. Selch MT, DeSalles AA, Kelly DF, Frighetto L, Vinters HV, Cabatan-Awang C, et al. Stereotactic radiotherapy for the treatment of lymphocytic hypophysitis. Report of two cases. J Neurosurg. 2003;99:591–6.
128. Ray DK, Yen CP, Vance ML, Laws ER, Lopes B, Sheehan JP. Gamma knife surgery for lymphocytic hypophysitis. J Neurosurg. 2010;112:118–21.
129. Ulfarsson E, Lindquist C, Roberts M, Rahn T, Lindquist M, Thoren M, et al. Gamma knife radiosurgery for craniopharyngiomas: long-term results in the first Swedish patients. J Neurosurg. 2002;97(5 Suppl):613–22.
130. Xu Z, Yen CP, Schlesinger D, Sheehan J. Outcomes of Gamma Knife surgery for craniopharyngiomas. J Neurooncol. 2011;104:305–13.
131. Chung WY, Pan DH, Shiau CY, Guo WY, Wang LW. Gamma knife radiosurgery for craniopharyngiomas. J Neurosurg. 2000;93 Suppl 3:47–56.
132. Kobayashi T, Kida Y, Mori Y, Hasegawa T. Long-term results of gamma knife surgery for the treatment of craniopharyngioma in 98 consecutive cases. J Neurosurg. 2005;103(6 Suppl):482–8.
133. Mokry M. Craniopharyngiomas: a six year experience with Gamma Knife radiosurgery. Stereotact Funct Neurosurg. 1999;72 Suppl 1:140–9.
134. Barua KK, Ehara K, Kohmura E, Tamaki N. Treatment of recurrent craniopharyngiomas. Kobe J Med Sci. 2003;49:123–32.
135. Chiou SM, Lunsford LD, Niranjan A, Kondziolka D, Flickinger JC. Stereotactic radiosurgery of residual or recurrent craniopharyngioma, after surgery, with or without radiation therapy. Neuro Oncol. 2001;3:159–66.
136. Prasad D, Steiner M, Steiner L. Gamma knife surgery for craniopharyngioma. Acta Neurochir (Wien). 1995;134:167–76.
137. Amendola BE, Wolf A, Coy SR, Amendola MA. Role of radiosurgery in craniopharyngiomas: a preliminary report. Med Pediatr Oncol. 2003;41:123–7.
138. Albright AL, Hadjipanayis CG, Lunsford LD, Kondziolka D, Pollack IF, Adelson PD. Individualized treatment of pediatric craniopharyngiomas. Childs Nerv Syst. 2005;21:649–54.
139. Yu X, Liu Z, Li S. Combined treatment with stereotactic intracavitary irradiation and gamma knife surgery for craniopharyngiomas. Stereotact Funct Neurosurg. 2000;75:117–22.
140. Yomo S, Hayashi M, Chernov M, Tamura N, Izawa M, Okada Y, et al. Stereotactic radiosurgery of residual or recurrent craniopharyngioma: new treatment concept using Leksell gamma knife model C with automatic positioning system. Stereotact Funct Neurosurg. 2009;87:360–7.
141. Gopalan R, Dassoulas K, Rainey J, Sherman JH, Sheehan JP. Evaluation of the role of Gamma Knife surgery in the treatment of craniopharyngiomas. Neurosurg Focus. 2008;24(5):E5.
142. Lee M, Kalani MY, Cheshier S, Gibbs IC, Adler JR, Chang SD. Radiation therapy and CyberKnife radiosurgery in the management of craniopharyngiomas. Neurosurg Focus. 2008;24(5):E4.
143. Niranjan A, Kano H, Mathieu D, Kondziolka D, Flickinger JC, Lunsford LD. Radiosurgery for craniopharyngioma. Int J Radiat Oncol Biol Phys. 2010;78:64–71.
144. Elliott RE, Jane Jr JA, Wisoff JH. Surgical management of craniopharyngiomas in children: meta-analysis and comparison of transcranial and transsphenoidal approaches. Neurosurgery. 2011;69: 630–43; discussion 643.
145. Sughrue ME, Yang I, Kane AJ, Fang S, Clark AJ, Aranda D, et al. Endocrinologic, neurologic, and visual morbidity after treatment for craniopharyngioma. J Neurooncol. 2011;101:463–76.
146. Veeravagu A, Lee M, Jiang B, Chang SD. The role of radiosurgery in the treatment of craniopharyngiomas. Neurosurg Focus. 2010;28(4):E11.

Part II

The Normal Pituitary Gland

The Normal Pituitary Gland

8

Gabriel Zada, M. Beatriz S. Lopes, Srinivasan Mukundan Jr., and Edward Laws Jr.

The normal pituitary gland is composed of the adenohypophysis (anterior pituitary), neurohypophysis (posterior pituitary), and pars intermedia.
The pituitary gland forms as a result of a superior outgrowth of oral ectoderm derived from the Rathke pouch (forming the adenohypophysis) joining with an inferior axonal outgrowth from the hypothalamus (forming the neurohypophysis).

The adenohypophysis (anterior pituitary) makes up a majority of the bulk of the gland and communicates with hypothalamic cells via a specialized portal venous system whose capillaries are interspersed with hormonally active cells. The adenohypophysis is composed of various cells that secrete one (or more) of six hormones:

- Lactotrophs (prolactin)
- Thyrotrophs (thyroid-stimulating hormone)
- Corticotrophs (adrenocorticotropic hormone)
- Somatotrophs (growth hormone)
- Gonadotrophs (luteinizing hormone and follicle-stimulating hormone)

The cellular organization of the adenohypophysis is such that the somatotrophs and lactotrophs are located in the lateral lobes of the anterior gland, and the corticotrophs and thyrotrophs are located medially in the mucoid wedge of the gland.

The neurohypophysis is composed of axonal extensions of hypothalamic cells that directly deliver antidiuretic hormone (ADH) and oxytocin to the cell endings.

G. Zada, MD, MS (✉)
Department of Neurological Surgery, Keck School of Medicine, University of Southern California, 1200 N State Street, #3300, Los Angeles, CA 90033, USA
e-mail: gzada@usc.edu

M.B.S. Lopes, MD, PhD
Department of Pathology (Neuropathology), University of Virginia School of Medicine, 1215 Lee Street, Room 3060–HEP, Charlottesville, VA 22908, USA
e-mail: msl2e@virginia.edu

S. Mukundan Jr., PhD, MD
Department of Radiology, Brigham and Women's Hospital, 75 Francis Street, Boston, MA 02115, USA
e-mail: smukundan@partners.org

E. Laws Jr., MD
Department of Neurosurgery, Brigham and Women's Hospital, 15 Francis Street, Boston, MA 02115, USA
e-mail: elaws@partners.org

G. Zada et al. (eds.), *Atlas of Sellar and Parasellar Lesions: Clinical, Radiologic, and Pathologic Correlations*, DOI 10.1007/978-3-319-22855-6_8

8.1 Imaging

The normal pituitary gland measures approximately 5 mm in height and 8 mm in width and is often larger in adult women than in men (Figs. 8.1 and 8.2) [1]. Pituitary gland height greater than 9 mm in women and 8 mm in men is rare in normal circumstances and may warrant further evaluation [1]. The size of the pituitary gland changes throughout life and fluctuates with normal physiologic conditions, including puberty, menstrual cycles, and pregnancy [2].

In men, the height of the pituitary gland remains somewhat constant following puberty. In women, the peak height of the normal pituitary gland occurs in the second to third decade of life, and the height of the gland may decrease thereafter [3].

On computed tomographic (CT) imaging, the normal pituitary gland is isodense to the brain and may appear homogeneous or heterogeneous [4]. Following magnetic resonance imaging (MRI) contrast administration, the normal gland usually enhances brightly.

Over 90 % of normal pituitary glands have flat or concave superior surfaces along the diaphragm sella [5]. The pituitary stalk (infundibulum) connects the gland to the hypothalamus and runs through the diaphragm sella; it should be seen on the midline.

The neurohypophysis appears as a "bright spot" on standard T1-weighted MRI in over 90 % of healthy participants [6].

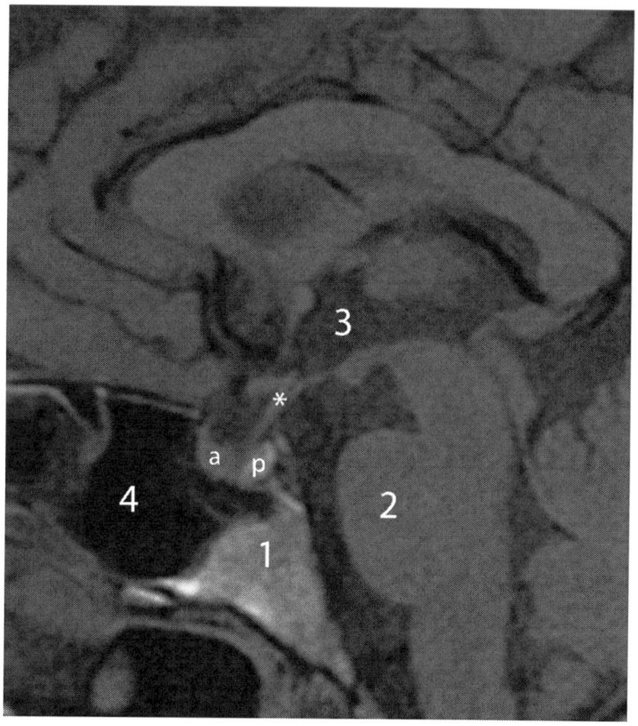

Fig. 8.1 Sagittal T1-weighted image without contrast. (*1*) clivus; (*2*) pons; (*3*) third ventricle; (*4*) sphenoid sinus; (*a*) anterior pituitary gland; (*p*) posterior pituitary gland; *asterisk* indicates pituitary stalk

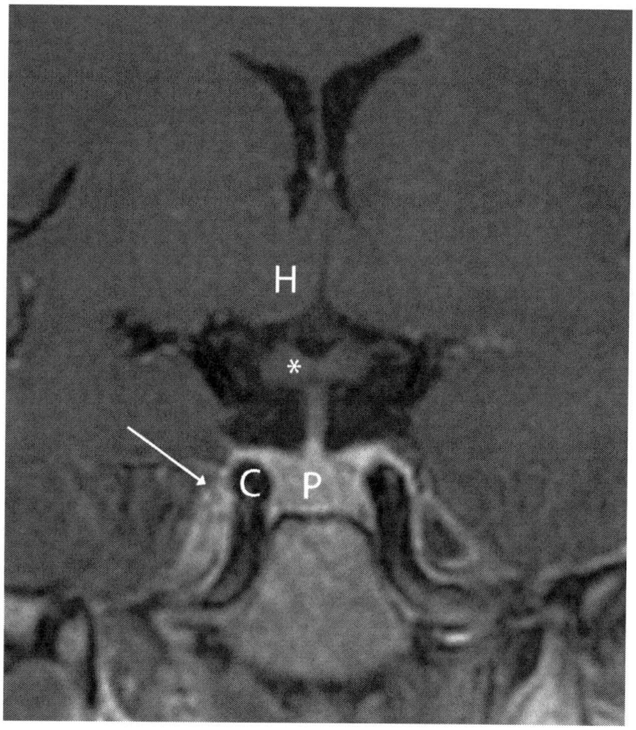

Fig. 8.2 Coronal T1-weighted image without contrast. (*P*) pituitary gland. (*C*) cavernous sinus; (*H*) hypothalamus; *asterisk* indicates optic chiasm

8.1.1 Sellar and Sphenoid Sinus Anatomy on MRI

Three general morphologies of the sellar floor have been described on sagittal MRI (Fig. 8.3) [7]:

- Prominent (sellar angle of <90°) in 25 % of people
- Curved (sellar angle 90–150°) in 63 % of people
- Flat (sellar angle >150°) in 11 % of people
- No floor (conchal sphenoid) in 1 % of people

In healthy adults, mean measurements on sagittal MRI of the following structures are as follows: sellar face length, 13.4 mm; sellar prominence, 3.0 mm; sellar angle, 112°; angle of tuberculum sellae, 112°; and sellar-clival angle, 117°. The average width of the normol sella is 12.7 mm [7].

A simple sphenoid sinus configuration, defined as having no septa, one vertical septum, or two symmetric vertical septa, is noted in 71 % of studies. In the other 29 % of people, an MRI shows a complex configuration, defined as two or more asymmetric septa, three or more septa of any kind, or the presence of a horizontal septum [7].

On MRI, the normal distance between the internal carotid arteries (ICAs) at the parasellar and midclivus levels are 16.2 and 18.5 mm, respectively [7].

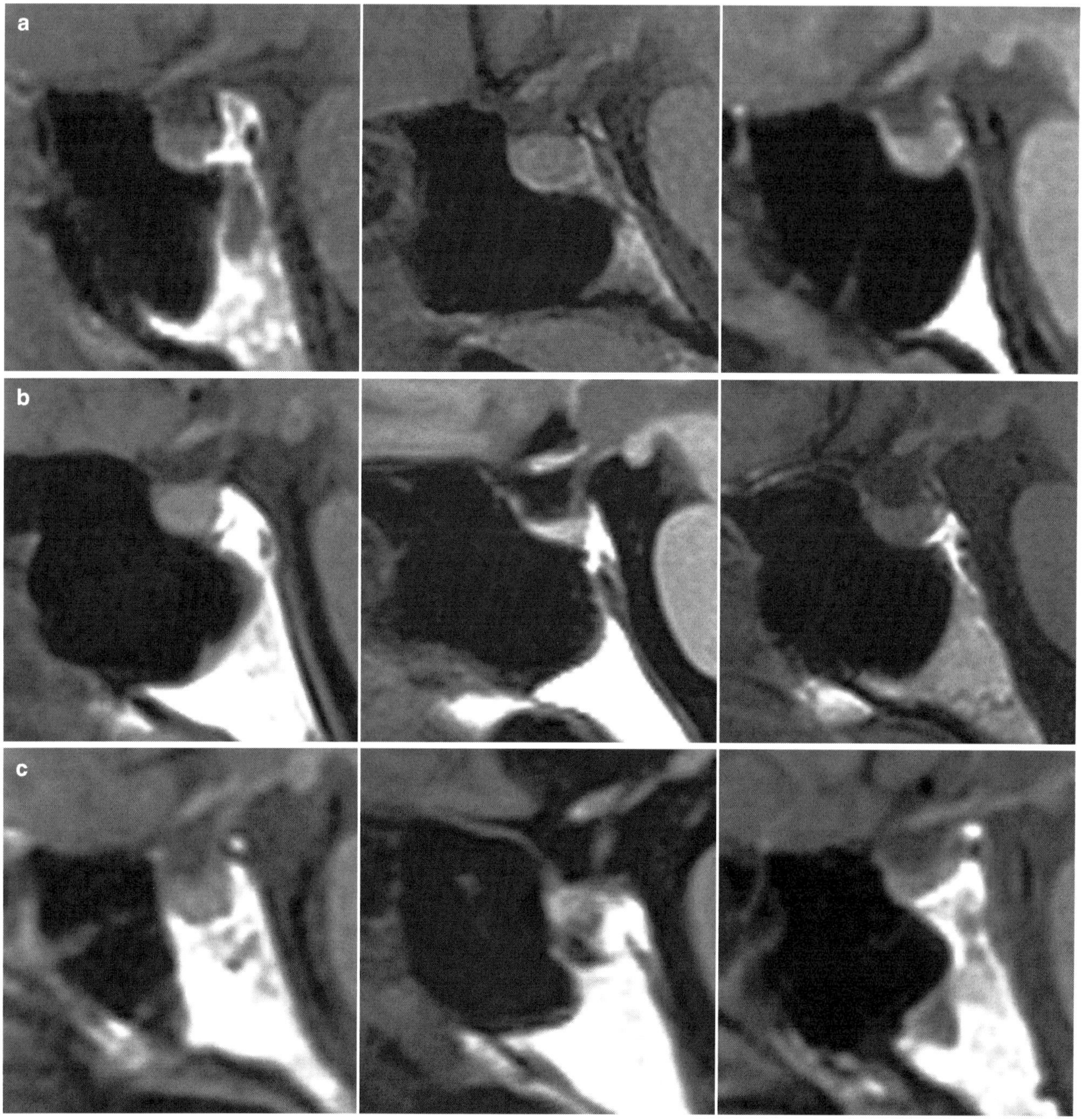

Fig. 8.3 Normal variants of sellar and pituitary morphology seen on sagittal post-contrast MRIs. (**a**) The top row depicts prominent sellar floor morphology that is easy to identify. (**b**) The middle row shows normal variants with a curved, intermediate morphology. (**c**) The bottom row shows examples of a "flat" sella with a partially pneumatized sphenoid sinus that is harder to identify intraoperatively (Adapted from Zada et al. [7]; with permission)

8.2 Histopathology

The normal pituitary gland consists of two distinct regions, the adenohypophysis and the neurohypophysis. Adenohypophyseal cells are derived from an extension of the oral ectoderm (Rathke pouch), while the neurohypophysis is derived from the floor of the diencephalon. The adenohypophysis includes the pars distalis, intermedia, and tuberalis. The neurohypophysis consists of the infundibulum, the pituitary stalk, and the posterior lobe.

A normal anterior pituitary gland retains a delicate acinar pattern that can often be seen when using a reticulin stain (Fig. 8.4d). Pituitary adenomas rarely retain this characteristic, whereas patients with pituitary hyperplasia often show a retained acinar pattern (although enlarged).

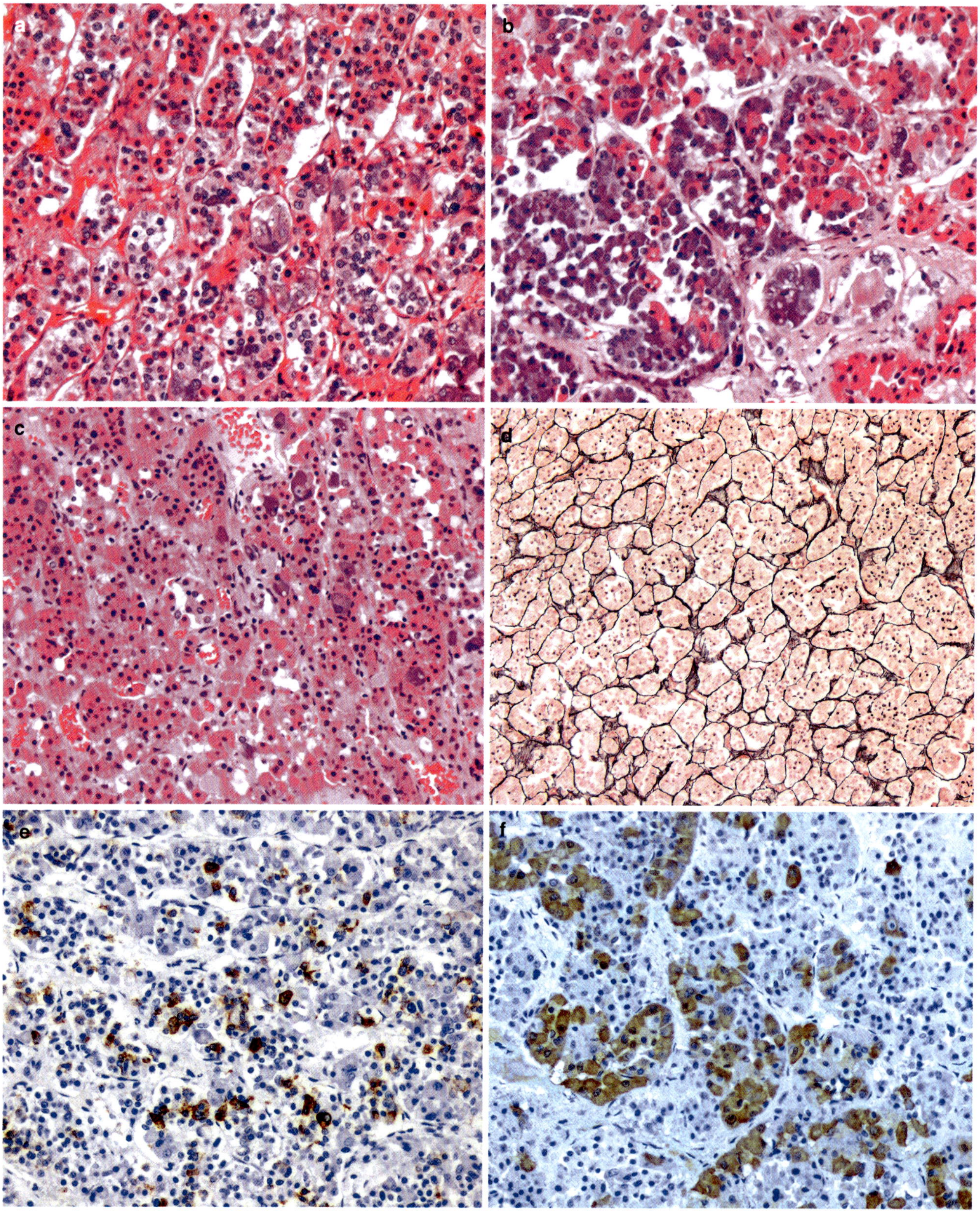

Fig 8.4 Anterior pituitary gland. (**a**) Low magnification of the anterior pituitary shows a mixed population of chromophobic, acidophilic, and basophilic cells by H&E staining. However, the different neuroendocrine cells show a preferential location in the anterior gland. Basophils are most numerous in the central or mucoid wedge (**b**), while acidophils are most numerous in the lateral wings (**c**). The different cell types are arranged in acinar formations surrounded by a rich capillary network and connective tissue that can be highlighted by reticulin stain (**d**). The several hormone-producing cells are distinctive by immunostains against the specific hormones as prolactin (**e**) and growth hormone (**f**). Note the different pattern of immunoreaction of the neuroendocrine cells; while lactotroph cells show focal and sparse immunoreaction (**e**), somatotroph cells are densely granulated cells with immunoreaction of the entire cytoplasm (**f**)

8.3 The Adenohypophysis

Historically, anterior pituitary tissue cells were classified as acidophilic (Fig. 8.4c) (somatotroph and lactotroph cells), basophilic (Fig. 8.4b) (corticotroph, thyrotroph, and gonadotroph cells), or chromophobic (thyrotroph, and gonadotroph cells), depending on their histochemical properties (Fig. 8.4a–c).

Since the 1960s, cell-specific radiolabeling assays have allowed more accurate classification of adenohypophyseal cells. The composition of the anterior pituitary gland by cell type is as follows: somatotroph (50 %) (Fig. 8.4f), lactotroph (20 %) (Fig. 8.4e), corticotroph (20 %), thyrotroph (5 %), and gonadotroph (5 %).

8.4 The Neurohypophysis

The neurohypophysis is composed of hypothalamic-derived nonmyelinated axons (Fig. 8.5b) interspersed with specialized glial cells, the so-called pituicytes (Fig. 8.5c, d).

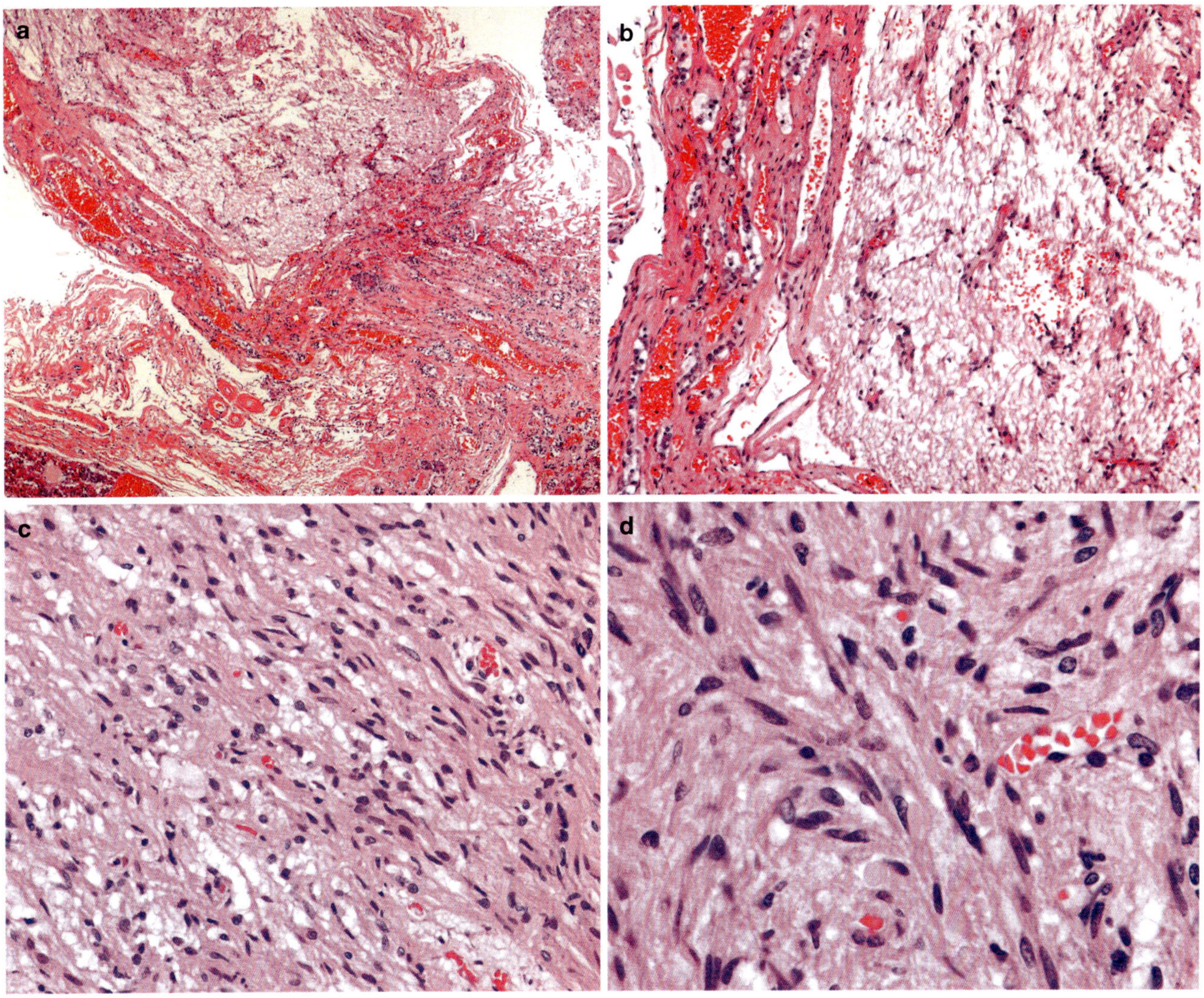

Fig 8.5 Pituitary stalk and posterior pituitary gland. The pituitary stalk is composed of the axons of neuronal cells from the hypothalamus surrounded by the modified glia, named pituicytes (**a**, **b**). Note that the stalk may be surrounded by projections of the anterior pituitary (**b**). The posterior lobe shows pituicytes with elongated nuclei dispersed within the neuropil of the neurohypophysis (**c**) and arranged in vague fascicles (**d**)

References

1. Suzuki M, Takashima T, Kadoya M, Konishi H, Kameyama T, Yoshikawa J, et al. Height of normal pituitary gland on MR imaging: age and sex differentiation. J Comput Assist Tomogr. 1990;14: 36–9.
2. Gonzalez JG, Elizondo G, Saldivar D, Nanez H, Todd LE, Villarreal JZ. Pituitary gland growth during normal pregnancy: an in vivo study using magnetic resonance imaging. Am J Med. 1988;85: 217–20.
3. Peyster RG, Adler LP, Viscarello RR, Hoover ED, Skarzynski J. CT of the normal pituitary gland. Neuroradiology. 1986;28:161–5.
4. Syvertsen A, Haughton VM, Williams AL, Cusick JF. The computed tomographic appearance of the normal pituitary gland and pituitary microadenomas. Radiology. 1979;133:385–91.
5. Brown SB, Irwin KM, Enzmann DR. CT characteristics of the normal pituitary gland. Neuroradiology. 1983;24:259–62.
6. Colombo N, Berry I, Kucharczyk J, Kucharczyk W, de Groot J, Larson T, et al. Posterior pituitary gland: appearance on MR images in normal and pathologic states. Radiology. 1987;165:481.
7. Zada G, Agarwalla PK, Mukundan Jr S, Dunn I, Golby AJ, Laws Jr ER. The neurosurgical anatomy of the sphenoid sinus and sellar floor in endoscopic transsphenoidal surgery. J Neurosurg. 2011;114: 1319–30.

Part III

Pituitary Hyperplasia

Pituitary Hyperplasia

9

Gabriel Zada, M. Beatriz S. Lopes, Srinivasan Mukundan Jr., and Edward Laws Jr.

9.1 Epidemiology and Clinical Presentation

Pituitary hyperplasia is nonneoplastic growth or enlargement of pituitary gland cells without a major qualitative change in cell biology. It is typically reversible if the inciting cause is corrected.

Pituitary hyperplasia has a wide spectrum of underlying etiologies, pathological findings, and clinical presentations, so it is often underdiagnosed or misdiagnosed. It may be physiologic (related to pregnancy, lactation, or puberty), or it may be pathologic, resulting from primary hypothyroidism or secondary to ectopic secretion of hypothalamic-releasing hormones by neuroendocrine tumors. In rare cases, the gland enlargement may be great enough to cause mass effect on surrounding structures, presenting with headache, visual loss, amenorrhea/galactorrhea, hyperprolactinemia, and/or hypopituitarism [1–4].

Pituitary hyperplasia seldom requires surgical intervention; it comprises less than 1 % of major transsphenoidal series for pituitary pathology. It is often represented in surgical series because it was thought to be an adenoma, or the primary tumor (i.e., microadenoma) was not preserved during the surgical resection [5, 6].

9.2 Etiology and Incidence

Pituitary hyperplasia can arise from any cells of the adenohypophysis. Its etiology and incidence vary according to cell type, as discussed below [6].

9.2.1 Lactotroph Hyperplasia

Hyperplasia of this type is commonly observed with pregnancy, lactation, or estrogen administration [7, 8]. "Pregnancy cells" are hyperplastic lactotrophs that progressively increase within the gland during pregnancy and ultimately make up 60–70 % of the adenohypophysis at term. Lactotroph hyperplasia may also occur in cases of pituitary stalk effect owing to compression from a mass lesion.

9.2.2 Thyrotroph Hyperplasia

This type of hyperplasia is well known to occur in cases of chronic primary hypothyroidism [9, 10]. It typically develops in women in the third or fourth decade of life. It is often noted to be associated with a level of thyroid-stimulating hormone (TSH) greater than 100 mIU/mL and a low free T4 level [9]. It may be associated with prolactin hyperplasia and hyperprolactinemia; in these patients it is frequently mistaken for a prolactinoma [1, 11].

G. Zada, MD, MS (✉)
Department of Neurological Surgery, Keck School of Medicine, University of Southern California, 1200 N State Street, #3300, Los Angeles, CA 90033, USA
e-mail: gzada@usc.edu

M.B.S. Lopes, MD, PhD
Department of Pathology (Neuropathology), University of Virginia School of Medicine, 1215 Lee Street, Room 3060–HEP, Charlottesville, VA 22908, USA
e-mail: msl2e@virginia.edu

S. Mukundan Jr., PhD, MD
Department of Radiology, Brigham and Women's Hospital, 75 Francis Street, Boston, MA 02115, USA
e-mail: smukundan@partners.org

E. Laws Jr., MD
Department of Neurosurgery, Brigham and Women's Hospital, 15 Francis Street, Boston, MA 02115, USA
e-mail: elaws@partners.org

G. Zada et al. (eds.), *Atlas of Sellar and Parasellar Lesions: Clinical, Radiologic, and Pathologic Correlations*, DOI 10.1007/978-3-319-22855-6_9

9.2.3 Corticotroph Hyperplasia

Corticotroph hyperplasia is a rare condition that can be associated with Cushing's disease or Cushing's syndrome (e.g., owing to ectopic steroid administration or hypercortisolemia) [12, 13]. It also may occur secondary to ectopic corticotropin-releasing hormone (CRH) secretion [14, 15].

9.2.4 Somatotroph Hyperplasia

Somatotroph hyperplasia is rarely encountered, usually in the setting of oversecretion of growth hormone-releasing hormone (GHRH) from a neuroendocrine tumor of nonpituitary origin, such as bronchial carcinoid, pancreatic islet cell tumor, medullary carcinoma of the thyroid, or pheochromocytoma [6].

Mammosomatotroph hyperplasia may present with gigantism or as part of the McCune-Albright syndrome [6, 16].

9.2.5 Gonadotroph Hyperplasia

Gonadotroph hyperplasia is exceedingly rare and is almost never a cause of pituitary disease [6].

9.3 Imaging

Gland enlargement secondary to hyperplasia is often mistaken for a pituitary adenoma, especially in the setting of hyperprolactinemia. Several imaging findings should suggest it as a diagnosis:

- Symmetric involvement of the pituitary gland with smooth contours [17]
- Homogeneous contrast enhancement (Figs. 9.1, 9.2, and 9.3)
- Pituitary stalk rarely deviated laterally
- May demonstrate suprasellar extension with upward bowing of the diaphragma sellae and, in rare cases, compression of the optic chiasm

Parasellar and infrasellar invasion are extremely rare.

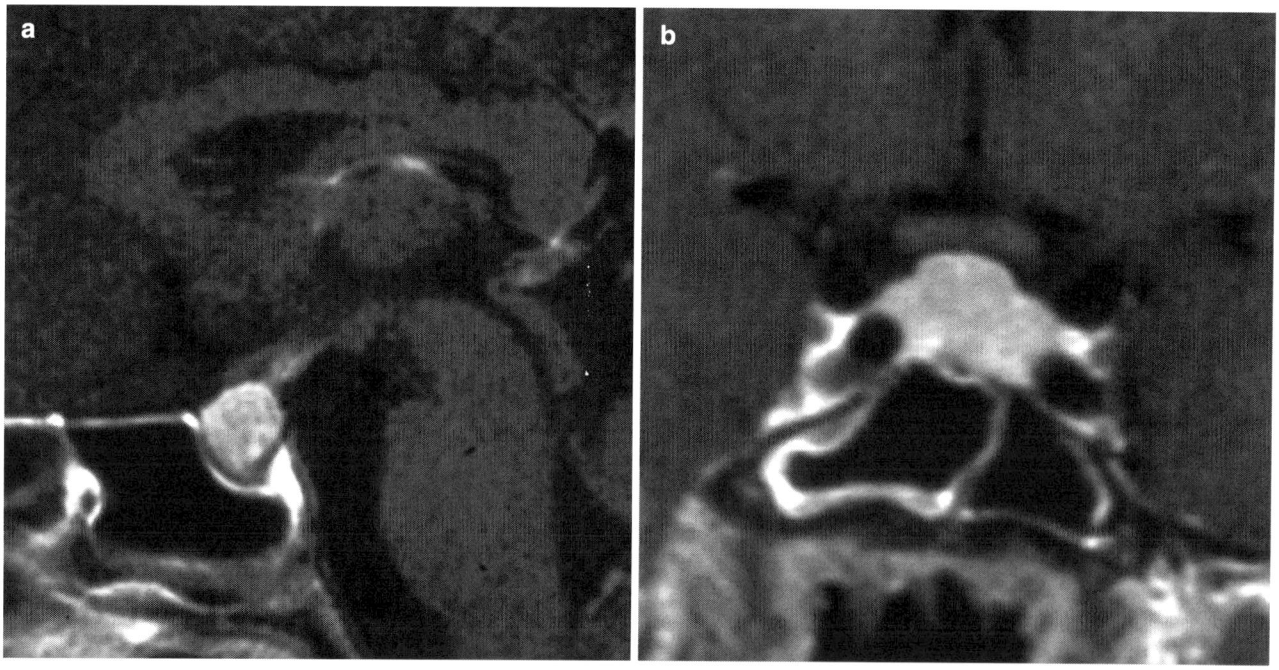

Fig. 9.1 (**a**) Sagittal T1-weighted image post gadolinium contrast enhancement. (**b**) Coronal T1-weighted image post gadolinium contrast enhancement. The pituitary gland exhibits homogeneous enhancement with a convex upper margin and a craniocaudal measurement exceeding 1 cm. No focal mass or hypoenhancement is seen

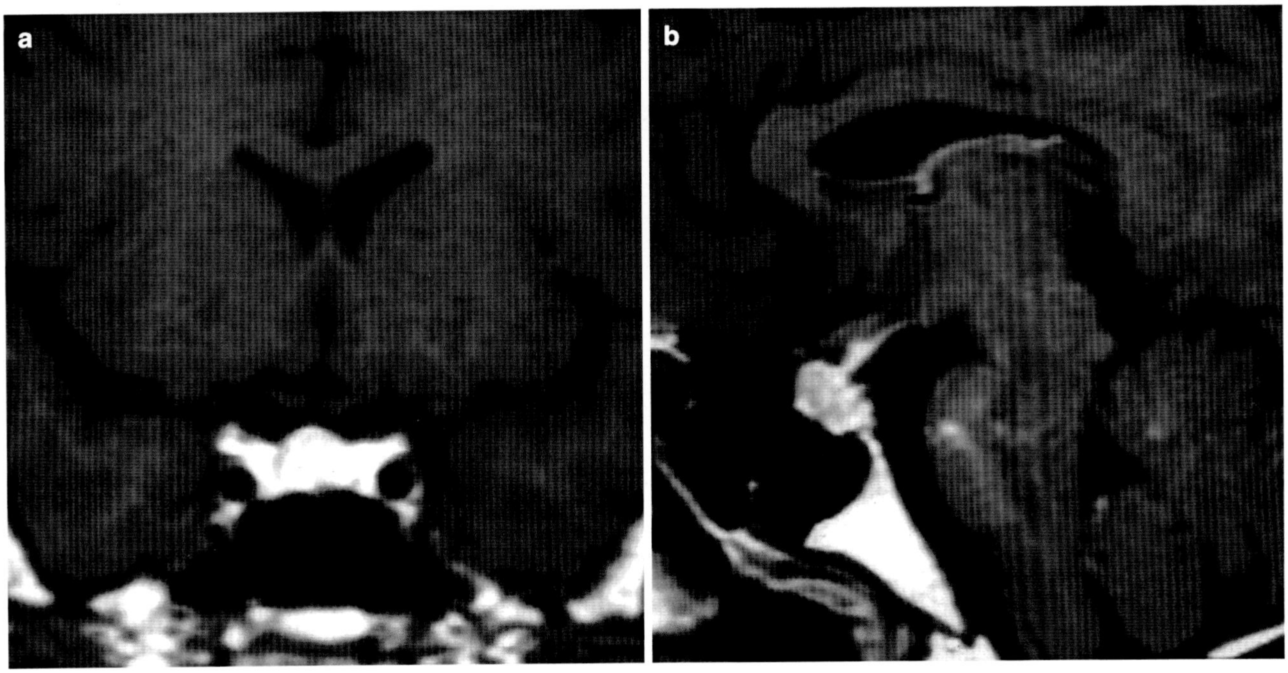

Fig. 9.2 (**a**) Coronal T1-weighted image post gadolinium contrast enhancement. (**b**) Sagittal T1-weighted image post gadolinium contrast enhancement. The pituitary gland exhibits homogeneous enhancement with a convex upper margin and craniocaudal measurement exceeding 1 cm. No focal mass or hypoenhancement is seen

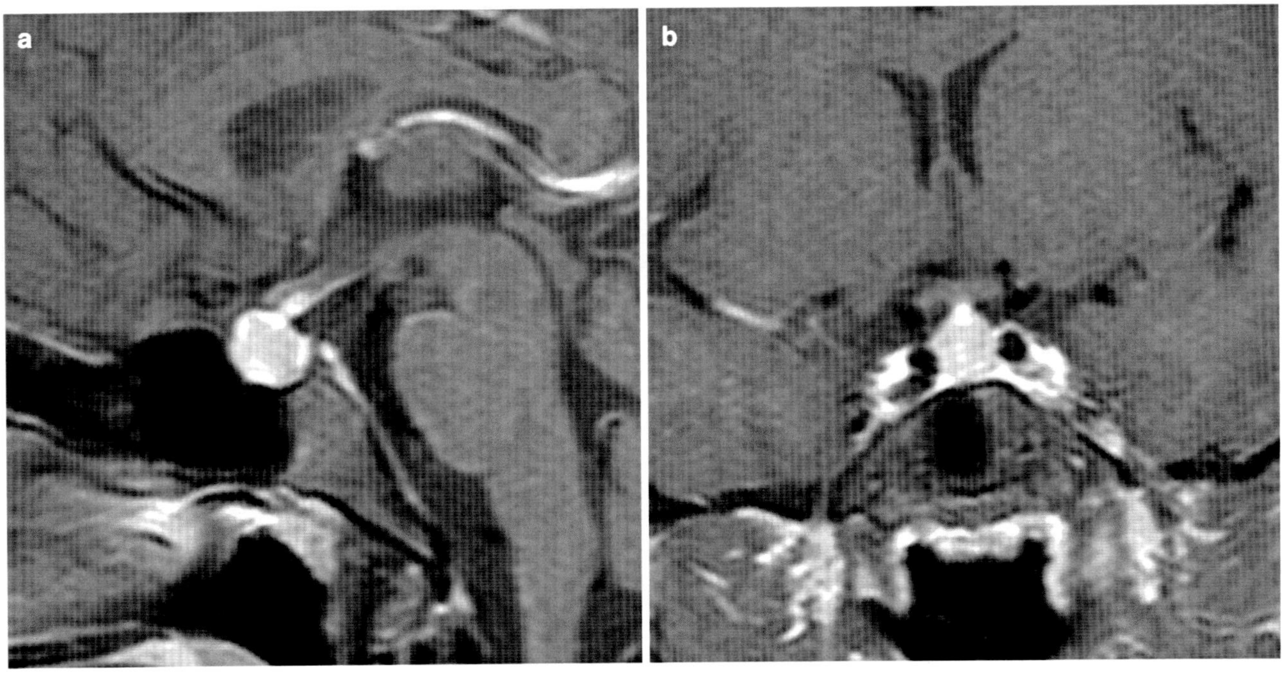

Fig. 9.3 (**a**) Sagittal T1-weighted image post gadolinium contrast enhancement. (**b**) Coronal T1-weighted image post gadolinium contrast enhancement. The pituitary gland exhibits homogeneous enhancement with a convex upper margin and craniocaudal measurement exceeding 1 cm. No focal mass or hypoenhancement is seen

9.4 Histopathology

It may be difficult to differentiate pituitary hyperplasia from an adenoma. The reticulin stain can often be used to help this differentiation [18]. In hyperplasia, the normal acinar structure of the pituitary gland is maintained but it is enlarged, whereas adenomas typically demonstrate disruption of the reticular acinar structure.

Histopathology may demonstrate diffuse or nodular hyperplasia, typically identifiable with a silver/reticulin stain [6]. In diffuse hyperplasia, an increase in the size of glandular cells and acini is seen throughout the gland, without disruption of the acinar network [18] (Fig. 9.4). Nodular hyperplasia appears as a local, nodular growth of pituitary cells, with enlargement and possible disruption of the acinar network. Thyrotroph hyperplasia is diffuse in 69 % of cases and nodular in 25 % [10]. Lactotroph hyperplasia is generally of the diffuse type [6].

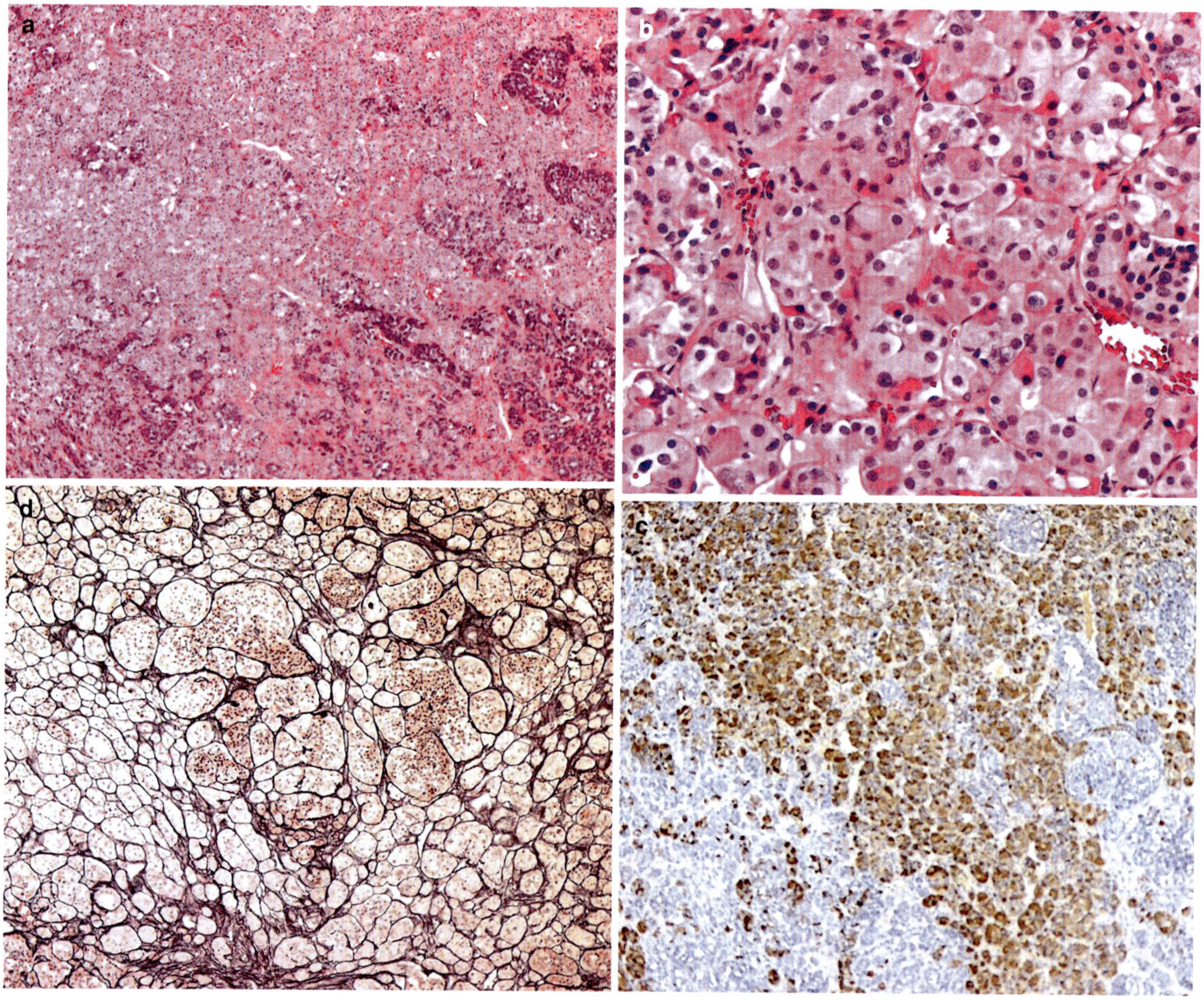

Fig. 9.4 Surgical specimen from a patient with a history of hypothyroidism and a nonfunctioning adenoma found incidentally after a trauma to the head. (**a**, **b**) In addition to a null-cell adenoma (*not shown*), the adjacent normal gland showed expansion of the acini, which were composed mostly of acidophilic cells. (**c**) Reticulin stain emphasized expansion of the acini as compared with the normal pituitary pattern. (**d**) Immunostain for thyroid-stimulating hormone (TSH) confirmed the expansion of the thyrotroph cell population due to uncontrolled hypothyroidism

9.5 Clinical Management

When clinical and imaging characteristics lead to suspicion of pituitary hyperplasia, the underlying hormonal cause should be sought. If the inciting cause is identified and treated, pituitary hyperplasia is typically reversible. For example, thyrotroph hyperplasia is generally reversible following treatment with thyroid hormone replacement [9]. Lactotroph hyperplasia is partially reversible following pregnancy or lactation. Nulliparous women have less massive pituitary glands than multiparous women [19].

In the rare cases when mass effect results in severe headache, visual loss, or panhypopituitarism, surgical intervention for tissue diagnosis and decompression may be indicated.

References

1. Grubb MR, Chakeres D, Malarkey WB. Patients with primary hypothyroidism presenting as prolactinomas. Am J Med. 1987;83:765–9.
2. Yamamoto K, Saito K, Takai T, Naito M, Yoshida S. Visual field defects and pituitary enlargement in primary hypothyroidism. J Clin Endocrinol Metab. 1983;57:283–7.
3. Inoue T, Hotta A, Awai M, Tanihara H. Loss of vision due to a physiologic pituitary enlargement during normal pregnancy. Graefes Arch Clin Exp Ophthalmol. 2007;245:1049–51.
4. Simsek E, Simsek T, Savas-Erdeve S, Erdogmus B, Dosoglu M. Pituitary hyperplasia mimicking pituitary macroadenoma in two adolescent patients with long-standing primary hypothyroidism: case reports and review of literature. Turk J Pediatr. 2009;51:624–30.
5. Saeger W, Ludecke DK, Buchfelder M, Fahlbusch R, Quabbe HJ, Petersenn S. Pathohistological classification of pituitary tumors: 10 years of experience with the German Pituitary Tumor Registry. Eur J Endocrinol. 2007;156:203–16.
6. Horvath E, Kovacs K, Scheithauer BW. Pituitary hyperplasia. Pituitary. 1999;1:169–79.
7. Scheithauer BW, Kovacs KT, Randall RV, Ryan N. Effects of estrogen on the human pituitary: a clinicopathologic study. Mayo Clin Proc. 1989;64:1077–84.
8. Scheithauer BW, Sano T, Kovacs KT, Young Jr WF, Ryan N, Randall RV. The pituitary gland in pregnancy: a clinicopathologic and immunohistochemical study of 69 cases. Mayo Clin Proc. 1990;65:461–74.
9. Joshi AS, Woolf PD. Pituitary hyperplasia secondary to primary hypothyroidism: a case report and review of the literature. Pituitary. 2005;8:99–103.
10. Scheithauer BW, Kovacs K, Randall RV, Ryan N. Pituitary gland in hypothyroidism. Histologic and immunocytologic study. Arch Pathol Lab Med. 1985;109:499–504.
11. Khalil A, Kovacs K, Sima AA, Burrow GN, Horvath E. Pituitary thyrotroph hyperplasia mimicking prolactin-secreting adenoma. J Endocrinol Invest. 1984;7:399–404.
12. Schnall AM, Kovacs K, Brodkey JS, Pearson OH. Pituitary Cushing's disease without adenoma. Acta Endocrinol (Cop). 1980;94:297–303.
13. Lloyd RV, Chandler WF, McKeever PE, Schteingart DE. The spectrum of ACTH-producing pituitary lesions. Am J Surg Pathol. 1986;10:618–26.
14. Carey RM, Varma SK, Drake Jr CR, Thorner MO, Kovacs K, Rivier J, Vale W. Ectopic secretion of corticotropin-releasing factor as a cause of Cushing's syndrome. A clinical, morphologic, and biochemical study. N Engl J Med. 1984;311:13–20.
15. Schteingart DE, Lloyd RV, Akil H, Chandler WF, Ibarra-Perez G, Rosen SG, Ogletree R. Cushing's syndrome secondary to ectopic corticotropin-releasing hormone-adrenocorticotropin secretion. J Clin Endocrinol Metab. 1986;63:770–5.
16. Zimmerman D, Young Jr WF, Ebersold MJ, Scheithauer BW, Kovacs K, Horvath E, et al. Congenital gigantism due to growth hormone-releasing hormone excess and pituitary hyperplasia with adenomatous transformation. J Clin Endocrinol Metab. 1993;76:216–22.
17. Sarlis NJ, Brucker-Davis F, Doppman JL, Skarulis MC. MRI-demonstrable regression of a pituitary mass in a case of primary hypothyroidism after a week of acute thyroid hormone therapy. J Clin Endocrinol Metab. 1997;82:808–11.
18. Al-Brahim NY, Asa SL. My approach to pathology of the pituitary gland. J Clin Pathol. 2006;59:1245–53.
19. Asa SL, Penz G, Kovacs K, Ezrin C. Prolactin cells in the human pituitary. A quantitative immunocytochemical analysis. Arch Pathol Lab Med. 1982;106:360–3.

Part IV

Pituitary Adenomas

Nonfunctioning Pituitary Adenomas

10

Gabriel Zada, M. Beatriz S. Lopes, Srinivasan Mukundan Jr., and Edward Laws Jr.

10.1 Epidemiology and Clinical Presentation

- Nonfunctioning pituitary adenomas (NFPAs) are those that do not produce any functional pituitary hormones.
- They comprise 25–50 % of all surgically resected pituitary tumors and are the sellar tumors that are most frequently surgically resected [1–4].
- Because they do not secrete active hormones, NFPAs are more likely to present secondary to features of mass effect on surrounding structures. For this reason, they are typically larger than functional adenomas at the time of diagnosis.
- Presenting symptoms often include headache, visual field deficits, decreased libido, fatigue, and other features of hypopituitarism [3].
- The most frequent hormonal abnormalities associated with NFPAs are hypogonadism and hyperprolactinemia, followed by growth hormone deficiency [5].
- NFPAs frequently result in elevated serum prolactin levels due to pituitary "stalk effect." In the normal state, the hypothalamus inhibits the tonic secretion of prolactin from the adenohypophysis via dopamine release into the communicating portal system, which is a unique phenomenon among all the hypothalamic-pituitary hormonal axes. Any lesion causing compression and subsequent dysfunction of this communication may result in oversecretion of prolactin, typically in the range of 30–200 ng/mL.
- Early compression of the inferior optic chiasm from NFPAs emerging from within the sella typically produces visual field deficits in the superior temporal quadrants (superior quadrantanopsia) prior to full bitemporal hemianopsia. Testing visual fields with a red pin or formal visual field examination (i.e., Humphrey visual field test) is a good way to assess for early peripheral field loss [6].

G. Zada, MD, MS (✉)
Department of Neurological Surgery, Keck School of Medicine, University of Southern California, 1200 N State Street, #3300, Los Angeles, CA 90033, USA
e-mail: gzada@usc.edu

M.B.S. Lopes, MD, PhD
Department of Pathology (Neuropathology), University of Virginia School of Medicine, 1215 Lee Street, Room 3060–HEP, Charlottesville, VA 22908, USA
e-mail: msl2e@virginia.edu

S. Mukundan Jr., PhD, MD
Department of Radiology, Brigham and Women's Hospital, 75 Francis Street, Boston, MA 02115, USA
e-mail: smukundan@partners.org

E. Laws Jr., MD
Department of Neurosurgery, Brigham and Women's Hospital, 15 Francis Street, Boston, MA 02115, USA
e-mail: elaws@partners.org

G. Zada et al. (eds.), *Atlas of Sellar and Parasellar Lesions: Clinical, Radiologic, and Pathologic Correlations*, DOI 10.1007/978-3-319-22855-6_10

10.2 Diagnosis

10.2.1 Imaging

- NFPAs are frequently large masses with a "dumbbell," "hourglass," or "snowman" shape; they are isointense on T1- and T2-weighted MR imaging.
- At the time of diagnosis, 95 % of symptomatic NFPAs are macroadenomas [4].
- Their average maximal diameter at time of presentation is slightly more than 2 cm [3].
- NFPAs typically demonstrate homogeneous contrast enhancement, but they may have intratumoral cystic or hemorrhagic components.
- The typical pattern of extension is superiorly through the plane of the diaphragma sella. NFPAs often demonstrate cavernous sinus and infrasellar extension as well.
- Giant NFPAs may demonstrate superior invasion into the ventricular system or lateral invasion into the middle fossa or deep frontal lobes.
- Figs. 10.1, 10.2, 10.3, 10.4, 10.5, 10.6, 10.7, 10.8, 10.9, 10.10, 10.11, 10.12, and 10.13.

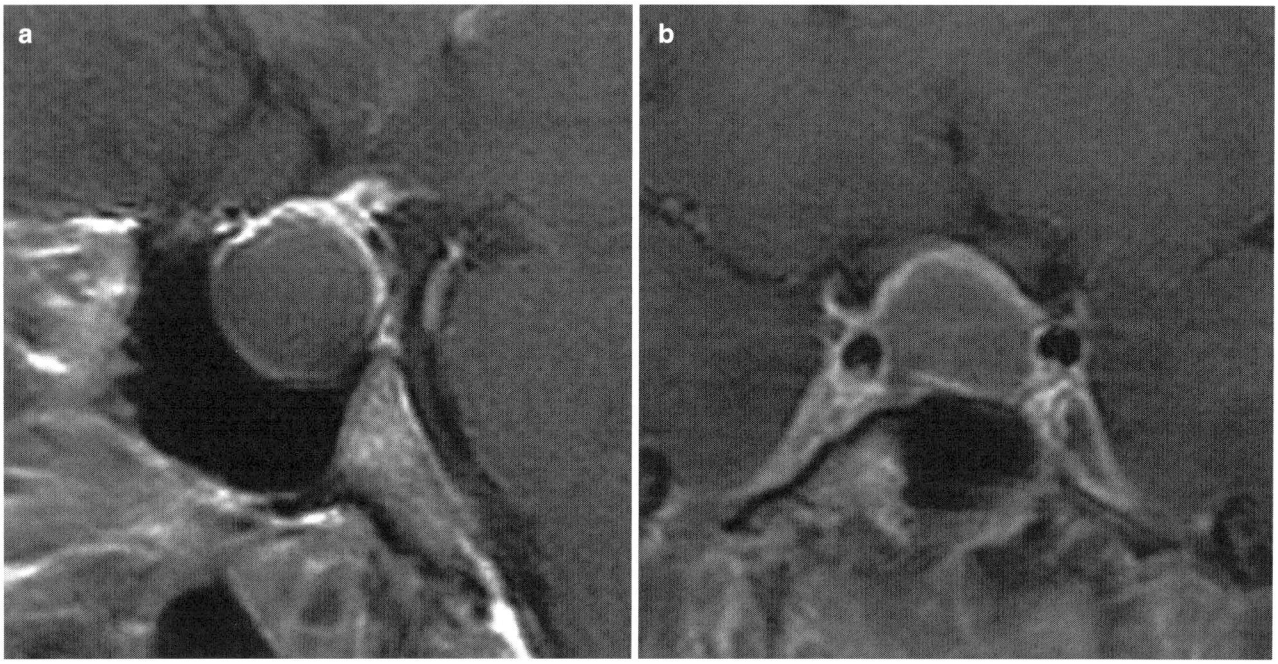

Fig. 10.1 Nonfunctioning pituitary adenoma. (**a**) Sagittal T1-weighted post-gadolinium image. (**b**) Coronal T1-weighted post-gadolinium image. A hypoenhancing sellar mass remodels the sellar floor and abuts the cavernous internal carotid arteries without encasement. The normal gland appears along the superior aspect of the mass. The pituitary stalk is elevated

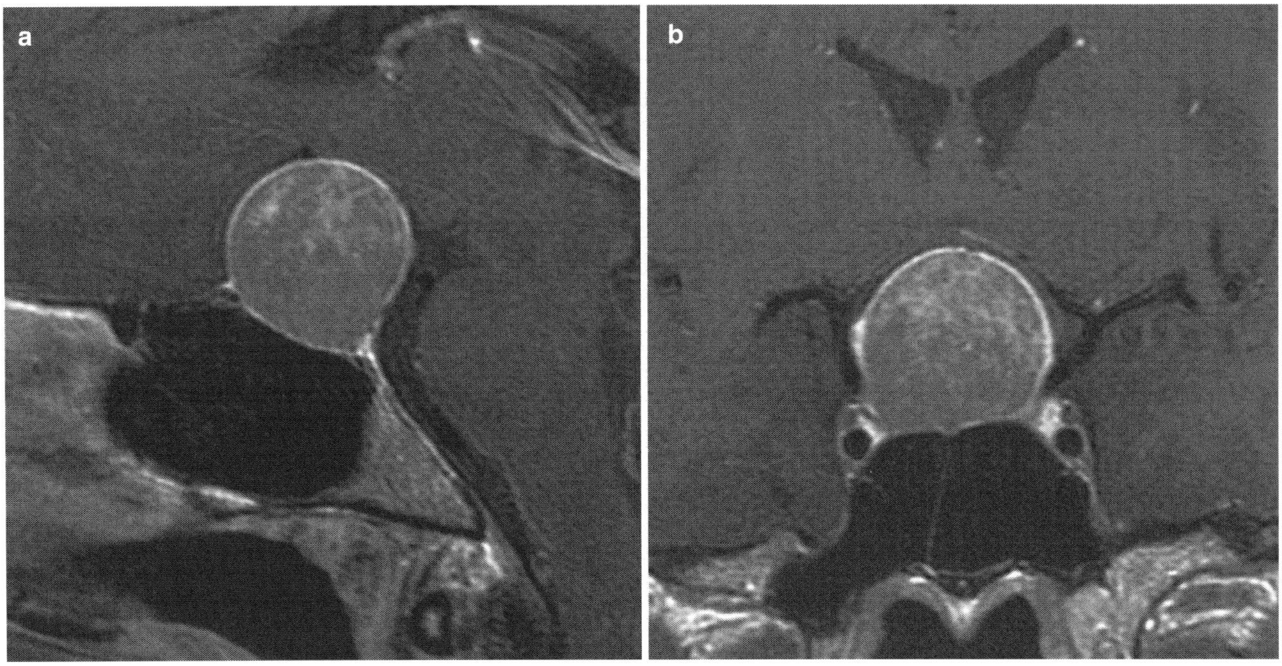

Fig. 10.2 Nonfunctioning pituitary adenoma. (**a**) Sagittal T1-weighted post-gadolinium image. (**b**) Coronal T1-weighted post-gadolinium image. There is a heterogeneous, predominantly hypoenhancing sellar mass with remodeling of the sellar floor and suprasellar extension with elevation of the optic chiasm

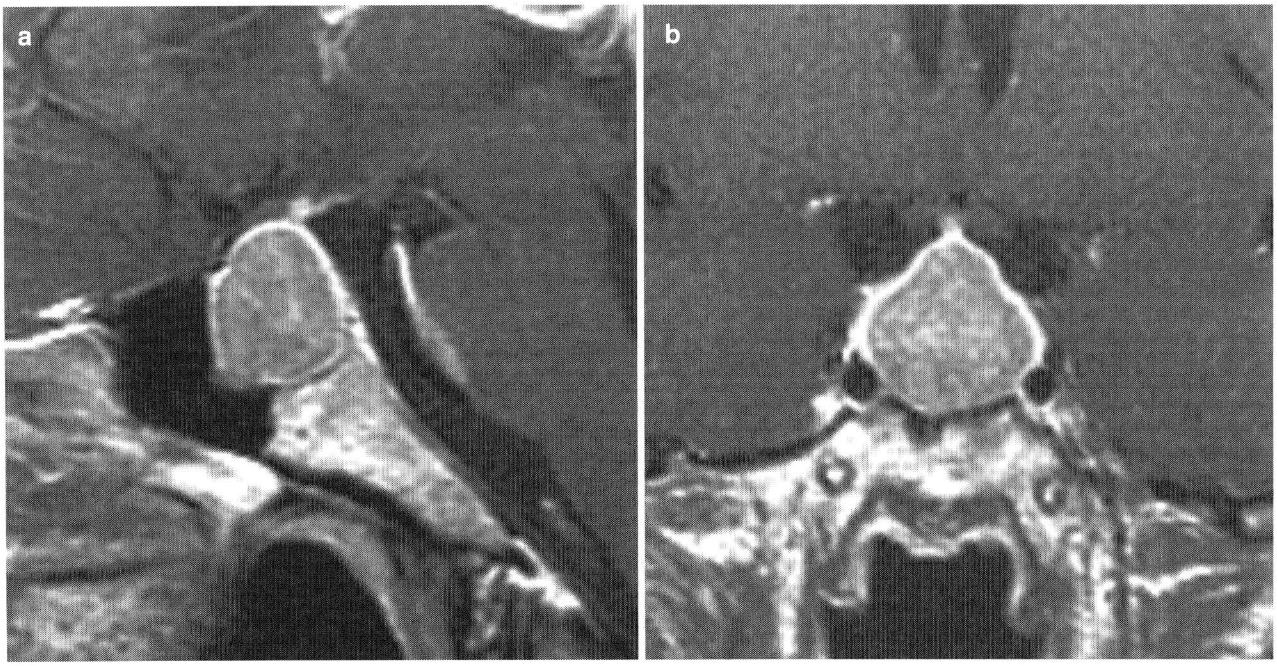

Fig. 10.3 Nonfunctioning pituitary adenoma. (**a**) Sagittal T1-weighted post-gadolinium image. (**b**) Coronal T1-weighted post-gadolinium image. A hypoenhancing sellar mass abuts the cavernous internal carotid arteries without encasement. There is suprasellar extension but no significant mass effect on the optic chiasm

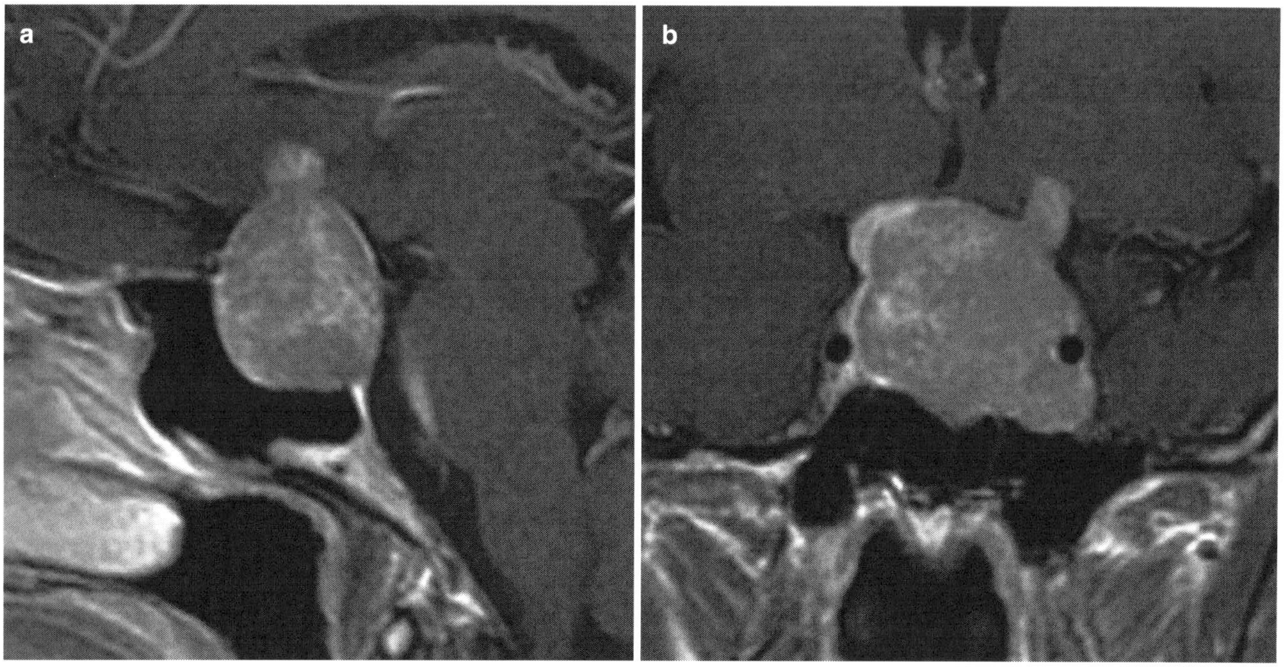

Fig. 10.4 Nonfunctioning pituitary adenoma. (**a**) Sagittal T1-weighted post-gadolinium image. (**b**) Coronal T1-weighted post-gadolinium image. There is a hypoenhancing sellar mass with remodeling of the sellar floor. The mass encases the left cavernous internal carotid artery, suggestive of cavernous invasion. The image also shows suprasellar extension with elevation of the optic chiasm, with a small nodular component contacting the left hypothalamus. The normal gland appears along the superior right aspect of the mass

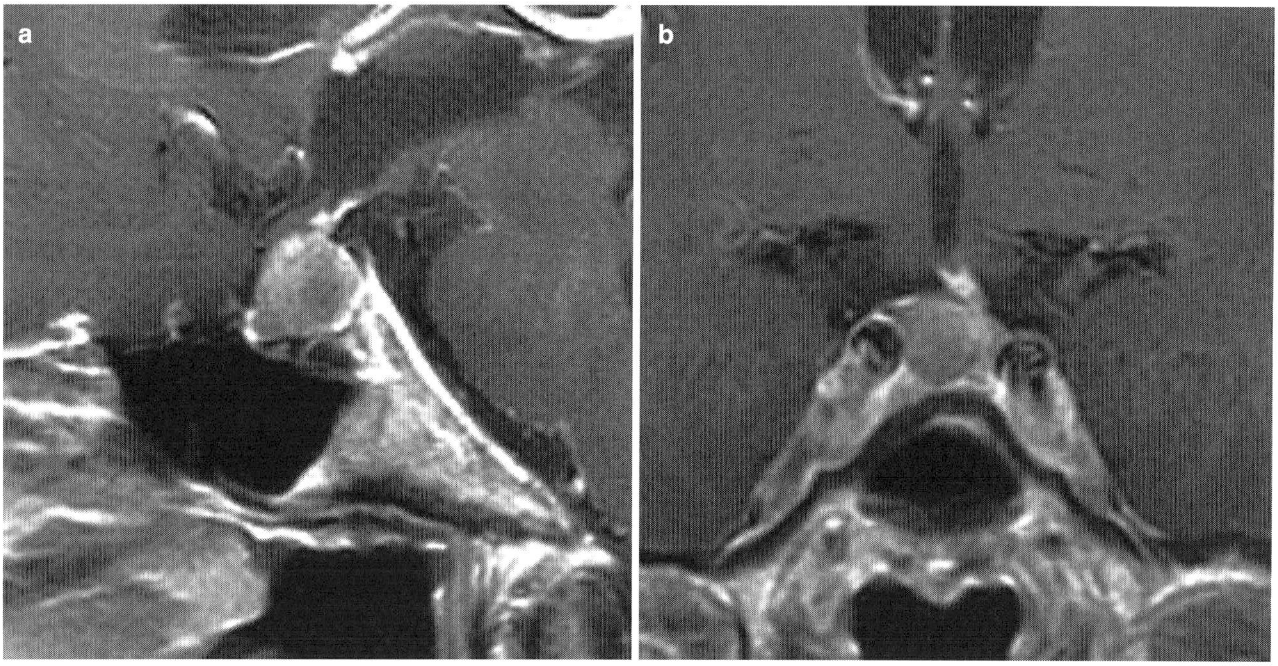

Fig. 10.5 Nonfunctioning pituitary adenoma. (**a**) Sagittal T1-weighted post-gadolinium image. (**b**) Coronal T1-weighted post-gadolinium image. There is a hypoenhancing sellar mass abutting the right cavernous internal carotid artery without encasement. The pituitary stalk is deviated to the left

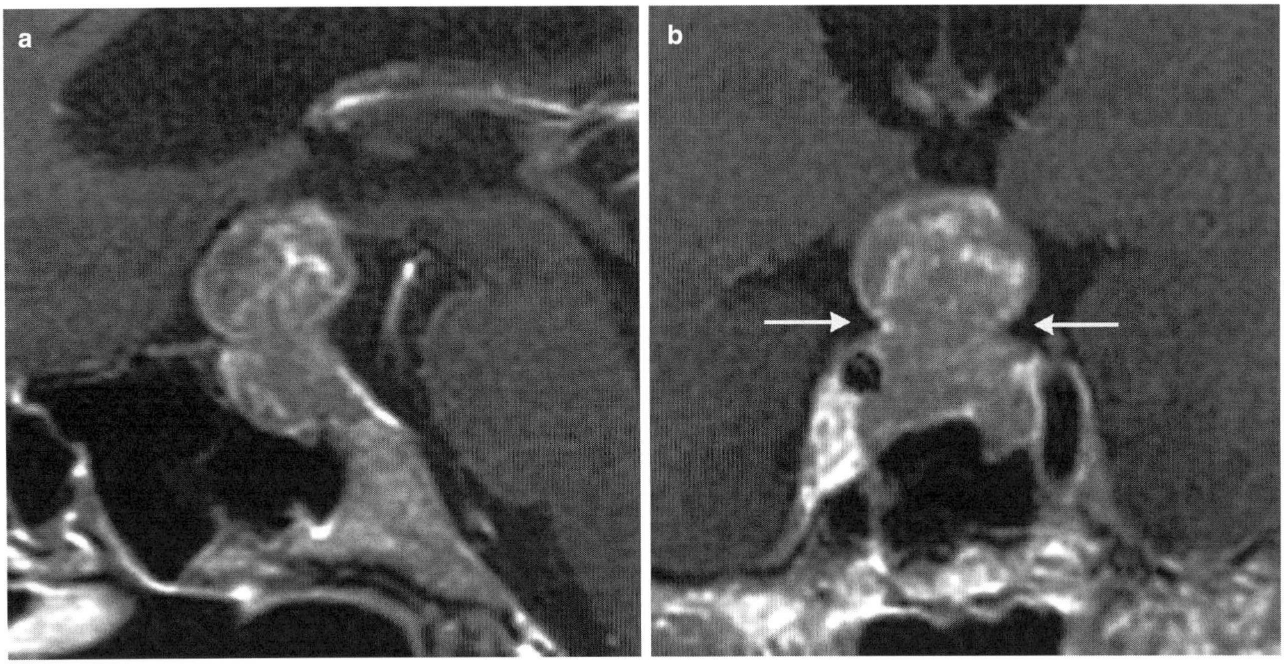

Fig. 10.6 Nonfunctioning pituitary adenoma. (**a**) Sagittal T1-weighted post-gadolinium image. (**b**) Coronal T1-weighted post-gadolinium image. A hypoenhancing sellar mass remodels the sellar floor with a nodular component extending to the suprasellar compartment. The mass demonstrates a "snowman" appearance with a waist indicating the level of dural defect or dural thinning (*white arrows*). The optic chiasm is likely to be superiorly displaced. The mass abuts the cavernous internal carotid arteries without encasement

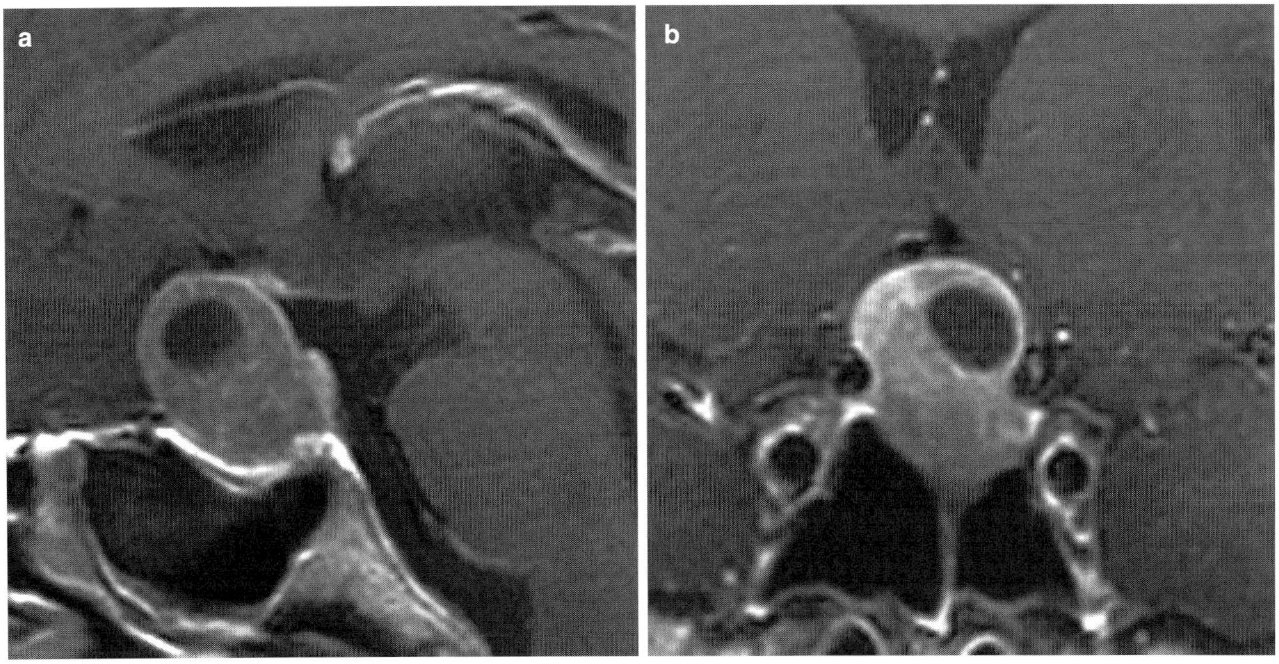

Fig. 10.7 Nonfunctioning pituitary adenoma. (**a**) Sagittal T1-weighted post-gadolinium image. (**b**) Coronal T1-weighted post-gadolinium image. There is a hypoenhancing sellar mass with remodeling of the sellar floor and a partly cystic component extending to the suprasellar compartment. The optic chiasm is superiorly displaced

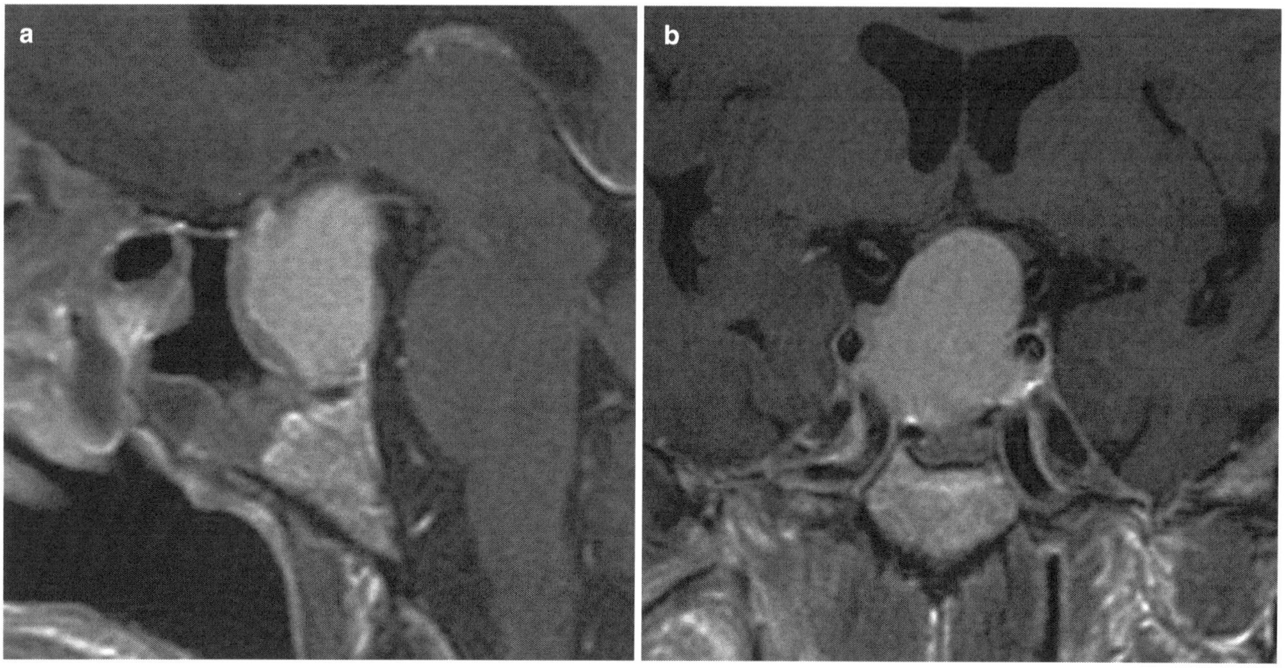

Fig. 10.8 Nonfunctioning pituitary adenoma. (**a**) Sagittal T1-weighted post-gadolinium image. (**b**) Coronal T1-weighted post-gadolinium image. A hypoenhancing sellar mass remodels the sellar floor and extends to the suprasellar compartment, displacing the optic chiasm superiorly. The mass abuts the cavernous internal carotid arteries without encasement

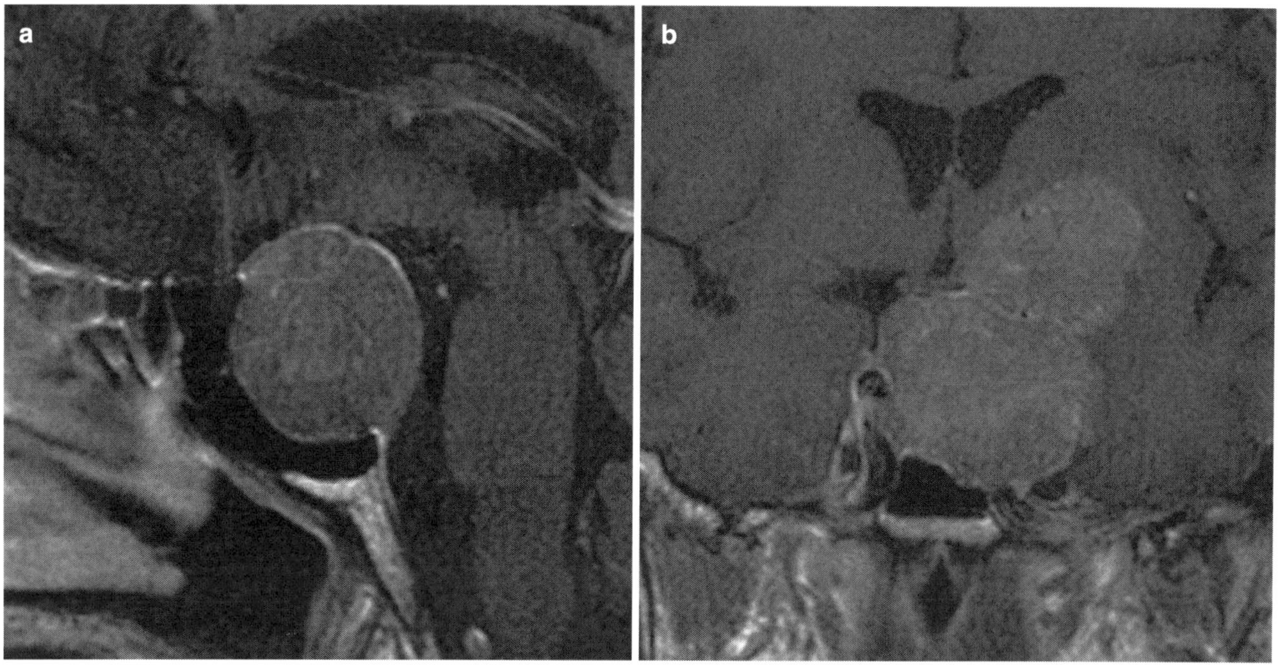

Fig. 10.9 Nonfunctioning pituitary adenoma. (**a**) Sagittal T1-weighted post-gadolinium image. (**b**) Coronal T1-weighted post-gadolinium image. There is a hypoenhancing sellar mass with remodeling of the sellar floor and a nodular component extending to the left suprasellar compartment impressing on the left hypothalamus. The mass extends to the left cavernous sinus, lateral to the cavernous internal carotid artery. On the right, the mass abuts the right cavernous internal carotid artery without definite encasement

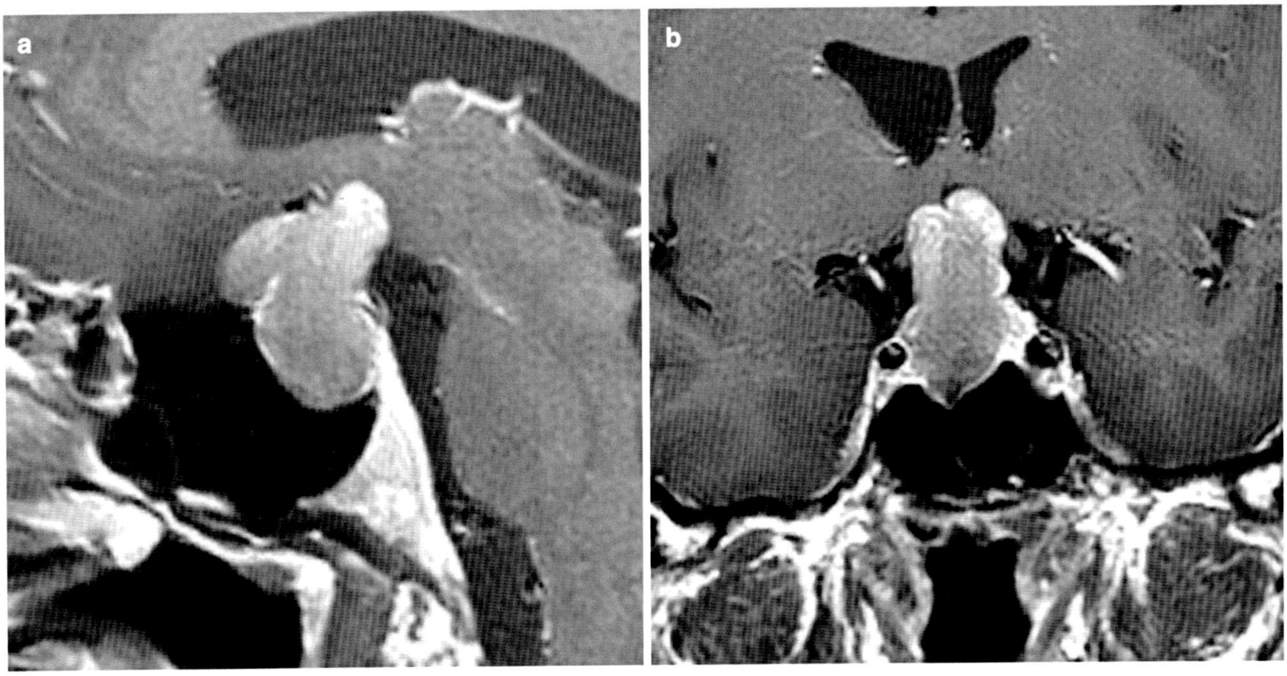

Fig. 10.10 Nonfunctioning pituitary adenoma. (**a**) Sagittal T1-weighted post-gadolinium image. (**b**) Coronal T1-weighted post-gadolinium image. A hypoenhancing sellar/suprasellar mass contacts the hypothalamus and displaces optic chiasm superiorly. The mass abuts the right cavernous internal carotid artery without encasement

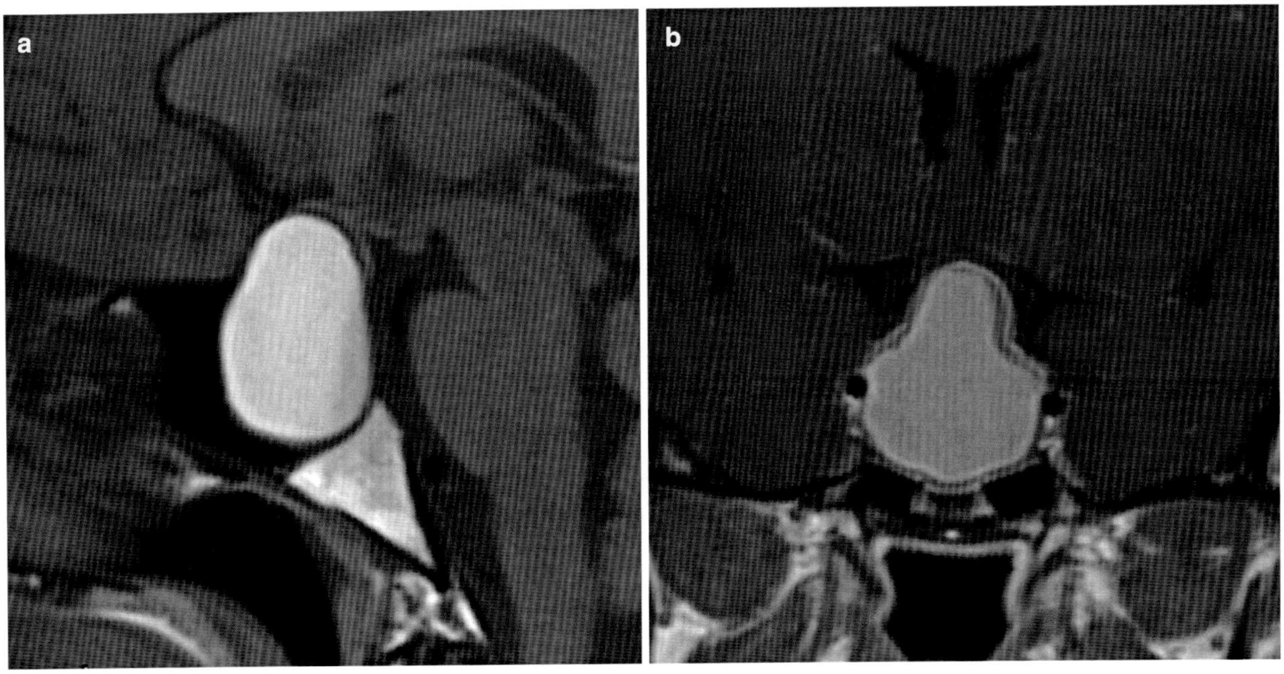

Fig. 10.11 Nonfunctioning pituitary adenoma. (**a**) Sagittal T1-weighted pre-gadolinium image. (**b**) Coronal T1-weighted post-gadolinium image. There is a peripherally enhancing sellar mass containing T1 hyperintense content, with remodeling of the sellar floor and a component extending to the suprasellar compartment contacting the hypothalamus. The optic chiasm is superiorly displaced. The mass abuts the cavernous internal carotid arteries without encasement

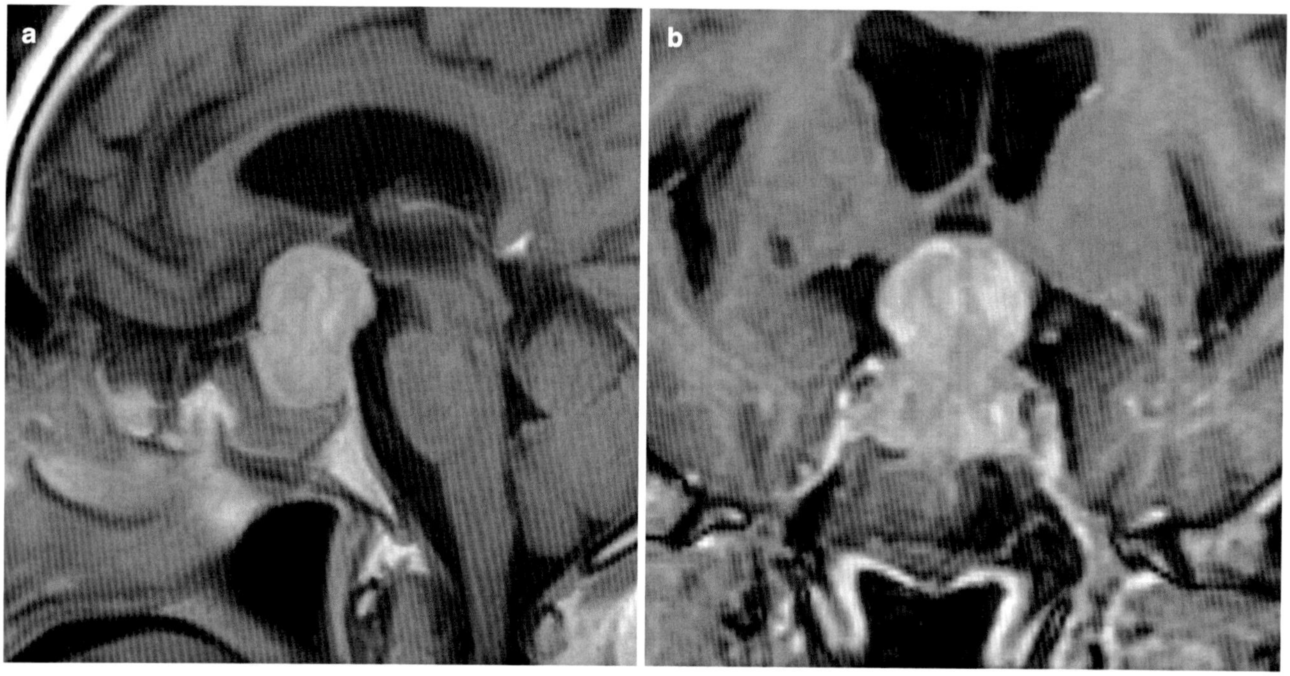

Fig. 10.12 Nonfunctioning pituitary adenoma. (**a**) Sagittal T1-weighted post-gadolinium image. (**b**) Coronal T1-weighted post-gadolinium image. A hypoenhancing sellar/suprasellar mass contacts the hypothalamus and displaces the optic chiasm superiorly. The mass abuts the right cavernous internal carotid artery without encasement

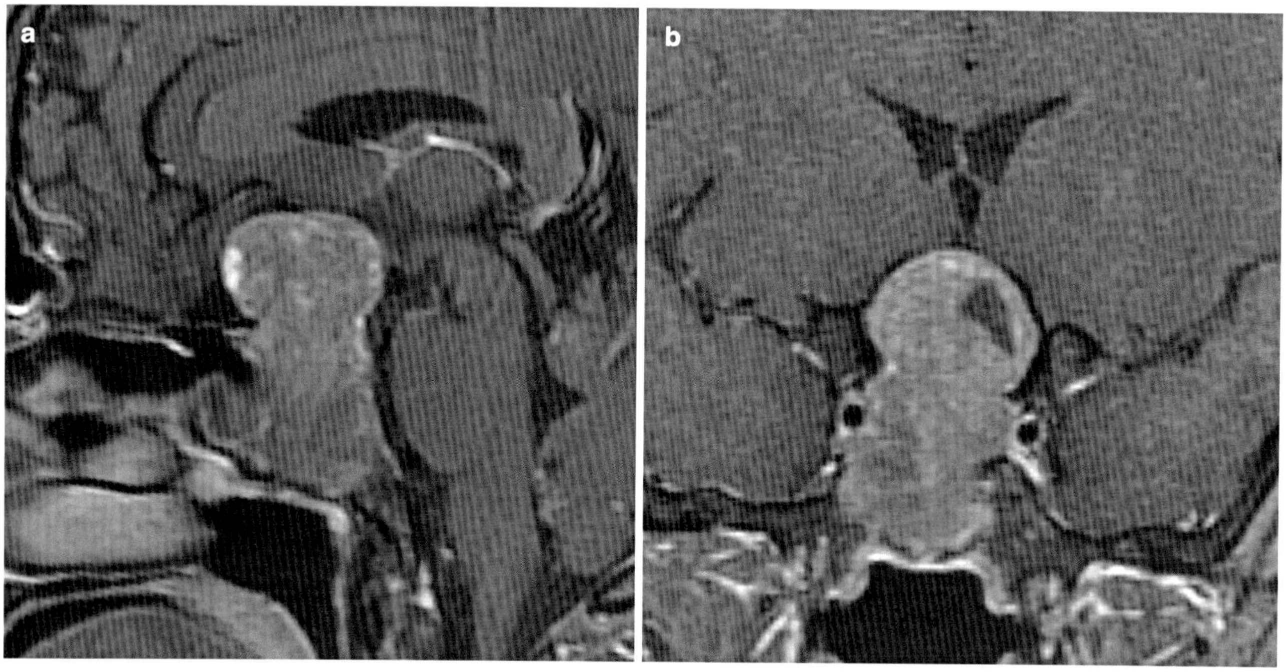

Fig. 10.13 Nonfunctioning pituitary adenoma. (**a**) Sagittal T1-weighted post-gadolinium image. (**b**) Coronal T1-weighted post-gadolinium image. There is a heterogeneously enhancing sellar mass with erosion of the sellar floor and a nodular component extending to the suprasellar compartment, contacting the hypothalamus. The optic chiasm is superiorly displaced. The mass abuts the right cavernous internal carotid artery and possibly invades the right cavernous sinus

10.2.2 Histopathology

- In 40–50 % of cases, NFPAs demonstrate immunoreactivity for gonadotrope-secreting cells, but it is exceedingly rare for them to secrete functional follicle-stimulating hormone (FSH) or luteinizing hormone (LH) causing clinically apparent changes [4, 7–9]. (*See* the later section on gonadotroph adenomas.)
- Silent FSH/LH adenomas are the most common subtype of surgically resected NFPA. They comprise large cells with a sinusoidal or sheetlike growth pattern that may be interrupted by pseudorosettes and pseudopapillae. Most adenomas stain for both FSH and LH, followed by FSH alone and finally LH alone. Many NFPAs also stain for the alpha subunit [4, 10].
- Null-cell adenomas do not stain for any of the anterior pituitary hormone immunostains (Fig. 10.14). They are composed of small to medium cells in sinusoidal or diffuse growth patterns. Chromogranin A is typically strongly expressed and can be used to differentiate them from other intrasellar neoplasms [4, 10].
- Tumors staining positive for any hormonal subtype may be "silent." They comprise 12.6 % of all pituitary adenomas. The most common of these are silent-ACTH (adrenocorticotropic hormone) adenomas, followed by plurihormonal tumors and then silent prolactinomas [4].
- Null-cell adenomas are more likely to be atypical adenomas than are silent-gonadotropin adenomas.

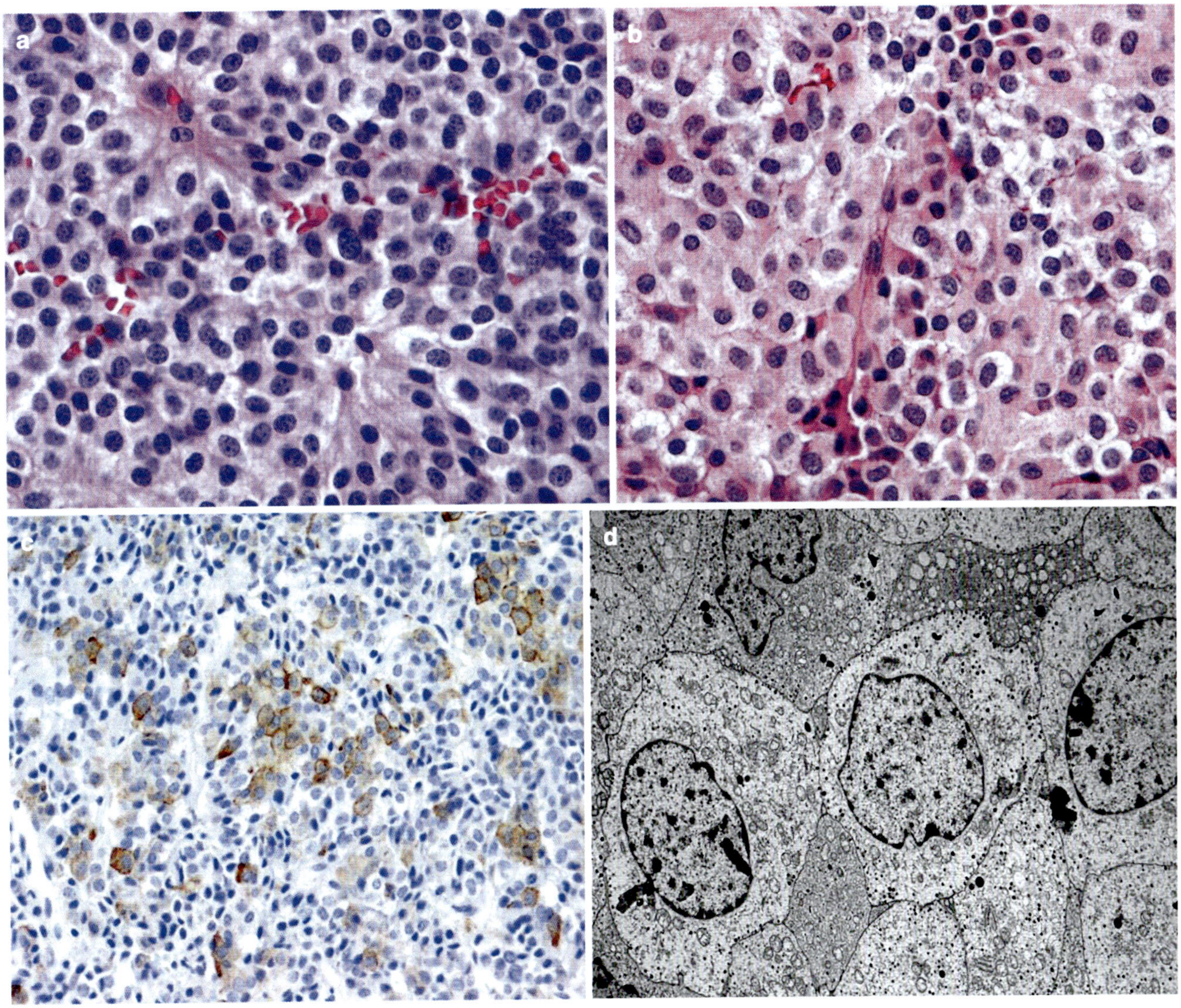

Fig. 10.14 Null-cell adenoma. (**a**) Null-cell adenomas are usually composed of chromophobic cells arranged in a diffuse or solid growth pattern. (**b**) Oncocytic changes are not unusual in these adenomas. (**c**) Although the great majority of null-cell adenomas are immunonegative for any pituitary hormones, focal immunostain for the α-subunit of glycoproteins may be seen. (**d**) Ultrastructural studies reveal sparse numbers of small, neurosecretory granules with lack of differentiation of any adenohypophyseal specific cell type

10.3 Clinical Management

10.3.1 Surgery

- Indications for surgery typically include visual loss, severe headaches, panhypopituitarism, or the presence of a macroadenoma (diameter ≥10 mm).
- Patients with smaller, incidentally discovered, asymptomatic macroadenomas that abut the optic chiasm may not require initial surgical intervention, but should undergo initial formal visual field testing and thorough endocrine evaluations. They may be monitored with biannual visual examinations and serial MR imaging if conservative rather than surgical management is in the patient's best interest [11].
- Transsphenoidal surgery has been the mainstay treatment of NFPAs for decades, providing excellent outcomes in the majority of cases.
- Giant adenomas with significant suprasellar or lateral extension may require staged or simultaneous transsphenoidal and transcranial approaches in order to achieve maximal tumor debulking [12, 13].
- Improvement in endocrine function has been reported in approximately 30 % of patients following surgical resection of NFPAs [14].
- The majority of patients with preoperative visual loss will have improved vision following surgery [15, 16].
- For intrasellar macroadenomas, rates of total surgical resection range from 80 to 95 % [17].
- Reported total resection rates for larger or invasive nonfunctioning macroadenomas have generally been between 35 and 60 %, depending on the size and the degree of surrounding tumor invasion [5, 17, 18].
- Recurrence following total resection has been reported in 5–27 % of patients [2, 3, 5, 15, 18–21].

10.3.2 Adjunctive Radiation Therapy and Radiosurgery

- Postoperative radiation has demonstrated improved long-term tumor control in patients with subtotal tumor resection, but it is associated with risks including hypopituitarism, visual loss, and formation of new tumors [18].
- Stereotactic radiosurgery has demonstrated tumor growth control rates in the range of 88–97 %, with acceptable risk profiles [22–26].
- The typical dose used to treat residual or recurrent NFPAs in the parasellar region is 15–16 Gy delivered to the 50 % isodose line [24, 27].

10.3.3 Hypopituitarism and Hormonal Replacement

- The incidence of postoperative hypopituitarism following transsphenoidal resection of NFPAs has been reported to be 12–44 % [28, 29] .
- At many pituitary centers, an incidence rate of 3–5 % for new anterior hypopituitarism is an achievable goal.
- Patients with macroadenomas or pituitary apoplexy often already have hypopituitarism upon presentation; however, requiring primary correction of several hormonal axes before treatment is initiated:
  - Replacement of the ACTH-cortisol axis is typically achieved with hydrocortisone or prednisone. Two daily doses at physiological levels are generally sufficient.
  - Oral levothyroxine is typically used to replace thyroid hormone deficiency.
  - The growth hormone (GH) axis can be replaced in the form of a daily injection of recombinant human growth hormone.
  - Multiple testosterone replacement preparations are available, including intramuscular injections, buccal mucosal patches, and topical patches or gels.
  - Patients with diabetes insipidus from stalk or posterior gland dysfunction may require oral or intranasal vasopressin (DDAVP), but this entity occurs much more commonly in a transient setting following surgical treatment for pituitary lesions.

References

1. Sanno N, Teramoto A, Osamura RY, Horvath E, Kovacs K, Lloyd RV, Scheithauer BW. Pathology of pituitary tumors. Neurosurg Clin N Am. 2003;14:25–39.
2. Fahlbusch R, Buchfelder M, Honegger J, Nomikos P. Nonfunctional pituitary adenomas. In: Krisht AF, Tindall GT, editors. Pituitary disorders: comprehensive management. Baltimore: Lippincott Williams & Wilkins; 1999. p. 281–5.
3. Ebersold MJ, Quast LM, Laws Jr ER, Scheithauer B, Randall RV. Long-term results in transsphenoidal removal of nonfunctioning pituitary adenomas. J Neurosurg. 1986;64:713–9.
4. Saeger W, Ludecke DK, Buchfelder M, Fahlbusch R, Quabbe HJ, Petersenn S. Pathohistological classification of pituitary tumors: 10 years of experience with the German Pituitary Tumor Registry. Eur J Endocrinol. 2007;156:203–16.
5. Ferrante E, Ferraroni M, Castrignano T, Menicatti L, Anagni M, Reimondo G, et al. Non-functioning pituitary adenoma database: a useful resource to improve the clinical management of pituitary tumors. Eur J Endocrinol. 2006;155:823–9.
6. Patten JP. Neurological differential diagnosis. 2nd ed. London: Springer; 1996.

7. Black PM, Hsu DW, Klibanski A, Kliman B, Jameson JL, Ridgway EC, et al. Hormone production in clinically nonfunctioning pituitary adenomas. J Neurosurg. 1987;66:244–50.
8. Saccomanno K, Gil del Alamo P, Bassetti M, Reza-Elahi F, Spada A. In vitro detection of glycoprotein production and secretion by human nonfunctioning pituitary adenomas. J Endocrinol Invest. 1993;16:109–15.
9. Yamada S, Asa SL, Kovacs K, Muller P, Smyth HS. Analysis of hormone secretion by clinically nonfunctioning human pituitary adenomas using the reverse hemolytic plaque assay. J Clin Endocrinol Metab. 1989;68:73–80.
10. Al-Brahim NY, Asa SL. My approach to pathology of the pituitary gland. J Clin Pathol. 2006;59:1245–53.
11. Molitch ME, Russell EJ. The pituitary "incidentaloma". Ann Intern Med. 1990;112:925–31.
12. Alleyne Jr CH, Barrow DL, Oyesiku NM. Combined transsphenoidal and pterional craniotomy approach to giant pituitary tumors. Surg Neurol. 2002;57:380–90; discussion 390.
13. Saito K, Kuwayama A, Yamamoto N, Sugita K. The transsphenoidal removal of nonfunctioning pituitary adenomas with suprasellar extensions: the open sella method and intentionally staged operation. Neurosurgery. 1995;36:668–75; discussion 675–6.
14. Nomikos P, Ladar C, Fahlbusch R, Buchfelder M. Impact of primary surgery on pituitary function in patients with non-functioning pituitary adenomas -- a study on 721 patients. Acta Neurochir (Wien). 2004;146:27–35.
15. Ciric I, Mikhael M, Stafford T, Lawson L, Garces R. Transsphenoidal microsurgery of pituitary macroadenomas with long-term follow-up results. J Neurosurg. 1983;59:395–401.
16. Trautmann JC, Laws Jr ER. Visual status after transsphenoidal surgery at the Mayo Clinic, 1971–1982. Am J Ophthalmol. 1983;96: 200–8.
17. Zada G, Kelly DF, Cohan P, Wang C, Swerdloff R. Endonasal transsphenoidal approach for pituitary adenomas and other sellar lesions: an assessment of efficacy, safety, and patient impressions. J Neurosurg. 2003;98:350–8.
18. Chang EF, Zada G, Kim S, Lamborn KR, Quinones-Hinojosa A, Tyrrell JB, et al. Long-term recurrence and mortality after surgery and adjuvant radiotherapy for nonfunctional pituitary adenomas. J Neurosurg. 2008;108:736–45.
19. Bradley KM, Adams CB, Potter CP, Wheeler DW, Anslow PJ, Burke CW. An audit of selected patients with non-functioning pituitary adenoma treated by transsphenoidal surgery without irradiation. Clin Endocrinol (Oxf). 1994;41:655–9.
20. Dekkers OM, Pereira AM, Roelfsema F, Voormolen JH, Neelis KJ, Schroijen MA, et al. Observation alone after transsphenoidal surgery for nonfunctioning pituitary macroadenoma. J Clin Endocrinol Metab. 2006;91:1796–801.
21. Jane Jr JA, Laws Jr ER. The surgical management of pituitary adenomas in a series of 3,093 patients. J Am Coll Surg. 2001;193:651–9.
22. Losa M, Valle M, Mortini P, Franzin A, da Passano CF, Cenzato M, et al. Gamma knife surgery for treatment of residual nonfunctioning pituitary adenomas after surgical debulking. J Neurosurg. 2004;100:438–44.
23. Pollock BE, Carpenter PC. Stereotactic radiosurgery as an alternative to fractionated radiotherapy for patients with recurrent or residual nonfunctioning pituitary adenomas. Neurosurgery. 2003;53: 1086–91; discussion 1091–4.
24. Sheehan JP, Kondziolka D, Flickinger J, Lunsford LD. Radiosurgery for residual or recurrent nonfunctioning pituitary adenoma. J Neurosurg. 2002;97:408–14.
25. Wowra B, Stummer W. Efficacy of gamma knife radiosurgery for nonfunctioning pituitary adenomas: a quantitative follow up with magnetic resonance imaging-based volumetric analysis. J Neurosurg. 2002;97:429–32.
26. Iwai Y, Yamanaka K, Yoshioka K. Radiosurgery for nonfunctioning pituitary adenomas. Neurosurgery. 2005;56:699–705.
27. Sheehan JP, Kondziolka D, Flickinger J, Lunsford LD. Radiosurgery for nonfunctioning pituitary adenoma. Neurosurg Focus. 2003;14:e9.
28. Petruson B, Jakobsson KE, Elfverson J, Bengtsson BA. Five-year follow-up of nonsecreting pituitary adenomas. Arch Otolaryngol Head Neck Surg. 1995;121:317–22.
29. Nielsen EH, Lindholm J, Laurberg P, Bjerre P, Christiansen JS, Hagen C, et al. Nonfunctioning pituitary adenoma: incidence, causes of death and quality of life in relation to pituitary function. Pituitary. 2007;10:67–73.

Prolactinomas

11

Gabriel Zada, M. Beatriz S. Lopes, Srinivasan Mukundan Jr., and Edward Laws Jr.

11.1 Epidemiology and Clinical Presentation

- Prolactinomas are the most commonly occurring functional pituitary adenomas, accounting for 40 % of all pituitary adenomas [1].
- In surgical series, however, they typically comprise a smaller proportion of tumors (approximately 8–10 %) because medical management is often successful [2].
- In women, prolactinomas typically present with amenorrhea, oligomenorrhea, infertility, and/or galactorrhea. When galactorrhea accompanies amenorrhea, the incidence of a prolactinoma is about 70–80 % [3].
- In men, the typical presentation is decreased libido and/or sexual dysfunction.
- Increased body fat is associated with hyperprolactinemia in men and women.
- Chronic hyperprolactinemia may result in osteoporosis [4].
- In adolescents, prolactinomas may cause delayed puberty.
- Other causes of hyperprolactinemia (e.g., stalk effect, medications, pregnancy, hypothyroidism) should always be ruled out.

11.2 Diagnosis

11.2.1 Imaging

- Imaging of prolactinomas is similar to imaging of NFPAs (Figs. 11.1, 11.2, 11.3, 11.4, and 11.5).

11.2.2 Histopathology

- Figure 11.6 shows several histopathologic characteristics of prolactin (PRL) cell adenomas, including central nuclei with delicate chromatin, microcalcifications, and focal PRL immunoreactivity in the tumor cells despite treatment.

G. Zada, MD, MS (✉)
Department of Neurological Surgery, Keck School of Medicine, University of Southern California, 1200 N State Street, #3300, Los Angeles, CA 90033, USA
e-mail: gzada@usc.edu

M.B.S. Lopes, MD, PhD
Department of Pathology (Neuropathology), University of Virginia School of Medicine, 1215 Lee Street, Room 3060–HEP, Charlottesville, VA 22908, USA
e-mail: msl2e@virginia.edu

S. Mukundan Jr., PhD, MD
Department of Radiology, Brigham and Women's Hospital, 75 Francis Street, Boston, MA 02115, USA
e-mail: smukundan@partners.org

E. Laws Jr., MD
Department of Neurosurgery, Brigham and Women's Hospital, 15 Francis Street, Boston, MA 02115, USA
e-mail: elaws@partners.org

G. Zada et al. (eds.), *Atlas of Sellar and Parasellar Lesions: Clinical, Radiologic, and Pathologic Correlations*, DOI 10.1007/978-3-319-22855-6_11

11.3 Clinical Management

11.3.1 Endocrinological Diagnosis

- A serum prolactin level greater than 200 ng/mL is typically indicative of a prolactin-secreting adenoma [5].
- Moderately elevated levels (<200 ng/mL) require correlation to the size of the tumor, as they may represent a stalk compression effect rather than a prolactinoma.
- Microprolactinomas also may have prolactin levels in the range of 30–200 ng/mL [1]. It should also be noted that various physiological states (e.g., pregnancy and breastfeeding) and a wide variety of medications (e.g., antipsychotics) may elevate the serum prolactin level.
- Clinicians must beware of the "hook effect" phenomenon, in which an excessively high serum prolactin level results in a laboratory value that is significantly lower than the actual value, secondary to the presence of excessive antigen [6]. This effect can be avoided if serial dilution testing of serum samples is carried out for all macroadenomas that are suspected of being prolactinomas.
- Macroprolactinemia is another diagnostic pitfall, in which macroprolactin, a biologically inactive form of prolactin with a high molecular mass, is detected by standard immunoassays. The presence of macroprolactin may lead to misdiagnosis in as many as 10 % of all reported instances of biochemical hyperprolactinemia, so it should be included in the differential diagnosis of hyperprolactinemia [7]. Gel filtration chromatography remains the gold standard for diagnosing macroprolactinemia.

11.3.2 Medical Treatment

- Prolactinomas usually can be treated successfully with medical management.
- Dopamine agonists (DAs) are the first line of therapy, with bromocriptine and cabergoline being the two most commonly used agents.
- Cabergoline is more potent than bromocriptine and therefore requires dosing less frequently (usually twice a week).
- DAs are effective in normalizing serum prolactin levels in 85–90 % of cases [1, 8].
- DAs are effective in reducing tumor size in the majority of patients; tumors may shrink up to 80 % within 6 weeks of medication use [9].
- Successful treatment accompanied by rapid tumor shrinkage has been reported to result in cerebrospinal fluid leaks, however, which often require surgical repair [10].
- For women desiring to become pregnant, bromocriptine therapy may be initiated and then discontinued once the patient is known to be pregnant [11].
- Women treated successfully for prolactinomas with DAs have a pregnancy rate as high as the general population of age-matched women [12].
- Prolactinomas may be resistant to DAs in 6–25 % of patients [1, 13, 14].
- DA-resistant prolactinomas, especially in men, tend to be highly invasive and vascular tumors. Medical treatment for DA-resistant prolactinomas often includes estrogen receptor antagonists and temozolomide [15].
- Valvular heart disease (tricuspid regurgitation) may develop with high doses of cabergoline. Practitioners should remain mindful of this adverse effect [16].
- Some patients can be weaned off medical treatment following successful hormonal remission and tumor disappearance on imaging studies [17].

11.3.3 Surgical Management

- There are several indications for surgical management of prolactinomas:
  - DA-resistant prolactinoma [14]
  - Visual loss or other neurological signs requiring decompression and not responding to early DA therapy
  - Intolerance of DA medications
  - Desire for fertility and tumor removal in women of childbearing age
- Surgical remission is defined by normalization of serum prolactin.
- A postoperative day 1 serum prolactin level of less than 10 ng/mL is highly predictive of long-term remission [18].
- Long-term remission rates following surgery are 50–60 % for all lesions and 80–90 % for microadenomas [18–20].
- Radiosurgery as an adjunctive modality is effective for normalization of serum prolactin in 25 % of patients and for tumor control in 89–100 % of patients with prolactinomas [21, 22].
- Recurrence of hyperprolactinemia has been reported in up to one third of patients following hormonal remission; it may occur more than a decade after remission [20, 23].

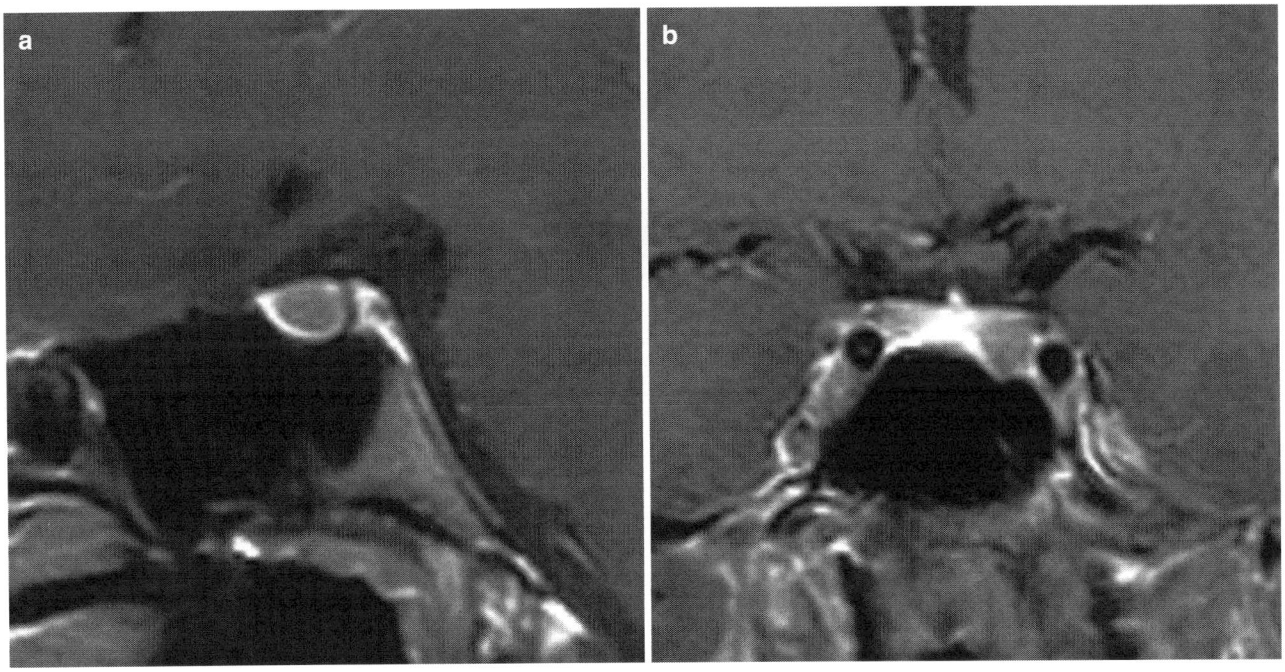

Fig. 11.1 Prolactinoma. (**a**) Sagittal T1-weighted post-gadolinium image. (**b**) Coronal T1-weighted post-gadolinium image. A small, hypoenhancing sellar mass is present in the left aspect of the sella. The mass abuts the left cavernous internal carotid artery without encasement

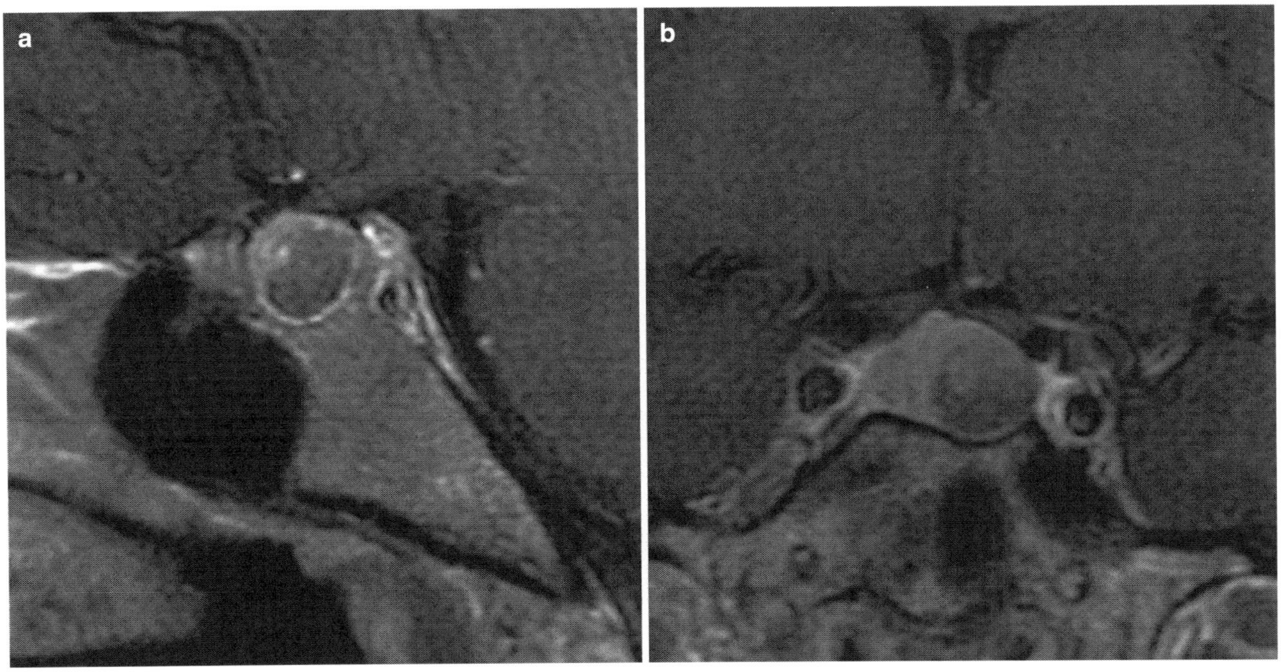

Fig. 11.2 Prolactinoma. (**a**) Sagittal T1-weighted post-gadolinium image. (**b**) Coronal T1-weighted post-gadolinium image. There is a hypoenhancing sellar mass in the left aspect of the sella, with erosion of the left sellar floor. The mass abuts the left cavernous internal carotid artery without encasement. There is mild elevation and rightward deviation of the pituitary stalk

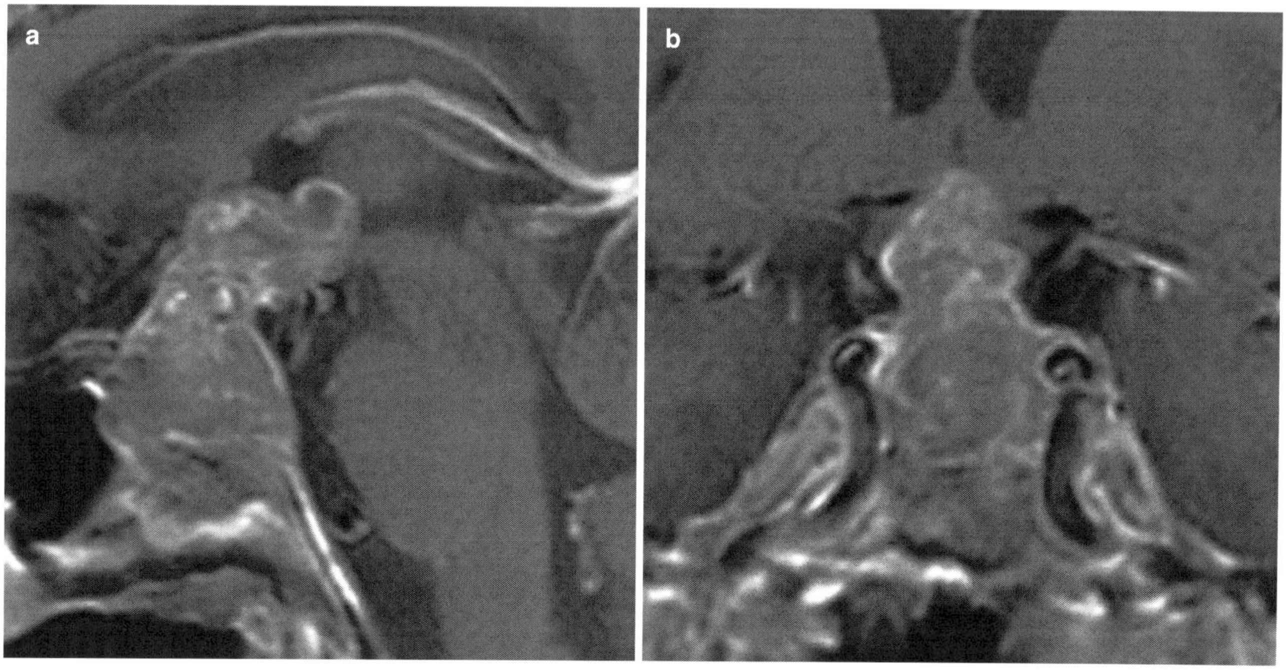

Fig. 11.3 Prolactinoma. (**a**) Sagittal T1-weighted post-gadolinium image. (**b**) Coronal T1-weighted post-gadolinium image. A heterogeneously enhancing sellar mass shows suprasellar extension and erosion of the sellar floor. The irregular, nodular suprasellar component extends to the floor of the third ventricle, contacting the hypothalamus. The mass abuts the cavernous internal carotid arteries without encasement

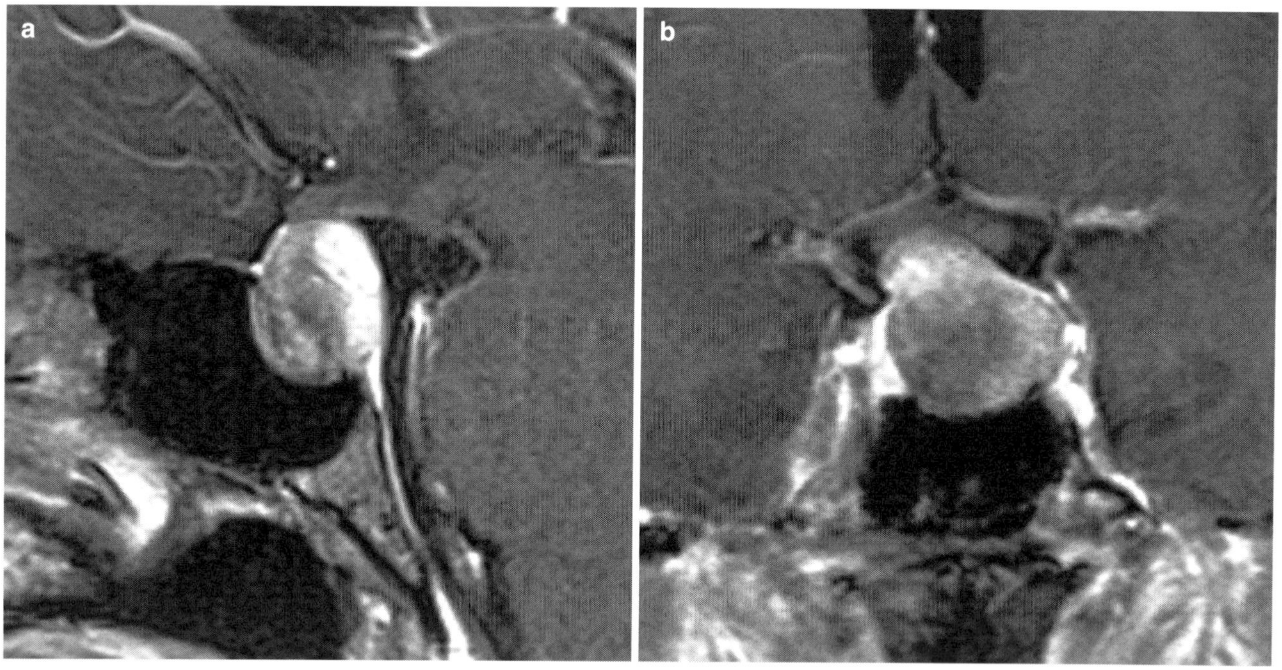

Fig. 11.4 Prolactinoma. (**a**) Sagittal T1-weighted post-gadolinium image. (**b**) Coronal T1-weighted post-gadolinium image. There is a hypoenhancing sellar mass with suprasellar extension and remodeling of the sellar floor. The mass abuts the left cavernous internal carotid artery without encasement. The mass also contacts the optic chiasm without significant displacement

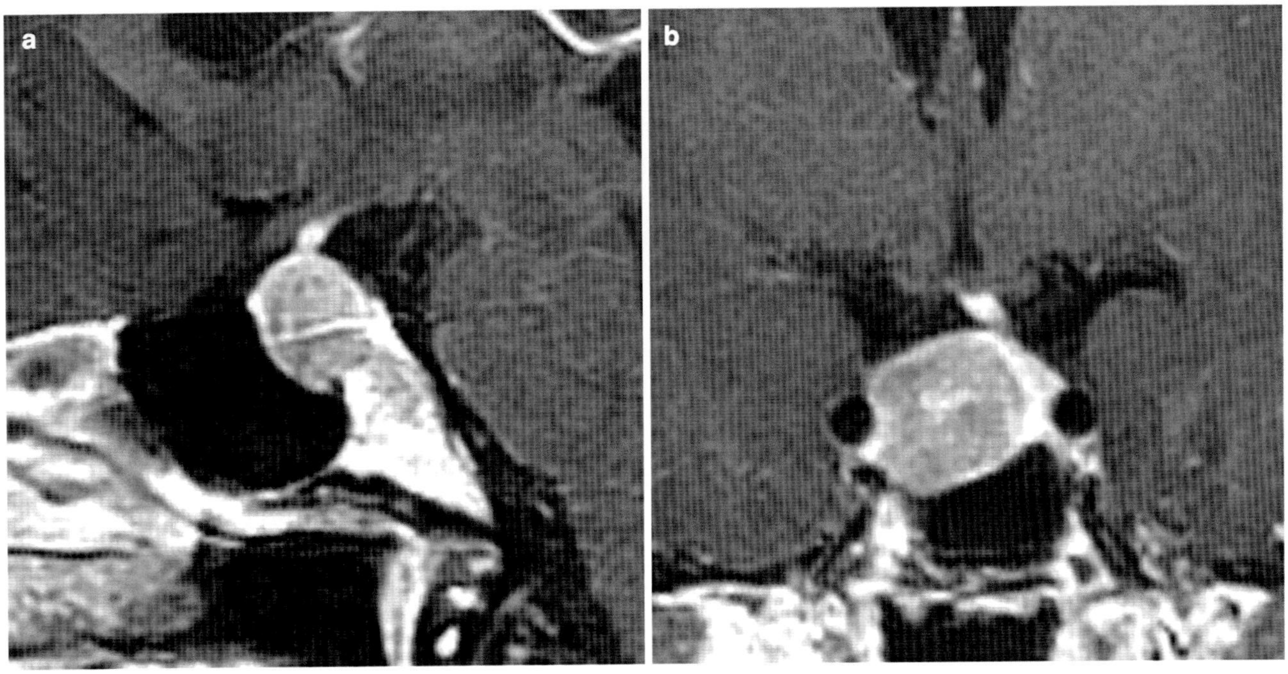

Fig. 11.5 Prolactinoma. (**a**) Sagittal T1-weighted post-gadolinium image. (**b**) Coronal T1-weighted post-gadolinium image. A hypoenhancing sellar mass is located in the right aspect of the sella, with erosion of the left sellar floor. The mass abuts the right cavernous internal carotid artery without encasement. There is leftward deviation of the pituitary stalk

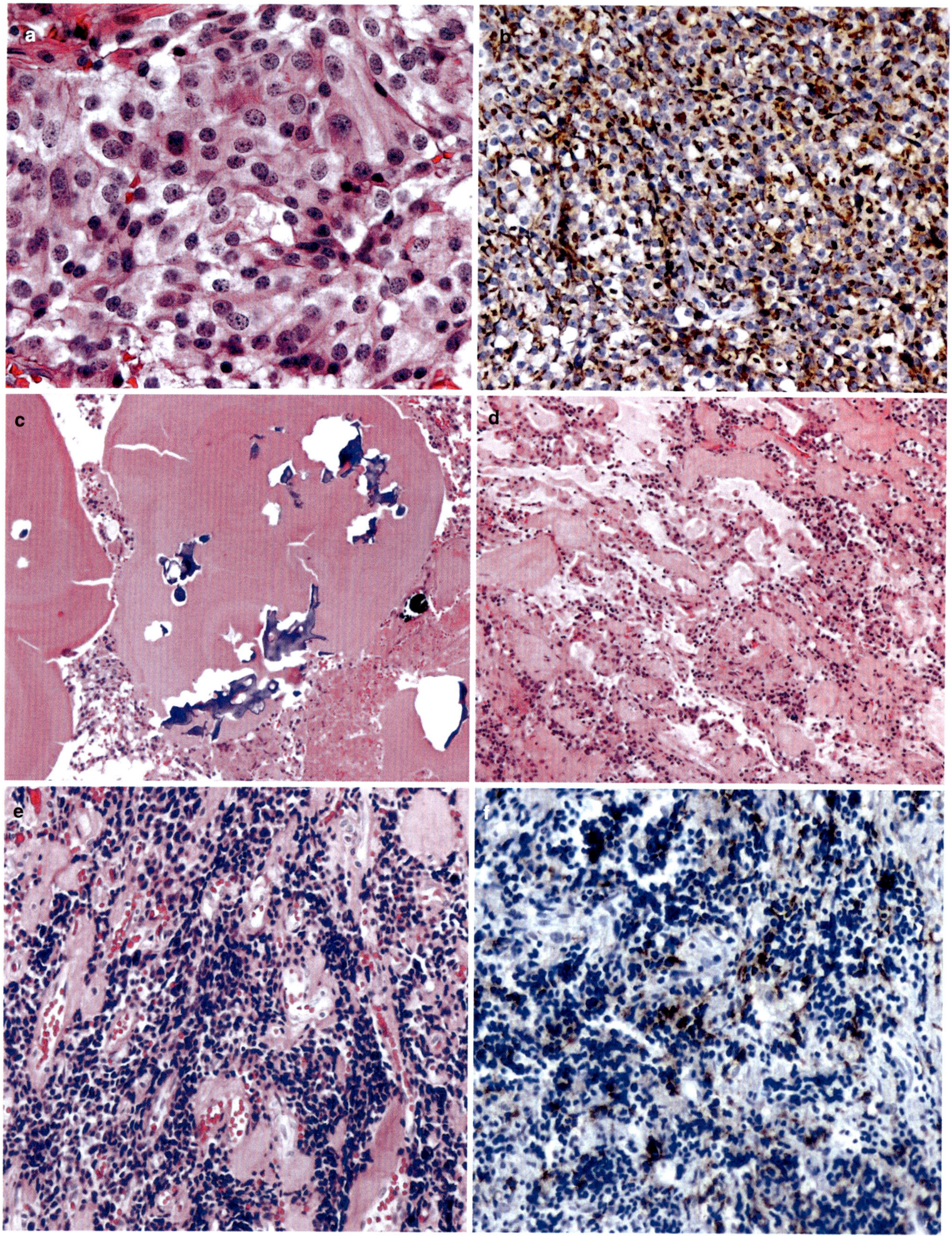

Fig. 11.6 Prolactin (PRL)-secreting adenoma. (**a**) PRL cell adenoma showing chromophobic-to-acidophilic cytoplasm and central nuclei with delicate chromatin. (**b**) PRL immunoreactivity is typically seen in a paranuclear location. (**c**) Microcalcifications are commonly seen in these tumors. (**d**, **e**) Prolactinomas may display variable degrees of shrinkage of the tumor cells and interstitial fibrosis after medical treatment. (**f**) Despite treatment, PRL immunoreactivity is focally seen in the tumor cells

References

1. Liu JK, Couldwell WT. Contemporary management of prolactinomas. Neurosurg Focus. 2004;16:E2.
2. Saeger W, Ludecke DK, Buchfelder M, Fahlbusch R, Quabbe HJ, Petersenn S. Pathohistological classification of pituitary tumors: 10 years of experience with the German pituitary tumor registry. Eur J Endocrinol. 2007;156:203–16.
3. Franks S, Murray MA, Jequier AM, Steele SJ, Nabarro JD, Jacobs HS. Incidence and significance of hyperprolactinaemia in women with amenorrhea. Clin Endocrinol (Oxf). 1975;4:597–607.
4. Duntas LH. Prolactinomas in children and adolescents--consequences in adult life. J Pediatr Endocrinol Metab. 2001;14:1227–32; discussion 1261–2.
5. Randall RV, Scheithauer BW, Laws Jr ER, Abboud CF, Ebersold MJ, Kao PC. Pituitary adenomas associated with hyperprolactinemia: a clinical and immunohistochemical study of 97 patients operated on transsphenoidally. Mayo Clin Proc. 1985;60:753–62.
6. Frieze TW, Mong DP, Koops MK. "Hook effect" in prolactinomas: case report and review of literature. Endocr Pract. 2002;8:296–303.
7. Smith TP, Kavanagh L, Healy ML, McKenna TJ. Technology insight: measuring prolactin in clinical samples. Nat Clin Pract Endocrinol Metab. 2007;3:279–89.
8. Weiss MH, Wycoff RR, Yadley R, Gott P, Feldon S. Bromocriptine treatment of prolactin-secreting tumors: surgical implications. Neurosurgery. 1983;12:640–2.
9. Vance ML, Thorner MO. Prolactinomas. Endocrinol Metab Clin North Am. 1987;16:731–53.
10. Lam G, Mehta V, Zada G. Spontaneous and medically induced cerebrospinal fluid leakage in the setting of pituitary adenomas: review of the literature. Neurosurg Focus. 2012;32:E2.
11. Molitch ME. Management of prolactinomas during pregnancy. J Reprod Med. 1999;44:1121–6.
12. Skrabanek P, McDonald D, Meagher D, de Valera E, Carroll C, Lanigan O, Powell D. Clinical course and outcome of thirty-five pregnancies in infertile hyperprolactinemic women. Fertil Steril. 1980;33:391–5.
13. Hamilton DK, Vance ML, Boulos PT, Laws ER. Surgical outcomes in hyporesponsive prolactinomas: analysis of patients with resistance or intolerance to dopamine agonists. Pituitary. 2005;8:53–60.
14. Vroonen L, Jaffrain-Rea ML, Petrossians P, Tamagno G, Chanson P, Vilar L, et al. Prolactinomas resistant to standard doses of cabergoline: a multicenter study of 92 patients. Eur J Endocrinol. 2012;167:651–62.
15. Oh MC, Aghi MK. Dopamine agonist-resistant prolactinomas. J Neurosurg. 2011;114:1369–79.
16. Colao A, Galderisi M, Di Sarno A, Pardo M, Gaccione M, D'Andrea M, et al. Increased prevalence of tricuspid regurgitation in patients with prolactinomas chronically treated with cabergoline. J Clin Endocrinol Metab. 2008;93:3777–84. doi:10.1210/jc.2007-1403.
17. Colao A, Savastano S. Medical treatment of prolactinomas. Nat Rev Endocrinol. 2011;7:267–78.
18. Amar AP, Couldwell WT, Chen JC, Weiss MH. Predictive value of serum prolactin levels measured immediately after transsphenoidal surgery. J Neurosurg. 2002;97:307–14.
19. Zada G, Kelly DF, Cohan P, Wang C, Swerdloff R. Endonasal transsphenoidal approach for pituitary adenomas and other sellar lesions: an assessment of efficacy, safety, and patient impressions. J Neurosurg. 2003;98:350–8.
20. Kreutzer J, Buslei R, Wallaschofski H, Hofmann B, Nimsky C, Fahlbusch R, Buchfelder M. Operative treatment of prolactinomas: indications and results in a current consecutive series of 212 patients. Eur J Endocrinol. 2008;158:11–8.
21. Pouratian N, Sheehan J, Jagannathan J, Laws Jr ER, Steiner L, Vance ML. Gamma knife radiosurgery for medically and surgically refractory prolactinomas. Neurosurgery. 2006;59:255–66.
22. Tanaka S, Link MJ, Brown PD, Stafford SL, Young Jr WF, Pollock BE. Gamma knife radiosurgery for patients with prolactin-secreting pituitary adenomas. World Neurosurg. 2010;74:147–52.
23. Primeau V, Raftopoulos C, Maiter D. Outcomes of transsphenoidal surgery in prolactinomas: improvement of hormonal control in dopamine agonist-resistant patients. Eur J Endocrinol. 2012;166:779–86.

Somatotroph (GH) Adenomas

12

Gabriel Zada, M. Beatriz S. Lopes,
Srinivasan Mukundan Jr., and Edward Laws Jr.

12.1 Epidemiology and Clinical Presentation

- Growth hormone (GH)–secreting pituitary adenomas (GH adenomas) result in the clinical syndromes of gigantism and acromegaly.
- More than 90 % of patients with acromegaly have a pituitary adenoma [1].
- GH adenomas comprise approximately 15 % of surgically resected pituitary adenomas [2–4].
- The annual incidence of acromegaly has been calculated to be 3–4 cases per 1 million people, with a prevalence of 40–60 cases per million people [5].
- Increased GH secretion results in increased liver production of insulin-like growth factor-1 (IGF-I), which mediates the systemic effects of GH.
- Acromegaly is associated with multiple physical features and symptoms, including increased soft tissue edema, enlargement of the hands and feet, frontal bossing, coarse facial features, prognathism, acral growth, skin tags, snoring, and hyperhidrosis.
- Among the associated medical conditions are hypertension, diabetes mellitus, carpal tunnel syndrome, arthropathy, osteoarthritis, obstructive sleep apnea, colon polyps/cancer, cardiac hypertrophy, cardiomyopathy, and pulmonary disease.
- The clinical presentation may be more subtle in older patients [6].
- Uncontrolled acromegaly is a life-threatening condition that has been associated with decreased survival. Of deaths related to acromegaly, 60 % are accounted for by cardiovascular disease, 25 % by respiratory disease, and 15 % by malignancies [7–9].

G. Zada, MD, MS (✉)
Department of Neurological Surgery, Keck School of Medicine, University of Southern California, 1200 N State Street, #3300, Los Angeles, CA 90033, USA
e-mail: gzada@usc.edu

M.B.S. Lopes, MD, PhD
Department of Pathology (Neuropathology), University of Virginia School of Medicine, 1215 Lee Street, Room 3060–HEP, Charlottesville, VA 22908, USA
e-mail: msl2e@virginia.edu

S. Mukundan Jr., PhD, MD
Department of Radiology, Brigham and Women's Hospital, 75 Francis Street, Boston, MA 02115, USA
e-mail: smukundan@partners.org

E. Laws Jr., MD
Department of Neurosurgery, Brigham and Women's Hospital, 15 Francis Street, Boston, MA 02115, USA
e-mail: elaws@partners.org

G. Zada et al. (eds.), *Atlas of Sellar and Parasellar Lesions: Clinical, Radiologic, and Pathologic Correlations*,
DOI 10.1007/978-3-319-22855-6_12

12.2 Diagnosis

12.2.1 Endocrinological Diagnosis

- An initial screening test consists of a serum GH and IGF-I level.
- The serum IGF-I level provides better correlation of the disease state in acromegaly, and early normalization of IGF-I correlates with restoration of a normal life expectancy [5, 10].
- IGF-I levels are age and sex specific, requiring appropriate correlation with the particular laboratory's normal ranges.
- An oral glucose tolerance test (OGTT) is the gold standard test used to confirm the diagnosis or its remission. An oral glucose load of 75 g is given and serum GH levels are subsequently monitored for up to 120 min afterward. A nadir GH level greater than 1 ng/L during an OGTT is generally consistent with a diagnosis of acromegaly.

12.2.2 Imaging

- GH adenomas typically originate in the lateral aspect of the gland and are likely to demonstrate patterns of infrasellar extension with invasion of the sellar floor and clivus (Figs. 12.1, 12.2, 12.3, 12.4, 12.5, 12.6, 12.7, 12.8, 12.9, 12.10, 12.11, 12.12, and 12.13) [11, 12].
- A variety of bone and soft tissue changes are commonly identified in acromegalic patients, including hypertrophic nasal turbinates, conchae bullosae, enlarged (hyperpneumatized) paranasal sinuses, and thickened bony anatomy [13].
- GH adenomas are typically isointense on T1- and T2-weighted MR imaging [11].
- Most GH adenomas (86 %) are macroadenomas at the time of diagnosis [2].
- Acromegalic patients often have tortuous or ectatic internal carotid arteries with increased caliber, making their identification during surgical treatment of paramount importance [13].

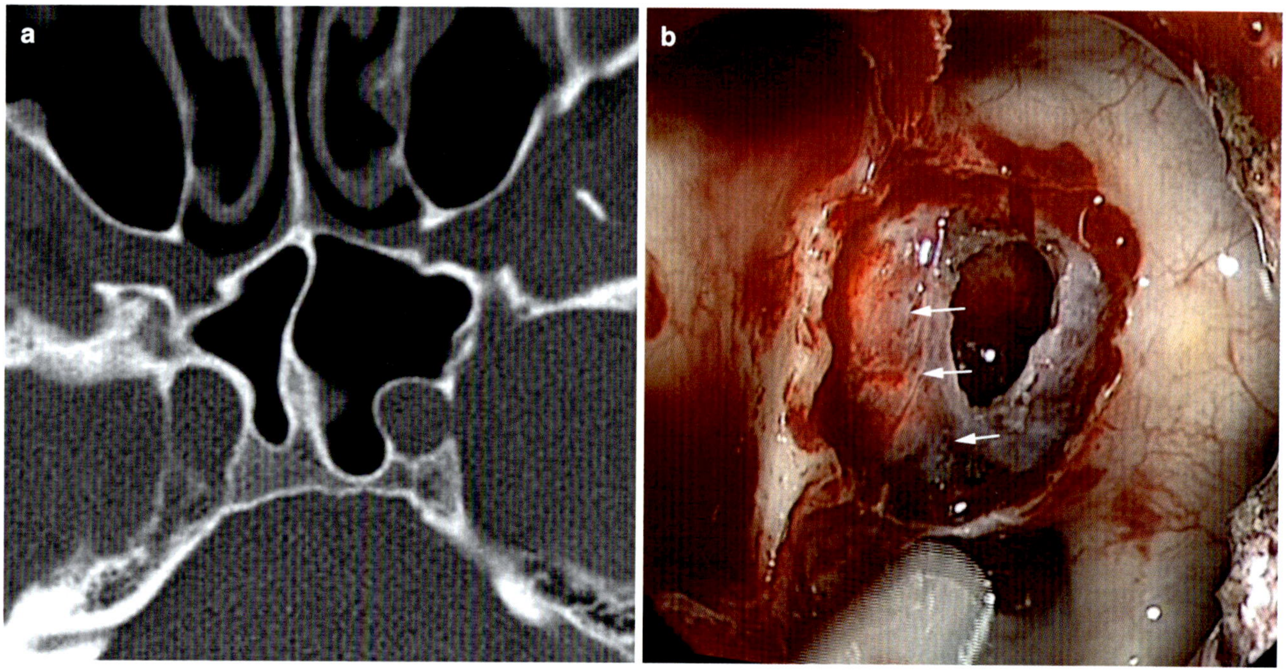

Fig. 12.1 Growth hormone (GH)–secreting adenoma. (**a**) Axial noncontrast CT scan with bony windowing. (**b**) Intraoperative endoscopic photo. The CT scan shows the large caliber and prominence of the internal carotid arteries, which demonstrate ectasia and tortuosity with extension into the sella (*white arrows*). Adapted from Zada et al. with permission [13]

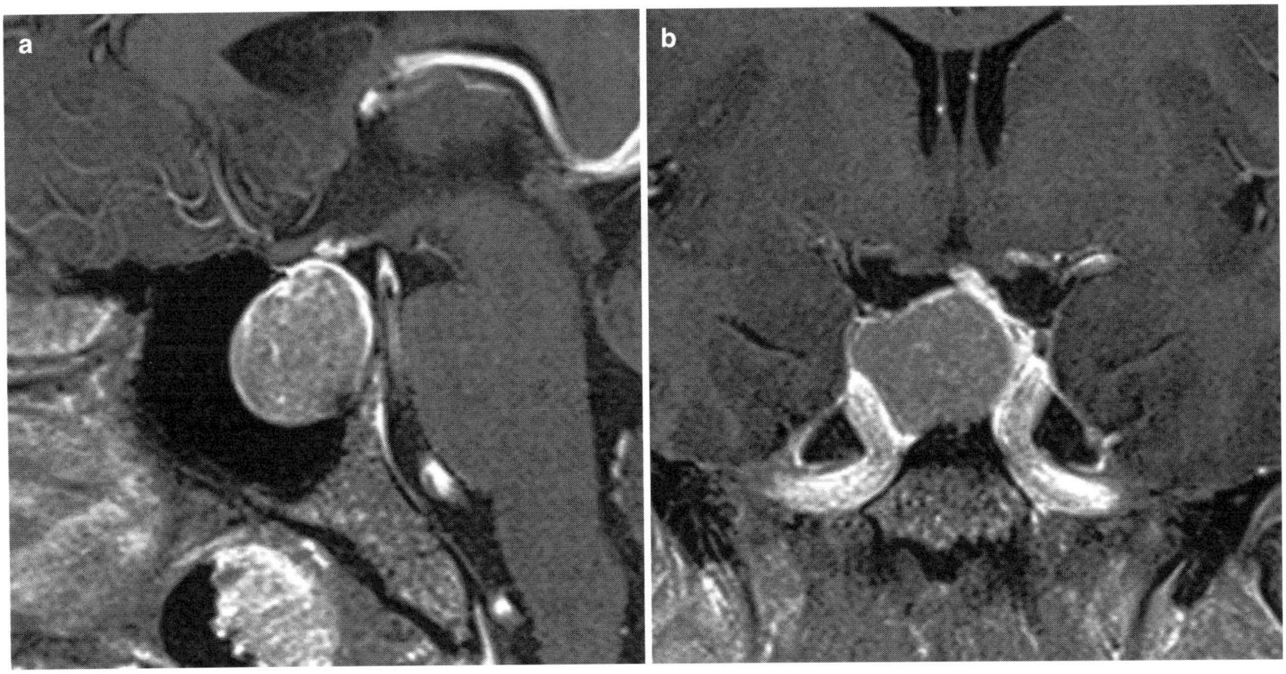

Fig. 12.2 GH adenoma. (**a**) Sagittal T1-weighted post-gadolinium image. (**b**) Coronal T1-weighted post-gadolinium image. An expansile sellar/suprasellar mass abuts the right cavernous internal carotid artery, and there is remodeling of the sellar floor. The pituitary stalk is elevated and deviated to the left

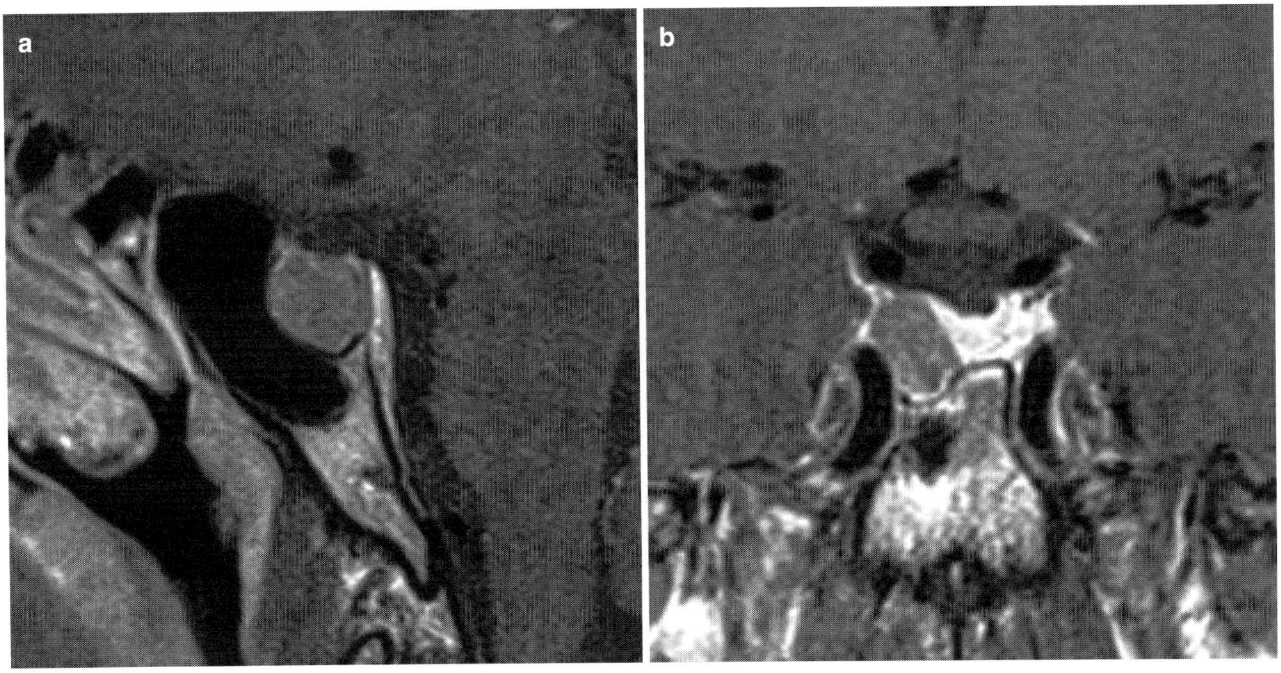

Fig. 12.3 GH adenoma. (**a**) Sagittal T1-weighted post-gadolinium image. (**b**) Coronal T1-weighted post-gadolinium image. A hypoenhancing mass presents in the *right* aspect of the sella abutting the right cavernous internal carotid artery without encasement. There is erosion of the right sellar floor

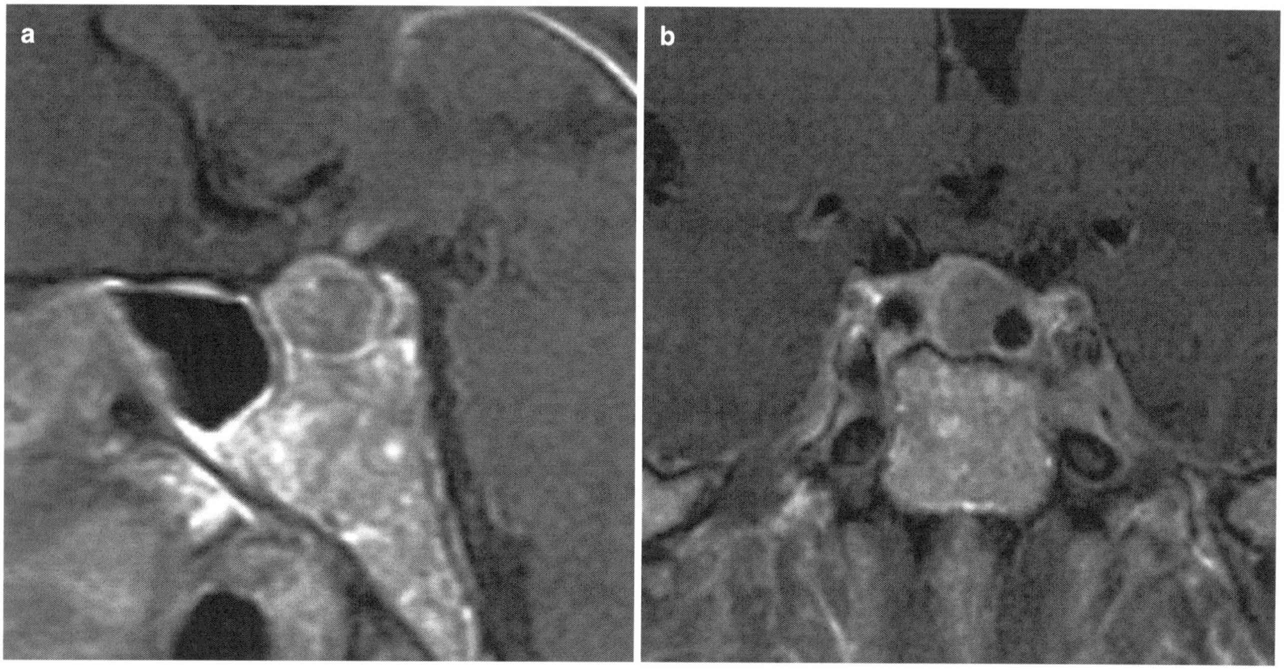

Fig. 12.4 GH adenoma. (**a**) Sagittal T1-weighted post-gadolinium image. (**b**) Coronal T1-weighted post-gadolinium image. A hypoenhancing mass is located in the left aspect of the sella, abutting the left cavernous internal carotid artery without encasement

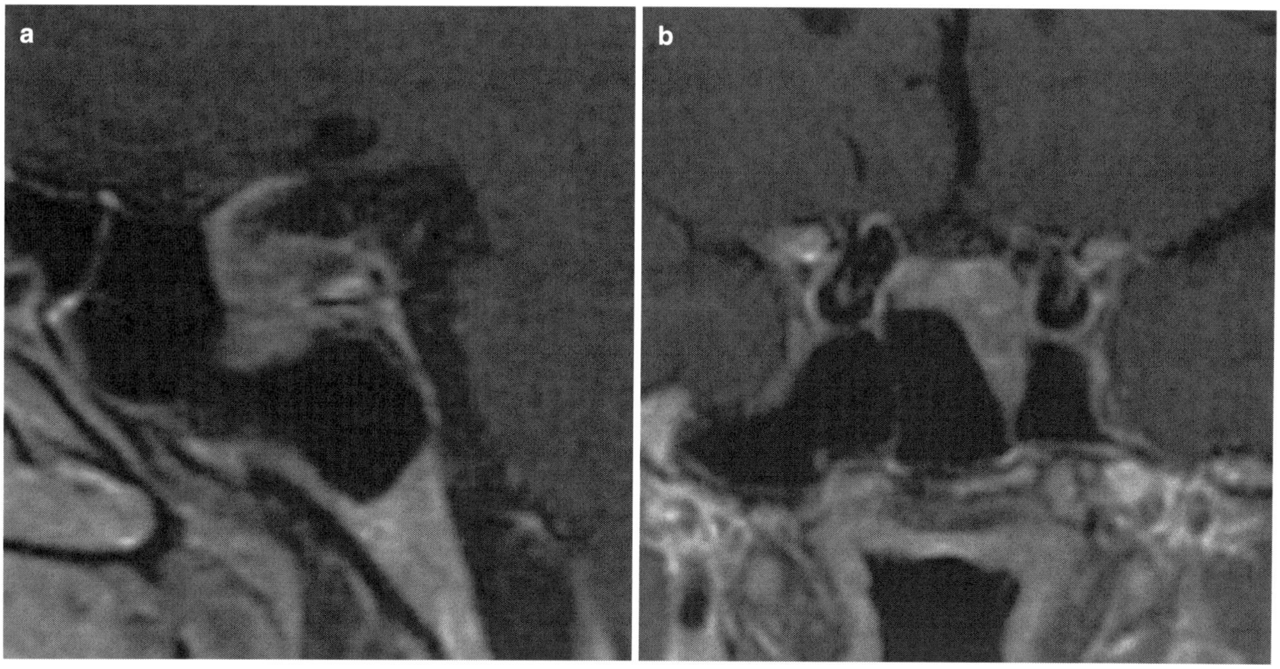

Fig. 12.5 GH adenoma. (**a**) Sagittal T1-weighted post-gadolinium image. (**b**) Coronal T1-weighted post-gadolinium image. Within the sella there is a heterogeneous, predominantly hypoenhancing mass causing erosion of the sellar floor. The mass contacts the left cavernous internal carotid artery without evidence of invasion

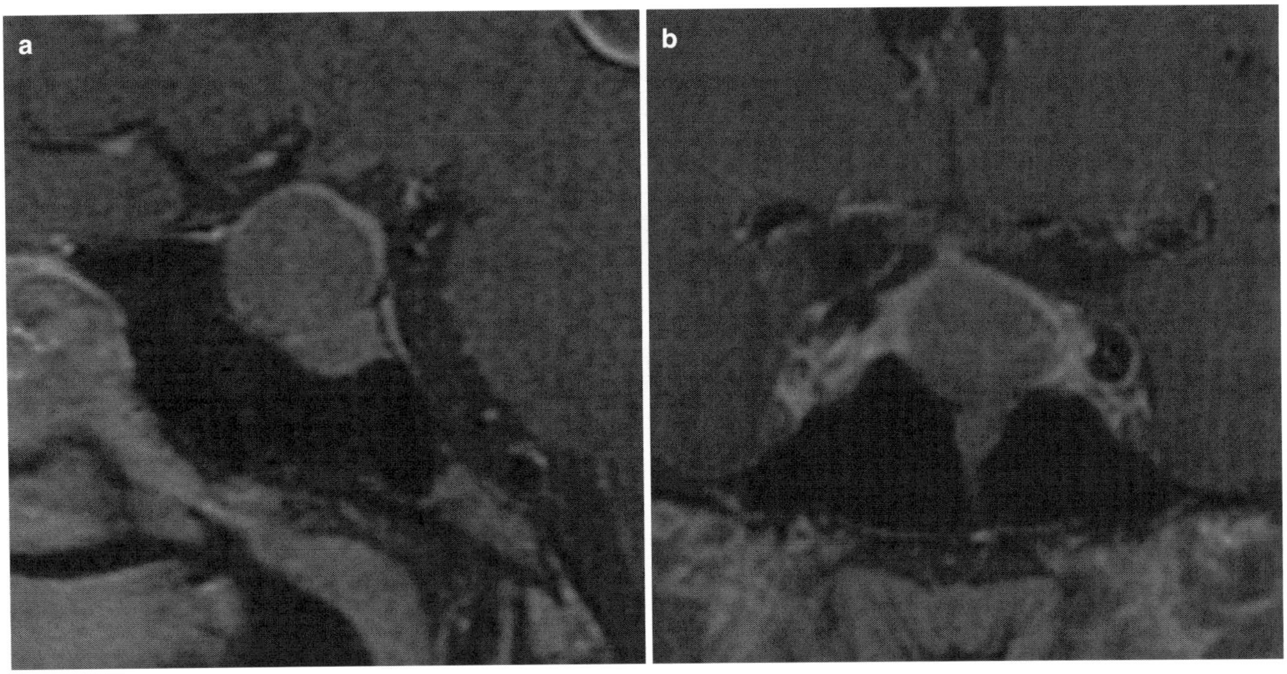

Fig. 12.6 GH adenoma. (**a**) Sagittal T1-weighted post-gadolinium image. (**b**) Coronal T1-weighted post-gadolinium image. There is a hypoenhancing mass in the sella causing erosion of the sellar floor and suprasellar extension without contacting the optic chiasm

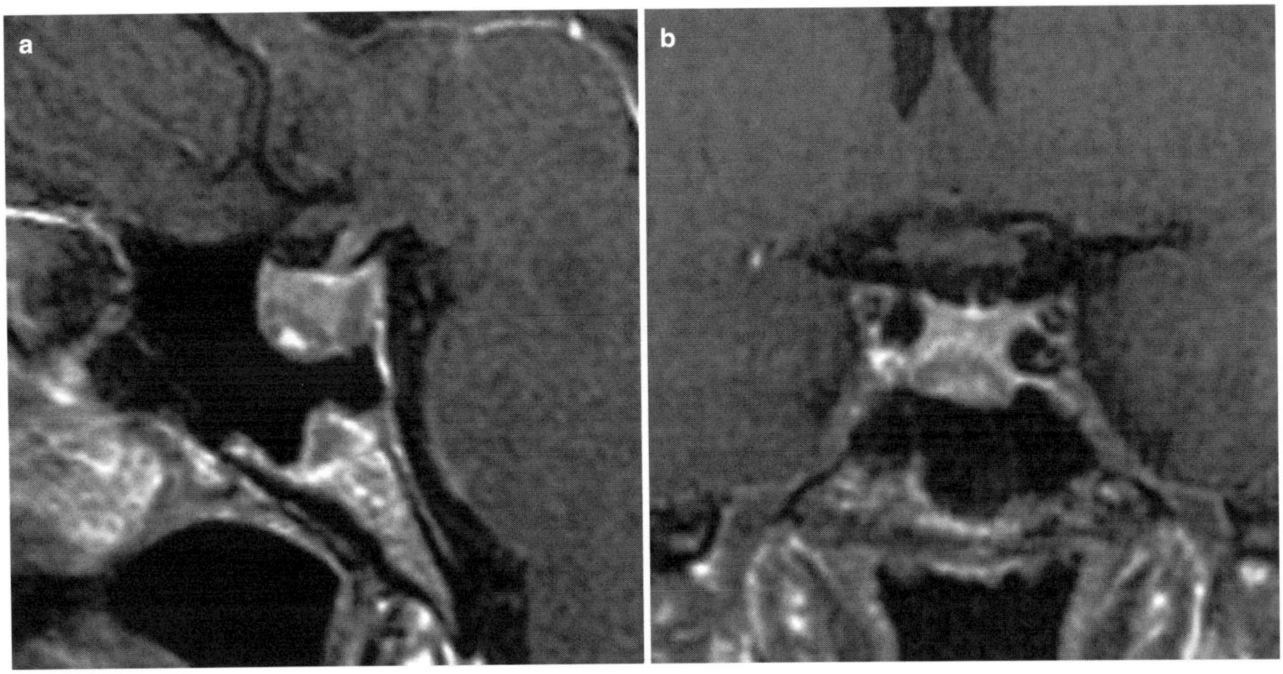

Fig. 12.7 GH adenoma. (**a**) Sagittal T1-weighted post-gadolinium image. (**b**) Coronal T1-weighted post-gadolinium image. A small, hypoenhancing mass is seen in the inferior anterior aspect of the sella, causing mild erosion of the sellar floor

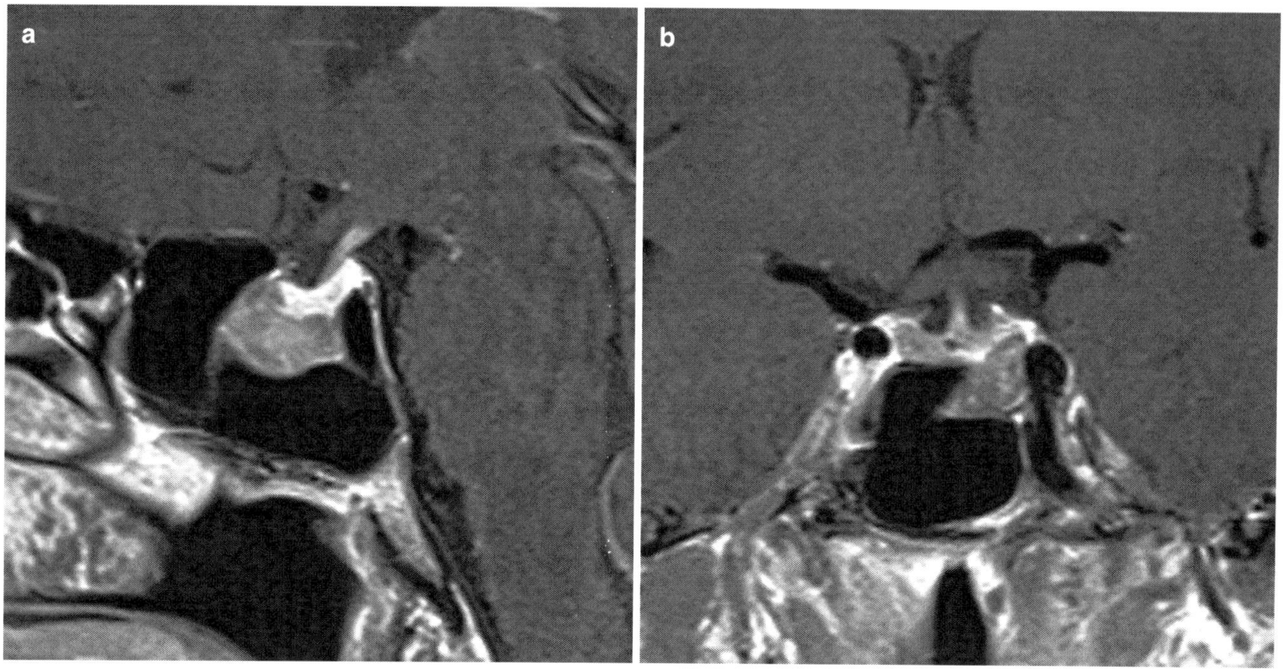

Fig. 12.8 GH adenoma. (**a**) Sagittal T1-weighted post-gadolinium image. (**b**) Coronal T1-weighted post-gadolinium image. There is a hypoenhancing mass in the left inferior aspect of the sella, causing erosion of the sellar floor. The mass contacts the left cavernous internal carotid artery without evidence of invasion of the left cavernous sinus

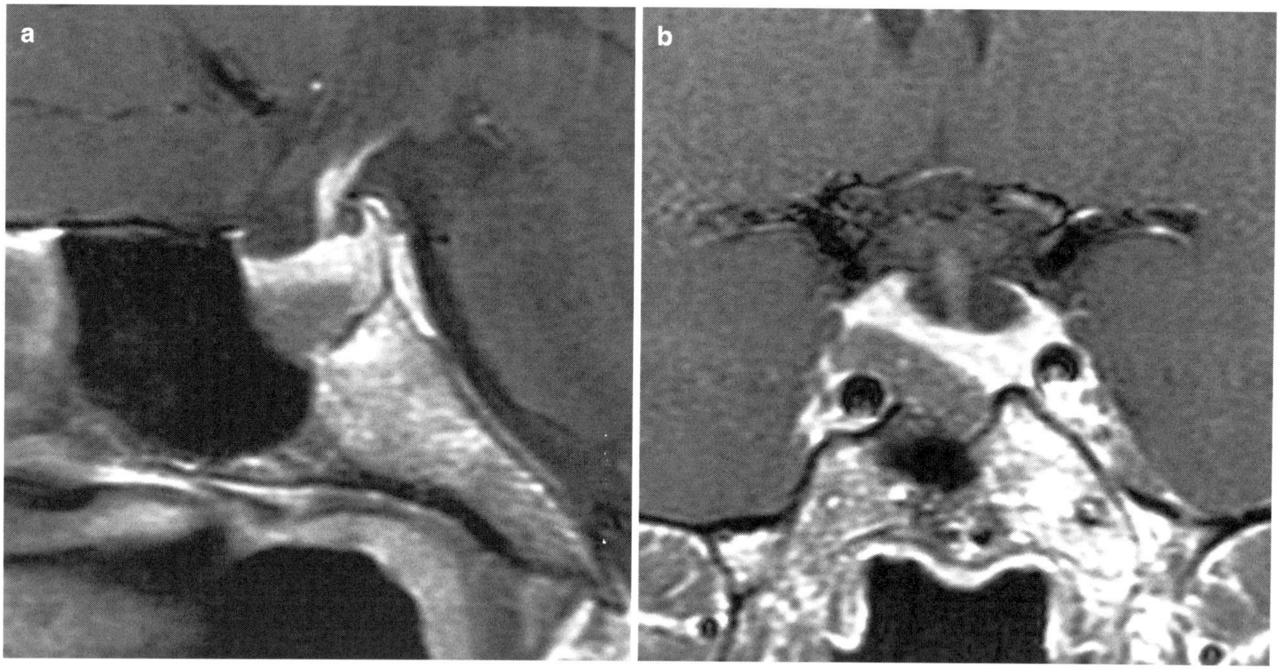

Fig. 12.9 GH adenoma. (**a**) Sagittal T1-weighted post-gadolinium image. (**b**) Coronal T1-weighted post-gadolinium image. There is a hypoenhancing mass located in the right inferior aspect of the sella, causing erosion of the sellar floor. The mass abuts the right cavernous internal carotid artery without evidence of encasement

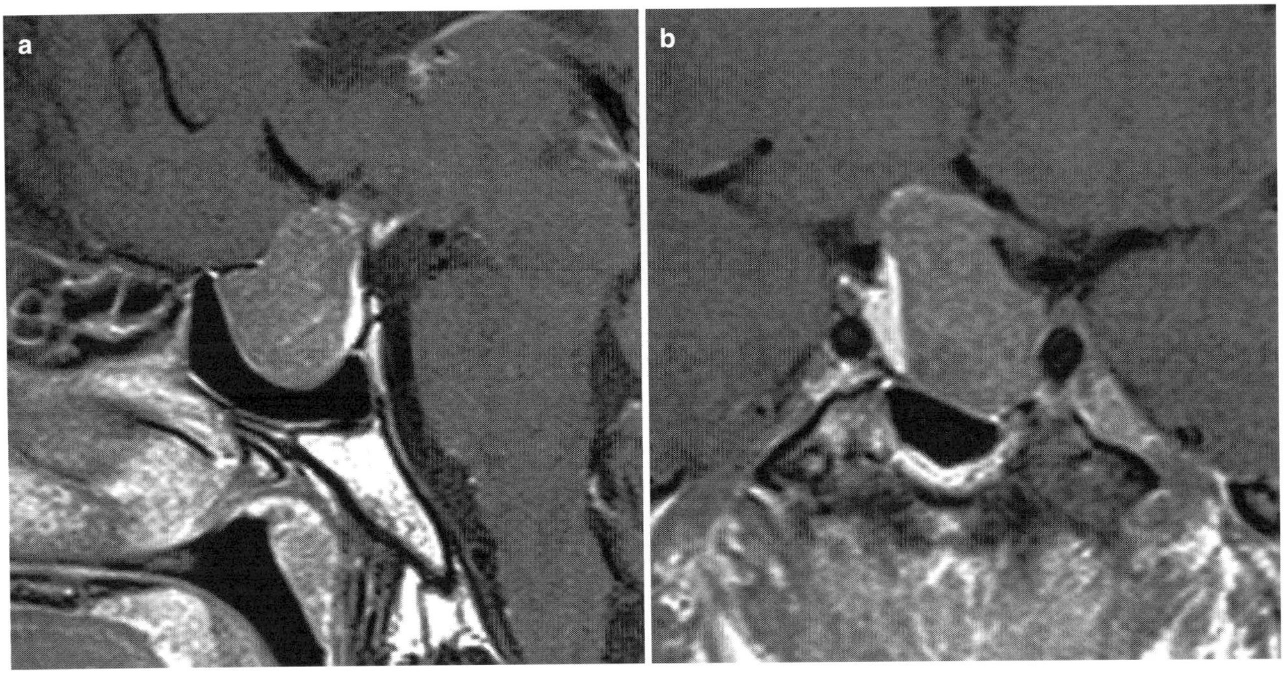

Fig. 12.10 GH adenoma. (**a**) Sagittal T1-weighted post-gadolinium image. (**b**) Coronal T1-weighted post-gadolinium image. There is a heterogeneously enhancing sellar mass with suprasellar extension. The mass abuts the left cavernous internal carotid artery without definite invasion of the left cavernous sinus. There is erosion of the left sellar floor. Superiorly, the mass abuts the right hypothalamus. Normal pituitary glandular tissue is seen along the right aspect of the sella

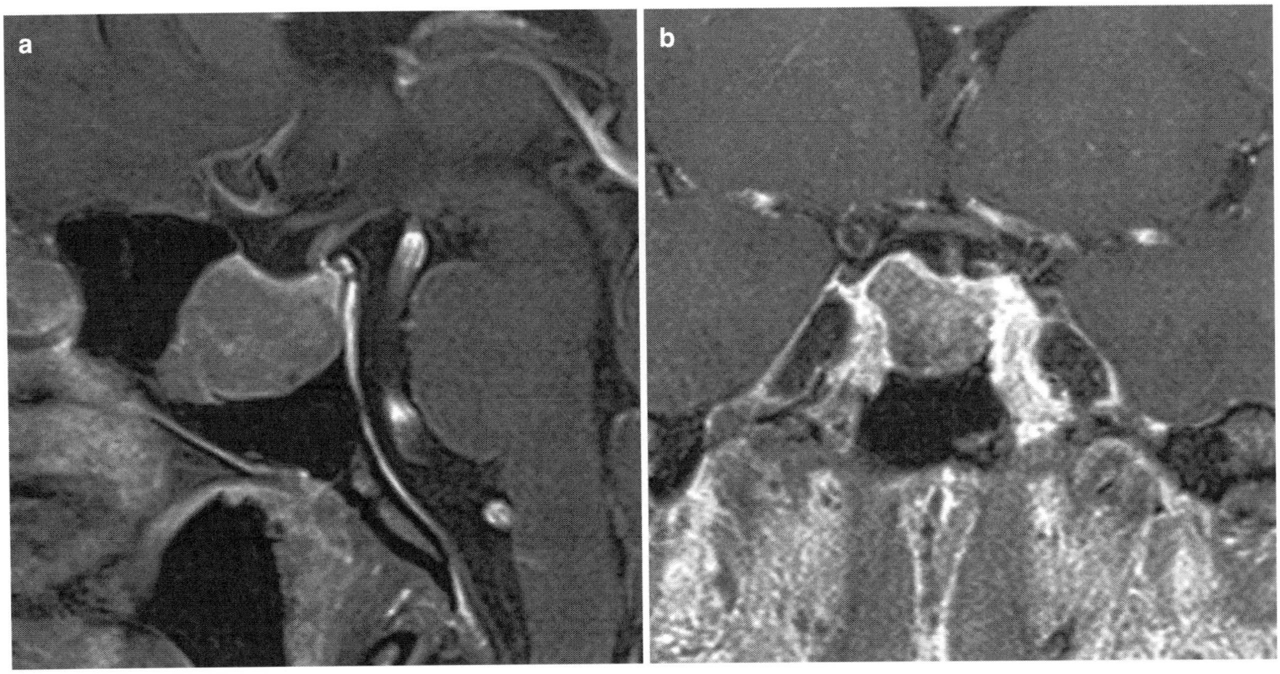

Fig. 12.11 GH adenoma. (**a**) Sagittal T1-weighted post-gadolinium image. (**b**) Coronal T1-weighted post-gadolinium image. There is a hypoenhancing sellar mass with erosion of the sellar floor. The mass abuts the bilateral cavernous internal carotid arteries without encasement

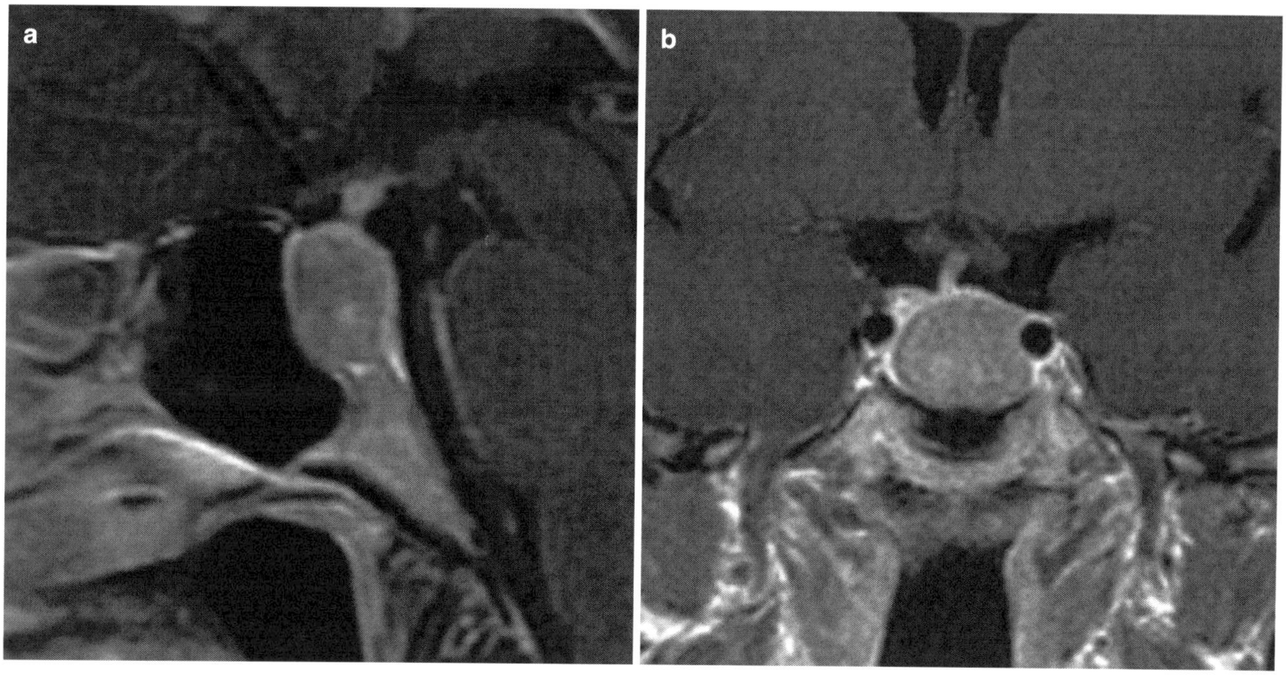

Fig. 12.12 GH adenoma. (**a**) Sagittal T1-weighted post-gadolinium image. (**b**) Coronal T1-weighted post-gadolinium image. A hypoenhancing sellar mass erodes the sellar floor and abuts the left cavernous internal carotid artery without encasement. The pituitary stalk is mildly deviated to the right, with normal gland flattened in the superior right aspect of the sella

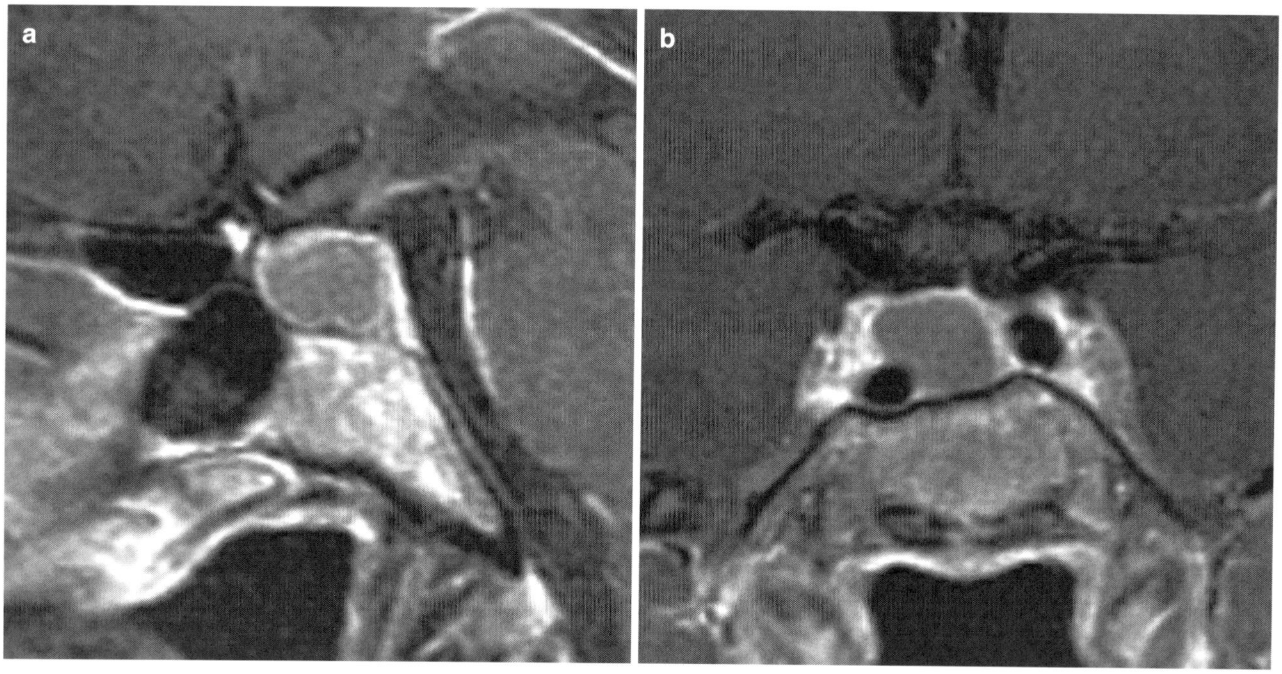

Fig. 12.13 GH adenoma. (**a**) Sagittal T1-weighted post-gadolinium image. (**b**) Coronal T1-weighted post-gadolinium image. There is a hypoenhancing sellar mass in the right aspect of the sella, contacting the right cavernous internal carotid artery without encasement

12.2.3 Histopathology

- Approximately two thirds of GH adenomas are densely granulated adenomas; the other third are sparsely granulated [2, 14].
- Densely granulated GH adenomas are characterized by medium- to large-sized cells with slight pleomorphism and a strong, diffuse staining pattern for GH (Fig. 12.14).
- Sparsely granulated GH adenomas are frequently pleomorphic, with fibrous bodies, a region of perinuclear clearing, and typically weaker immunoreactivity for GH stain (Fig. 12.15) [2]. Fibrous bodies in the cytoplasm can be stained with CAM 5.2 [14].
- Dural invasion has been noted in over 50 % of GH adenomas [2].
- Associated tumor subtypes are those composed of both GH and PRL cells, the mammosomatotroph cell adenoma, and the acidophil stem cell adenoma.
- GH/PRL tumors may be more primitive subtypes; they are more likely to be atypical adenomas than pure GH tumors [15].

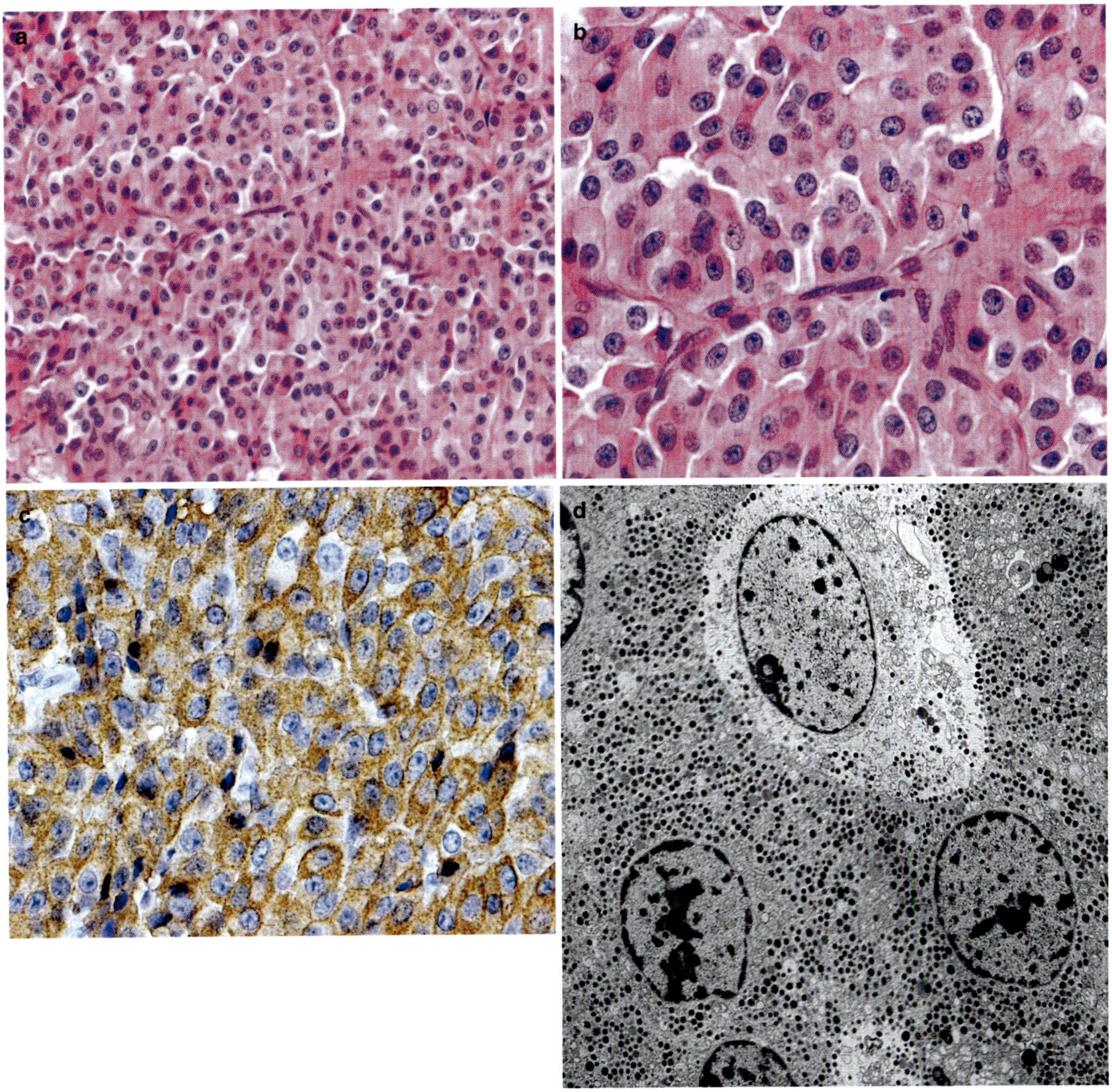

Fig. 12.14 GH adenoma. (**a**, **b**) Densely granulated GH cell adenomas show large cells with eosinophilic, granular cytoplasm and a central nucleus with prominent nucleoli. (**c**) On immunohistochemistry, the tumor shows intense and diffuse staining for GH. (**d**) Densely granulated GH cell adenoma exhibits well-developed organelles and abundant, large secretory granules at the ultrastructural level

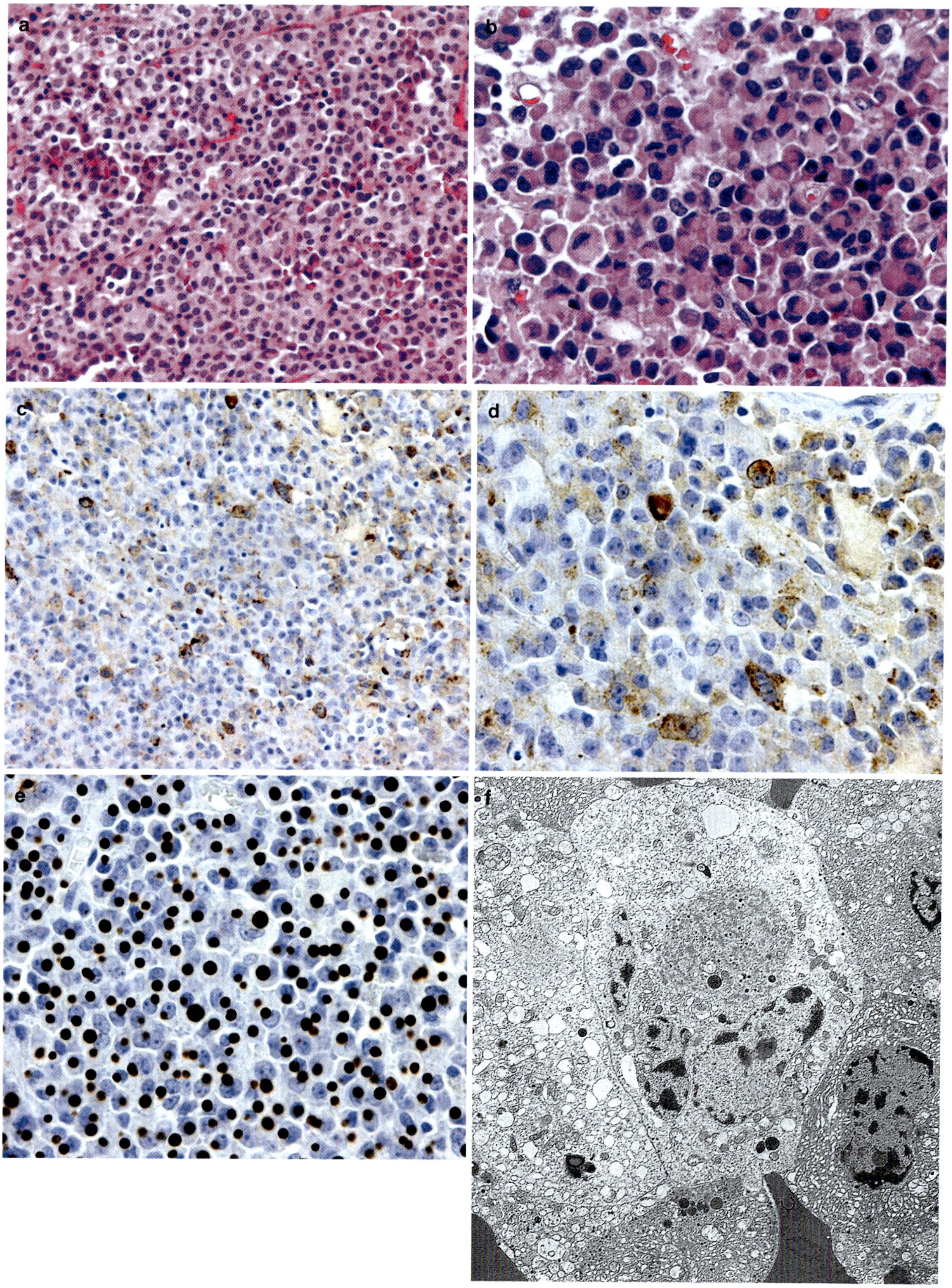

Fig. 12.15 GH adenoma. (**a**) Sparsely granulated GH cell adenomas have a more chromophobic appearance of the cells, with slight granular cytoplasm. (**b**) Characteristically, the tumors have a paranuclear eosinophilic inclusion called "fibrous bodies." (**c**, **d**) Immunohistochemistry for GH shows more focal staining within the cell that is less prominent than in densely granulated adenomas. (**e**) Cytokeratin (CAM 5.2) histochemistry highlights the paranuclear "fibrous body" seen in sparsely granulated GH adenomas. (**f**) At ultrastructure, sparsely granulated GH adenomas display sparse secretory granules and the characteristic "fibrous bodies"

12.3 Clinical Management

- The overall goal of multimodal treatment for acromegaly is the reduction of tumor mass effect and biochemical normalization of IGF-1 and GH levels [8, 16].

12.3.1 Medical Management

- Primary medical treatment typically consists of somatostatin receptor ligands (SRLs), the most notable ones being octreotide and lanreotide.
  - Octreotide has been reported to normalize GH and IGF-I levels in 34–70 % of patients over a 10-year period.
  - Significant tumor volume reduction may occur in 50–75 % of patients [8, 17].
  - Common adverse effects include cramping and diarrhea.
- In patients with refractory GH-secreting adenomas, especially those with mammosomatotroph subtypes, dopamine agonists (DAs) may provide normalization of the IGF-I level in 35–50 % of patients receiving combination therapy (DA and SRL) [17].
- Pegvisomant, a GH receptor antagonist, is a newer agent that acts by inhibiting the production of IGF-I:
  - IGF-1 normalization is reported in 80–97 % of patients [17, 18].
  - Liver dysfunction has occurred in approximately 25 % of patients and requires serial monitoring [8].
  - Infrequently, the size of GH-secreting adenomas has been reported to increase following administration of pegvisomant, owing to a compensatory somatotroph hypertrophy from the reduction of systemic IGF-I in the feedback mechanism [19].
  - Combination therapy using an SRL and pegvisomant has proven to be more effective in many cases [20].
- Routine colonoscopy screening is recommended for all acromegalic patients [21].

12.3.2 Surgical Treatment

- Transsphenoidal surgery is the most common approach for GH adenomas, with excellent resection and safety profiles [4].
- Variations in bony and soft tissue structures, such as thickened bone, boggy nasal mucosa, and excessive nasal polyps, may pose challenges for microscopic or endoscopic transsphenoidal surgery in some patients with severe acromegaly [13].
- Intraoperatively, GH-secreting adenomas tend to have a whiter color and softer consistency than other adenomas (Fig. 12.16).
- The gold standard definition of remission is a normalized IGF-I level obtained 2–3 months following surgery and a GH level less than 1 ng/mL following an OGTT [8, 22].
- A serum GH level less than 2 ng/mL on postoperative day 1 serves as an early marker for long-term remission (98 % predictive) [23].
- More pronounced fluid diuresis in the first 48 h following surgery has been correlated with lower postoperative GH levels [24].
- For GH-secreting tumors confined to the intrasellar space, reported surgical long-term remission rates have ranged from 75 to 95 % [4, 8].
- For invasive GH-secreting macroadenomas, remission rates have been reported to be 40–60 % [3, 4].
- The ability to achieve hormonal remission following transsphenoidal surgery is often limited by tumor size (i.e., macroadenomas ≥10 mm in diameter), the degree of extrasellar extension (particularly lateral into the cavernous sinuses), and high preoperative serum GH concentrations (≥45 ng/mL) [3, 25, 26].
- Disease recurrence has been reported in 8–20 % of patients with up to 10 years of follow-up; it was more likely when tumors invaded the parasellar dura or bone [23, 27, 28].

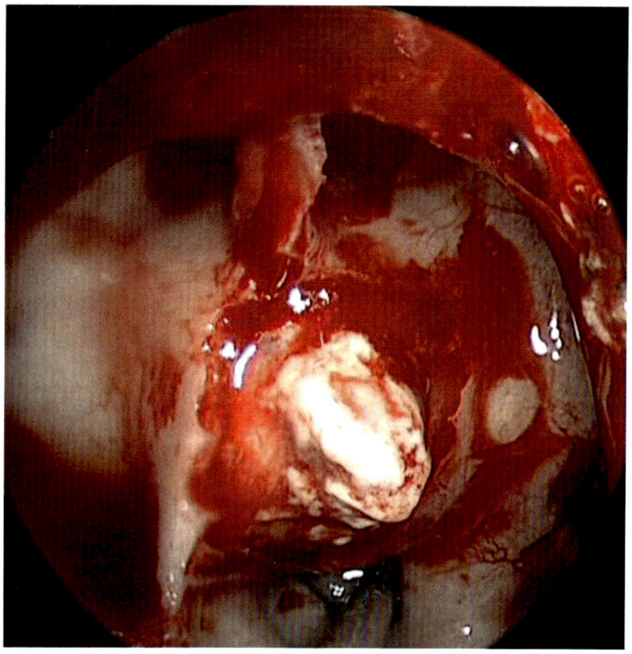

Fig. 12.16 Intraoperative endoscopic photo showing resection of a GH adenoma and its characteristic white color

12.3.3 Radiosurgical Management

- Fractionated or single fraction stereotactic radiosurgery is an effective adjunctive modality for achieving tumor control and potential biochemical remission in patients with residual or recurrent tumor burden.
- Stereotactic radiosurgery has been effective in achieving hormonal remission in approximately 50 % of patients following initial surgical resection, and tumor volume control has been achieved in over 90 % of patients [16, 29].

References

1. Melmed S. Acromegaly pathogenesis and treatment. J Clin Invest. 2009;119:3189–202.
2. Saeger W, Ludecke DK, Buchfelder M, Fahlbusch R, Quabbe HJ, Petersenn S. Pathohistological classification of pituitary tumors: 10 years of experience with the German Pituitary Tumor Registry. Eur J Endocrinol. 2007;156:203–16.
3. Zada G, Kelly DF, Cohan P, Wang C, Swerdloff R. Endonasal transsphenoidal approach for pituitary adenomas and other sellar lesions: an assessment of efficacy, safety, and patient impressions. J Neurosurg. 2003;98:350–8.
4. Laws ER. Surgery for acromegaly: evolution of the techniques and outcomes. Rev Endocr Metab Disord. 2008;9:67–70.
5. Cordero RA, Barkan AL. Current diagnosis of acromegaly. Rev Endocr Metab Disord. 2008;9:13–9.
6. Bush ZM, Vance ML. Management of acromegaly: is there a role for primary medical therapy? Rev Endocr Metab Disord. 2008;9:83–94.
7. Colao A, Ferone D, Marzullo P, Lombardi G. Systemic complications of acromegaly: epidemiology, pathogenesis, and management. Endocr Rev. 2004;25:102–52.
8. Melmed S, Colao A, Barkan A, Molitch M, Grossman AB, Kleinberg D, et al. Guidelines for acromegaly management: an update. J Clin Endocrinol Metab. 2009;94:1509–17.
9. Dekkers OM, Biermasz NR, Pereira AM, Romijn JA, Vandenbroucke JP. Mortality in acromegaly: a metaanalysis. J Clin Endocrinol Metab. 2008;93:61–7.
10. Swearingen B, Barker 2nd FG, Katznelson L, Biller BM, Grinspoon S, Klibanski A, et al. Long-term mortality after transsphenoidal surgery and adjunctive therapy for acromegaly. J Clin Endocrinol Metab. 1998;83:3419–26.
11. Marro B, Zouaoui A, Sahel M, Crozat N, Gerber S, Sourour N, et al. MRI of pituitary adenomas in acromegaly. Neuroradiology. 1997;39:394–9.
12. Zada G, Lin N, Laws Jr ER. Patterns of extrasellar extension in growth hormone-secreting and nonfunctional pituitary macroadenomas. Neurosurg Focus. 2010;29:E4.
13. Zada G, Cavallo LM, Esposito F, Fernandez-Jimenez JC, Tasiou A, De Angelis M, et al. Transsphenoidal surgery in patients with acromegaly: operative strategies for overcoming technically challenging anatomical variations. Neurosurg Focus. 2010;29:E8.
14. Al-Brahim NY, Asa SL. My approach to pathology of the pituitary gland. J Clin Pathol. 2006;59:1245–53.
15. Zada G, Woodmansee WW, Ramkissoon S, Amadio J, Nose V, Laws Jr ER. Atypical pituitary adenomas: incidence, clinical characteristics, and implications. J Neurosurg. 2011;114:336–44.
16. Marquez Y, Tuchman A, Zada G. Surgery and radiosurgery for acromegaly: a review of indications, operative techniques, outcomes, and complications. Int J Endocrinol. 2012;2012:386401. doi:10.1155/2012/386401.

17. Carmichael JD, Bonert VS. Medical therapy: options and uses. Rev Endocr Metab Disord. 2008;9:71–81.
18. Hodish I, Barkan A. Long-term effects of pegvisomant in patients with acromegaly. Nat Clin Pract Endocrinol Metab. 2008;4: 324–32.
19. Frohman LA, Bonert V. Pituitary tumor enlargement in two patients with acromegaly during pegvisomant therapy. Pituitary. 2007;10: 283–9.
20. Feenstra J, de Herder WW, ten Have SM, van den Beld AW, Feelders RA, Janssen JA, van der Lely AJ. Combined therapy with somatostatin analogues and weekly pegvisomant in active acromegaly. Lancet. 2005;365:1644–6.
21. Jenkins PJ, Fairclough PD, Richards T, Lowe DG, Monson J, Grossman A, et al. Acromegaly, colonic polyps and carcinoma. Clin Endocrinol (Oxf). 1997;47:17–22.
22. Carmichael JD, Bonert VS, Mirocha JM, Melmed S. The utility of oral glucose tolerance testing for diagnosis and assessment of treatment outcomes in 166 patients with acromegaly. J Clin Endocrinol Metab. 2009;94:523–7.
23. Krieger MD, Couldwell WT, Weiss MH. Assessment of long-term remission of acromegaly following surgery. J Neurosurg. 2003;98:719–24.
24. Zada G, Sivakumar W, Fishback D, Singer PA, Weiss MH. Significance of postoperative fluid diuresis in patients undergoing transsphenoidal surgery for growth hormone-secreting pituitary adenomas. J Neurosurg. 2010;112:744–9.
25. Clayton RN, Stewart PM, Shalet SM, Wass JA. Pituitary surgery for acromegaly. Should be done by specialists. BMJ. 1999;319:588–9.
26. Salaun C, Foubert L, Vialatou M, Kujas M, Turpin G. Prognostic factors in the surgical management of acromegaly. Ann Med Interne (Paris). 1999;150:195–8.
27. Laws ER, Vance ML, Thapar K. Pituitary surgery for the management of acromegaly. Horm Res. 2000;53:71–5.
28. Kreutzer J, Vance ML, Lopes MB, Laws Jr ER. Surgical management of GH-secreting pituitary adenomas: an outcome study using modern remission criteria. J Clin Endocrinol Metab. 2001;86:4072–7.
29. Yang I, Kim W, De Salles A, Bergsneider M. A systematic analysis of disease control in acromegaly treated with radiosurgery. Neurosurg Focus. 2010;29:E13.

13 Corticotroph (ACTH) Adenomas

Gabriel Zada, M. Beatriz S. Lopes,
Srinivasan Mukundan Jr., and Edward Laws Jr.

13.1 Epidemiology and Clinical Presentation

- Cushing's disease (CD) caused by an adrenocorticotropic (ACTH)-secreting pituitary adenoma accounts for 80 % of newly diagnosed cases of Cushing's syndrome.
- Functioning ACTH-staining adenomas comprise approximately 14 % of all surgically resected pituitary adenomas [1–3].
- Silent ACTH adenomas are discussed in chapter 14 and are nonfunctioning tumors with positive ACTH immunoreactivity and no clinical evidence of Cushing's disease or Nelson's syndrome.
- Patients with ACTH hypersecretion may present with Cushing's syndrome or Nelson's syndrome.
- Cushing's disease is more common in women than in men (8:1); it typically develops in the third and fourth decades of life [4].
- The disease may also manifest in children and adolescents and comprises a larger proportion of all pituitary adenoma subtypes in pediatric patients than in adults [5, 6].
- Typical symptoms and physical findings in CD include acne, hirsutism or hair loss, weight gain, lipodystrophy, moon facies, skin bruising, abdominal striae, insomnia, amenorrhea, and short-term memory and cognitive deficits.
- Among the associated medical conditions are diabetes mellitus, hypertension, osteoporosis, and arthralgia.
- Also commonly occurring are psychological disturbances such as anxiety, depression, insomnia, psychosis, or euphoria.
- Nelson's syndrome occurs in patients with ACTH-secreting adenomas who have undergone bilateral adrenalectomy.
  - These patients subsequently develop increased secretion of corticotropin-releasing hormone (CRH) and ACTH, typically 1–4 years after adrenalectomy [7, 8].
  - Patients classically present with a characteristic bronzing of the skin due to expression of pro-opiomelanocortin (POMC), frequent enlargement of the residual pituitary adenoma, and elevated serum ACTH levels (typically >200 ng/L) [8].
  - Hyperpigmentation frequently occurs on the extensor surfaces, knuckles, gingivae, scars, and areola.
  - In modern series, hyperpigmentation has been reported in 42 % of patients, owing to improved surveillance with laboratory and imaging studies [9].

G. Zada, MD, MS (✉)
Department of Neurological Surgery, Keck School of Medicine, University of Southern California, 1200 N State Street, #3300, Los Angeles, CA 90033, USA
e-mail: gzada@usc.edu

M.B.S. Lopes, MD, PhD
Department of Pathology (Neuropathology), University of Virginia School of Medicine, 1215 Lee Street, Room 3060–HEP, Charlottesville, VA 22908, USA
e-mail: msl2e@virginia.edu

S. Mukundan Jr., PhD, MD
Department of Radiology, Brigham and Women's Hospital, 75 Francis Street, Boston, MA 02115, USA
e-mail: smukundan@partners.org

E. Laws Jr., MD
Department of Neurosurgery, Brigham and Women's Hospital, 15 Francis Street, Boston, MA 02115, USA
e-mail: elaws@partners.org

G. Zada et al. (eds.), *Atlas of Sellar and Parasellar Lesions: Clinical, Radiologic, and Pathologic Correlations*, DOI 10.1007/978-3-319-22855-6_13

13.2 Diagnosis

- If clinical suspicion for Cushing's syndrome exists, one of several screening tests for hypercortisolism should be performed. These include a nighttime salivary cortisol test, a 24-h urinary free cortisol test, a 1-mg overnight dexamethasone suppression test (DST), or a longer low-dose DST (0.5 mg every 6 h for 48 h) [10].
- A second test for hypercortisolemia is preferable to confirm a diagnosis of Cushing's syndrome, followed by a serum ACTH level to differentiate ACTH-dependent from ACTH-independent hypercortisolemia.
- The majority of patients will have ACTH-dependent Cushing's syndrome. In these patients, an MRI of the sella with contrast administration should be performed next. MRI may be negative in as many as 30 % of cases of CD despite the presence of a small pituitary ACTH microadenoma, however, and additional modalities may therefore be required to establish the diagnosis.

13.2.1 Imaging

- In patients with CD, 85–87 % have microadenomas and 13–15 % have macroadenomas [1, 11].
- Invasion occurs in 13–25 % of cases [11].
- Patients with Nelson's syndrome frequently have invasive macroadenomas.
- Compared with a normal pituitary gland, ACTH adenomas may be hyperintense on T2 imaging; they are typically hypoenhancing on T1 imaging following contrast administration (Figs. 13.1, 13.2, 13.3, 13.4, 13.5, and 13.6) [12].
- Dynamic contrast MRI has been reported to provide a diagnostic advantage for small microadenomas in selected cases [13].
- Spoiled gradient recalled acquisition with thin-slice imaging has been reported to substantially improve imaging resolution and diagnosis of small microadenomas [14].
- MRI may be negative in a small proportion of cases despite the presence of a pituitary microadenoma.

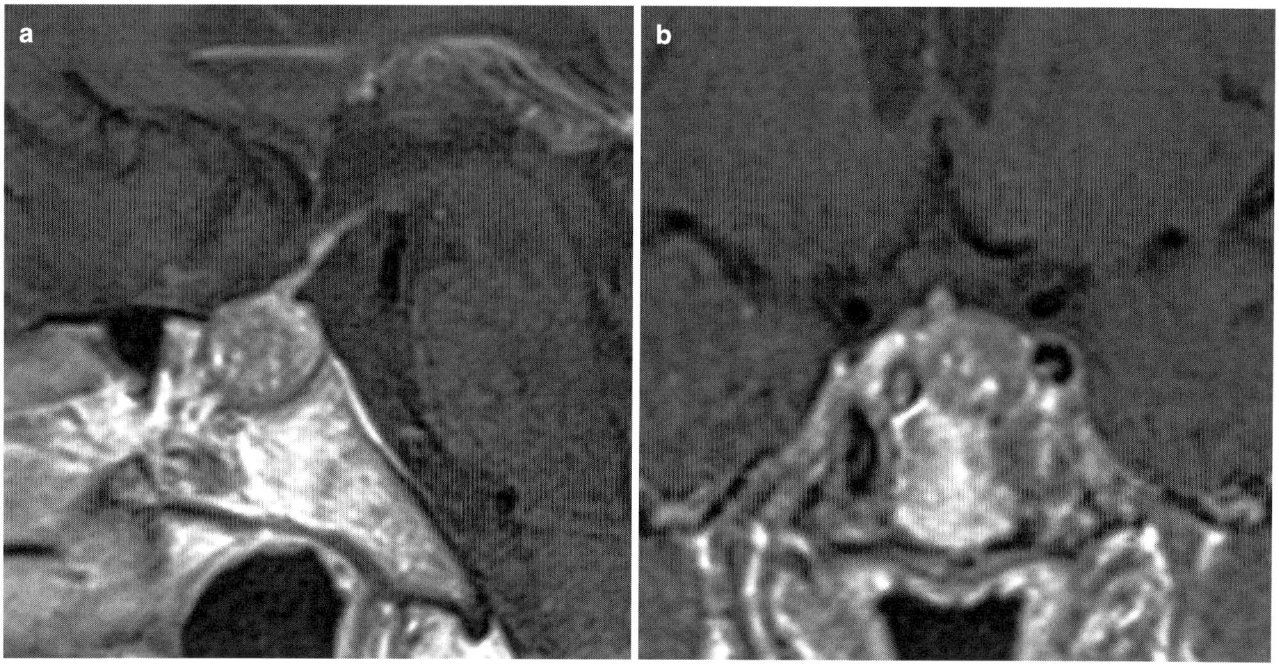

Fig. 13.1 ACTH adenoma. (**a**) Sagittal T1-weighted post-gadolinium image. (**b**) Coronal T1-weighted post-gadolinium image. The pituitary gland is enlarged, with heterogeneous enhancement and nodular erosion of the left sellar floor. The pituitary stalk is mildly deviated to the right

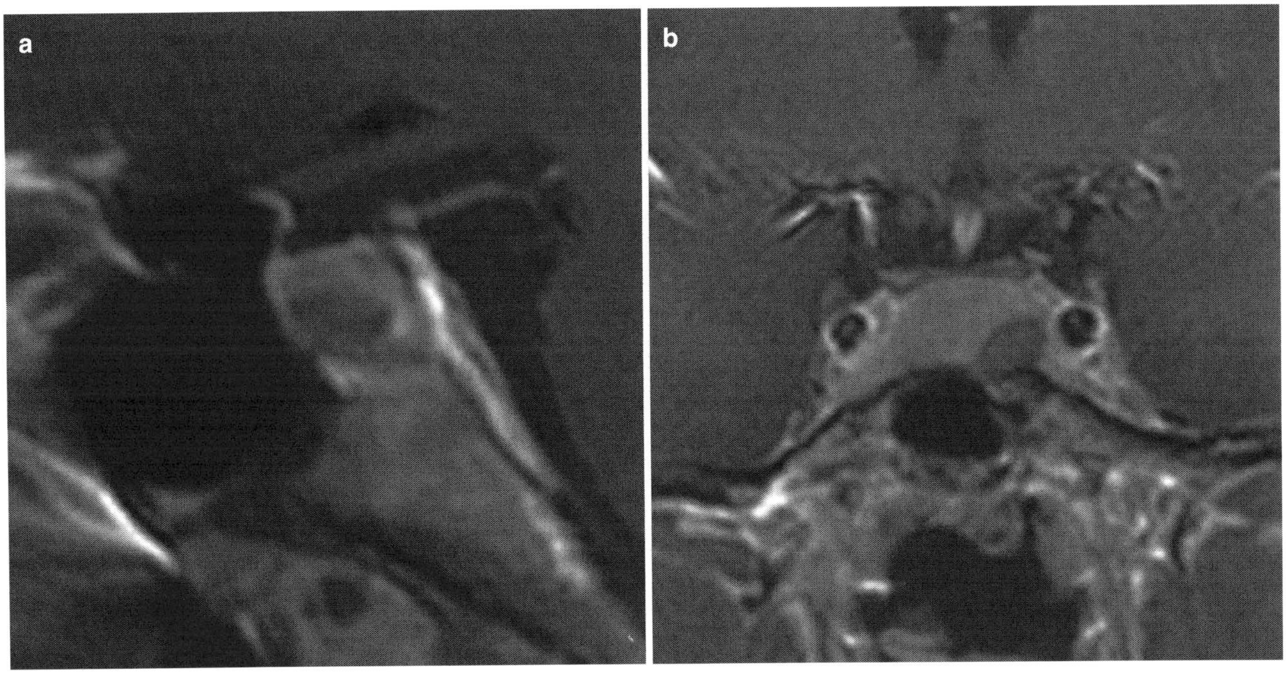

Fig. 13.2 Adrenocorticotropic hormone (ACTH)–secreting adenoma. (**a**) Sagittal T1-weighted post-gadolinium image. (**b**) Coronal T1-weighted post-gadolinium image. A focal hypoenhancing mass presents in the left inferior aspect of the pituitary gland. The mass appears separate from the left cavernous internal carotid artery

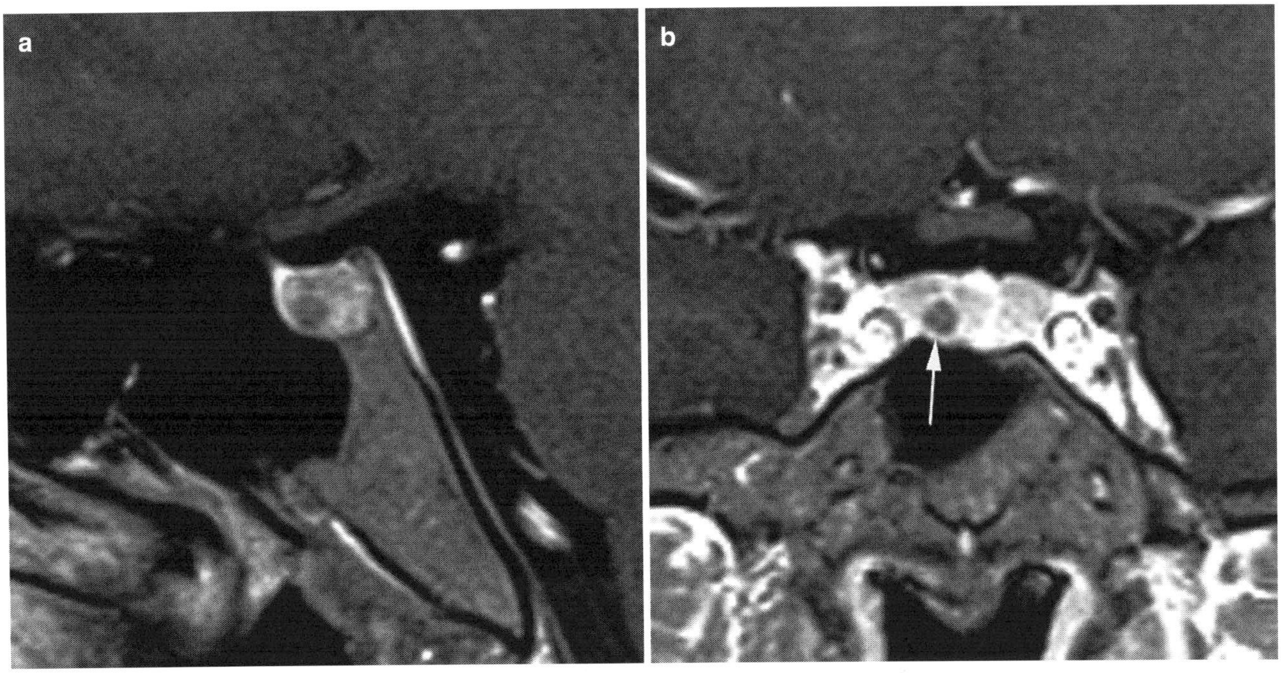

Fig. 13.3 ACTH adenoma. (**a**) Sagittal T1-weighted post-gadolinium image. (**b**) Coronal T1-weighted post-gadolinium image. There is a small, hypoenhancing mass (*white arrow*) in the inferior aspect of the pituitary gland right to midline

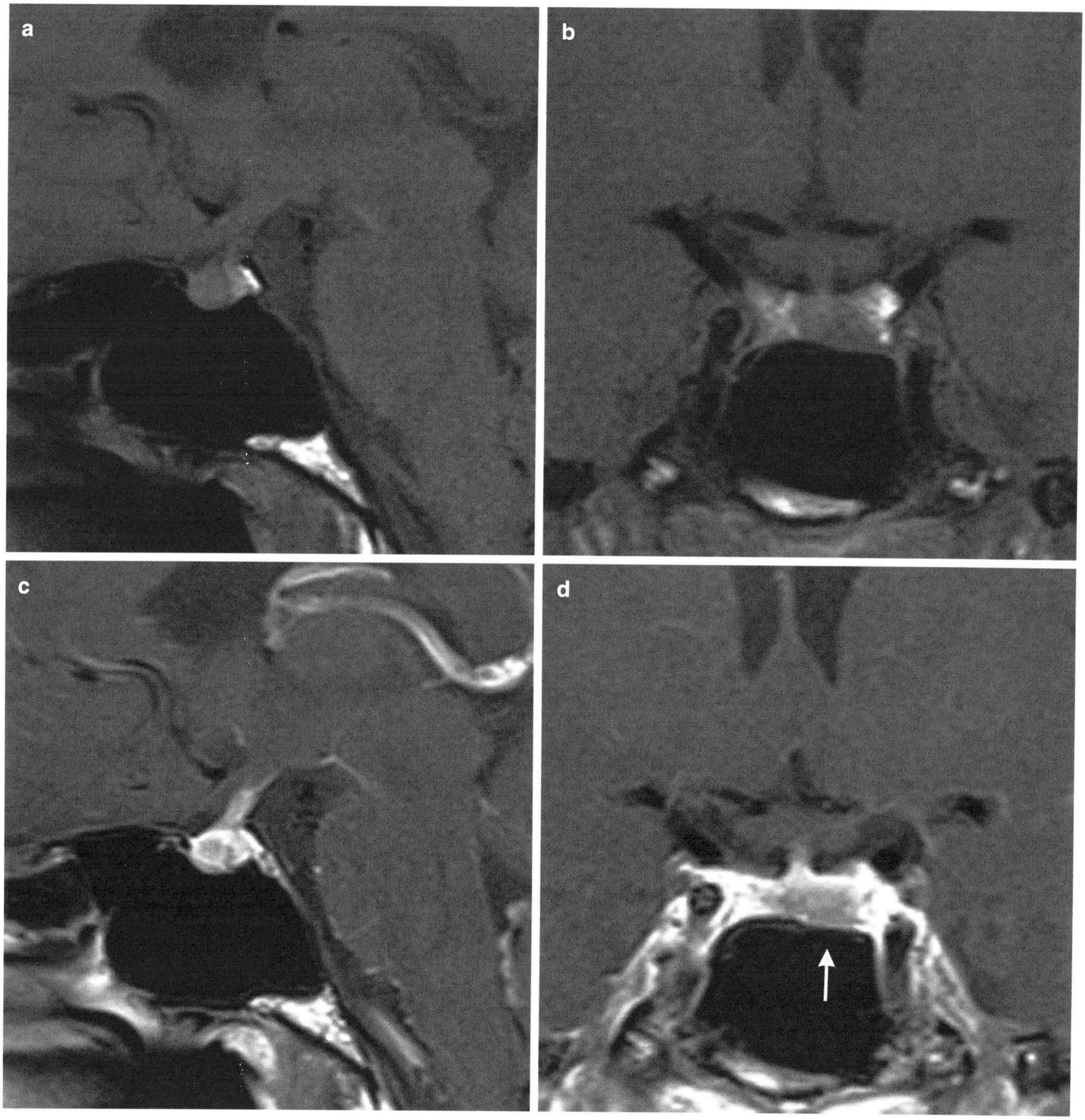

Fig. 13.4 ACTH adenoma. (**a**) Sagittal T1-weighted pre-gadolinium image. (**b**) Coronal T1-weighted pre-gadolinium image. (**c**) Sagittal T1-weighted post-gadolinium image. (**d**) Coronal T1-weighted post-gadolinium image. A hypoenhancing region is located in the inferior left aspect of the pituitary gland (*white arrow*), with subtle erosion of the sellar floor

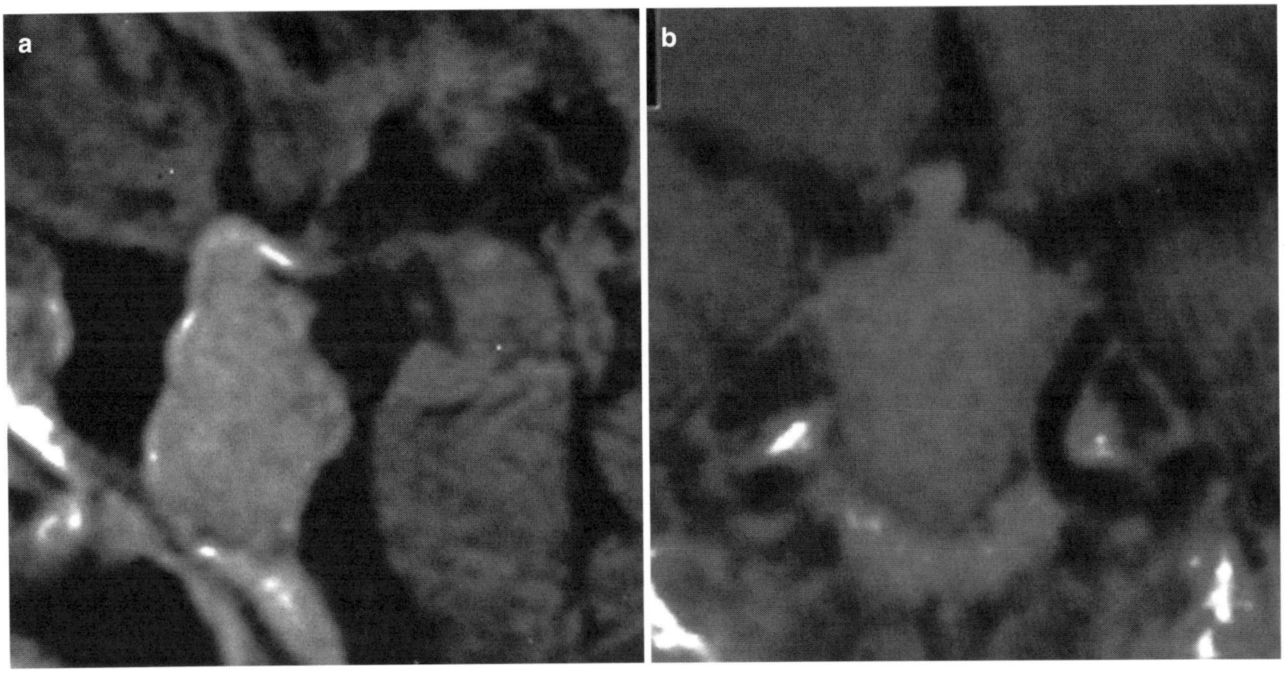

Fig. 13.5 ACTH adenoma. (**a**) Sagittal T1-weighted post-gadolinium image. (**b**) Coronal T1-weighted post-gadolinium image. There is an enhancing mass eroding the sellar floor, with suprasellar extension. The mass abuts the cavernous internal carotid arteries bilaterally

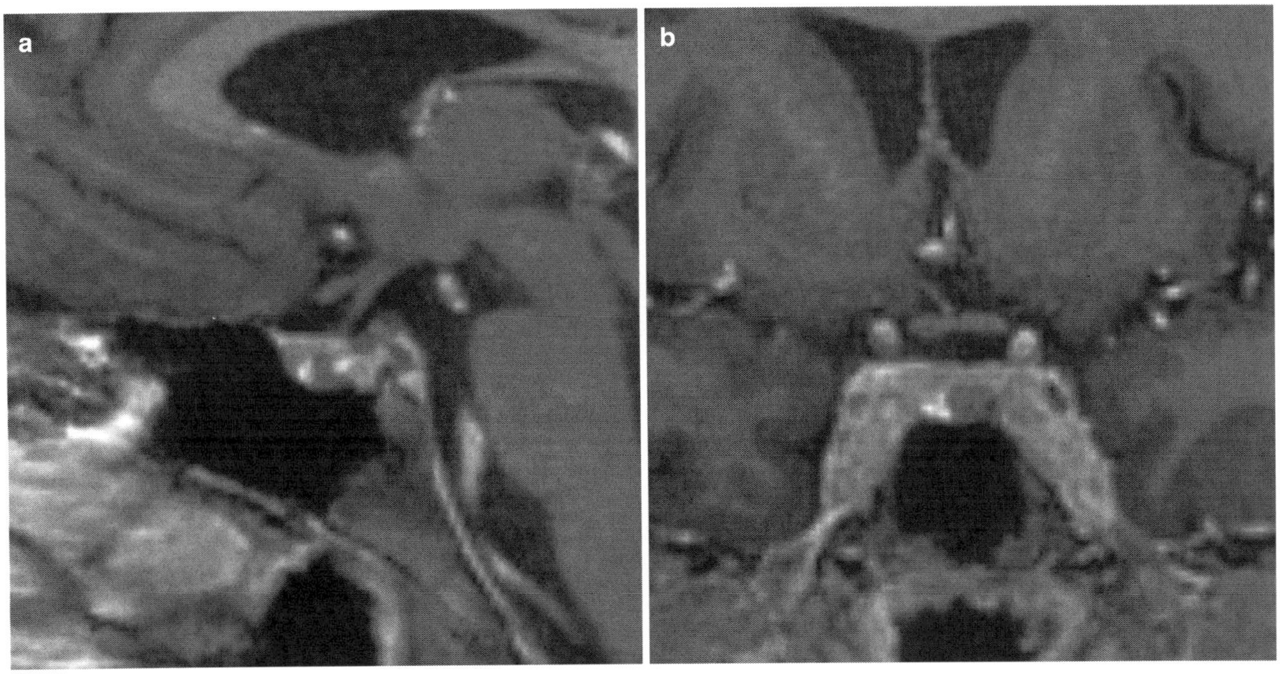

Fig. 13.6 ACTH adenoma. (**a**) Sagittal T1-weighted post-gadolinium image. (**b**) Coronal T1-weighted post-gadolinium image. A hypoenhancing mass is seen in the left inferior aspect of the pituitary gland

13.2.2 Inferior Petrosal Sinus Sampling

- In some cases, inferior petrosal sinus sampling (IPSS) may be performed to confirm the diagnosis of central ACTH secretion and CD or in the event of suspected CD with a negative MRI.
- IPSS offers a sensitivity and specificity of 92–100 % for the diagnosis of CD.
- Following administration of CRH, ACTH levels are serially measured from both inferior petrosal sinuses, cavernous sinuses, and the inferior vena cava in order to calculate central–peripheral gradients and lateralization measurements.
- The accuracy of diagnosing the laterality of the tumor is 84 % if the measured ACTH level on one side is more than 1.4 times greater than the level on the other side [15–18].

13.2.3 Histopathology

- Corticotroph (ACTH) adenomas show positive immunoreactivity for ACTH immunostain and periodic acid–Schiff (PAS) [1].
  - Densely granulated (basophilic) ACTH adenomas (50 %) are strongly PAS and CAM 5.2 positive.
  - Sparsely granulated (chromophobic) ACTH adenomas are weakly PAS positive and have more frequent cellular pleomorphism.
- "Crooke's hyaline change" refers to a reactive process in adenohypophyseal cells in the setting of chronic hypercortisolemia. The presence of Crooke's hyaline change without an adenoma has been reported in up to 1.8 % of all sellar lesions, possibly due to intraoperative loss of a microadenoma specimen [1].
- "Crooke's cell adenoma" refers to a corticotroph adenoma displaying larger number of cells with Crooke's hyaline change (Fig. 13.7).
  - These tumors have been reported to account for less than 1 % of pituitary adenomas [1].
  - They are characterized by cellular pleomorphism and positive immunostaining for ACTH, PAS, and CAM 5.2 (which stains intracellular keratin) [19].
- Multiple ACTH adenomas have been reported in patients with Cushing's disease [20].

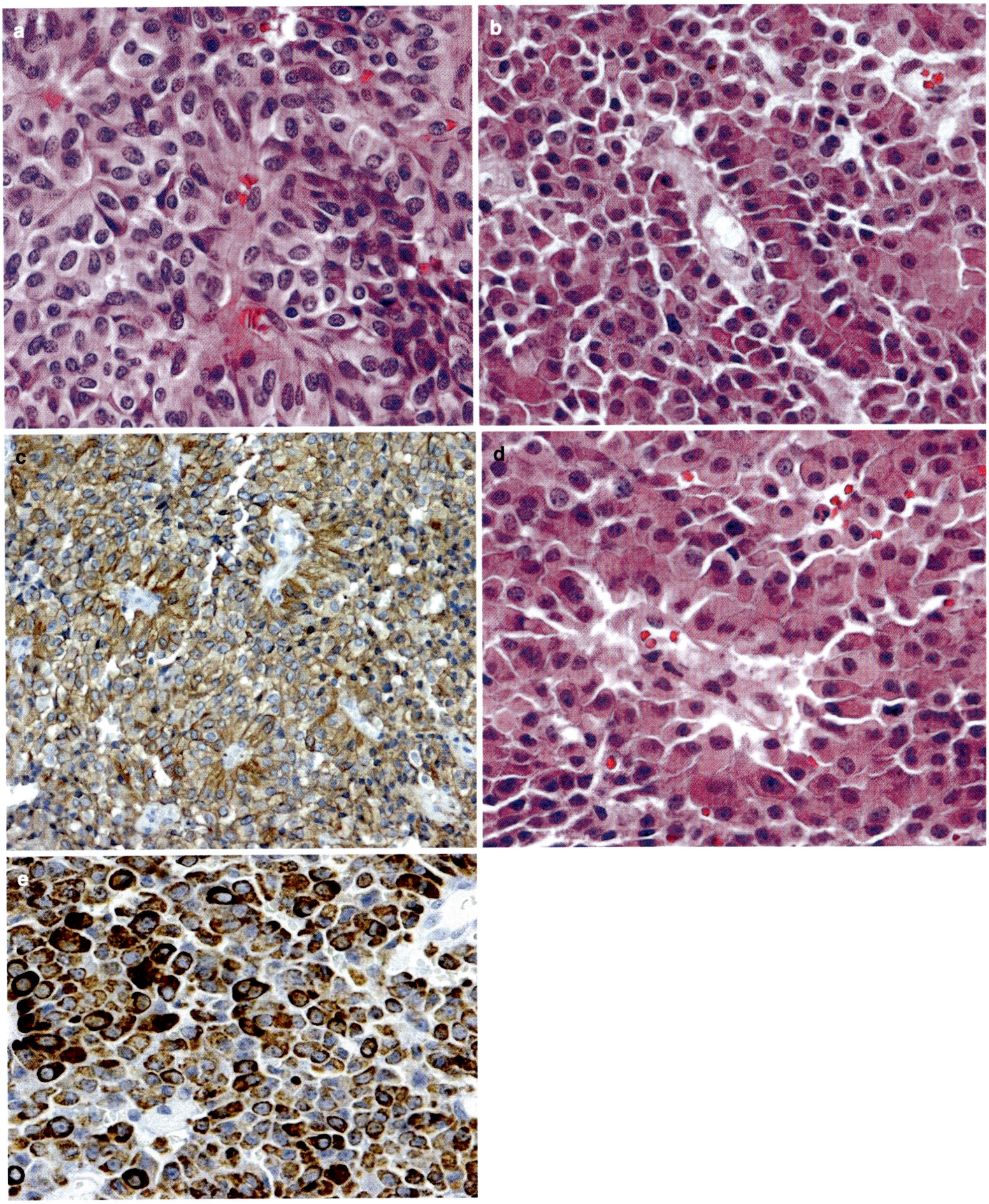

Fig. 13.7 ACTH adenoma. (**a**) Corticotroph (ACTH) cell adenomas are composed of large cells with angular, amphophilic to basophilic cytoplasm and large pleomorphic nuclei. (**b**) A tile-like arrangement of cells is sometimes seen. (**c**) Intense ACTH immunoreactivity in a papillary corticotroph adenoma. (**d**) A special variant of corticot roph adenomas has an increased accumulation of hyaline bundles in the cytoplasm, characterizing Crooke's changes. (**e**) These so-called Crooke's adenomas show extensive immunoreactivity of the cells, with CAM 5.2 cytokeratin highlighting the Crooke's changes. (**f–g**) Crooke's changes are commonly seen in the normal corticotroph cells of the adjacent pituitary as seen by H&E stain (**f**) or by the negative reaction of the cytoplasmic hyaline material on ACTH immunostain (**g**)

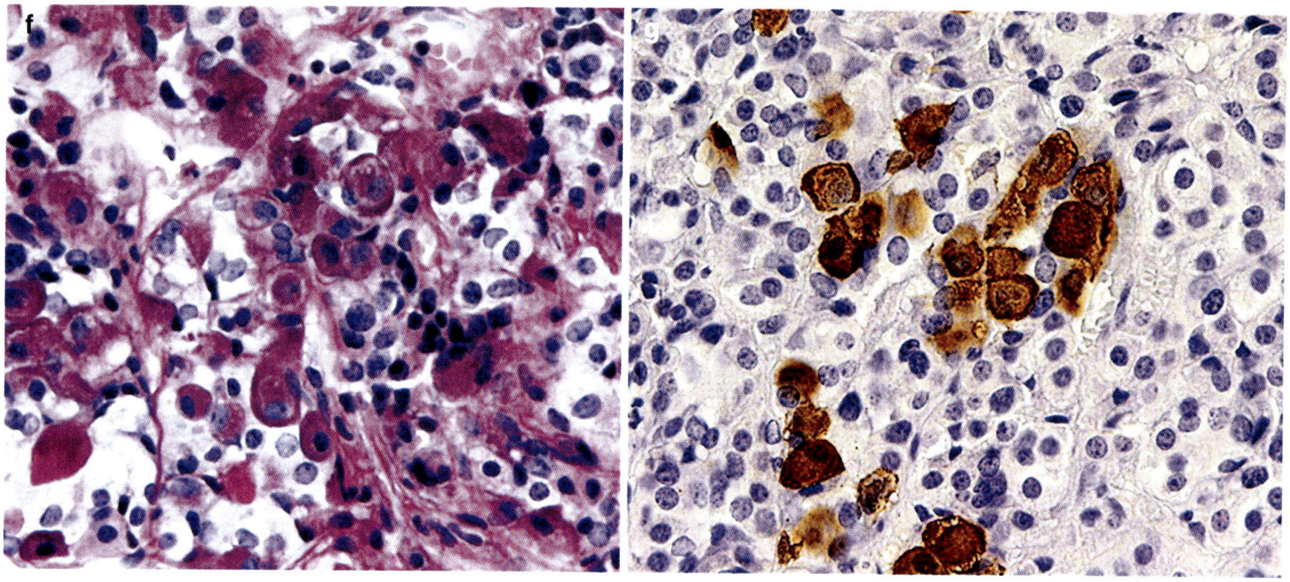

Fig. 13.7 (continued)

13.3 Clinical Management

- Surgery remains the primary option for patients with CD. Following exhaustive surgical management, multimodal therapy may be required for patients with persistent hypercortisolemia who do not obtain hormonal remission. Adjunctive treatments following surgical management for CD include radiosurgery and radiotherapy, medical therapy, and bilateral adrenalectomy.

13.3.1 Surgical Management

- The primary treatment for CD remains surgical resection.
- Endoscopic techniques may provide improved visualization, especially in cases that are MRI negative.
- During surgery, a wide exposure of the entire sella and pituitary gland is routinely performed, even in cases of lateralized microadenomas, in order to survey the entire gland.
- Extracapsular dissection of pituitary microadenomas should be attempted when a pseudocapsule exists [21].
- Following tumor resection, the remainder of the gland is inspected thoroughly for evidence of additional tumors, as multiple ACTH adenomas have been reported in CD patients [20].
- During the first several days after surgical resection, cortisol levels are typically evaluated every 6 h until a nadir cortisol level (optimally <2 μg/dL) is reached [22]. Replacement therapy (i.e., hydrocortisone) may be initiated at this time, especially if the patient becomes symptomatic [23].
- Parenteral (intravenous) hydrocortisone replacement may be transiently required if oral medications are not tolerated because of nausea and vomiting.
- Successful surgical remission in Cushing's disease is defined as a normal (or preferably subnormal) postoperative 24-h urinary free cortisol level. In Nelson's syndrome, a normalized ACTH level defines endocrinological remission.
- An overnight low-dose DST may be performed on postoperative day 3; a cortisol level less than 3 μg/dL may be used to predict remission in over 90 % of patients [24].
- If cortisol levels do not reach subnormal levels following surgery, immediate reoperation and gland reexploration should be considered, especially if histopathology was negative for tumor.
- Delayed endocrinological remission, with a mean time to remission of 38 days, has been reported in 5.6 % of patients following surgery and is associated with higher recurrence rates [25].
- In patients without early remission, early reoperation (within 60 days), usually for hemihypophysectomy or total hypophysectomy, has resulted in remission in 38–67 % [26, 27].
- Rates of remission following transsphenoidal surgery for ACTH-producing tumors have been reported to be 70–90 % for patients with noninvasive microadenomas and approximately 25–50 % for patients with invasive macroadenomas [2, 26, 28, 29].
- Recurrence occurs in approximately 17 % of patients achieving initial remission [3].
- The median time to recurrence is 3–5 years, but recurrence can occur more than a decade after initial remission [3, 26].

13.3.2 Medical Management

- Medical management of CD remains somewhat limited.
- Inhibitors of adrenal steroid synthesis, such as the antifungal agent ketoconazole, have been reported to reduce serum cortisol levels in approximately 70 % of patients, but significant adverse effects have been associated with this medication and other inhibitors of adrenal steroid synthesis. These effects include gastrointestinal distress, gynecomastia, decreased libido, and impotence. In addition, hepatotoxicity has been reported in up to 12 % of patients, mandating frequent liver function laboratory assessments [30].
- Cortisol receptor antagonists such as mifepristone (RU-486) are currently being evaluated as potential medical agents for CD. Mifepristone is a glucocorticoid receptor blocker that blunts the effects of cortisol despite raising cortisol levels. Adverse effects include an increased risk of adrenal insufficiency and hypokalemia [31–33].
- Second-line agents such as metyrapone and mitotane may result in more significant toxicity and are infrequently used.
- Pasireotide (SOM230) is a somatostatin analogue with higher specificity for the somatostatin receptor subtype 5. Pasireotide inhibits ACTH release at the level of the pituitary adenoma, but it may worsen hyperglycemia. In clinical trials, it decreased 24-h urinary free cortisol (UFC) levels in 76 % of patients and offered sustained normalization of UFC in up to 25 % [34, 35].

13.3.3 Stereotactic Radiosurgery

- Stereotactic fractionated or single-session radiosurgery is commonly utilized as an adjunctive treatment for residual disease, with typical marginal isodose levels of 18–25 Gy, depending on the tumor volume and proximity to surrounding structures.
- Long-term tumor control is achieved in more than 95 % of patients following Gamma Knife radiosurgery for ACTH adenomas [36].
- Hormonal remission has been reported in up to 54–70 % following Gamma Knife radiosurgery, but remission may take 1–2 years to achieve following radiosurgical treatment [28, 36].
- New hypopituitarism after Gamma Knife radiosurgery for CD was reported in 36 % of patients [36].
- Radiosurgery also can be used to target a portion of the pituitary gland in patients with MRI-negative CD.

13.3.4 Bilateral Adrenalectomy

- Bilateral adrenalectomy remains a viable option for patients with refractory or progressive CD.
- Remission from CD has been reported in 80–100 % of patients undergoing this procedure.
- Improved quality of life has been reported by 89 % of patients following bilateral adrenalectomy for CD [37].
- Nelson's disease develops in approximately 30 % of patients following a bilateral adrenalectomy; it is associated with aggressive, invasive macroadenomas.

References

1. Saeger W, Ludecke DK, Buchfelder M, Fahlbusch R, Quabbe HJ, Petersenn S. Pathohistological classification of pituitary tumors: 10 years of experience with the German Pituitary Tumor Registry. Eur J Endocrinol. 2007;156:203–16.
2. Zada G, Kelly DF, Cohan P, Wang C, Swerdloff R. Endonasal transsphenoidal approach for pituitary adenomas and other sellar lesions: an assessment of efficacy, safety, and patient impressions. J Neurosurg. 2003;98:350–8.
3. Patil CG, Prevedello DM, Lad SP, Vance ML, Thorner MO, Katznelson L, Laws Jr ER. Late recurrences of Cushing's disease after initial successful transsphenoidal surgery. J Clin Endocrinol Metab. 2008;93:358–62.
4. Mindermann T, Wilson CB. Age-related and gender-related occurrence of pituitary adenomas. Clin Endocrinol (Oxf). 1994;41:359–64.
5. Savage MO, Storr HL, Chan LF, Grossman AB. Diagnosis and treatment of pediatric Cushing's disease. Pituitary. 2007;10:365–71.
6. Kanter AS, Diallo AO, Jane Jr JA, Sheehan JP, Asthagiri AR, Oskouian RJ, et al. Single-center experience with pediatric Cushing's disease. J Neurosurg. 2005;103:413–20.
7. Gil-Cardenas A, Herrera MF, Diaz-Polanco A, Rios JM, Pantoja JP. Nelson's syndrome after bilateral adrenalectomy for Cushing's disease. Surgery. 2007;141:147–51; discussion 151–2.
8. Banasiak MJ, Malek AR. Nelson syndrome: comprehensive review of pathophysiology, diagnosis, and management. Neurosurg Focus. 2007;23:E13.
9. Kelly PA, Samandouras G, Grossman AB, Afshar F, Besser GM, Jenkins PJ. Neurosurgical treatment of Nelson's syndrome. J Clin Endocrinol Metab. 2002;87:5465–9.
10. Nieman LK, Biller BM, Findling JW, Newell-Price J, Savage MO, Stewart PM, Montori VM. The diagnosis of Cushing's syndrome: an Endocrine Society Clinical Practice Guideline. J Clin Endocrinol Metab. 2008;93:1526–40.
11. Scheithauer BW, Kovacs KT, Laws Jr ER, Randall RV. Pathology of invasive pituitary tumors with special reference to functional classification. J Neurosurg. 1986;65:733–44.
12. Jagannathan J, Sheehan JP, Jane Jr JA. Evaluation and management of Cushing syndrome in cases of negative sellar magnetic resonance imaging. Neurosurg Focus. 2007;23:E3.
13. Kucharczyk W, Bishop JE, Plewes DB, Keller MA, George S. Detection of pituitary microadenomas: comparison of dynamic keyhole fast spin-echo, unenhanced, and conventional contrast-enhanced MR imaging. AJR Am J Roentgenol. 1994;163:671–9.
14. Batista D, Courkoutsakis NA, Oldfield EH, Griffin KJ, Keil M, Patronas NJ, Stratakis CA. Detection of adrenocorticotropin-secreting pituitary adenomas by magnetic resonance imaging in children and adolescents with Cushing disease. J Clin Endocrinol Metab. 2005;90:5134–40.
15. Lad SP, Patil CG, Laws Jr ER, Katznelson L. The role of inferior petrosal sinus sampling in the diagnostic localization of Cushing's disease. Neurosurg Focus. 2007;23:E2.
16. Oldfield EH, Doppman JL, Nieman LK, Chrousos GP, Miller DL, Katz DA, et al. Petrosal sinus sampling with and without corticotropin-releasing hormone for the differential diagnosis of Cushing's syndrome. N Engl J Med. 1991;325:897–905.
17. Kaltsas GA, Giannulis MG, Newell-Price JD, Dacie JE, Thakkar C, Afshar F, et al. A critical analysis of the value of simultaneous inferior petrosal sinus sampling in Cushing's disease and the occult ectopic adrenocorticotropin syndrome. J Clin Endocrinol Metab. 1999;84:487–92.
18. Bonelli FS, Huston 3rd J, Carpenter PC, Erickson D, Young Jr WF, Meyer FB. Adrenocorticotropic hormone-dependent Cushing's syndrome: sensitivity and specificity of inferior petrosal sinus sampling. AJNR Am J Neuroradiol. 2000;21:690–6.

19. Al-Brahim NY, Asa SL. My approach to pathology of the pituitary gland. J Clin Pathol. 2006;59:1245–53.
20. Meij BP, Lopes MB, Vance ML, Thorner MO, Laws Jr ER. Double pituitary lesions in three patients with Cushing's disease. Pituitary. 2000;3:159–68.
21. Jagannathan J, Smith R, DeVroom HL, Vortmeyer AO, Stratakis CA, Nieman LK, Oldfield EH. Outcome of using the histological pseudocapsule as a surgical capsule in Cushing disease. J Neurosurg. 2009;111:531–9.
22. Esposito F, Dusick JR, Cohan P, Moftakhar P, McArthur D, Wang C, et al. Clinical review: early morning cortisol levels as a predictor of remission after transsphenoidal surgery for Cushing's disease. J Clin Endocrinol Metab. 2006;91:7–13.
23. Biller BM, Grossman AB, Stewart PM, Melmed S, Bertagna X, Bertherat J, et al. Treatment of adrenocorticotropin-dependent Cushing's syndrome: a consensus statement. J Clin Endocrinol Metab. 2008;93:2454–62.
24. Chen JC, Amar AP, Choi S, Singer P, Couldwell WT, Weiss MH. Transsphenoidal microsurgical treatment of Cushing disease: postoperative assessment of surgical efficacy by application of an overnight low-dose dexamethasone suppression test. J Neurosurg. 2003;98:967–73.
25. Valassi E, Biller BM, Swearingen B, Pecori Giraldi F, Losa M, Mortini P, et al. Delayed remission after transsphenoidal surgery in patients with Cushing's disease. J Clin Endocrinol Metab. 2010;95: 601–10.
26. Kelly DF. Transsphenoidal surgery for Cushing's disease: a review of success rates, remission predictors, management of failed surgery, and Nelson's Syndrome. Neurosurg Focus. 2007; 23:E5.
27. Locatelli M, Vance ML, Laws ER. Clinical review: the strategy of immediate reoperation for transsphenoidal surgery for Cushing's disease. J Clin Endocrinol Metab. 2005;90:5478–82.
28. Laws ER, Reitmeyer M, Thapar K, Vance ML. Cushing's disease resulting from pituitary corticotrophic microadenoma. Treatment results from transsphenoidal microsurgery and gamma knife radiosurgery. Neurochirurgie. 2002;48:294–9.
29. Nakane T, Kuwayama A, Watanabe M, Takahashi T, Kato T, Ichihara K, Kageyama N. Long term results of transsphenoidal adenomectomy in patients with Cushing's disease. Neurosurgery. 1987;21:218–22.
30. Engelhardt D, Weber MM. Therapy of Cushing's syndrome with steroid biosynthesis inhibitors. J Steroid Biochem Mol Biol. 1994;49:261–7.
31. Basina M, Liu H, Hoffman AR, Feldman D. Successful long-term treatment of Cushing disease with mifepristone (RU486). Endocr Pract. 2012;18:e114–20.
32. Carmichael JD, Fleseriu M. Mifepristone: is there a place in the treatment of Cushing's disease? Endocrine. 2013;44:20–32.
33. Fleseriu M, Biller BM, Findling JW, Molitch ME, Schteingart DE, Gross C. Mifepristone, a glucocorticoid receptor antagonist, produces clinical and metabolic benefits in patients with Cushing's syndrome. J Clin Endocrinol Metab. 2012;97: 2039–49.
34. Boscaro M, Ludlam WH, Atkinson B, Glusman JE, Petersenn S, Reincke M, et al. Treatment of pituitary-dependent Cushing's disease with the multireceptor ligand somatostatin analog pasireotide (SOM230): a multicenter, phase II trial. J Clin Endocrinol Metab. 2009;94:115–22.
35. Colao A, De Block C, Gaztambide MS, Kumar S, Seufert J, Casanueva FF. Managing hyperglycemia in patients with Cushing's disease treated with pasireotide: medical expert recommendations. Pituitary. 2014;17:180–6.
36. Sheehan JP, Xu Z, Salvetti DJ, Schmitt PJ, Vance ML. Results of gamma knife surgery for Cushing's disease. J Neurosurg. 2013; 119:1486–92.
37. Thompson SK, Hayman AV, Ludlam WH, Deveney CW, Loriaux DL, Sheppard BC. Improved quality of life after bilateral laparoscopic adrenalectomy for Cushing's disease: a 10-year experience. Ann Surg. 2007;245:790–4.

Silent Corticotroph (ACTH) Adenomas

14

Gabriel Zada, M. Beatriz S. Lopes, Srinivasan Mukundan Jr., and Edward Laws Jr.

14.1 Epidemiology and Clinical Presentation

- Silent ACTH tumors are a unique subgroup of nonfunctioning tumors that demonstrate strong immunoreactivity for ACTH, yet rarely cause hormonal excess of cortisol (Cushing's disease).
- The serum ACTH may be normal or mildly elevated [1].
- These tumors are more common in female patients [2].
- Their clinical presentation is similar to the presentation of macroadenomas, including headache, visual loss, panhypopituitarism, and amenorrhea/galactorrhea.
- A relatively high incidence of hemorrhagic infarction (33 %) has been reported [2].

14.2 Diagnosis

14.2.1 Imaging

- Silent ACTH adenomas are typically aggressive and invasive macroadenomas [3, 4].
- Extrasellar extension is identified in 93 % of tumors [2].
- Invasion of surrounding structures occurs in 82 % of lesions [5].
- Figs. 14.1, 14.2, 14.3, and 14.4.

14.2.2 Histopathology

- Silent ACTH adenomas may be densely granulated (Type I) or sparsely granulated (Type II) [6].
- The tumors demonstrate immunoreactivity for ACTH and are variably positive for periodic acid–Schiff and beta-endorphin immunostains [1].

G. Zada, MD, MS (✉)
Department of Neurological Surgery, Keck School of Medicine, University of Southern California, 1200 N State Street, #3300, Los Angeles, CA 90033, USA
e-mail: gzada@usc.edu

M.B.S. Lopes, MD, PhD
Department of Pathology (Neuropathology), University of Virginia School of Medicine, 1215 Lee Street, Room 3060–HEP, Charlottesville, VA 22908, USA
e-mail: msl2e@virginia.edu

S. Mukundan Jr., PhD, MD
Department of Radiology, Brigham and Women's Hospital, 75 Francis Street, Boston, MA 02115, USA
e-mail: smukundan@partners.org

E. Laws Jr., MD
Department of Neurosurgery, Brigham and Women's Hospital, 15 Francis Street, Boston, MA 02115, USA
e-mail: elaws@partners.org

G. Zada et al. (eds.), *Atlas of Sellar and Parasellar Lesions: Clinical, Radiologic, and Pathologic Correlations*,
DOI 10.1007/978-3-319-22855-6_14

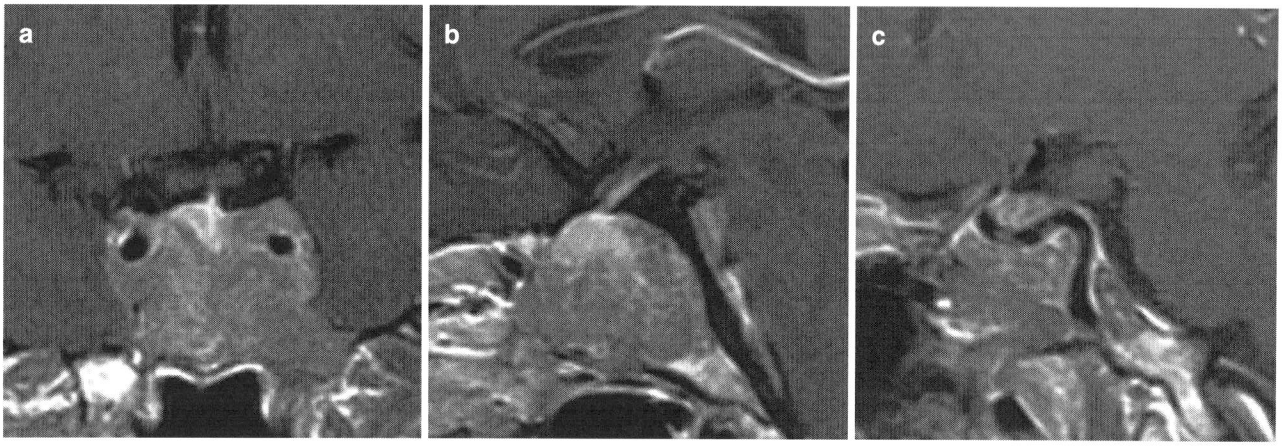

Fig. 14.1 Silent corticotroph (ACTH) adenoma. (**a**, **b**) Sagittal T1-weighted post-gadolinium image. (**c**) Coronal T1-weighted post-gadolinium image. There is a large, heterogeneously enhancing sellar mass with suprasellar extension and encasement of bilateral cavernous internal carotid arteries suggestive of invasion. There is erosion of the clivus. The normal pituitary gland appears along the superior margin of the mass

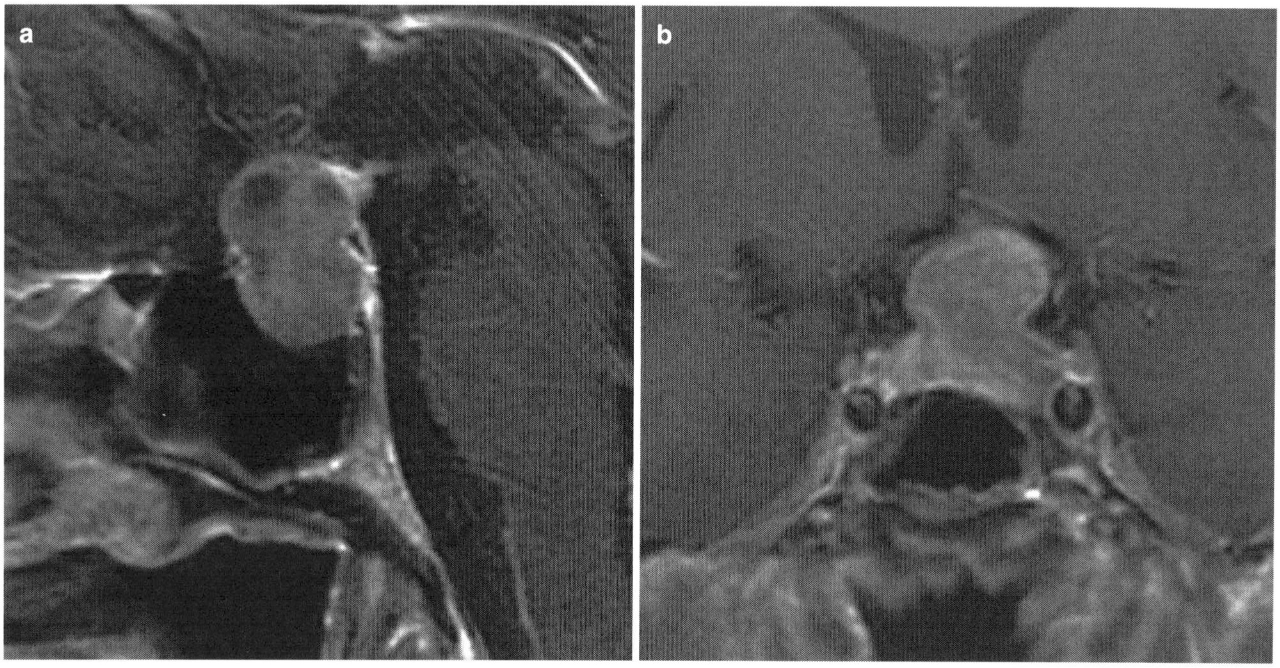

Fig. 14.2 Silent corticotroph (ACTH) adenoma. (**a**) Sagittal T1-weighted post-gadolinium image. (**b**) Coronal T1-weighted post-gadolinium image. A heterogeneously enhancing sellar/suprasellar mass contacts the left cavernous internal carotid artery without encasement. The optic chiasm is elevated by the mass

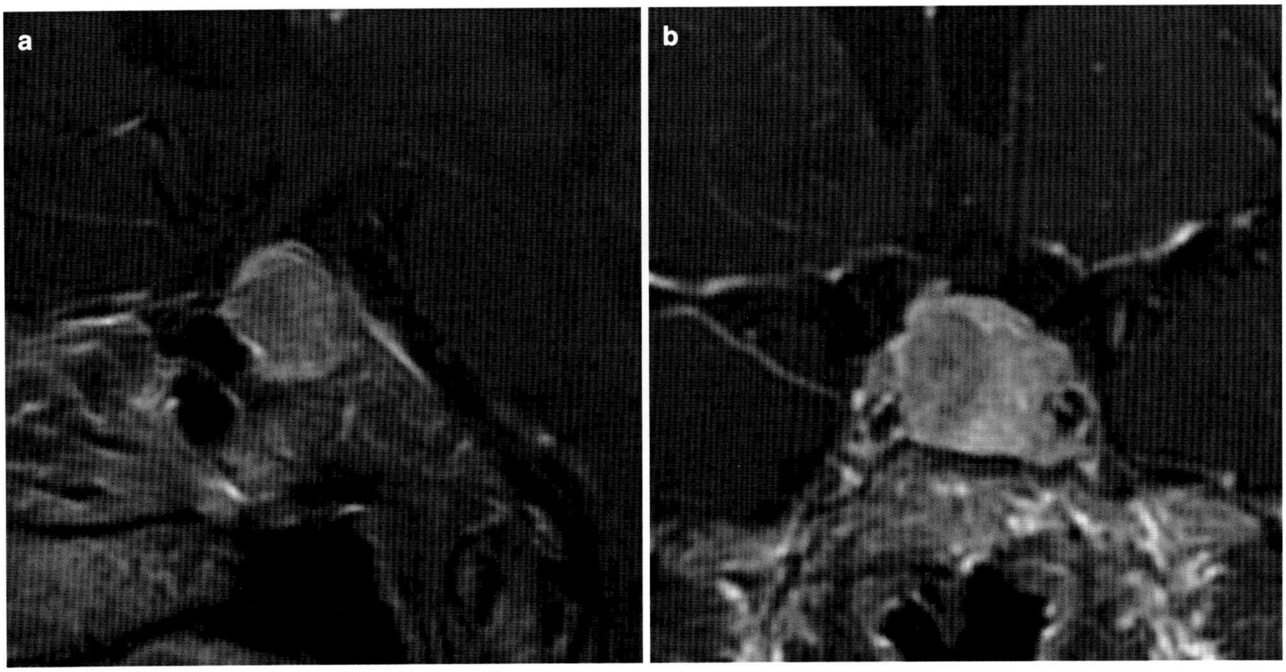

Fig. 14.3 Silent corticotroph (ACTH) adenoma. (**a**) Sagittal T1-weighted post-gadolinium image. (**b**) Coronal T1-weighted post-gadolinium image. A heterogeneously enhancing sellar mass contacts bilateral cavernous internal carotid arteries with possible encasement on the left. The normal pituitary gland appears along the superior margin of the mass, with the stalk deviated to the right

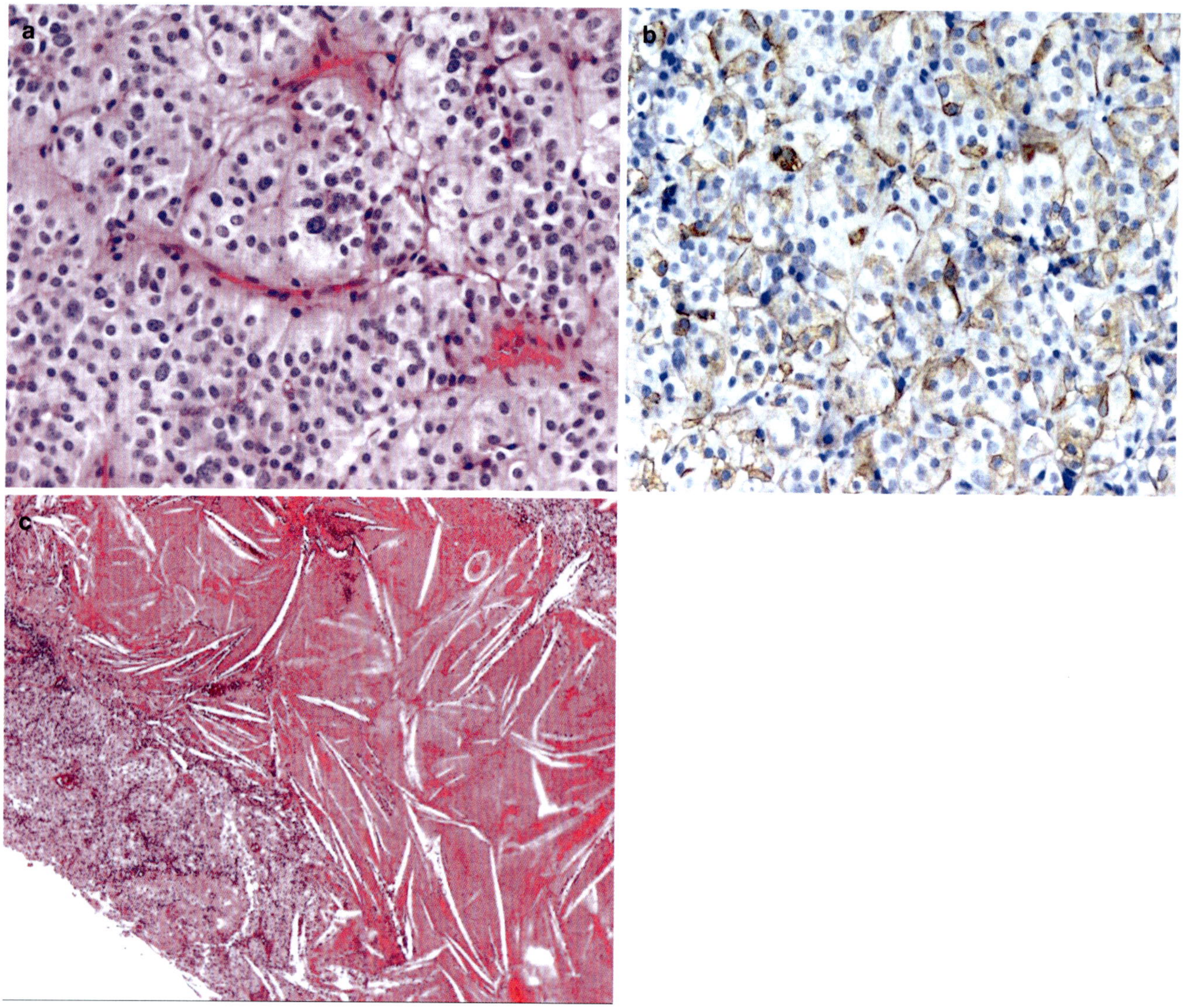

Fig. 14.4 Silent corticotroph (ACTH) adenoma that presented clinically as a nonfunctioning adenoma. (**a**) A chromophobic adenoma exhibiting a diffuse growth pattern. (**b**) Despite lack of clinical symptoms, this adenoma shows immunopositivity for ACTH. (**c**) The same adenoma displays a large area of previous hemorrhage with accumulation of cholesterol clefts. Silent corticotroph adenomas show a high tendency for hemorrhage and/or apoplexy, which may be the presenting symptom in about one third of patients

14.3 Clinical Management

- Surgical resection remains the mainstay of treatment.
- Long-term recurrence rates (typically 30–54 % in most series) are generally as high or higher than for other nonfunctioning adenomas [1, 2, 8].
- Recurrence typically occurs much earlier than for other nonfunctioning adenomas [7].
- Patients with silent ACTH adenomas require vigilant long-term follow-up.
- Radiosurgery may be beneficial for postoperative adjunctive treatment of residual tumor.
- A potential for transformation to functional tumors with hormonal excess and Cushing's disease has been reported at later stages in their natural history [9, 10].

References

1. Scheithauer BW, Jaap AJ, Horvath E, Kovacs K, Lloyd RV, Meyer FB, et al. Clinically silent corticotroph tumors of the pituitary gland. Neurosurgery. 2000;47:723–9; discussion 729–30.
2. Webb KM, Laurent JJ, Okonkwo DO, Lopes MB, Vance ML, Laws Jr ER. Clinical characteristics of silent corticotrophic adenomas and creation of an internet-accessible database to facilitate their multi-institutional study. Neurosurgery. 2003;53:1076–84; discussion 1084–5.
3. Alahmadi H, Lee D, Wilson JR, Hayhurst C, Mete O, Gentili F, et al. Clinical features of silent corticotroph adenomas. Acta Neurochir (Wien). 2012;154:1493–8.
4. Saeger W, Ludecke DK, Buchfelder M, Fahlbusch R, Quabbe HJ, Petersenn S. Pathohistological classification of pituitary tumors: 10 years of experience with the German Pituitary Tumor Registry. Eur J Endocrinol. 2007;156:203–16.
5. Scheithauer BW, Kovacs KT, Laws Jr ER, Randall RV. Pathology of invasive pituitary tumors with special reference to functional classification. J Neurosurg. 1986;65:733–44.
6. Kovacs K, Horvath E. Tumors of the pituitary gland. Washington, DC: Armed Forces Institute of Pathology; 1986;21:150–64.
7. Cooper O, Ben-Shlomo A, Bonert V, Bannykh S, Mirocha J, Melmed S. Silent corticogonadotroph adenomas: clinical and cellular characteristics and long-term outcomes. Horm Cancer. 2010;1:80–92.
8. Bradley KJ, Wass JA, Turner HE. Non-functioning pituitary adenomas with positive immunoreactivity for ACTH behave more aggressively than ACTH immunonegative tumours but do not recur more frequently. Clin Endocrinol (Oxf). 2003;58:59–64.
9. Baldeweg SE, Pollock JR, Powell M, Ahlquist J. A spectrum of behaviour in silent corticotroph pituitary adenomas. Br J Neurosurg. 2005;19:38–42.
10. Psaras T, Honegger J, Buslei R, Saeger W, Klein D, Capper D, et al. Atypical type II silent corticotrophic adenoma developing into Cushing's disease upon second recurrence. Exp Clin Endocrinol Diabetes. 2007;115:610–5.

Thyrotroph (TSH) Adenomas

15

Gabriel Zada, M. Beatriz S. Lopes, Srinivasan Mukundan Jr., and Edward Laws Jr.

15.1 Epidemiology and Clinical Presentation

- Pituitary adenomas that secrete functional thyroid-stimulating hormone (TSH or thyrotropin) are uncommonly encountered lesions, comprising approximately 1–2 % of all pituitary adenomas.
- TSH adenomas can result in the classic symptoms and signs associated with hyperthyroidism, including weight loss, tachycardia, palpitations, hypertension, intolerance to heat, tremor, loss of libido, nausea/vomiting, and diarrhea.
- They have also been associated with Graves' disease.
- TSH oversecretion with hyperthyroidism occurs in approximately 40–80 % of tumors; the remainder are clinically silent.
- TSH adenomas also may occur in the setting of primary hypothyroidism with thyrotroph hyperplasia and neoplastic conversion.
- In the past, TSH adenomas often have been misdiagnosed as primary hyperthyroidism, with a significant proportion of patients undergoing thyroid ablation procedures prior to the diagnosis of a pituitary adenoma [1].
- Some TSH adenomas (plurihormonal pituitary adenomas) may also secrete other functional hormones [8].

G. Zada, MD, MS (✉)
Department of Neurological Surgery, Keck School of Medicine, University of Southern California, 1200 N State Street, #3300, Los Angeles, CA 90033, USA
e-mail: gzada@usc.edu

M.B.S. Lopes, MD, PhD
Department of Pathology (Neuropathology), University of Virginia School of Medicine, 1215 Lee Street, Room 3060–HEP, Charlottesville, VA 22908, USA
e-mail: msl2e@virginia.edu

S. Mukundan Jr., PhD, MD
Department of Radiology, Brigham and Women's Hospital, 75 Francis Street, Boston, MA 02115, USA
e-mail: smukundan@partners.org

E. Laws Jr., MD
Department of Neurosurgery, Brigham and Women's Hospital, 15 Francis Street, Boston, MA 02115, USA
e-mail: elaws@partners.org

G. Zada et al. (eds.), *Atlas of Sellar and Parasellar Lesions: Clinical, Radiologic, and Pathologic Correlations*, DOI 10.1007/978-3-319-22855-6_15

15.2 Diagnosis

- The diagnosis of a functional TSH-secreting adenoma is supported by elevated free thyroid hormone levels and inappropriately elevated or normal (nonsuppressed) TSH levels.

15.2.1 Imaging

- Imaging characteristics of TSH adenomas are similar to those described for other functioning adenomas (Figs. 15.1 and 15.2), except that most tend to be invasive macroadenomas [1, 6, 9].

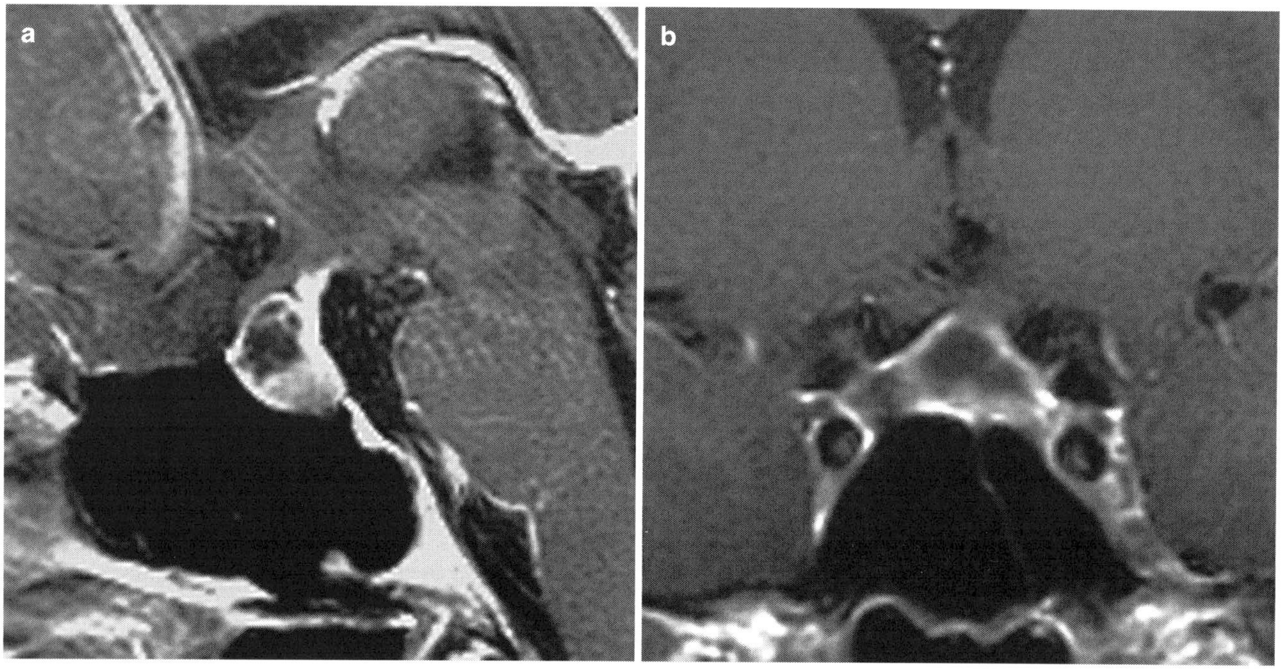

Fig. 15.1 Thyrotroph (TSH) adenoma. (**a**) Sagittal T1-weighted post-gadolinium image. (**b**) Coronal T1-weighted post-gadolinium image. A cystic, enhancing mass is present in the superior anterior part of the sella. There is no encasement of bilateral cavernous internal carotid arteries. The mass contacts the optic chiasm without significant displacement

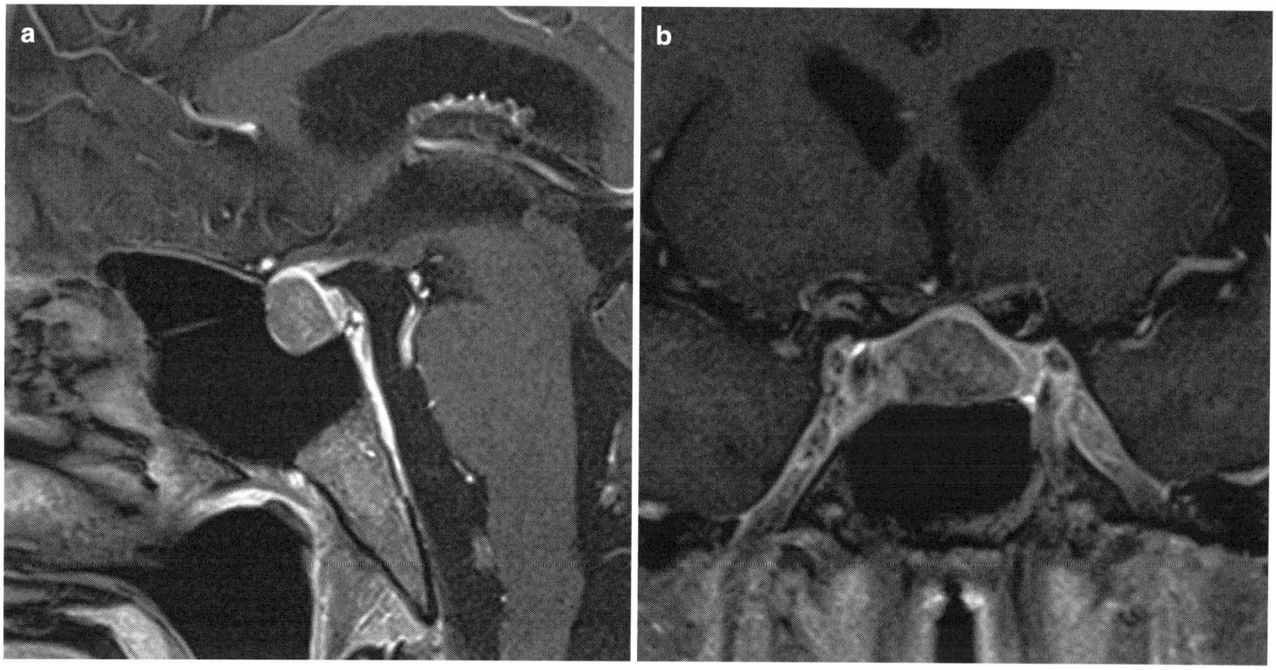

Fig. 15.2 TSH adenoma. (**a**) Sagittal T1-weighted post-gadolinium image. (**b**) Coronal T1-weighted post-gadolinium image. A hypoenhancing mass is located in the right aspect of the sella, contacting the right cavernous internal carotid artery without encasement. The mass contacts the optic chiasm without significant displacement

15.2.2 Histopathology

- These tumors are differentiated via expression of thyrotroph embryonic factor (TEF) and GATA-2 transcription factors [10].
- Histopathologically, medium-sized, elongated chromophobic cells are observed, with sinusoidal growth pattern, partial PAS immunoreactivity, and globular inclusions (Fig. 15.3) [2].
- They frequently demonstrate immunoreactivity for TSH and the alpha-subunit [1].
- These tumors have been reported to have a relatively high rate of atypical features [6].

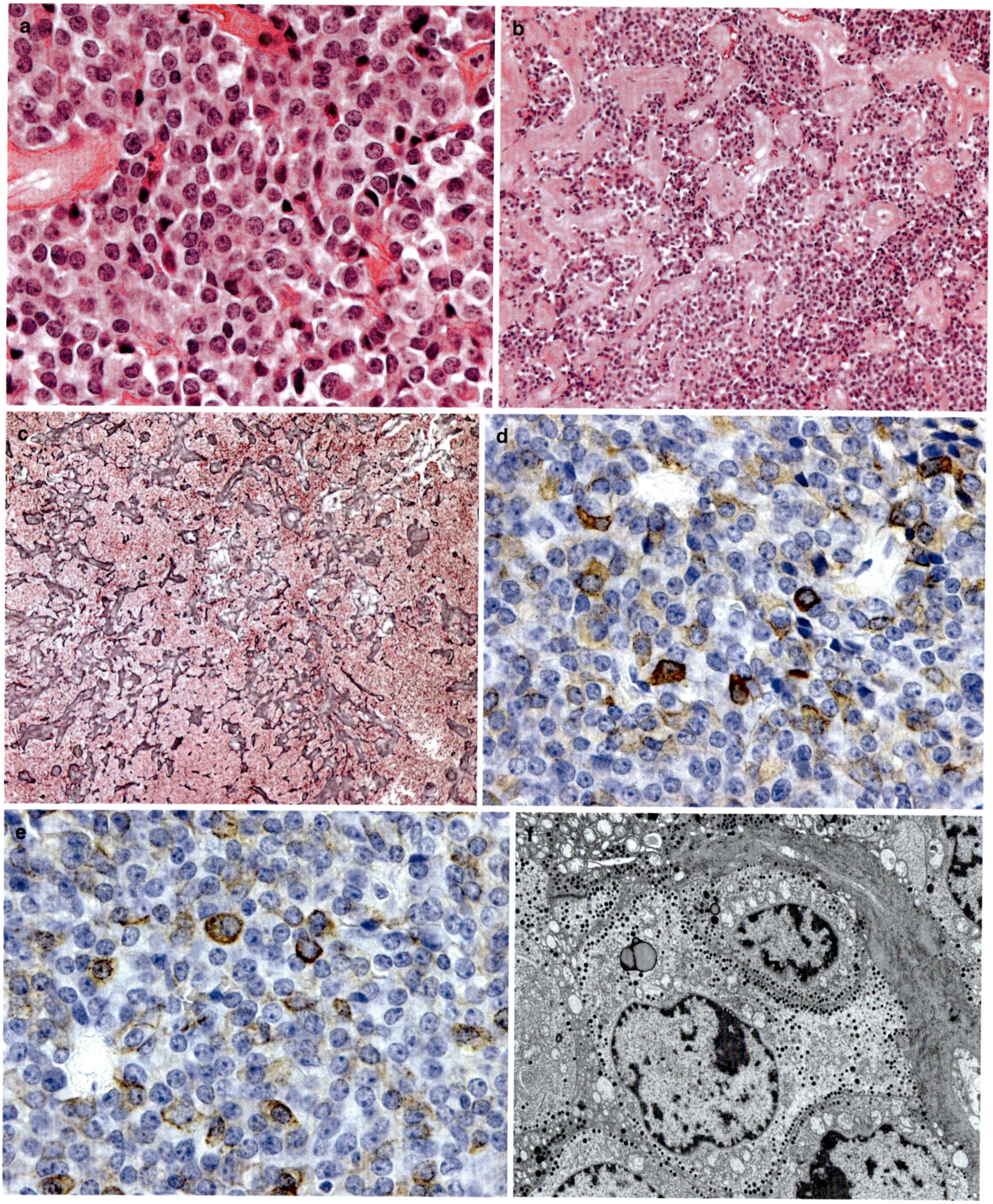

Fig. 15.3 TSH adenoma. (**a**) This TSH cell adenoma shows small to medium cells with chromophobic to acidophilic cytoplasm and central nuclei with delicate chromatin. Increased stromal fibrosis seen on H&E stain (**b**) and highlighted by reticulin staining (**c**) is commonly seen in these adenomas. Immunostains for thyroid-stimulating hormone (TSH) may show variable intensity (**d**), and reactivity for the α-subunit of the glycoproteins (**e**) is commonly seen. The ultrastructure of thyrotroph cell adenomas shows angular cells with rich subcellular organelles and the presence of small, dense secretory granules displayed near the plasmalemma (**f**)

15.3 Clinical Management

- For control of unresectable tumors, somatostatin analogues are effective in decreasing excess TSH secretion [11]. Pretreatment with octreotide has been reported to result in tumor shrinkage prior to surgical resection [9, 12].
- Gross total resection with hormonal remission has been reported in approximately 50–60 % of patients—a rate that can be improved with adjunctive radiation or radiosurgery [1, 4, 9].
- At surgery, TSH adenomas are often firm in texture.
- Undetectable TSH levels on postoperative day 7 are highly predictive of hormonal remission.
- Normal thyroid function alone does not accurately predict long-term remission; MRI findings and TSH suppression following T3 administration should also be assessed [8].
- A majority of patients will require thyroid replacement (i.e., levothyroxine) following successful surgery [1].
- Close endocrinological and neuroimaging monitoring for recurrence is warranted in all patients following surgery.

References

1. Clarke MJ, Erickson D, Castro MR, Atkinson JL. Thyroid-stimulating hormone pituitary adenomas. J Neurosurg. 2008;109:17–22.
2. Saeger W, Ludecke DK, Buchfelder M, Fahlbusch R, Quabbe HJ, Petersenn S. Pathohistological classification of pituitary tumors: 10 years of experience with the German Pituitary Tumor Registry. Eur J Endocrinol. 2007;156:203–16.
3. Zada G, Kelly DF, Cohan P, Wang C, Swerdloff R. Endonasal transsphenoidal approach for pituitary adenomas and other sellar lesions: an assessment of efficacy, safety, and patient impressions. J Neurosurg. 2003;98:350–8.
4. Laws ER, Vance ML, Jane Jr JA. TSH adenomas. Pituitary. 2006;9:313–5.
5. Koriyama N, Nakazaki M, Hashiguchi H, Aso K, Ikeda Y, Kimura T, et al. Thyrotropin-producing pituitary adenoma associated with Graves' disease. Eur J Endocrinol. 2004;151:587–94.
6. Marucci G, Faustini-Fustini M, Righi A, Pasquini E, Frank G, Agati R, Foschini MP. Thyrotropin-secreting pituitary tumours: significance of "atypical adenomas" in a series of 10 patients and association with Hashimoto thyroiditis as a cause of delay in diagnosis. J Clin Pathol. 2009;62:455–9.
7. Scheithauer BW, Kovacs K, Randall RV, Ryan N. Pituitary gland in hypothyroidism. Histologic and immunocytologic study. Arch Pathol Lab Med. 1985;109:499–504.
8. Losa M, Giovanelli M, Persani L, Mortini P, Faglia G, Beck-Peccoz P. Criteria of cure and follow-up of central hyperthyroidism due to thyrotropin-secreting pituitary adenomas. J Clin Endocrinol Metab. 1996;81:3084–90.
9. Sanno N, Teramoto A, Osamura RY. Long-term surgical outcome in 16 patients with thyrotropin pituitary adenoma. J Neurosurg. 2000;93:194–200.
10. Al-Brahim NY, Asa SL. My approach to pathology of the pituitary gland. J Clin Pathol. 2006;59:1245–53.
11. Polak M, Bertherat J, Li JY, Kujas M, Le Dafniet M, Weizani H, et al. A human TSH-secreting adenoma: endocrine, biochemical and morphological studies. Evidence of somatostatin receptors by using quantitative autoradiography. Clinical and biological improvement by SMS 201–995 treatment. Acta Endocrinol (Copenh). 1991;124:479–86.
12. Kole MK, Goldman J, Rock JP. TSH-secreting pituitary adenoma: current management and review. Skull Base Surg. 1997;7:89–93.

Gonadotroph Adenomas

16

Gabriel Zada, M. Beatriz S. Lopes,
Srinivasan Mukundan Jr., and Edward Laws Jr.

16.1 Epidemiology and Clinical Presentation

- Pituitary adenomas that hypersecrete functional follicle-stimulating hormone (FSH) and/or luteinizing hormone (LH) are extremely rare.
- Although many nonfunctioning pituitary adenomas demonstrate positive immunoreactivity for FSH and LH, the overwhelming majority of these tumors are clinically silent [1], as discussed previously in chapter 10.
- In women, functional gonadotroph adenomas may cause ovarian stimulation syndrome with enlarged ovaries, pelvic pain, galactorrhea, and/or menstrual abnormalities [2, 3]. Levels of circulating estradiol are typically elevated.
- In men, excess levels of serum testosterone with testicular enlargement have been reported.
- In boys, precocious puberty has been reported.
- Functioning gonadotroph adenomas are often plurihormonal tumors, which may co-secrete TSH, prolactin, and/or GH.
- Exacerbation of disease has been reported with administration of gonadotropin-releasing hormone agonists such as leuprolide [4].

16.2 Diagnosis

16.2.1 Imaging

- Imaging characteristics of gonadotroph adenomas are similar to those described for other functioning adenomas.

16.2.2 Histopathology

- Adenomas may demonstrate immunoreactivity for FSH, LH, or both, and invariably for the gonadotrophic transcription factor SF-1.
- Many of these adenomas will also demonstrate immunoreactivity for the alpha-subunit (Fig. 16.1) [5].
- Electron microscopy may demonstrate different structural features in the adenomas of men versus those of women. Gonadotroph adenomas in men resemble null-cell adenomas, with poorly or moderately developed cytoplasmic organelles. In women, tumors tend to be well differentiated, with distinctive vesicular dilatation of the Golgi complex ("honeycomb Golgi") [6].

G. Zada, MD, MS (✉)
Department of Neurological Surgery, Keck School of Medicine,
University of Southern California, 1200 N State Street, #3300,
Los Angeles, CA 90033, USA
e-mail: gzada@usc.edu

M.B.S. Lopes, MD, PhD
Department of Pathology (Neuropathology),
University of Virginia School of Medicine,
1215 Lee Street, Room 3060–HEP,
Charlottesville, VA 22908, USA
e-mail: msl2e@virginia.edu

S. Mukundan Jr., PhD, MD
Department of Radiology, Brigham and Women's Hospital,
75 Francis Street, Boston, MA 02115, USA
e-mail: smukundan@partners.org

E. Laws Jr., MD
Department of Neurosurgery, Brigham and Women's Hospital,
15 Francis Street, Boston, MA 02115, USA
e-mail: elaws@partners.org

G. Zada et al. (eds.), *Atlas of Sellar and Parasellar Lesions: Clinical, Radiologic, and Pathologic Correlations*,
DOI 10.1007/978-3-319-22855-6_16

16.3 Clinical Management

- As with most functional pituitary adenomas, transsphenoidal surgical resection remains the mainstay of treatment.
- Dopamine agonist therapy (cabergoline or bromocriptine) has been reported to be an effective medical treatment for a subset of these tumors [7].
- Successful treatment with a gonadotropin-releasing hormone antagonist also has been reported [8].
- Resolution of ovarian hyperstimulation, reduction of ovary size, and successful pregnancy have been reported following effective treatment.
- Gonadotropin-releasing hormone agonists should be avoided in these patients, as they may promote tumor growth [9, 10].

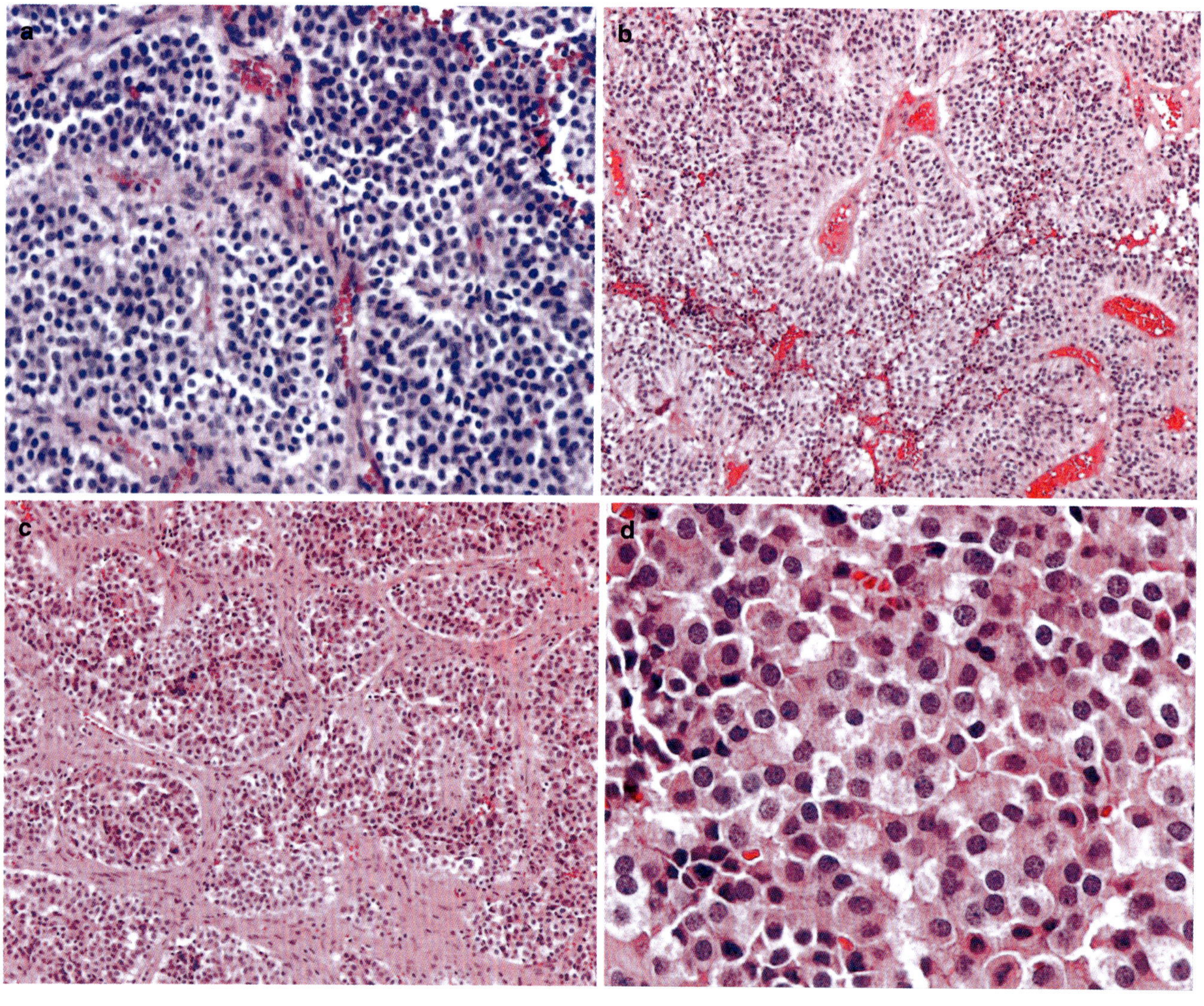

Fig. 16.1 Gonadotropin-secreting adenoma. Gonadotropin-secreting adenomas or gonadotroph cell adenomas are characteristically chromophobic tumors (**a**) with diverse histopathological arrangements. Tumors may have papillary arrangements (**b**), nested arrangements (**c**), and focal oncocytic appearance (**d**). Gonadotroph adenomas show variable immunoreactivity for follicle-stimulating hormone (FSH) (**e**), luteinizing hormone (LH) (**f**), and the alpha-subunit of glycoproteins (**g**). Gonadotroph cell adenomas are mostly composed of well-differentiated, elongated cells with a degree of cellular polarity at the ultrastructure level. Secretory granules are small and tend to be located at the periphery of the cytoplasm (**h**)

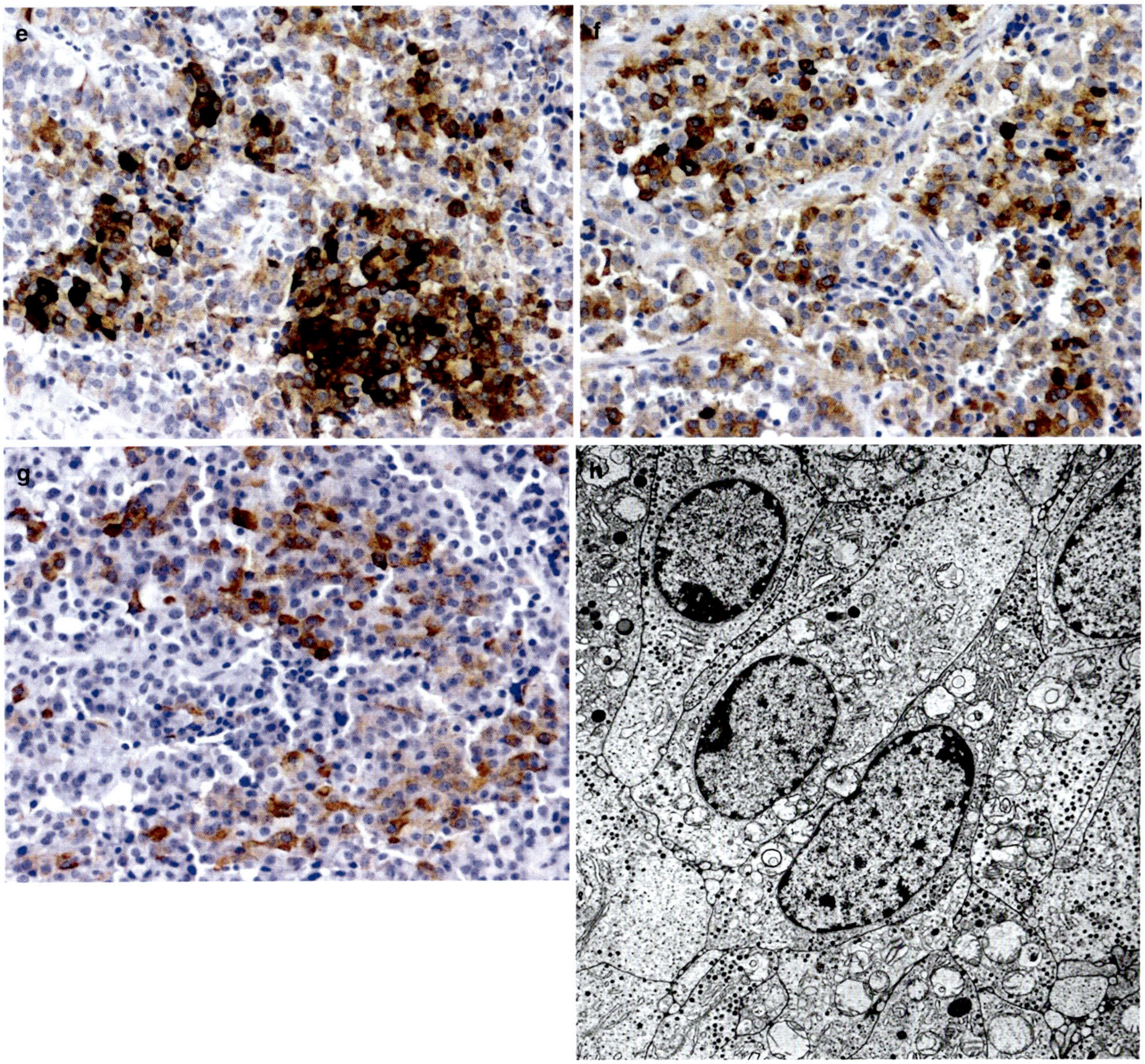

Fig. 16.1 (continued)

References

1. Young Jr WF, Scheithauer BW, Kovacs KT, Horvath E, Davis DH, Randall RV. Gonadotroph adenoma of the pituitary gland: a clinicopathologic analysis of 100 cases. Mayo Clin Proc. 1996;71:649–56.
2. Valimaki MJ, Tiitinen A, Alfthan H, Paetau A, Poranen A, Sane T, Stenman UH. Ovarian hyperstimulation caused by gonadotroph adenoma secreting follicle-stimulating hormone in a 28-year-old woman. J Clin Endocrinol Metab. 1999;84:4204–8.
3. Cooper O, Geller JL, Melmed S. Ovarian hyperstimulation syndrome caused by an FSH-secreting pituitary adenoma. Nat Clin Pract Endocrinol Metab. 2008;4:234–8.
4. Castelbaum AJ, Bigdeli H, Post KD, Freedman MF, Snyder PJ. Exacerbation of ovarian hyperstimulation by leuprolide reveals a gonadotroph adenoma. Fertil Steril. 2002;78:1311–3.
5. Al-Shraim M, Scheithauer BW, Horvath E, Kovacs K, Smyth H, Coire C, et al. Plurihormonal gonadotroph cell pituitary adenoma: report of a unique case. Clin Neuropathol. 2009;28:182–7.
6. Horvath E, Kovacs K. Gonadotroph adenomas of the human pituitary: sex-related fine-structural dichotomy. A histologic, immunocytochemical, and electron-microscopic study of 30 tumors. Am J Pathol. 1984;117:429–40.
7. Knoepfelmacher M, Danilovic DL, Rosa Nasser RH, Mendonca BB. Effectiveness of treating ovarian hyperstimulation syndrome with cabergoline in two patients with gonadotropin-producing pituitary adenomas. Fertil Steril. 2006;86:e715–8.
8. Garmes HM, Grassiotto OR, Fernandes YB, Queiroz Lde S, Vassalo J, de Oliveira DM, Benetti-Pinto CL. A pituitary adenoma secreting follicle-stimulating hormone with ovarian hyperstimulation: treatment using a gonadotropin-releasing hormone antagonist. Fertil Steril. 2012;97:231–4.
9. Reznik Y, Chapon F, Lahlou N, Deboucher N, Mahoudeau J. Pituitary apoplexy of a gonadotroph adenoma following gonadotrophin releasing hormone agonist therapy for prostatic cancer. J Endocrinol Invest. 1997;20:566–8.
10. Macchia E, Simoncini T, Raffaelli V, Lombardi M, Iannelli A, Martino E. A functioning FSH-secreting pituitary macroadenoma causing an ovarian hyperstimulation syndrome with multiple cysts resected and relapsed after leuprolide in a reproductive-aged woman. Gynecol Endocrinol. 2012;28:56–9.

Pituitary Apoplexy

17

Gabriel Zada, M. Beatriz S. Lopes,
Srinivasan Mukundan Jr., and Edward Laws Jr.

17.1 Epidemiology and Clinical Presentation

- Pituitary apoplexy is a clinical diagnosis corresponding to the acute onset of pituitary hemorrhage or infarction. It should be differentiated from pituitary hemorrhage, which may be an asymptomatic or incidental finding.
- The clinical diagnosis is usually supported by imaging and pathological findings consistent with hemorrhage and/or infarction of a pituitary adenoma.
- Most series report an incidence of less than 5 % in patients with pituitary tumors, although apoplexy has been reported in up to 21 % of patients with nonfunctioning macroadenomas [1–4].
- The average age at clinical presentation is approximately 50 years.
- It occurs more commonly in men [1].
- Most patients (81 %) have no known history of a pituitary tumor at the time of clinical presentation [5].
- Factors that may predispose patients to pituitary apoplexy include surgery, pregnancy, anticoagulation or coagulopathy, or radiosurgery [6].
- At presentation with apoplexy, a sudden onset of headache may occur, which is frequently mistaken for subarachnoid hemorrhage.
- Various common symptoms and signs at presentation have been reported [2, 4, 5]:
  - Headache (87–92 %)
  - Hypopituitarism/fatigue (70–73 %)
  - Diminished visual acuity (50–56 %)
  - Cranial nerve paresis (45–54 %)
  - Visual field deficits (34 %)
  - Diminished level of consciousness (13–42 %)
  - Diabetes insipidus (8 %)
  - Hypopituitarism (especially hypocortisolemia) is the most life-threatening aspect of this condition. Panhypopituitarism occurs in up to 72 % of cases and should indicate immediate replacement therapy [2, 4].

G. Zada, MD, MS (✉)
Department of Neurological Surgery, Keck School of Medicine, University of Southern California, 1200 N State Street, #3300, Los Angeles, CA 90033, USA
e-mail: gzada@usc.edu

M.B.S. Lopes, MD, PhD
Department of Pathology (Neuropathology), University of Virginia School of Medicine, 1215 Lee Street, Room 3060–HEP, Charlottesville, VA 22908, USA
e-mail: msl2e@virginia.edu

S. Mukundan Jr., PhD, MD
Department of Radiology, Brigham and Women's Hospital, 75 Francis Street, Boston, MA 02115, USA
e-mail: smukundan@partners.org

E. Laws Jr., MD
Department of Neurosurgery, Brigham and Women's Hospital, 15 Francis Street, Boston, MA 02115, USA
e-mail: elaws@partners.org

G. Zada et al. (eds.), *Atlas of Sellar and Parasellar Lesions: Clinical, Radiologic, and Pathologic Correlations*, DOI 10.1007/978-3-319-22855-6_17

17.2 Diagnosis

17.2.1 Imaging

- The tumors involved are typically macroadenomas with sellar expansion and frequent cavernous sinus invasion.
- Imaging corroboration often shows evidence of acute or subacute hemorrhage that is typically hyperintense on T1 MR imaging.
- The tumor contents are often heterogeneous and appear mottled.
- A high degree of association with sphenoid sinus mucosal thickening has been reported [7].
- Partially cystic lesions may exhibit a fluid level on imaging.
- MRI findings of infarction and necrosis correlate with histopathological findings (Figs. 17.1, 17.2, 17.3, 17.4, 17.5, and 17.6) [8].

17.2.2 Histopathology

- Histopathological specimens demonstrate hemorrhagic infarction in 47 % of patients with clinical evidence of apoplexy, with simple infarction in 40 % and frank hemorrhage in 8 % [5].
- In some patients, no tumor is isolated because of the predominance of subacute blood products.
- In pituitary adenoma specimens from patients without clinical apoplexy, 14 % demonstrate microscopic evidence of necrosis, infarction, or hemorrhage [3].

17.3 Clinical Management

- Initial steps include administering corticosteroids early if suspicion of apoplexy exists.
- Correction of bleeding diathesis or reversal of anticoagulation should be performed, along with management of diabetes insipidus, which occurs in about 8 % of cases [5].
- Transsphenoidal surgery is effective in relieving symptoms and signs of mass effect in the majority of cases [4, 5].
- Conservative management has been successfully implemented in some cases of pituitary apoplexy [9, 10].
- Following surgical treatment, a good overall outcome is reported in up to 79 % of patients, with visual improvement in more than 90 % and improvement of oculomotor paresis in 85 % [2, 5].
- Postoperative hypopituitarism requires hormonal replacement in 83–95 % of patients.

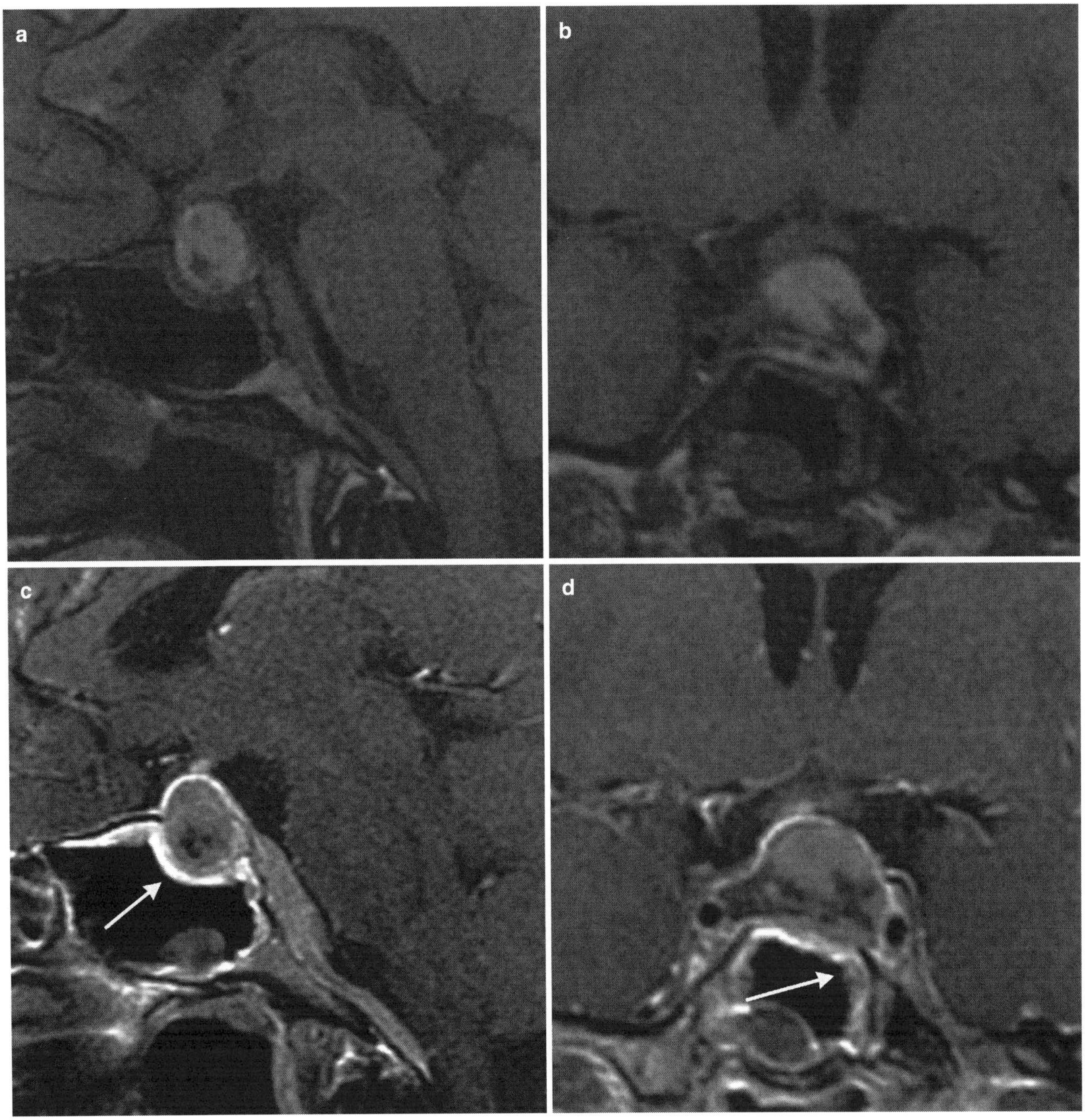

Fig. 17.1 Pituitary apoplexy. (**a**) Sagittal T1-weighted pre-gadolinium image. (**b**) Coronal T1-weighted pre-gadolinium image. (**c**) Sagittal T1-weighted post-gadolinium image. (**d**) Coronal T1-weighted post-gadolinium image. Within the sella, there is an expansile mass with heterogeneous signal intensity and areas of T1 hyperintensity that may represent proteinaceous materials or blood products. There is muco-periosteal thickening along the roof of the right sphenoid sinus (*white arrow*). The pituitary stalk is elevated and deviated to the right

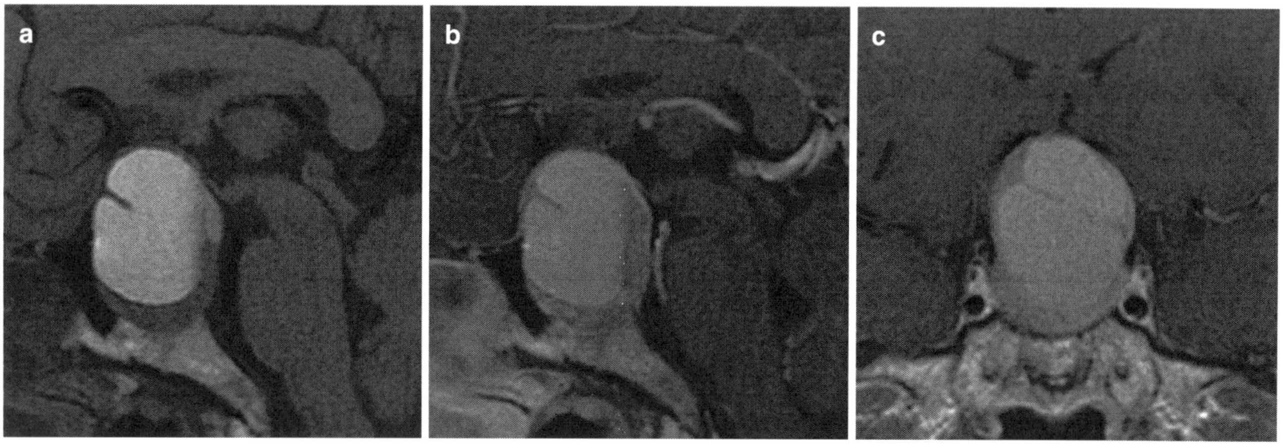

Fig. 17.2 Pituitary apoplexy. (**a**) Sagittal T1-weighted pre-gadolinium image. (**b**) Sagittal T1-weighted post-gadolinium image. (**c**) Coronal T1-weighted post-gadolinium image. Within the sella, there is a large sellar mass with suprasellar extension, containing a septated region of T1 hyperintensity that may represent proteinaceous materials or blood products. There is enhancing soft tissue along the periphery in the inferior and posterior aspect of the sella

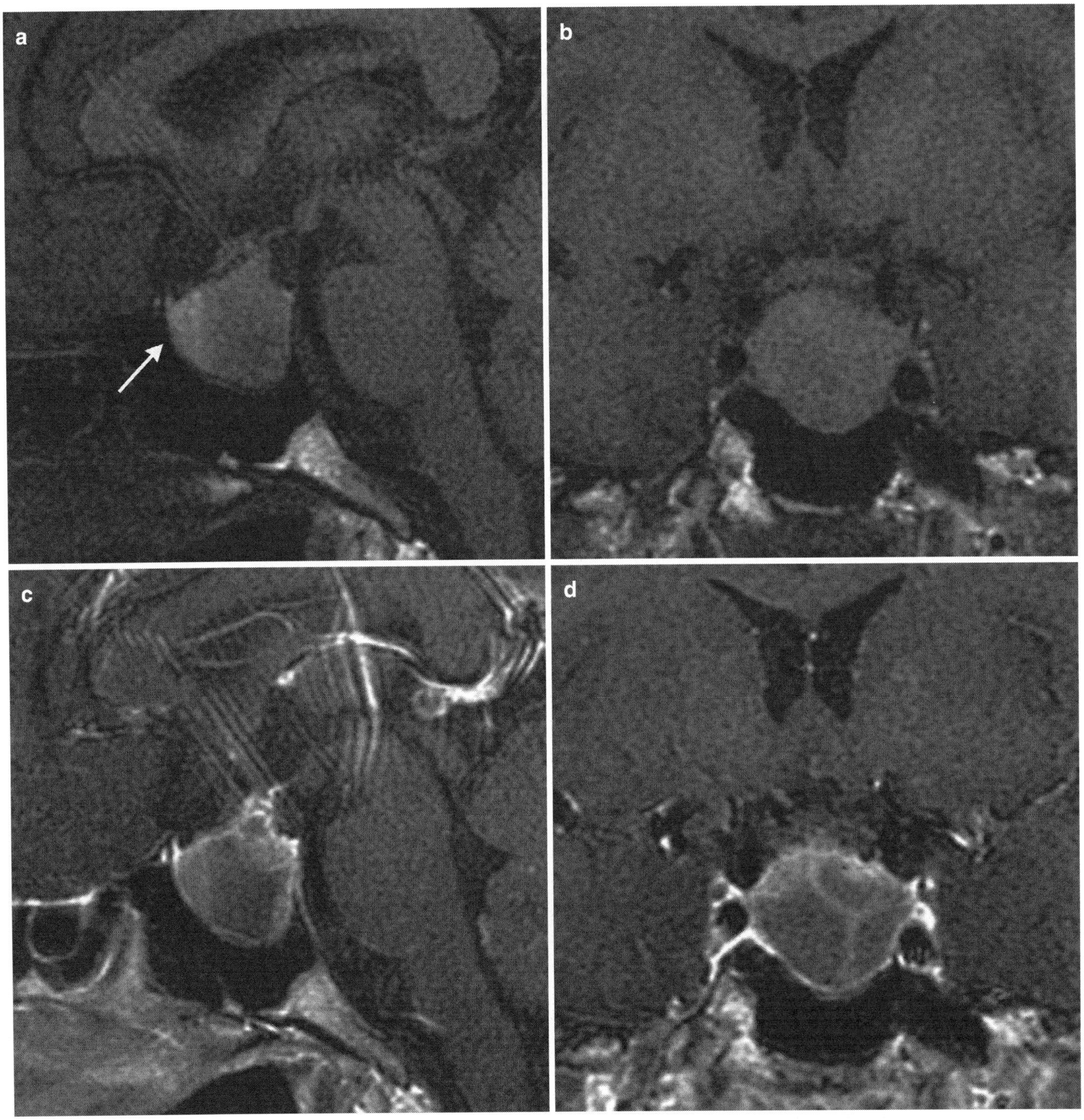

Fig. 17.3 Pituitary apoplexy. (**a**) Sagittal T1-weighted pre-gadolinium image. (**b**) Coronal T1-weighted pre-gadolinium image. (**c**) Sagittal T1-weighted post-gadolinium image. (**d**) Coronal T1-weighted post-gadolinium image. Within the sella, there is an expansile mass with layering T1 hyperintensity (*white arrow*), which may represent proteinaceous materials or blood products. Enhancing septations are seen within the mass. There is erosion of the sellar floor

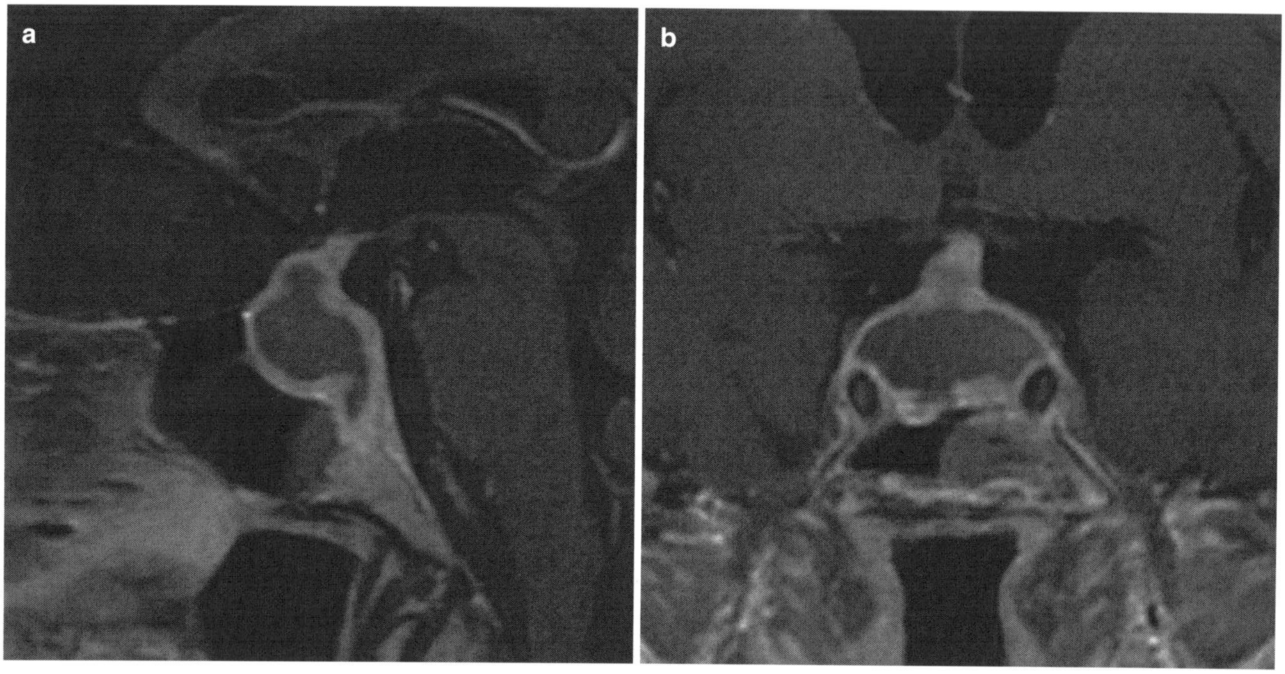

Fig. 17.4 Pituitary apoplexy. (**a**) Sagittal T1-weighted post-gadolinium image. (**b**) Coronal T1-weighted post-gadolinium image. Within the sella, there is an expansile mass with peripheral enhancement and central cyst or necrosis. Superiorly, the mass abuts the stalk without significant mass effect. There is erosion of the sellar floor. A mucous retention cyst is seen in the right sphenoid sinus

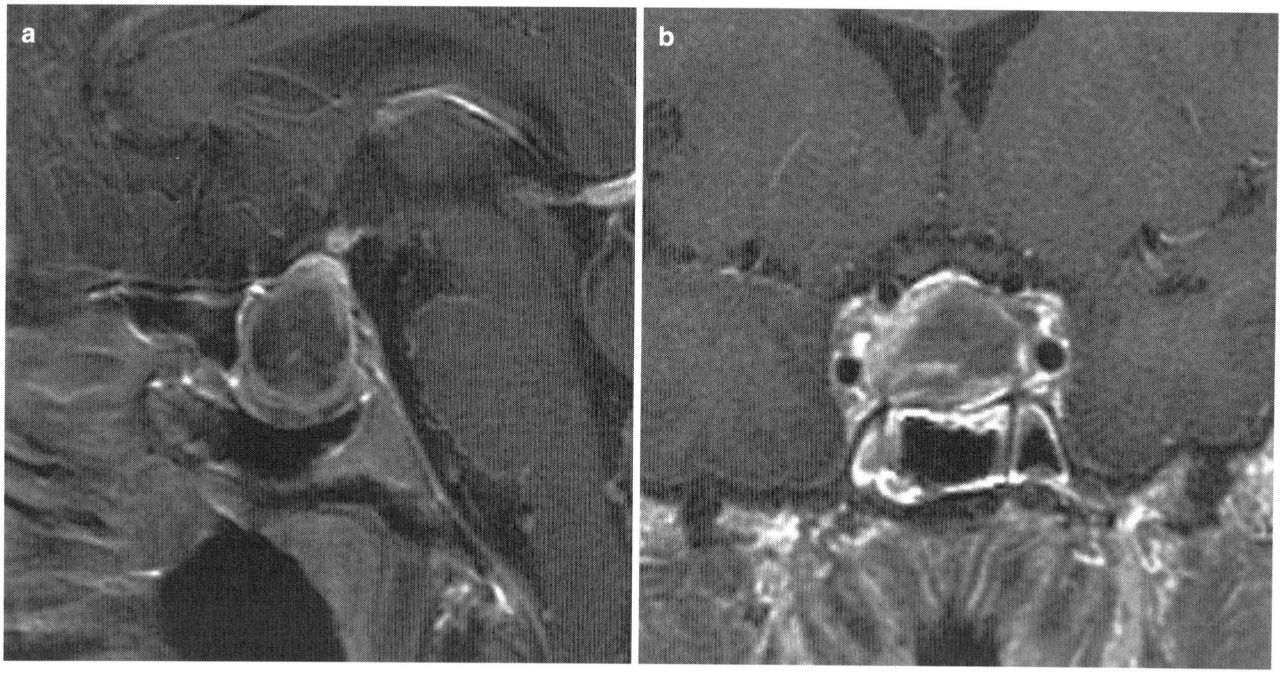

Fig. 17.5 Pituitary apoplexy. (**a**) Sagittal T1-weighted post-gadolinium image. (**b**) Coronal T1-weighted post-gadolinium image. Within the sella, there is a lobular, expansile mass with peripheral enhancement and central cyst or necrosis. The mass extends superiorly, abutting and mildly elevating the optic chiasm. There is erosion of the sellar floor and mucoperiosteal thickening along the roofs of the sphenoid sinuses

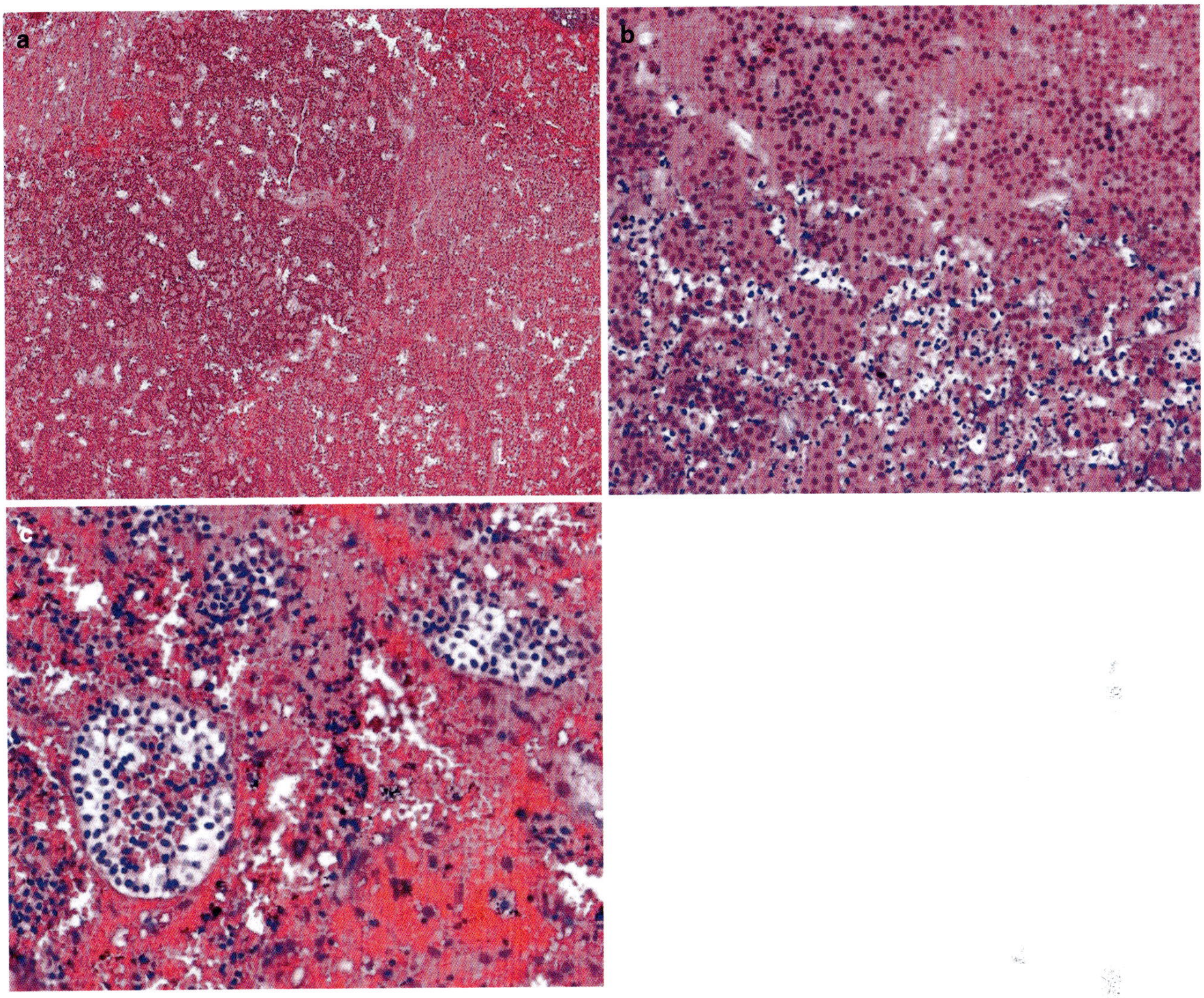

Fig. 17.6 Pituitary apoplexy. (**a**) An apoplectic pituitary adenoma showing extensive necrosis with nearly complete dissolution of the adenoma structure. (**b**) Note "ghost cells" within the necrosis. (**c**) Focal areas of remaining intact adenoma may be seen intermixed with the necrotic tumor

References

1. Nielsen EH, Lindholm J, Bjerre P, Christiansen JS, Hagen C, Juul S, et al. Frequent occurrence of pituitary apoplexy in patients with non-functioning pituitary adenoma. Clin Endocrinol (Oxf). 2006;64: 319–22.
2. Dubuisson AS, Beckers A, Stevenaert A. Classical pituitary tumour apoplexy: clinical features, management and outcomes in a series of 24 patients. Clin Neurol Neurosurg. 2007;109:63–70.
3. Bonicki W, Kasperlik-Zaluska A, Koszewski W, Zgliczynski W, Wislawski J. Pituitary apoplexy: endocrine, surgical and oncological emergency. Incidence, clinical course and treatment with reference to 799 cases of pituitary adenomas. Acta Neurochir (Wien). 1993;120:118–22.
4. Laws ER. Pituitary tumor apoplexy: a review. J Intensive Care Med. 2008;23:146–7.
5. Semple PL, Webb MK, de Villiers JC, Laws Jr ER. Pituitary apoplexy. Neurosurgery. 2005;56:65–72; discussion 72–3.
6. Semple PL, Jane Jr JA, Laws Jr ER. Clinical relevance of precipitating factors in pituitary apoplexy. Neurosurgery. 2007;61:956–61; discussion 961–2.
7. Agrawal B, Dziurzynski K, Salamat MS, Baskaya M. The temporal association of sphenoid sinus mucosal thickening on MR imaging with pituitary apoplexy. Turk Neurosurg. 2012;22:785–90.
8. Semple PL, Jane JA, Lopes MB, Laws ER. Pituitary apoplexy: correlation between magnetic resonance imaging and histopathological results. J Neurosurg. 2008;108:909–15.
9. Leyer C, Castinetti F, Morange I, Gueydan M, Oliver C, Conte-Devolx B, et al. A conservative management is preferable in milder forms of pituitary tumor apoplexy. J Endocrinol Invest. 2011;34:502–9.
10. Gruber A, Clayton J, Kumar S, Robertson I, Howlett TA, Mansell P. Pituitary apoplexy: retrospective review of 30 patients – is surgical intervention always necessary? Br J Neurosurg. 2006;20:379–85.

Atypical Pituitary Adenomas

18

Gabriel Zada, M. Beatriz S. Lopes, Srinivasan Mukundan Jr., and Edward Laws Jr.

18.1 Epidemiology and Clinical Presentation

- The World Health Organization (WHO) classifies atypical pituitary adenomas as having "atypical morphologic features suggestive of aggressive behavior such as invasive growth" [1].
- Other features seen in atypical adenomas include elevated mitotic index, a Ki-67 (MIB-1) labeling index greater than 3 %, and extensive nuclear immunoexpression for the p53 protein.
- These tumors have histopathological features that may correlate with increased rates of recurrence, invasion, and possibly malignant transformation.
- They comprise approximately 3–15 % of surgically resected pituitary adenomas [2–4].
- The mean age at presentation is 48 years.
- They are more common in women.
- These adenomas may be hormonally active or nonfunctioning.

18.2 Diagnosis

18.2.1 Imaging

- More than 90 % of atypical pituitary adenomas are macroadenomas [3].
- They may also occur as microadenomas, especially in Cushing's disease.
- Invasion on MRI is seen with 83 % of atypical adenomas (Figs. 18.1, 18.2, 18.3, 18.4, 18.5, 18.6, 18.7, 18.8, and 18.9), compared with 45 % of typical adenomas ($p = 0.004$) [3].
- Atypical GH-staining adenomas have a high propensity for infrasellar bony invasion through the sellar floor or into the clivus.

G. Zada, MD, MS (✉)
Department of Neurological Surgery,
Keck School of Medicine, University of Southern California,
1200 N State Street, #3300, Los Angeles, CA 90033, USA
e-mail: gzada@usc.edu

M.B.S. Lopes, MD, PhD
Department of Pathology (Neuropathology),
University of Virginia School of Medicine,
1215 Lee Street, Room 3060–HEP,
Charlottesville, VA 22908, USA
e-mail: msl2e@virginia.edu

S. Mukundan Jr., PhD, MD
Department of Radiology, Brigham and Women's Hospital,
75 Francis Street, Boston, MA 02115, USA
e-mail: smukundan@partners.org

E. Laws Jr., MD
Department of Neurosurgery, Brigham and Women's Hospital,
15 Francis Street, Boston, MA 02115, USA
e-mail: elaws@partners.org

G. Zada et al. (eds.), *Atlas of Sellar and Parasellar Lesions: Clinical, Radiologic, and Pathologic Correlations*,
DOI 10.1007/978-3-319-22855-6_18

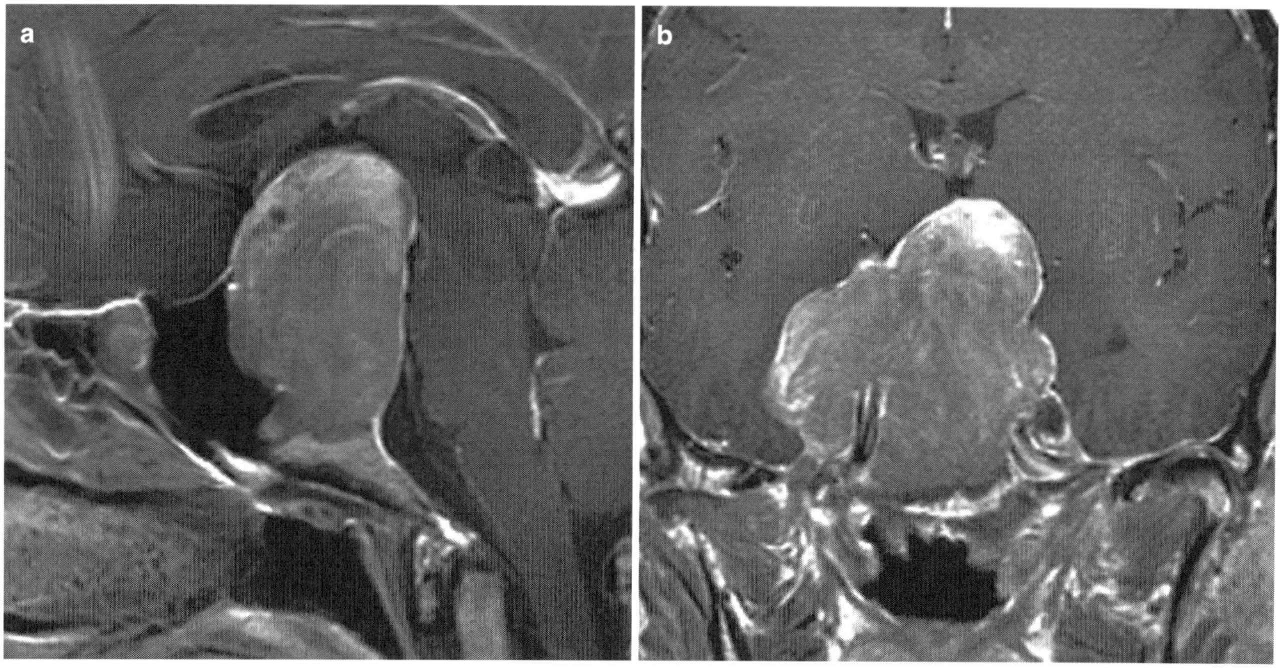

Fig. 18.1 Atypical pituitary adenoma. (**a**) Sagittal T1-weighted post-gadolinium image. (**b**) Coronal T1-weighted post-gadolinium image. A large, heterogeneously enhancing sellar mass demonstrates suprasellar extension and encasement of the right cavernous internal carotid artery, as well as erosion of the sellar floor. Superiorly, the mass has elevated the floor of the third ventricle, and the optic chiasm is likely elevated and compressed. Posteriorly, the mass effaces the prepontine cistern and mildly impresses on the pons. The sagittal image incidentally shows a small pineal cyst

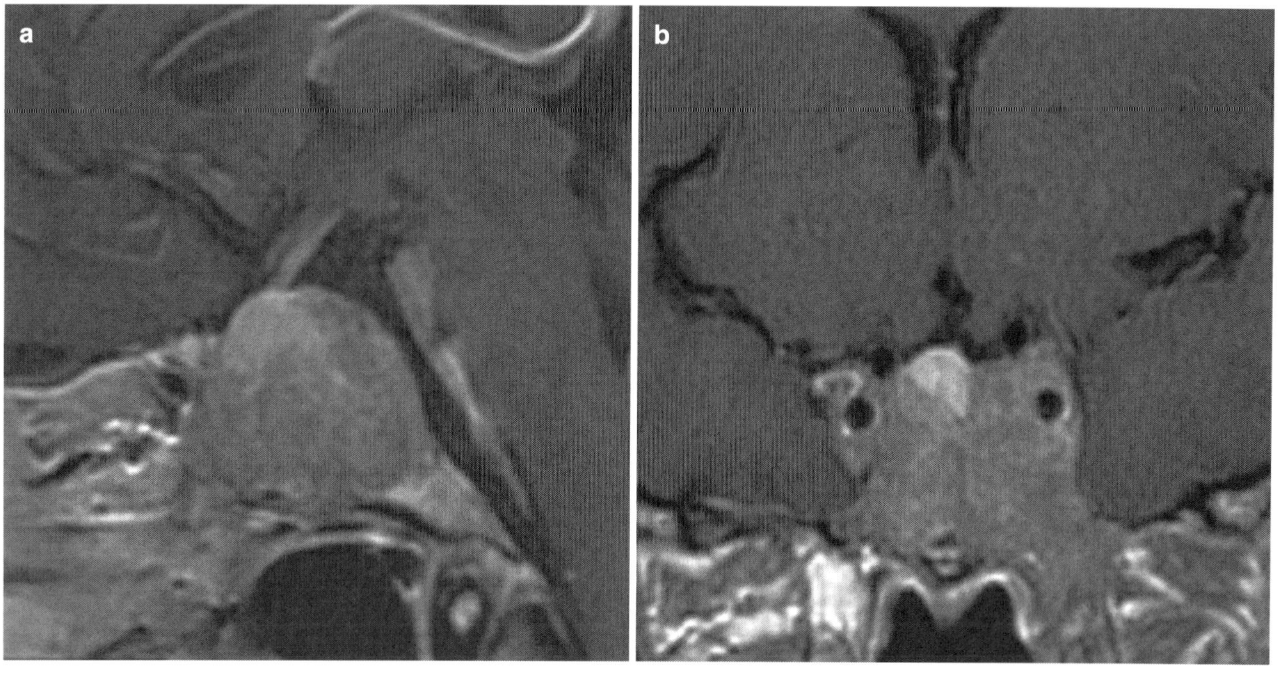

Fig. 18.2 Atypical pituitary adenoma. (**a**) Sagittal T1-weighted post-gadolinium image. (**b**) Coronal T1-weighted post-gadolinium image. A large, heterogeneously enhancing sellar mass encases the cavernous internal carotid arteries bilaterally, and there is erosion of the sellar floor. The normal pituitary glandular tissue is seen along the superior margin of the mass

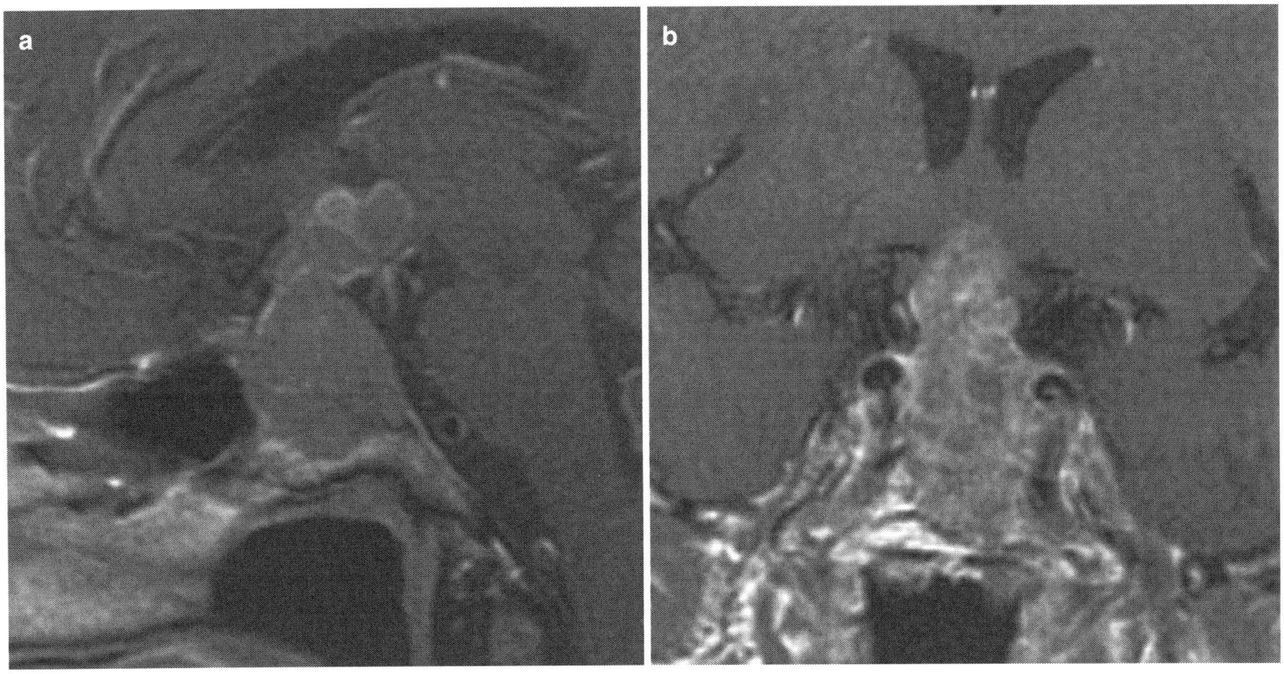

Fig. 18.3 Atypical pituitary adenoma. (**a**) Sagittal T1-weighted post-gadolinium image. (**a**) Coronal T1-weighted post-gadolinium image. There is a large, heterogeneously enhancing sellar mass with suprasellar extension. The mass abuts the cavernous internal carotid arteries without definite encasement. There is erosion of the sellar floor. Superiorly, the mass has elevated the floor of the third ventricle, and the optic chiasm is likely elevated and compressed

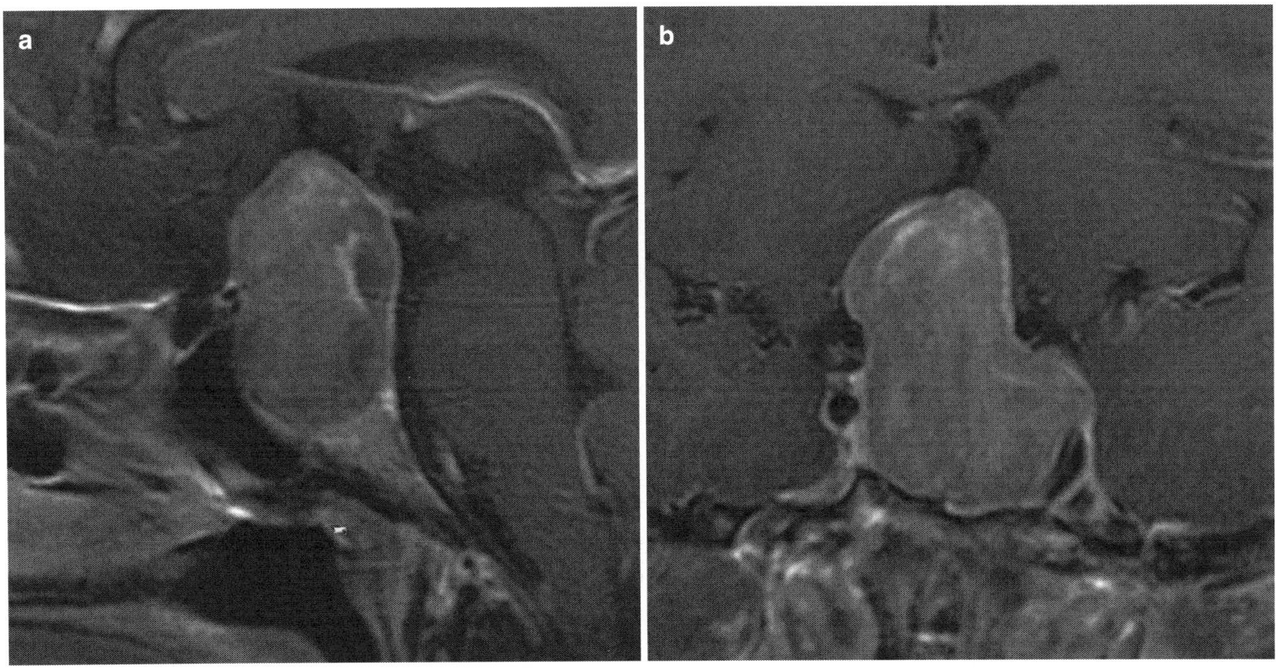

Fig. 18.4 Atypical pituitary adenoma. (**a**) Sagittal T1-weighted post-gadolinium image. (**b**) Coronal T1-weighted post-gadolinium image. A large, heterogeneously enhancing sellar/suprasellar mass abuts the cavernous internal carotid arteries, with possible invasion of the left cavernous sinus on the left. There is erosion of the sellar floor. Superiorly, the mass has elevated the lamina terminalis, and the optic chiasm is likely elevated and compressed

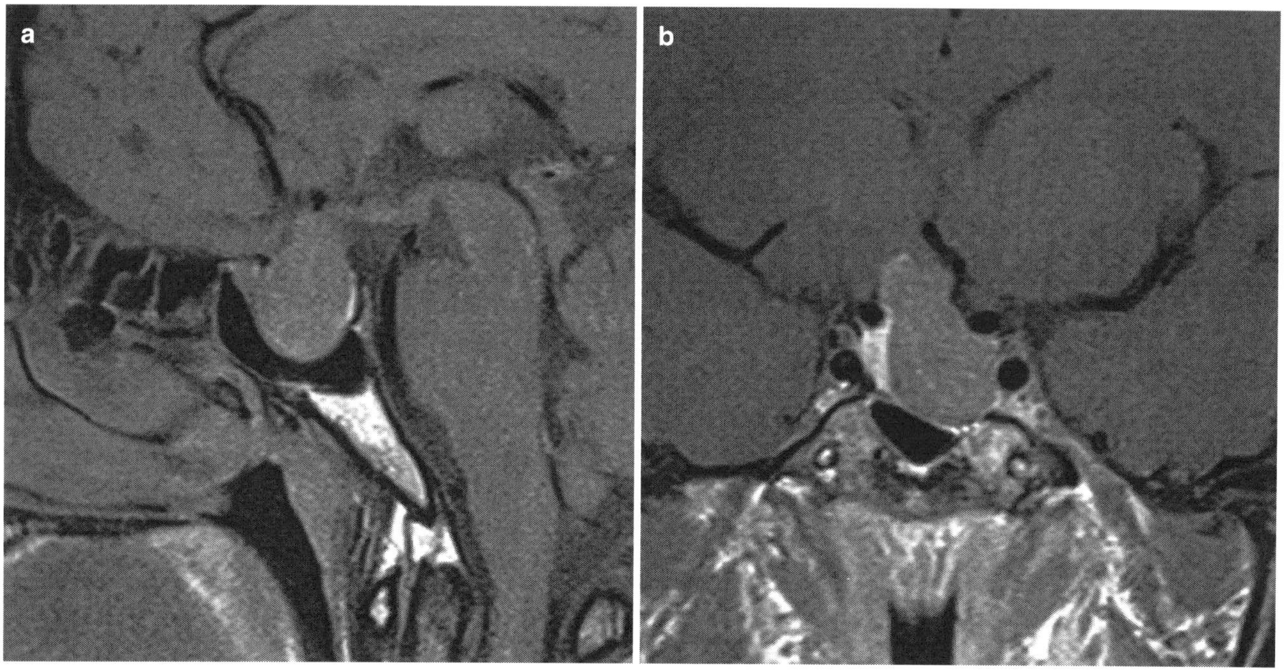

Fig. 18.5 Atypical pituitary adenoma. (**a**) Sagittal T1-weighted post-gadolinium image. (**b**) Coronal T1-weighted post-gadolinium image. There is a heterogeneously enhancing sellar mass with suprasellar extension. The mass abuts the left cavernous internal carotid artery without definite invasion of the left cavernous sinus. There is erosion of the left sellar floor. Superiorly, the mass abuts the right hypothalamus. The normal pituitary glandular tissue is seen along the right aspect of the sella

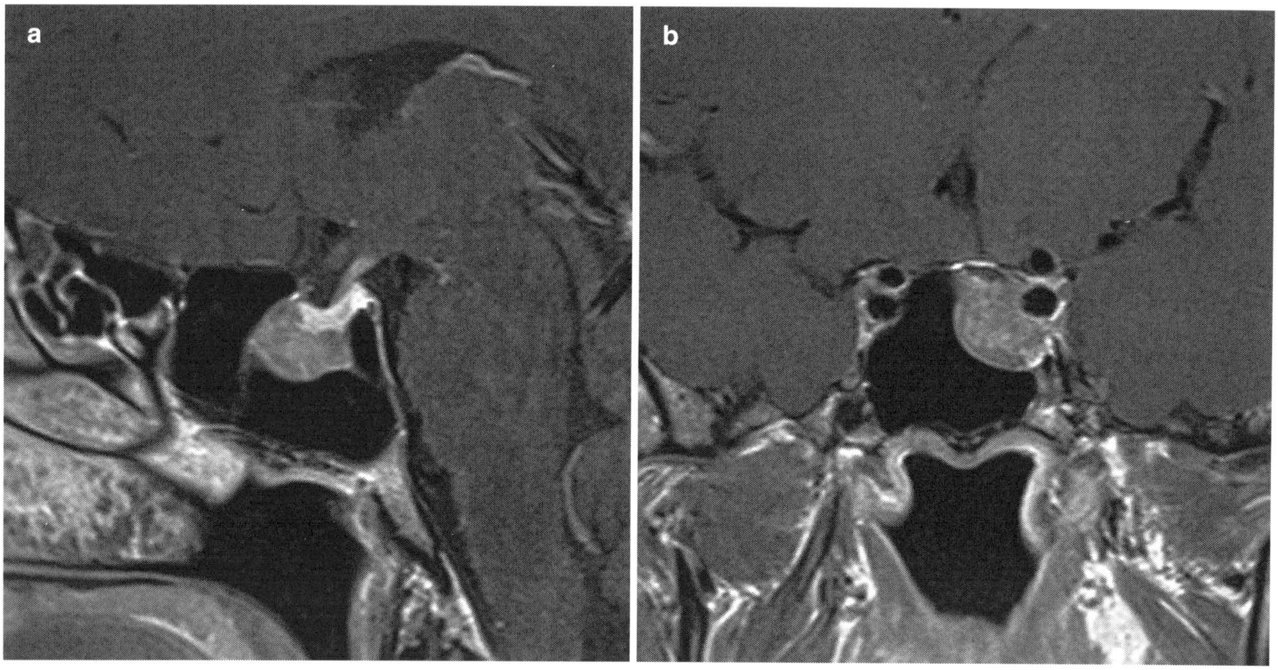

Fig. 18.6 Atypical pituitary adenoma. (**a**) Sagittal T1-weighted post-gadolinium image. (**b**) Coronal T1-weighted post-gadolinium image. An enhancing sellar mass in the left aspect of the sella abuts the left cavernous internal carotid artery without definite invasion of the left cavernous sinus. There is erosion of the left sellar floor. The normal pituitary glandular tissue is seen along the superior aspect of the mass

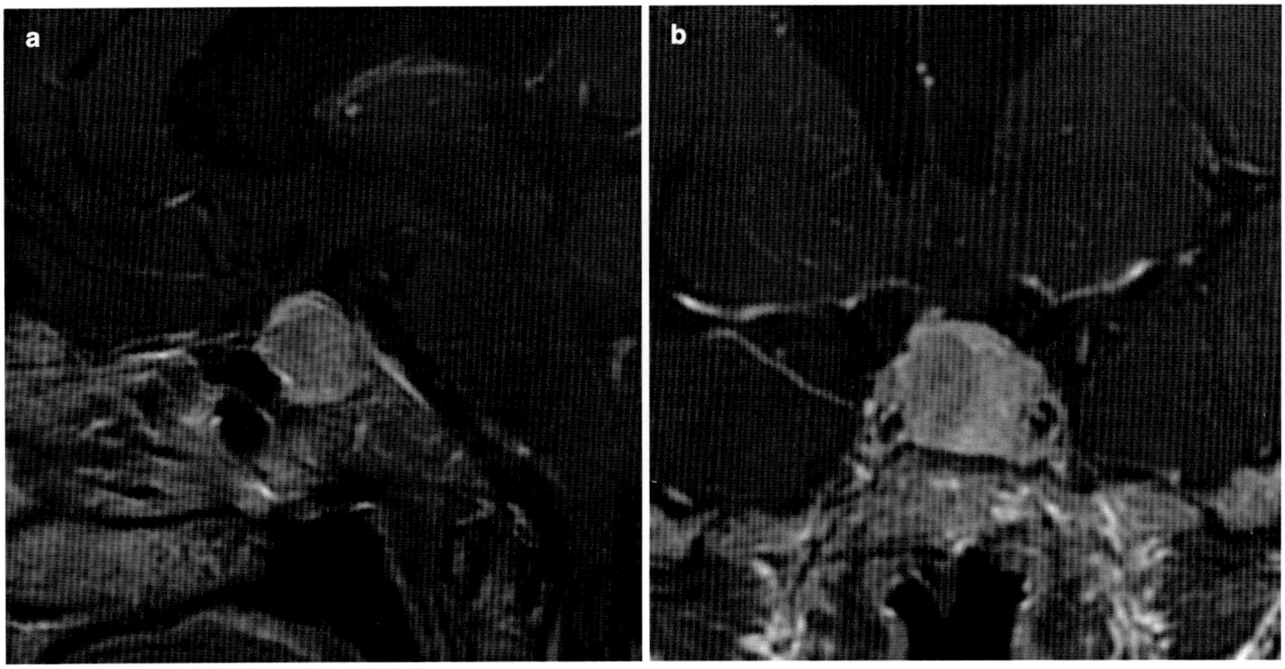

Fig. 18.7 Atypical pituitary adenoma. (**a**) Sagittal T1-weighted post-gadolinium image. (**b**) Coronal T1-weighted post-gadolinium image. There is an enhancing sellar mass in the sella, abutting the cavernous internal carotid arteries bilaterally without definite invasion of the cavernous sinuses. There is erosion of the left sellar floor. The normal pituitary glandular tissue is seen along the superior aspect of the mass

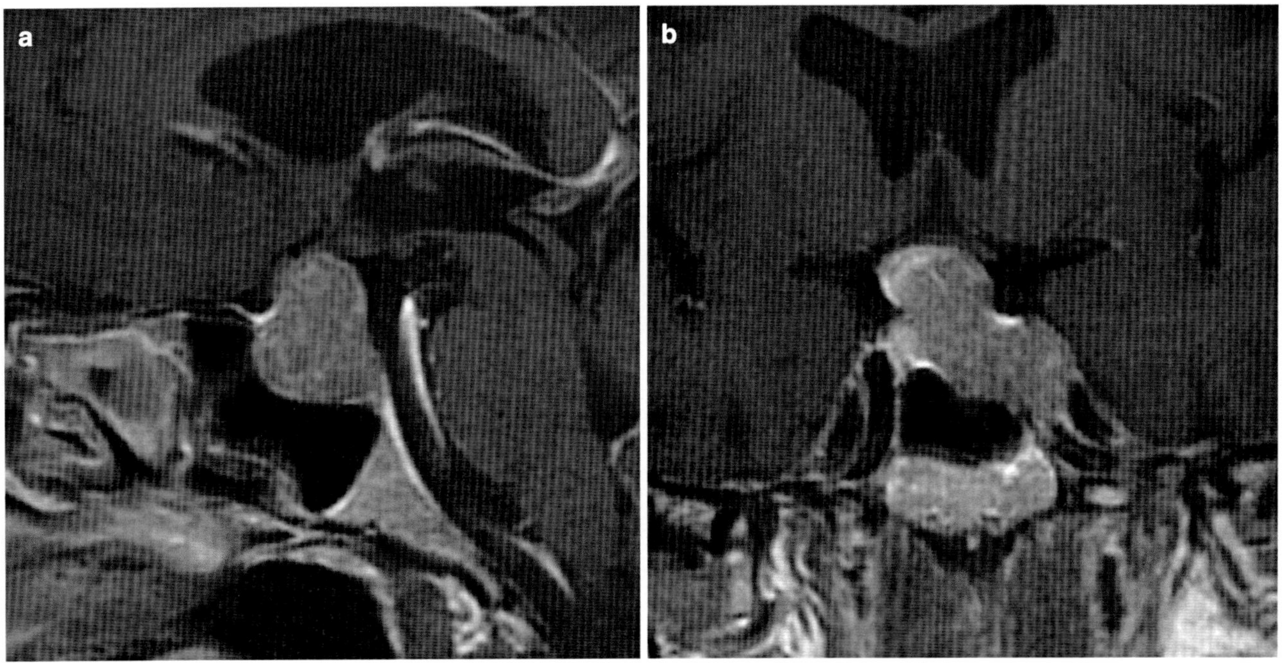

Fig. 18.8 Atypical pituitary adenoma. (**a**) Sagittal T1-weighted post-gadolinium image. (**b**) Coronal T1-weighted post-gadolinium image. A heterogeneously enhancing sellar/suprasellar mass shows left cavernous invasion with encasement of the left internal carotid artery. There is erosion of the sellar floor. Superiorly, the mass has elevated the optic chiasm. The normal pituitary glandular tissue is seen along the right superior aspect of the mass

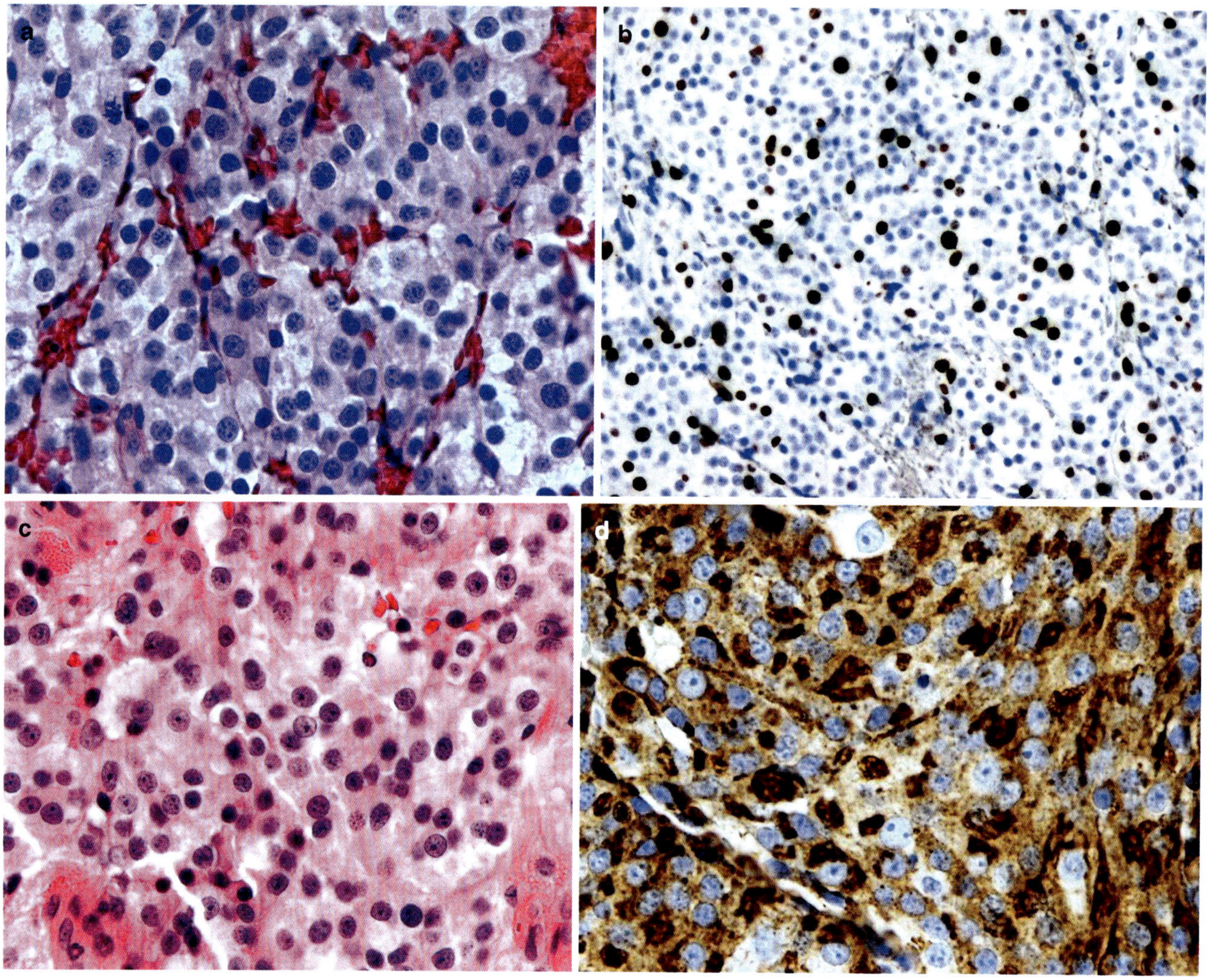

Fig. 18.9 Atypical pituitary adenoma. In this example of a prolactinoma, the tumor exhibits high mitotic index (**a**) and elevated proliferative index by Ki-67 (MIB-1) (**b**). Note that in this case, the adenoma shows only minimal cellular atypia (**c**) and has strong immunoreactivity for prolactin (**d**)

18.2.2 Histopathology

- The average MIB-1 labeling index in patients is 7 % with atypical PAs, but it may be higher than 20 % in some patients.
- Scattered or excessive p53 immunoreactivity is identified in all patients.
- All specimens demonstrate frequent mitoses and pleomorphism (Fig. 18.9).
- The most common tumor subtypes are nonfunctioning adenoma, GH-staining adenoma with prolactin immunopositivity, and ACTH-staining tumors (silent and active) [3].
- The mean Ki-67 growth fraction has been reported as 1.37 % in noninvasive adenomas, 4.66 % in invasive adenomas, and 11.91 % in carcinomas [5]
- p53 expression has been reported in 15.2 % of patients with invasive adenomas and 100 % of patients with carcinomas, but it has not been reported in any patients with noninvasive adenomas [6].
- Hyperacetylation of H3K9 may correlate with increased atypia and nuclear proliferation [7].

18.3 Clinical Management

- The diagnosis of atypical adenoma is a postsurgical diagnosis. Therefore, as in most cases of pituitary adenomas, transsphenoidal surgery is the standard management.
- Staged or simultaneous transsphenoidal and/or open craniotomy may be required for large, invasive macroadenomas that cannot be adequately debulked.
- As subtotal resection of invasive atypical tumors is common, many of these patients may require multimodality therapy utilizing adjunctive medical and or radiosurgical treatments.
- The long-term progression-free survival and the potential for malignant transformation are not yet known in this subtype of pituitary adenoma [8].
- It remains to be determined whether patients with atypical adenomas will have lower remission rates and higher recurrence rates or whether early adjunctive therapy such as radiosurgery will be indicated in this subgroup [8].

References

1. DeLellis R, Lloyd RV, Heitz P, Eng C, editors. World Health Organization classification of tumours: tumours of endocrine organs. Lyon: IARC Press; 2004.
2. Scheithauer BW, Gaffey TA, Lloyd RV, Sebo TJ, Kovacs KT, Horvath E, et al. Pathobiology of pituitary adenomas and carcinomas. Neurosurgery. 2006;59:341–53.
3. Zada G, Woodmansee WW, Ramkissoon S, Amadio J, Nose V, Laws Jr ER. Atypical pituitary adenomas: incidence, clinical characteristics, and implications. J Neurosurg. 2011;114:336–44.
4. Saeger W, Ludecke DK, Buchfelder M, Fahlbusch R, Quabbe HJ, Petersenn S. Pathohistological classification of pituitary tumors: 10 years of experience with the German Pituitary Tumor Registry. Eur J Endocrinol. 2007;156:203–16.
5. Thapar K, Kovacs K, Scheithauer BW, Stefaneanu L, Horvath E, Pernicone PJ, et al. Proliferative activity and invasiveness among pituitary adenomas and carcinomas: an analysis using the MIB-1 antibody. Neurosurgery. 1996;38:99–106; discussion 106–7.
6. Thapar K, Scheithauer BW, Kovacs K, Pernicone PJ, Laws Jr ER. p53 expression in pituitary adenomas and carcinomas: correlation with invasiveness and tumor growth fractions. Neurosurgery. 1996;38:765–70; discussion 770–1.
7. Ebrahimi A, Schittenhelm J, Honegger J, Schluesener HJ. Histone acetylation patterns of typical and atypical pituitary adenomas indicate epigenetic shift of these tumours. J Neuroendocrinol. 2011;23:525–30.
8. Laws Jr ER, Lopes MB. The new WHO classification of pituitary tumors: highlights and areas of controversy. Acta Neuropathol. 2006;111:80–1.

Pituitary Carcinoma

19

Gabriel Zada, M. Beatriz S. Lopes, Srinivasan Mukundan Jr., and Edward Laws Jr.

19.1 Epidemiology and Clinical Presentation

- The overwhelming majority of pituitary neoplasms remain benign and do not undergo malignant transformation.
- Pituitary carcinomas comprise less than 0.2 % of all surgically treated sellar lesions [1, 2].
- The mean age of patients at the time of diagnosis is 45–55 years [3, 4].
- Diagnosis by definition requires the presence of metastases either within or outside the central nervous system (CNS).
- Associated patterns of pituitary carcinoma metastases are as follows: only intra-CNS metastases are identified in 45 % of cases, only extra-CNS metastases in 39 %, and both in 16 % [3].
- Diagnosis of pituitary carcinoma often follows a prolonged treatment course (frequently with medical, surgical, and/or radiotherapy management) for a refractory adenoma. The median reported time from symptom onset to diagnosis of carcinoma is 5–7 years [3–7].
- Pituitary carcinoma is more likely to derive from functional endocrine tumors, especially prolactinomas and ACTH-secreting tumors (often with Nelson's syndrome) [2, 4, 8, 9].
- Levels of associated hormones such as GH, ACTH, and prolactin may be atypically elevated if metastases are present [3, 5].
- The atypical pituitary adenomas discussed in the previous section are a new entity (defined in the 2004 WHO classification [10]) and are thought to represent intermediate lesions with a high proclivity for malignant transformation. These have also been referred to as "carcinoma in situ."

19.2 Diagnosis

19.2.1 Imaging

- These highly invasive tumors often are associated with multiple metastases to the brain and spine (Figs. 19.1 and 19.2).

G. Zada, MD, MS (✉)
Department of Neurological Surgery,
Keck School of Medicine, University of Southern California,
1200 N State Street, #3300, Los Angeles, CA 90033, USA
e-mail: gzada@usc.edu

M.B.S. Lopes, MD, PhD
Department of Pathology (Neuropathology),
University of Virginia School of Medicine,
1215 Lee Street, Room 3060–HEP,
Charlottesville, VA 22908, USA
e-mail: msl2e@virginia.edu

S. Mukundan Jr., PhD, MD
Department of Radiology, Brigham and Women's Hospital,
75 Francis Street, Boston, MA 02115, USA
e-mail: smukundan@partners.org

E. Laws Jr., MD
Department of Neurosurgery, Brigham and Women's Hospital,
15 Francis Street, Boston, MA 02115, USA
e-mail: elaws@partners.org

G. Zada et al. (eds.), *Atlas of Sellar and Parasellar Lesions: Clinical, Radiologic, and Pathologic Correlations*,
DOI 10.1007/978-3-319-22855-6_19

- Intra-CNS metastases have been reported throughout the craniospinal axis, including the cerebrum, cerebellum, spinal cord, leptomeninges, and subarachnoid space [11].
- Strong contrast enhancement is usually present.
- Dural metastases can mimic meningiomas [11].
- The primary lesion in pituitary carcinoma and the metastases demonstrate a similar vascularity pattern [12].

19.2.2 Pathology

- Malignant features are usually observed, with a high frequency of cellular atypia and mitotic activity [13].
- Half of primary carcinoma tumors and the majority of metastases demonstrate nuclear pleomorphism and/or hyperchromasia [4].

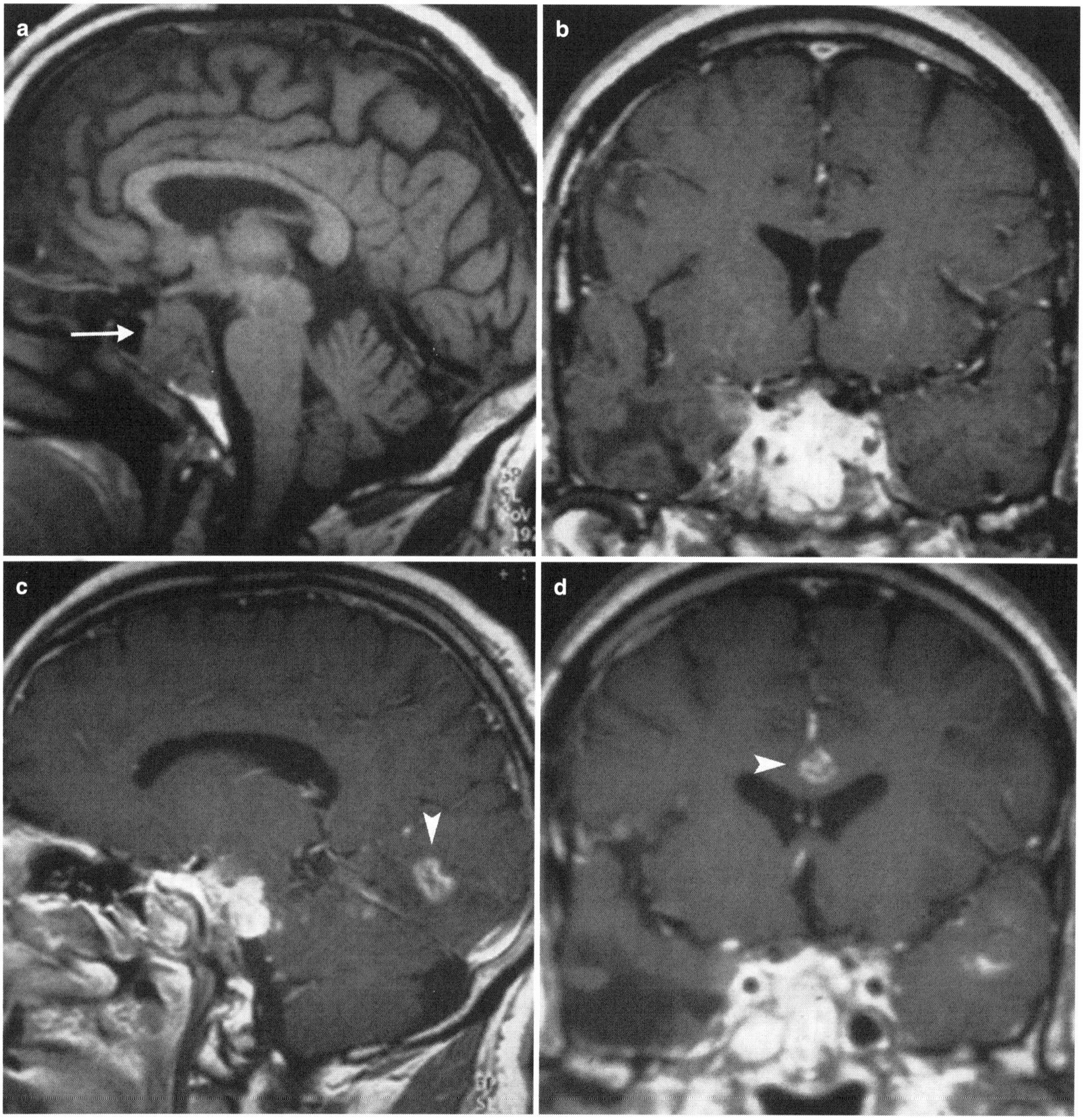

Fig. 19.1 Pituitary carcinoma. (**a**) Sagittal T1-weighted pre-gadolinium image. (**b**) Coronal T1-weighted post-gadolinium image. (**c**) Sagittal T1-weighted post-gadolinium image. (**d**) Coronal T1-weighted post-gadolinium image. There is a large, heterogeneously enhancing sellar mass with erosion of the sella, as well as suprasellar and retroclival extensions. The mass extends anteriorly to involve the sphenoid sinus (*arrow* in **a**). There are additional parenchymal enhancing masses in the occipital lobe and corpus callosum (*white arrowheads* in **c**, **d**). The pituitary stalk is elevated and deviated to the right

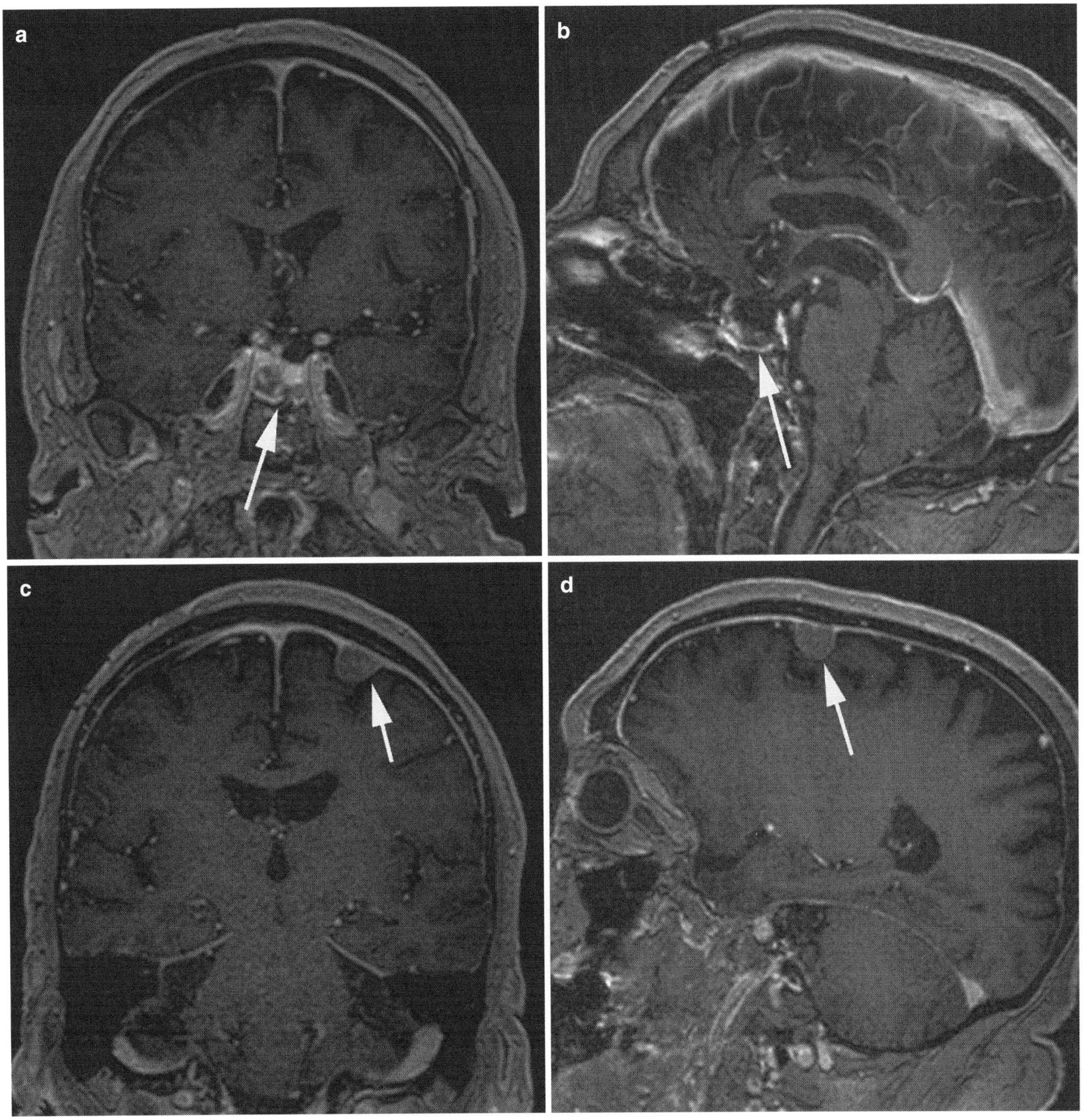

Fig. 19.2 Pituitary carcinoma. Coronal (**a**) and sagittal (**b**) T1-weighted post-gadolinium MRI in a patient with a treated atypical prolactinoma and a rising prolactin level. The sellar region (*arrow*) shows some residual tumor, postoperative changes, scar tissue, and radiation effects. Coronal (**c**) and sagittal (**d**) T1-weighted post-gadolinium MR images show a dura-based mass (*arrow*) consistent with pituitary carcinoma originating from a prolactinoma. The mass was verified histologically and subsequently resected surgically

- Pituitary carcinoma has been associated with a higher mitotic index, p53 immunoreactivity, and a higher MIB-1 labeling index [4, 9, 13–16].
- The mean MIB-1 index (reported as 8–11.9 % in metastatic pituitary carcinomas) is typically higher in the metastatic components [4, 13, 14].
- Pituitary carcinomas have been reported to occur in almost all cell types of pituitary tumors, although they most commonly develop in ACTH adenomas and prolactinomas [1, 3].
- Malignant features may be identified in atypical adenomas without the presence of metastases, but these features do not meet the qualification for the diagnosis of pituitary carcinoma [17].

19.3 Clinical Management

- Treatment is frequently palliative and consists of aggressive surgical resection followed by management with chemotherapy with or without radiotherapy or radiosurgery [4].
- In appropriate cases, medical therapy such as dopamine agonists and somatostatin analogs should be continued [12].
- According to some recent reports, temozolomide has demonstrated some efficacy in tumor control [18–20].
- Prognosis remains generally poor, however, with a mean survival time of 2–4 years; 33 % of patients do not survive 1 year beyond the time of diagnosis [4, 12].
- One case report described a patient who survived 33 years with pituitary carcinoma [5].

References

1. Saeger W, Ludecke DK, Buchfelder M, Fahlbusch R, Quabbe HJ, Petersenn S. Pathohistological classification of pituitary tumors: 10 years of experience with the German Pituitary Tumor Registry. Eur J Endocrinol. 2007;156:203–16.
2. Kaltsas GA, Nomikos P, Kontogeorgos G, Buchfelder M, Grossman AB. Clinical review: diagnosis and management of pituitary carcinomas. J Clin Endocrinol Metab. 2005;90:3089–99.
3. Kaltsas GA, Grossman AB. Malignant pituitary tumours. Pituitary. 1998;1:69–81.
4. Pernicone PJ, Scheithauer BW, Sebo TJ, Kovacs KT, Horvath E, Young Jr WF, et al. Pituitary carcinoma: a clinicopathologic study of 15 cases. Cancer. 1997;79:804–12.
5. Scheithauer BW, Randall RV, Laws Jr ER, Kovacs KT, Horvath E, Whitaker MD. Prolactin cell carcinoma of the pituitary. Clinicopathologic, immunohistochemical, and ultrastructural study of a case with cranial and extracranial metastases. Cancer. 1985;55:598–604.
6. Brown RL, Wollman R, Weiss RE. Transformation of a pituitary macroadenoma into to a corticotropin-secreting carcinoma over 16 years. Endocr Pract. 2007;13:463–71.
7. Lopes MB, Scheithauer BW, Schiff D. Pituitary carcinoma: diagnosis and treatment. Endocrine. 2005;28:115–21.
8. Gaffey TA, Scheithauer BW, Lloyd RV, Burger PC, Robbins P, Fereidooni F, et al. Corticotroph carcinoma of the pituitary: a clinicopathological study. Report of four cases. J Neurosurg. 2002;96:352–60.
9. Scheithauer BW, Fereidooni F, Horvath E, Kovacs K, Robbins P, Tews D, et al. Pituitary carcinoma: an ultrastructural study of eleven cases. Ultrastruct Pathol. 2001;25:227–42.
10. DeLellis R, Lloyd RV, Heitz P, Eng C, editors. World Health Organization classification of tumours: tumours of endocrine organs. Lyon: IARC Press; 2004.
11. Ragel BT, Couldwell WT. Pituitary carcinoma: a review of the literature. Neurosurg Focus. 2004;16, E7.
12. Matsuki M, Kaji Y, Matsuo M, Kobashi Y. MR findings of subarachnoid dissemination of a pituitary adenoma. Br J Radiol. 2000;73:783–5.
13. Thapar K, Yamada Y, Scheithauer B, Kovacs K, Yamada S, Stefaneanu L. Assessment of mitotic activity in pituitary adenomas and carcinomas. Endocr Pathol. 1996;7:215–21.
14. Scheithauer BW, Gaffey TA, Lloyd RV, Sebo TJ, Kovacs KT, Horvath E, et al. Pathobiology of pituitary adenomas and carcinomas. Neurosurgery. 2006;59:341–53.
15. Thapar K, Kovacs K, Scheithauer BW, Stefaneanu L, Horvath E, Pernicone PJ, et al. Proliferative activity and invasiveness among pituitary adenomas and carcinomas: an analysis using the MIB-1 antibody. Neurosurgery. 1996;38:99–106; discussion 106–7.
16. Thapar K, Scheithauer BW, Kovacs K, Pernicone PJ, Laws Jr ER. p53 expression in pituitary adenomas and carcinomas: correlation with invasiveness and tumor growth fractions. Neurosurgery. 1996;38:765–70; discussion 770–1.
17. Mamelak AN, Carmichael JD, Park P, Bannykh S, Fan X, Bonert HV. Atypical pituitary adenoma with malignant features. Pituitary. 2011;14:92–7.
18. Fadul CE, Kominsky AL, Meyer LP, Kingman LS, Kinlaw WB, Rhodes CH, et al. Long-term response of pituitary carcinoma to temozolomide. Report of two cases. J Neurosurg. 2006;105:621–6.
19. Lim S, Shahinian H, Maya MM, Yong W, Heaney AP. Temozolomide: a novel treatment for pituitary carcinoma. Lancet Oncol. 2006;7:518–20.
20. Bush ZM, Longtine JA, Cunningham T, Schiff D, Jane Jr JA, Vance ML, et al. Temozolomide treatment for aggressive pituitary tumors: correlation of clinical outcome with O(6)-methylguanine methyltransferase (MGMT) promoter methylation and expression. J Clin Endocrinol Metab. 2010;95:E280–90.

Ectopic Pituitary Adenomas

20

Gabriel Zada, M. Beatriz S. Lopes, Srinivasan Mukundan Jr., and Edward Laws Jr.

20.1 Epidemiology and Clinical Presentation

- Ectopic pituitary adenomas (EPAs) are rare tumors that develop outside the usual location in the sella turcica. They may arise in conjunction with, or separate from, congenital and developmental syndromes that involve pituitary agenesis and hypoplasia [1].
- EPAs may arise in the clivus, nasopharynx, sphenoid sinus, cavernous sinus, suprasellar region, and even the third ventricle [2–6].
- All varieties of pituitary adenomas have been reported to arise as ectopic tumors, with associated hypersecretion syndromes including Cushing's disease, acromegaly, hyperthyroidism, and hyperprolactinemia [2–4, 7, 8].
- The clinical presentation is highly variable and depends on the tumor's location, size, and pathological subtype.
- Some EPAs are thought to arise from aberrant cells located in the pars tuberalis above the diaphragma sella, infundibulum, or craniopharyngeal duct [9].

G. Zada, MD, MS (✉)
Department of Neurological Surgery,
Keck School of Medicine, University of Southern California,
1200 N State Street, #3300, Los Angeles, CA 90033, USA
e-mail: gzada@usc.edu

M.B.S. Lopes, MD, PhD
Department of Pathology (Neuropathology),
University of Virginia School of Medicine,
1215 Lee Street, Room 3060–HEP,
Charlottesville, VA 22908, USA
e-mail: msl2e@virginia.edu

S. Mukundan Jr., PhD, MD
Department of Radiology, Brigham and Women's Hospital,
75 Francis Street, Boston, MA 02115, USA
e-mail: smukundan@partners.org

E. Laws Jr., MD
Department of Neurosurgery, Brigham and Women's Hospital,
15 Francis Street, Boston, MA 02115, USA
e-mail: elaws@partners.org

G. Zada et al. (eds.), *Atlas of Sellar and Parasellar Lesions: Clinical, Radiologic, and Pathologic Correlations*,
DOI 10.1007/978-3-319-22855-6_20

20.2 Diagnosis

20.2.1 Imaging

- EPAs usually appear as well-circumscribed, heterogeneously enhancing masses that are isointense on T1-weighted imaging and isointense or hyperintense on T2-weighted imaging [10].
- By definition, EPAs have no communication with the sella (Fig. 20.1). In most cases, MRI can demonstrate an intact sellar floor and dura [11].
- An empty sella may be seen in conjunction with an EPA [1, 11–13].

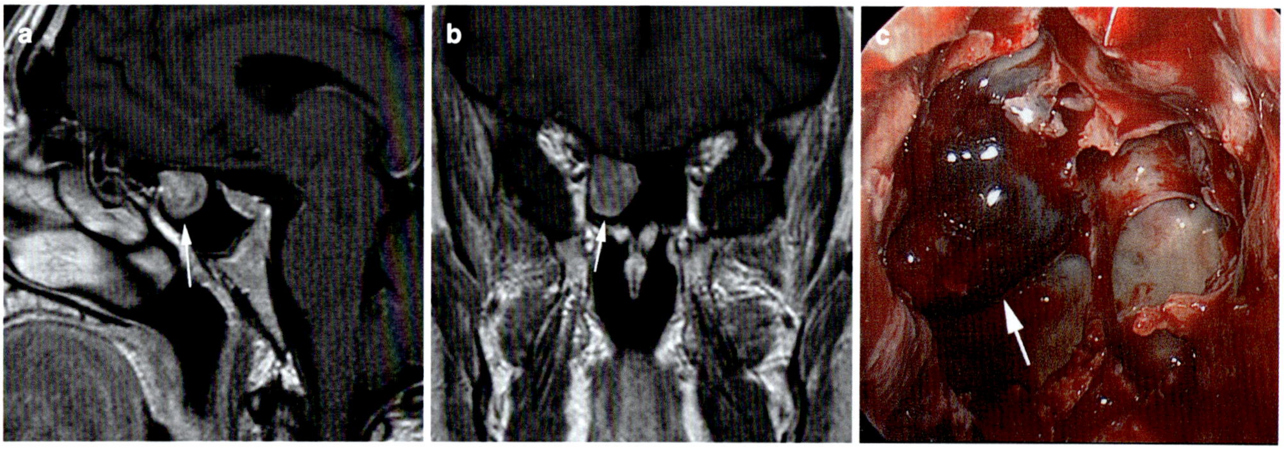

Fig. 20.1 Ectopic pituitary adenoma. (**a**) Sagittal T1-weighted post-gadolinium image. (**b**) Coronal T1-weighted post-gadolinium image. An enhancing lesion is located in the roof of the right sphenoid sinus (*white arrow*), anterior to the sella. The pituitary gland within the sella is normal in size. (**c**) Intraoperative photo taken via endoscopic endonasal approach (*white arrow*) showing the ectopic pituitary adenoma arising from the roof of the right sphenoid sinus

20.2.2 Histopathology

- Histopathological findings are similar to those seen in classic PAs. Immunostaining may show reactivity for any of the anterior pituitary hormone cell types.
- The MIB-1 labeling index in EPAs is usually less than 1 % [14].
- Malignant transformation of an EPA is rare, but it has been reported [15].
- Normal histology of the anterior pituitary gland can be seen along with the finding of an EPA [16].

20.3 Clinical Management

- EPAs are often mistaken for other tumors prior to pathological analysis, and a thorough endocrine work-up is not always performed. This work-up should be done as soon as possible (before or after surgery), to characterize the hormonal tumor profile.
- Resection depends on the location and the relationship of the tumor to surrounding neurovascular structures.
- Endoscopic endonasal techniques have been utilized to treat these tumors (Fig. 20.1c) [17].
- Suprasellar EPAs may be treated via craniotomy (typically pterional or subfrontal) or extended endonasal approaches.
- As with classic PAs, postoperative management is focused on normalization of hormonal hypersecretion syndromes and achieving tumor control with any combination of medications and adjunctive radiation-based therapy.
- Stereotactic radiosurgery may be used as needed to treat residual areas of EPAs.
- Sphenoid sinus EPAs recur in approximately 14 % of patients following tumor resection [14].

References

1. Das CJ, Seith A, Gamanagatti S, Goswami R. On the AJR viewbox. Ectopic pituitary adenoma with an empty sella. AJR Am J Roentgenol. 2006;186:1468–9.
2. Appel JG, Bergsneider M, Vinters H, Salamon N, Wang MB, Heaney AP. Acromegaly due to an ectopic pituitary adenoma in the clivus: case report and review of literature. Pituitary. 2012;15:S53–6.
3. Burch WM, Kramer RS, Kenan PD, Hammond CB. Cushing's disease caused by an ectopic pituitary adenoma within the sphenoid sinus. N Engl J Med. 1985;312:587–8.
4. Dyer EH, Civit T, Abecassis JP, Derome PJ. Functioning ectopic supradiaphragmatic pituitary adenomas. Neurosurgery. 1994;34:529–32; discussion 532.
5. Hata N, Inoue T, Katsuta T, Iwaki T. Ectopic pituitary adenoma in the cavernous sinus causing oculomotor nerve paresis – case report. Neurol Med Chir (Tokyo). 2003;43:399–403.
6. Kleinschmidt-DeMasters BK, Winston KR, Rubinstein D, Samuels MH. Ectopic pituitary adenoma of the third ventricle. Case report. J Neurosurg. 1990;72:139–42.
7. Collie RB, Collie MJ. Extracranial thyroid-stimulating hormone-secreting ectopic pituitary adenoma of the nasopharynx. Otolaryngol Head Neck Surg. 2005;133:453–4.
8. Cooper DS, Wenig BM. Hyperthyroidism caused by an ectopic TSH-secreting pituitary tumor. Thyroid. 1996;6:337–43.
9. Takahata T, Katayama Y, Tsubokawa T, Oshima H, Yoshino A. Ectopic pituitary adenoma occurring in the interpeduncular cistern. Case report. J Neurosurg. 1995;83:1092–4.
10. Slonim SM, Haykal HA, Cushing GW, Freidberg SR, Lee AK. MRI appearances of an ectopic pituitary adenoma: case report and review of the literature. Neuroradiology. 1993;35:546–8.
11. Yang BT, Chong VF, Wang ZC, Xian JF, Chen QH. Sphenoid sinus ectopic pituitary adenomas: CT and MRI findings. Br J Radiol. 2010;83:218–24.
12. Hong JF, Ding XH, Wang SS. Coexistence of ectopic pituitary adenoma and empty sella in a patient with acromegaly: a case report and review of literature. Neurol India. 2012;60:304–6.
13. Kusano Y, Horiuchi T, Oya F, Miyaoka Y, Oguchi K, Takemae T, Hongo K. Ectopic pituitary adenoma associated with an empty sella: a case report and review of the literature. J Neuroimaging. 2013;23:135–6.
14. Thompson LD, Seethala RR, Muller S. Ectopic sphenoid sinus pituitary adenoma (ESSPA) with normal anterior pituitary gland: a clinicopathologic and immunophenotypic study of 32 cases with a comprehensive review of the English literature. Head Neck Pathol. 2012;6:75–100.
15. Hosaka N, Kitajiri S, Hiraumi H, Nogaki H, Toki J, Yang G, et al. Ectopic pituitary adenoma with malignant transformation. Am J Surg Pathol. 2002;26:1078–82.
16. Lloyd RV, Chandler WF, Kovacs K, Ryan N. Ectopic pituitary adenomas with normal anterior pituitary glands. Am J Surg Pathol. 1986;10:546–52.
17. Alexander AA, Niktash N, Kardon DE, Sadeghi N. Ectopic nasopharyngeal pituitary adenoma resected with endoscopic technique. Ear Nose Throat J. 2008;87:E8–10.

Part V

Craniopharyngiomas and Other Epithelial Cystic Lesions of the Sellar Region

Craniopharyngiomas

21

Gabriel Zada, M. Beatriz S. Lopes, Srinivasan Mukundan Jr., and Edward Laws Jr.

21.1 Epidemiology and Clinical Presentation

- Craniopharyngiomas (CP) are benign, yet locally invasive, neoplasms typically arising as suprasellar and sellar lesions.
- CPs can arise anywhere along the vestiges of the stomodeal diverticulum and craniopharyngeal duct, most frequently in the region of the infundibulum [1–3].
- In rare cases, CPs have been reported to arise in less typical locations along the remnants of the primitive craniopharyngeal duct, including the nasopharynx or sphenoid bone, or as primary intraventricular lesions [3–6].
- Overall, CPs comprise approximately 3 % of all intracranial tumors, but this proportion is notably higher in the pediatric population (8–10 % of all pediatric brain tumors) [3, 7–9].
- The estimated incidence of craniopharyngiomas is 0.13 per 100,000 persons per year [10].
- CPs comprise approximately 3 % of surgically resected lesions in major transsphenoidal series [11, 12].
- Historically, CPs were said to present in a bimodal age distribution with peak ages at 5–14 years and then 50–74 years [10], but they could present in patients of any age. These statistics are outmoded, distorted by reports of pediatric data. Age-specific incidence in adults increases with age.
- The clinical presentation of CPs at any age frequently includes headache, visual loss, and hypopituitarism [1, 13].
- In children and adolescents, growth and sexual retardation, obesity, and hydrocephalus are frequently observed [7, 14, 15].
- Many patients with CPs suffer from chronic obesity, which is thought to develop secondary to hypothalamic dysfunction.
- Memory loss and cognitive deficits are more common findings in older patients [16].
- Diabetes insipidus occurs on presentation in 6–38 % of new cases [1, 17].

21.2 Imaging Features

- CPs are typically described as calcified, solid, and/or cystic lesions with a lobular shape and a diameter of 20–40 mm [18–21].
- Most arise within the suprasellar space, with 40–53 % of cases demonstrating some intrasellar involvement [7, 22].
- They occasionally extend into the anterior, middle, or posterior fossa and may invade the floor or walls of the third ventricle [19, 22].
- Hydrocephalus is observed in up to 38 % of surgical cases and is a more common finding in children [7, 20].

G. Zada, MD, MS (✉)
Department of Neurological Surgery,
Keck School of Medicine, University of Southern California,
1200 N State Street, #3300, Los Angeles, CA 90033, USA
e-mail: gzada@usc.edu

M.B.S. Lopes, MD, PhD
Department of Pathology (Neuropathology),
University of Virginia School of Medicine,
1215 Lee Street, Room 3060–HEP,
Charlottesville, VA 22908, USA
e-mail: msl2e@virginia.edu

S. Mukundan Jr., PhD, MD
Department of Radiology, Brigham and Women's Hospital,
75 Francis Street, Boston, MA 02115, USA
e-mail: smukundan@partners.org

E. Laws Jr., MD
Department of Neurosurgery, Brigham and Women's Hospital,
15 Francis Street, Boston, MA 02115, USA
e-mail: elaws@partners.org

G. Zada et al. (eds.), *Atlas of Sellar and Parasellar Lesions: Clinical, Radiologic, and Pathologic Correlations*,
DOI 10.1007/978-3-319-22855-6_21

21.2.1 Adamantinomatous Craniopharyngiomas

- On standard CT imaging, calcification is evident in 60 % of tumors; it is more common in pediatric cases and in the adamantinomatous subtype [1, 18, 20, 23].
- The majority of adamantinomatous CPs are mixed solid-cystic or predominantly cystic tumors with a lobulated appearance [18, 20, 23].
- On MRI, the solid elements are usually isointense or hypointense on T1-weighted images, exhibit inhomogeneous high intensity on T2-weighted images, and heterogeneously enhance following gadolinium administration [23, 24].
- The cystic elements of adamantinomatous CPs typically display a high intensity on T1-weighted images, high or mixed intensity on T2-weighted images, and contrast enhancement of the cyst wall.
- (Figs. 21.1, 21.2, 21.3, 21.4, 21.5, 21.6, 21.7, 21.8, 21.9, 21.10, and 21.11) [23].

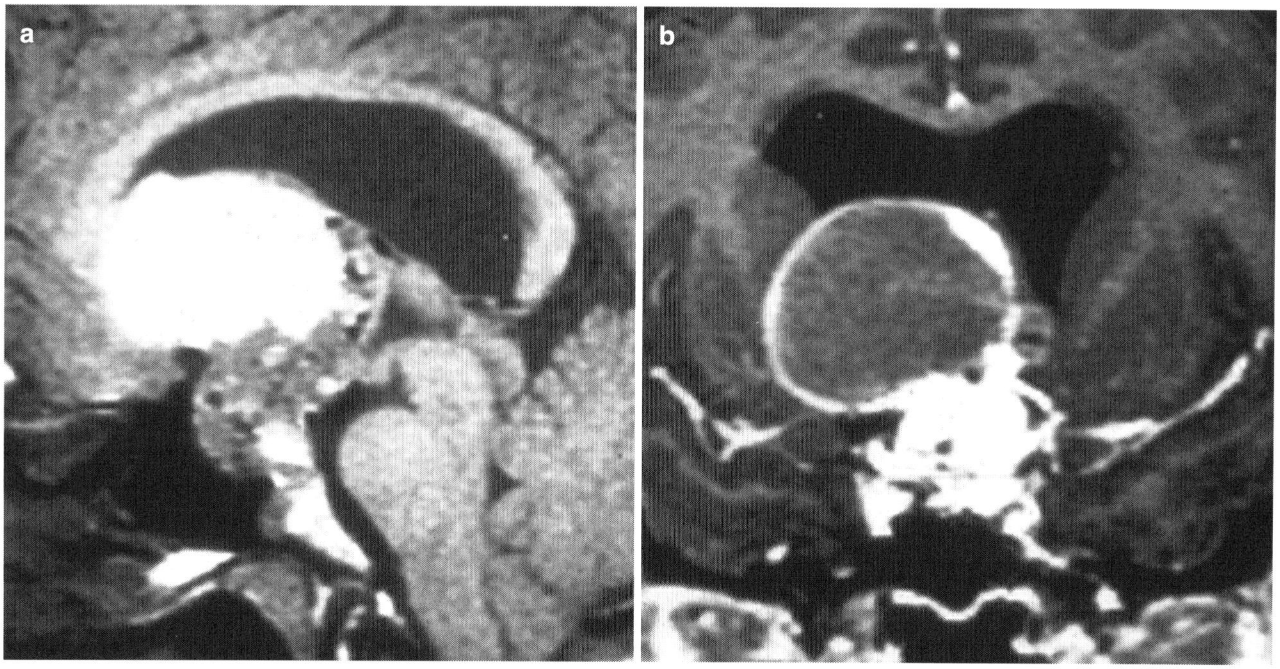

Fig. 21.1 (**a**) Sagittal T1-weighted pre-gadolinium image. (**b**) Coronal T1-weighted post-gadolinium image. A large mass with heterogeneous signal intensity is centered in the sella with a large cystic suprasellar component extending to the foramen of Monro causing hydrocephalus. There are also hypointense structures within the inferior sellar component of the lesion that may represent calcifications. The clivus is eroded

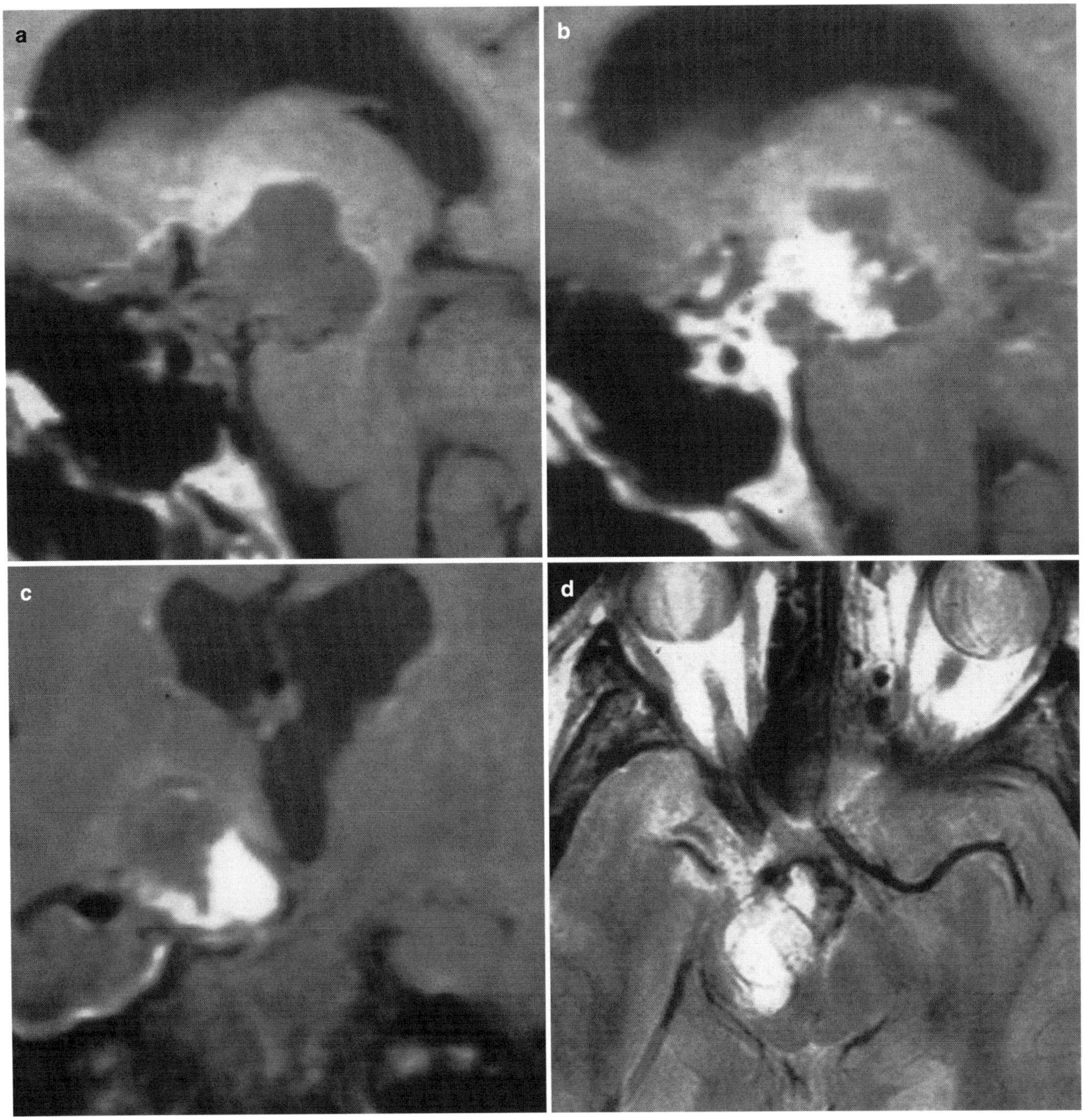

Fig. 21.2 (**a**) Sagittal T1-weighted pre-gadolinium image. (**b**) Sagittal T1-weighted post-gadolinium image. (**c**) Coronal T1-weighted pre-gadolinium image. (**d**) Axial T2-weighted image. There is a large mixed cystic and solid enhancing mass in the right suprasellar region impressing on the right hypothalamus. Posteriorly, the mass indents on the right midbrain

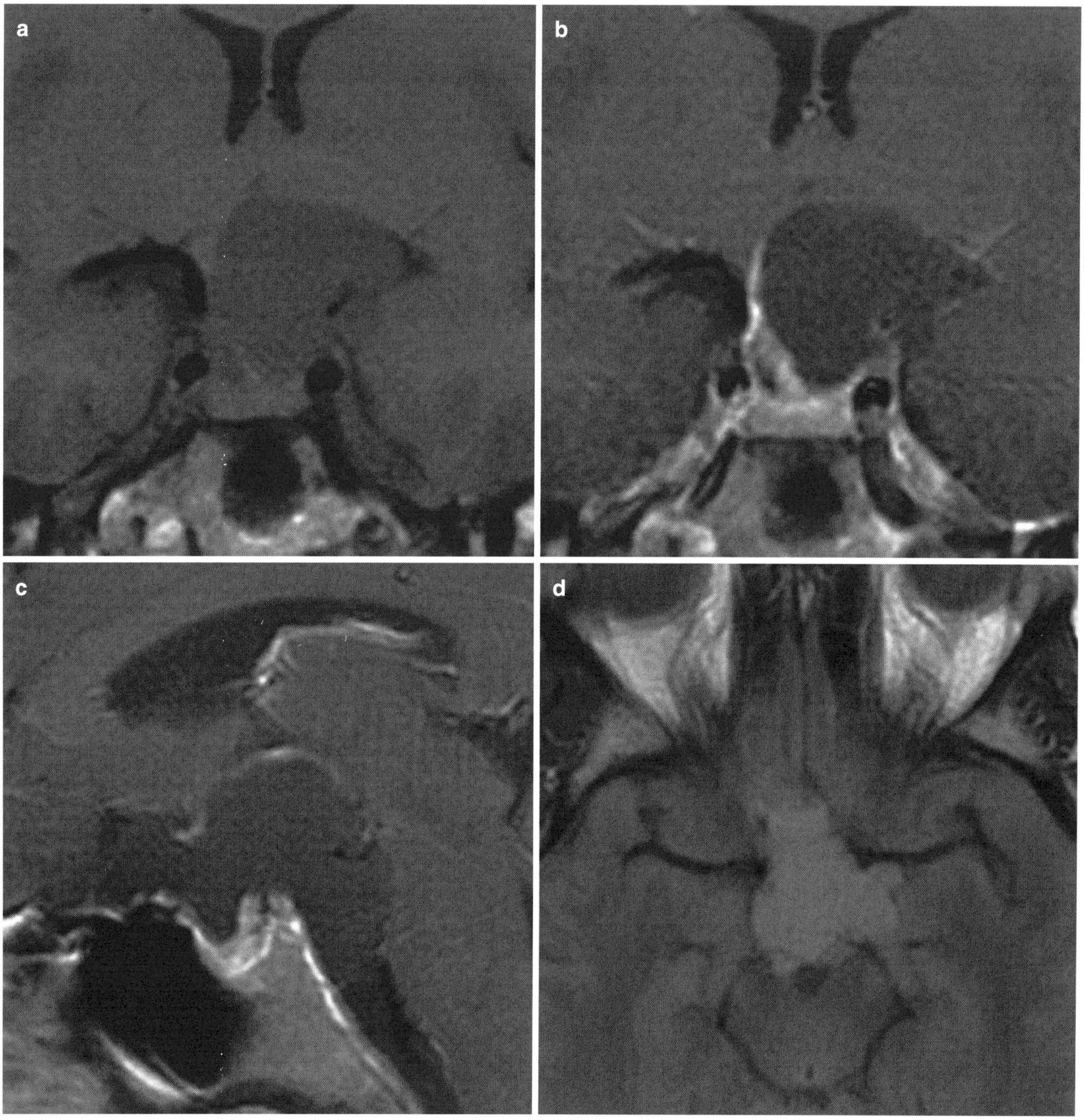

Fig. 21.3 (**a**) Coronal T1-weighted pre-gadolinium image. (**b**) Coronal T1-weighted post-gadolinium image. (**c**) Sagittal T1-weighted post-gadolinium image. (**d**) Axial *f*luid-*a*ttenuated *i*nversion *r*ecovery (FLAIR) image. A large cystic mass centers in the suprasellar region extending to the interpeduncular cistern. The content of the cystic component is slightly hyperintense on both T1-weighted and FLAIR images. The mass indents on the left hypothalamus. The pituitary gland is located in the sella inferior to the mass

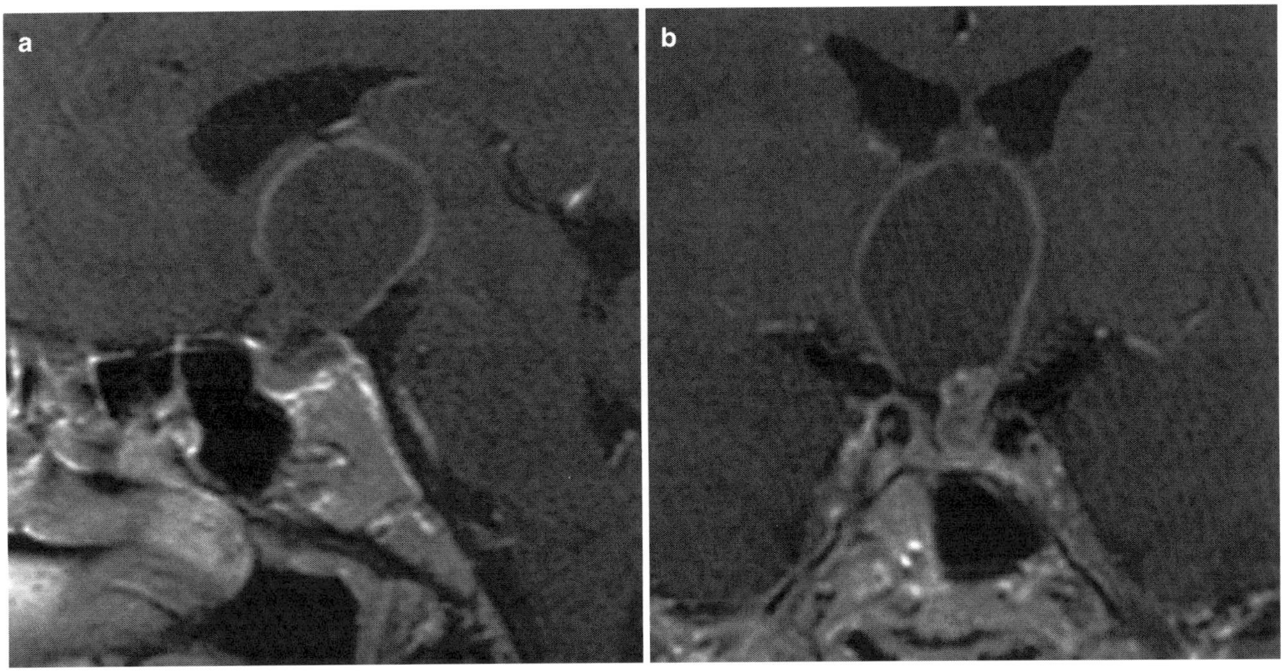

Fig. 21.4 (**a**) Sagittal T1-weighted post-gadolinium image. (**b**) Coronal T1-weighted post-gadolinium image. There is an enhancing sellar mass with a cystic suprasellar component extending to the root of the third ventricle

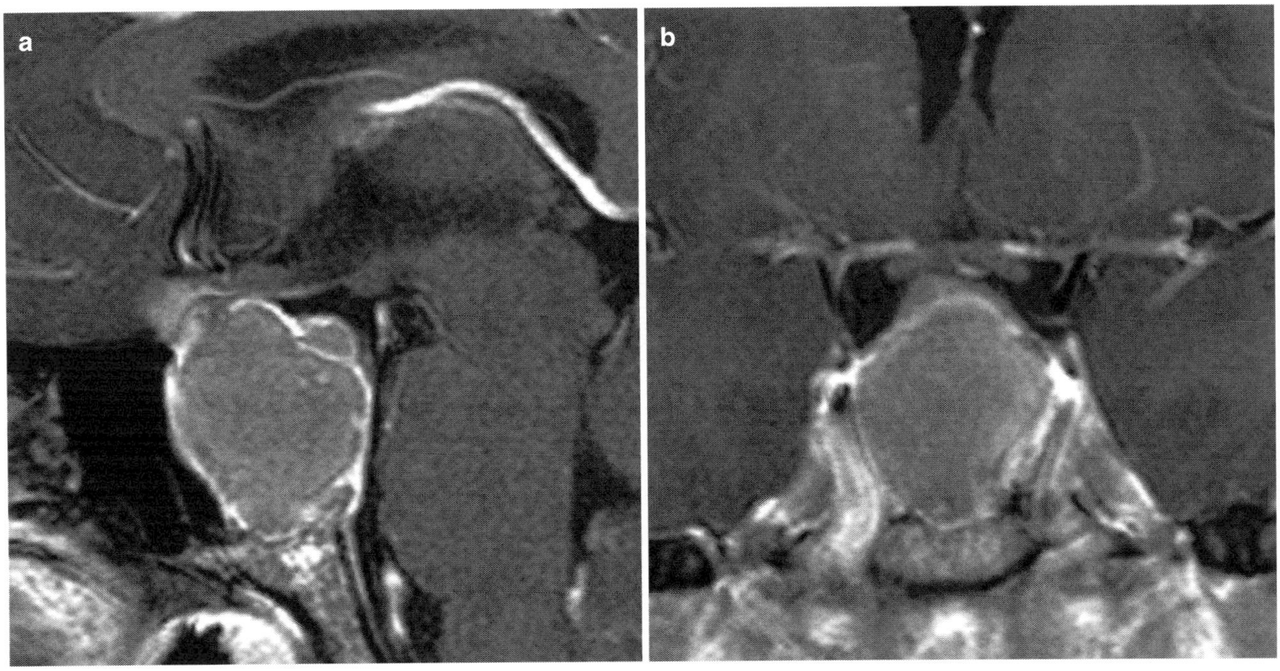

Fig. 21.5 (**a**) Sagittal T1-weighted post-gadolinium image. (**b**) Coronal T1-weighted post-gadolinium image. A heterogeneously enhancing sellar/suprasellar mass erodes the sellar floor and contacts the optic chiasm without significant displacement

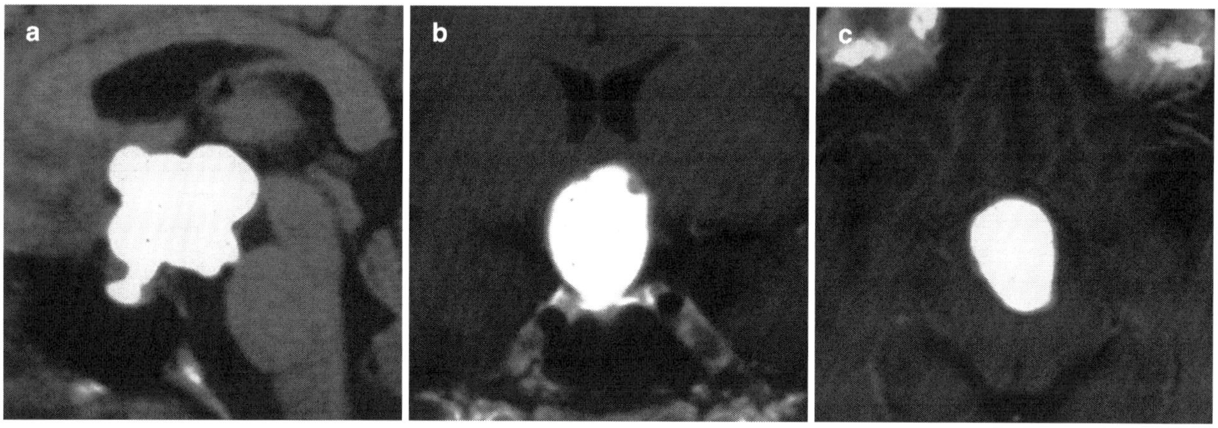

Fig. 21.6 (**a**) Sagittal T1-weighted pre-gadolinium image. (**b**) Coronal T1-weighted post-gadolinium image. (**c**) Axial T1-weighted post-gadolinium image. A lobulated cystic mass centers in the sellar and suprasellar regions. The content of the cystic component is hyperintense on T1-weighted images. The mass extends superiorly to the third ventricle and posteriorly to the interpeduncular cistern

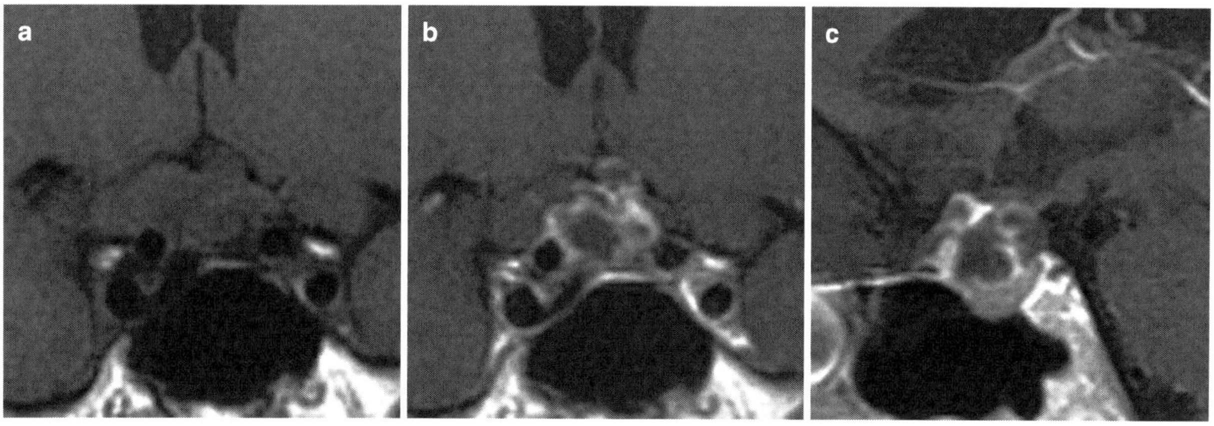

Fig. 21.7 (**a**) Coronal T1-weighted pre-gadolinium image. (**b**) Coronal T1-weighted post-gadolinium image. (**c**) Sagittal T1-weighted post-gadolinium image. There is a mixed cystic and solid enhancing mass in the sellar and suprasellar regions. There is remodeling of the sellar floor. The mass abuts the optic chiasm without significant displacement. There is no encasement of the cavernous internal carotid arteries

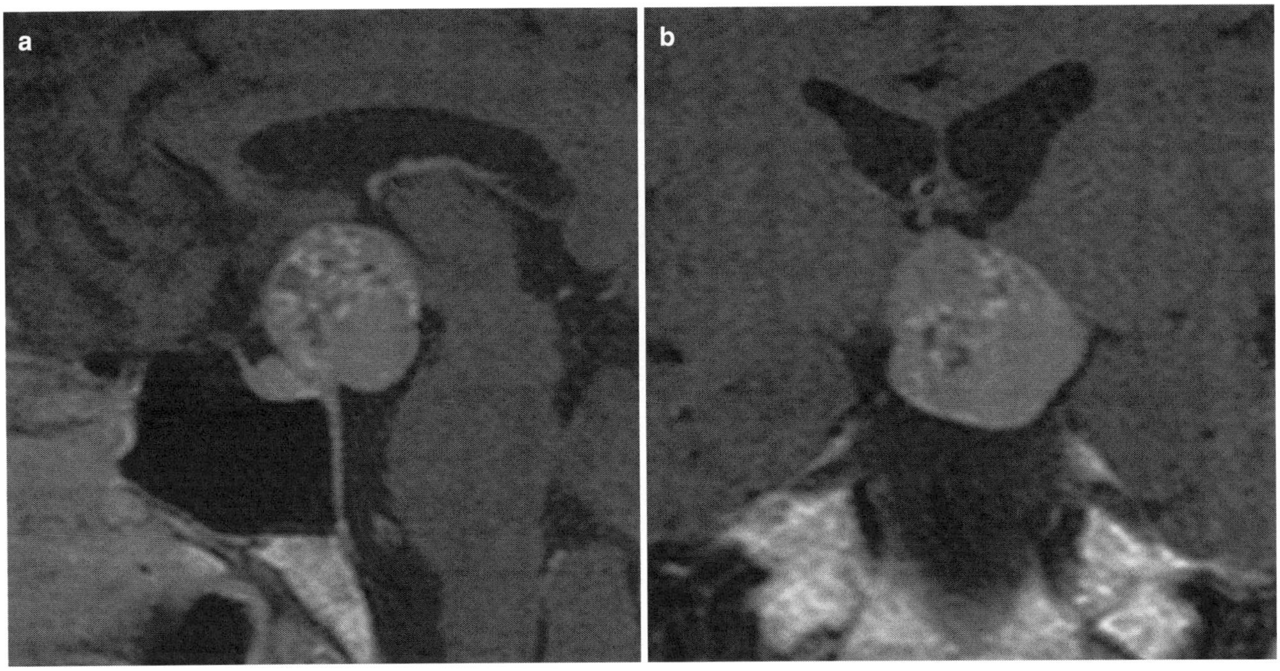

Fig. 21.8 (**a**) Sagittal T1-weighted post-gadolinium image. (**b**) Coronal T1-weighted post-gadolinium image. A suprasellar mass with heterogeneous signal intensity extends to the interpeduncular cistern and indents the hypothalami. The pituitary gland is located in the sella inferior to the mass

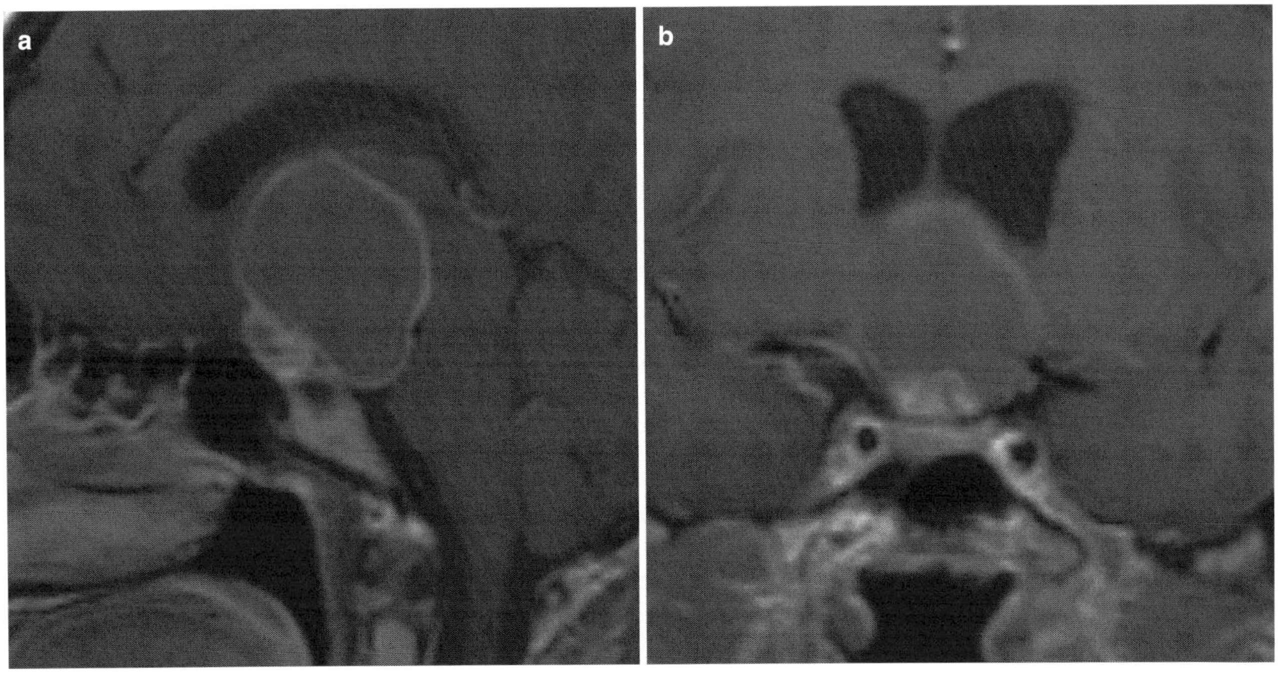

Fig. 21.9 (**a**) Sagittal T1-weighted post-gadolinium image. (**b**) Coronal T1-weighted post-gadolinium image. There is a suprasellar cystic mass extending to the interpeduncular cistern. The mass indents the hypothalamus. The pituitary gland is located in the sella inferior to the mass

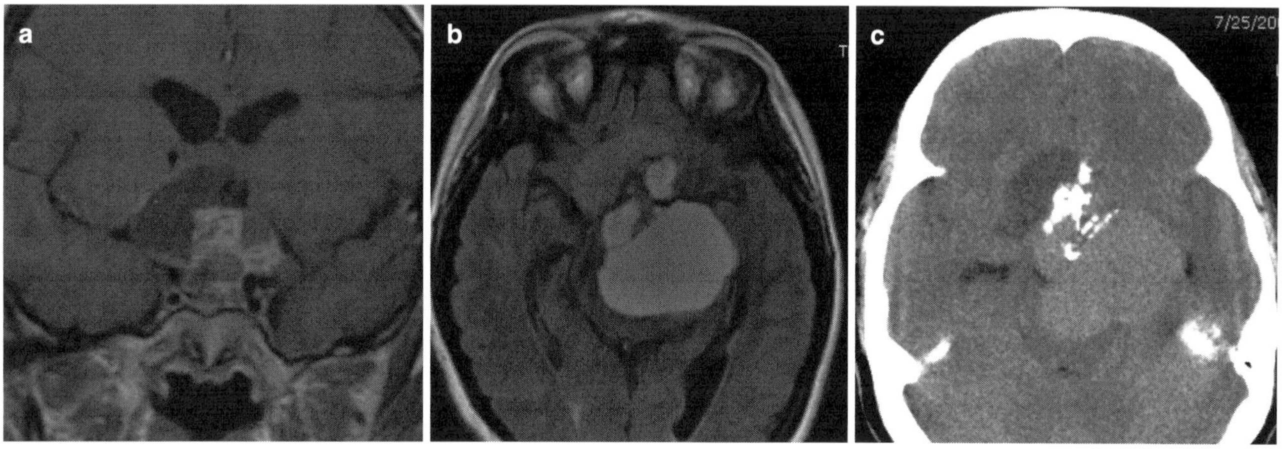

Fig. 21.10 (**a**) Coronal T1-weighted pre-gadolinium image. (**b**) Axial *f*luid-*a*ttenuated *i*nversion *r*ecovery (FLAIR) image. (**c**) Axial CT image. A large mixed cystic and solid enhancing sellar and suprasellar mass containing calcification impresses on the hypothalami and brainstem

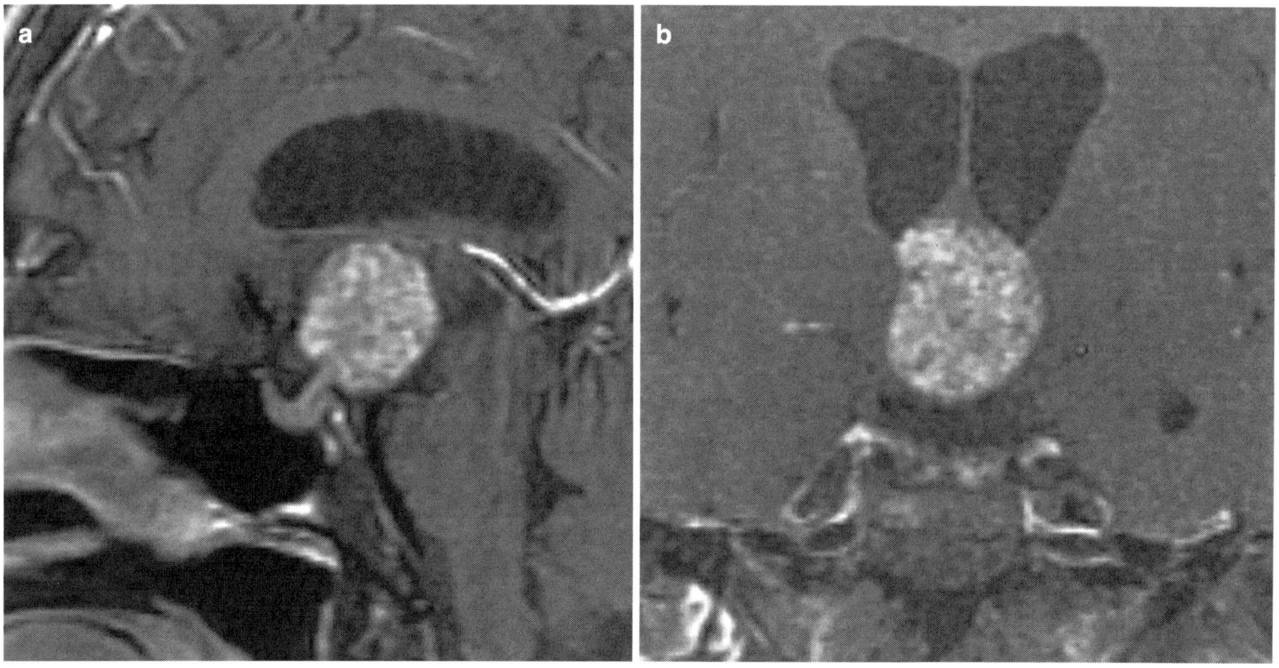

Fig. 21.11 (**a**) Sagittal T1-weighted post-gadolinium image. (**b**) Coronal T1-weighted post-gadolinium image. There is a mass with heterogeneous signal intensity in the suprasellar region anterior to the third ventricle and abutting the hypothalamus. The pituitary gland and stalk are visualized separately from the mass

21.2.2 Papillary Craniopharyngiomas

- The squamous-papillary subtype is found in approximately one third of adult CP cases and rarely shows calcification [4, 18, 20, 23].
- The majority of squamous-papillary CPs are predominantly solid or mixed solid-cystic tumors with a spherical shape. They usually exhibit low intensity on T1-weighted images, high intensity on T2-weighted images, and enhancement of the cyst wall after addition of gadolinium [4, 18, 23].
- The MRI appearance of the solid regions is frequently similar to those of the adamantinomatous variety (Figs. 21.12 and 21.13).

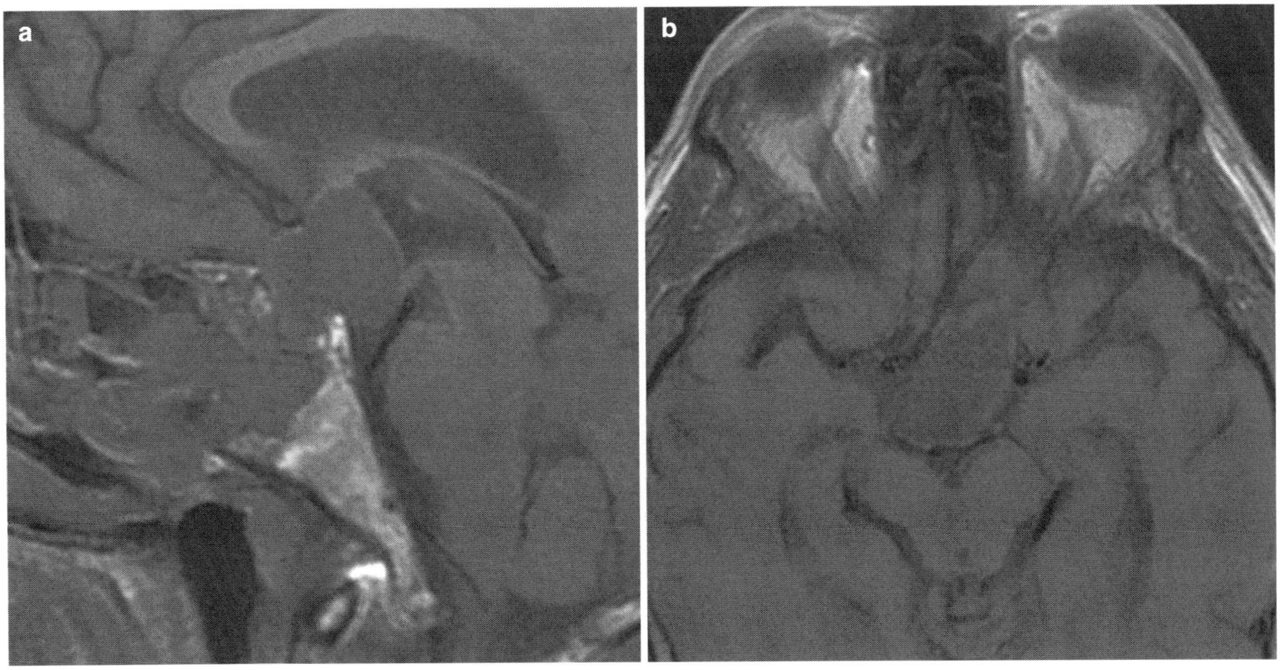

Fig. 21.12 (**a**) Sagittal T1-weighted pre-gadolinium image. (**b**) Axial T1-weighted pre-gadolinium image. A mass with heterogeneous signal intensity in the sellar/suprasellar region extends to the interpeduncular cistern. The lamina terminalis is posteriorly displaced. There is erosion of the sella

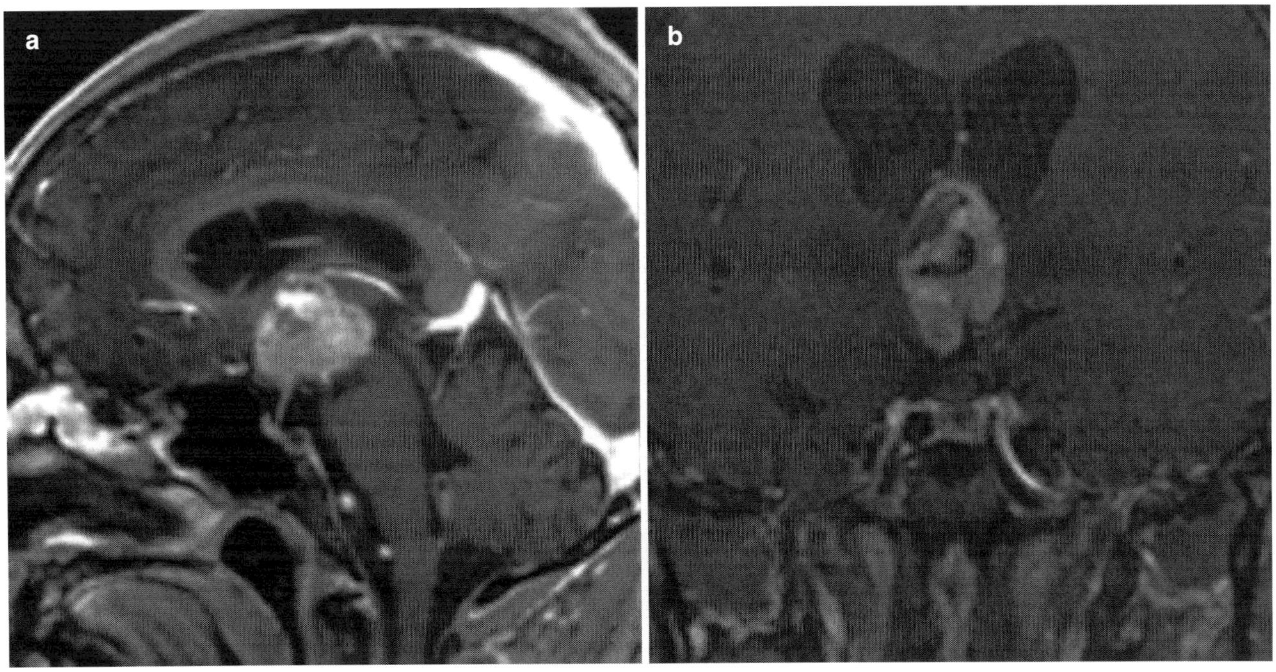

Fig. 21.13 Sagittal (**a**) and coronal (**b**) T1-weighted post-gadolinium imaging showing a large, heterogeneously enhancing papillary craniopharyngioma contained entirely within the third ventricle

21.3 Pathology

- Many authors have suggested that CPs and Rathke cleft cysts are related lesions representing two ends of a spectrum of similar disease entities originating from ectodermal remnants of Rathke's pouch [21, 25, 26].
- In addition to the two major pathological subtypes (adamantinomatous and papillary), several mixed or transitional forms also have been reported.
- Several investigators have argued that adamantinomatous and papillary CPs may represent two distinct entities that are located at opposing ends of a pathological continuum [20, 27].
- New molecular genetics data have shown that these tumors may have a different pathway of formation with mutually exclusive gene mutations. Mutations in the *CTNNB1* (β-catenin) gene are present in adamantinomatous craniopharyngiomas, whereas recurrent mutations in the *BRAF* gene are seen in papillary craniopharyngiomas [28].
- There have been rare reports of progression to malignancy, mainly in the adamantinomatous variety.

21.3.1 Adamantinomatous Craniopharyngiomas

- Adamantinomatous CPs are thought to arise from squamous embryonic rests and bear similarity to adamantinomas or ameloblastomas of the jaw, with the potential for enamel production.
- On gross examination, the cystic components are often described as having a characteristic "machine-oil" interior, containing desquamated squamous epithelium and comprising mainly keratin and cholesterol.
- The solid component has a rubbery texture and may contain foci of calcifications or even bone.
- Histologically, the tumors are characterized by cystic formations of stratified epithelium with a palisading arrangement of basal cells, intermixed with nodular strands of solid and cystic epithelium, which in turn undergo transition to loose tissue termed stellate reticulum and "wet keratin" (Fig. 21.14).
- The nodular masses of "wet keratin" are distinctive and diagnostic of the adamantinomatous variant.
- Extensive fibrosis and xanthogranulomatous reaction with chronic inflammation and cholesterol clefts with a giant cell reaction may be prominent.
- CPs may compress or invade the brain parenchyma, producing variable gliosis and occasional Rosenthal fiber formation that may mimic pilocytic astrocytoma.

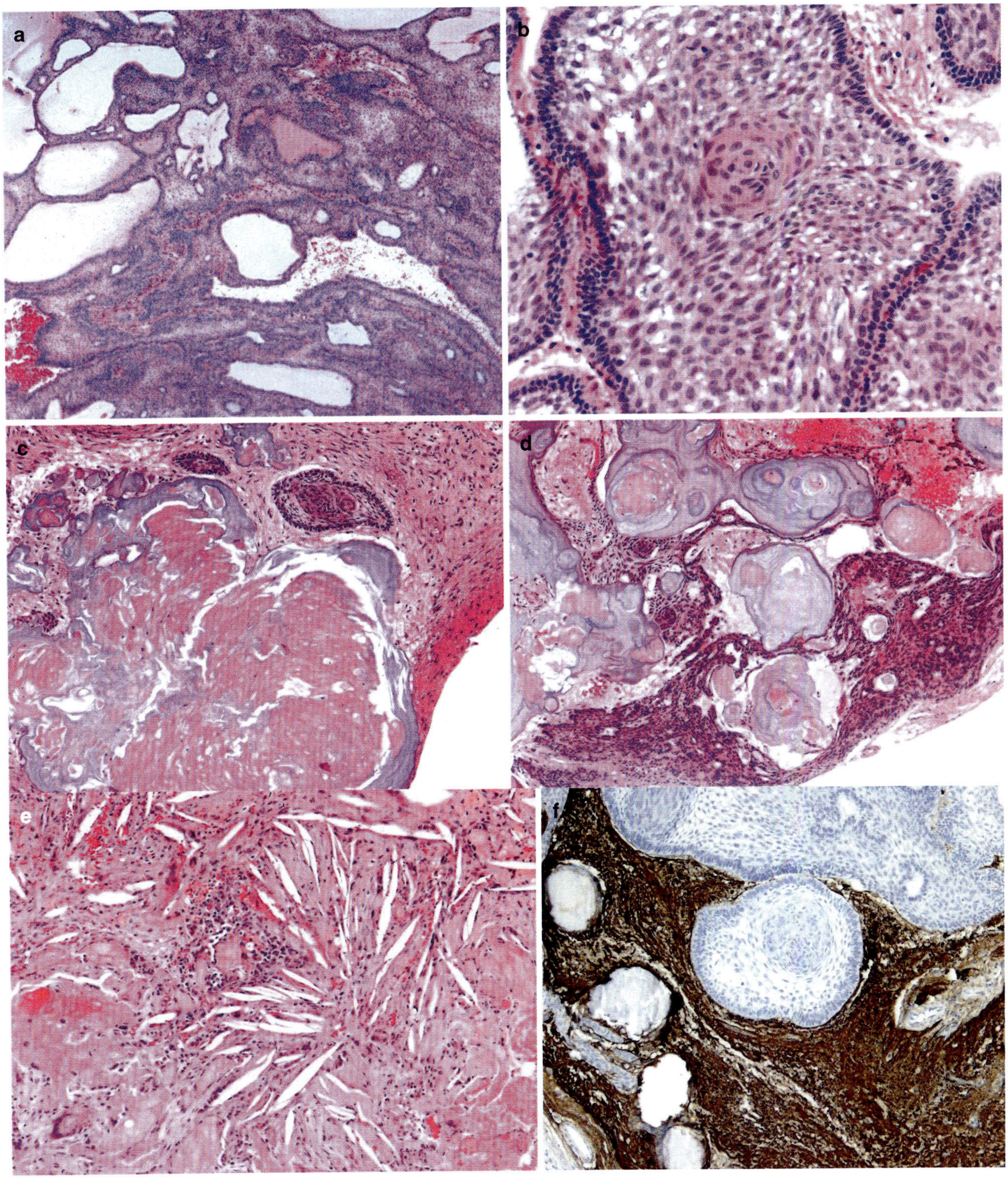

Fig. 21.14 Adamantinomatous craniopharyngioma (CP). Adamantinomatous CP typically shows a stratified epithelium with a palisading arrangement of the basal cells that mature into large, flat cells within a loose stroma (hematoxylin and eosin [H&E] stain) (**a**, **b**). One of the most characteristic features of adamantinomatous CP is the formation of "wet keratin" consisting of ghost keratinocytes with no nuclei (**c**). Adamantinomatous CP exhibits cystic formation (**a**) and calcifications (**d**). Reactive inflammatory reaction is commonly seen, with xanthomatous changes including the presence of large macrophages and cholesterol cleft accumulation (**e**). Intense gliosis in the adjacent brain parenchyma can be mistaken for low-grade glioma and highlighted by GFAP immunostain (**f**)

21.3.2 Papillary Craniopharyngiomas

- Papillary CPs are more common in adults (14–50 % of CPs in adults, compared with 2 % in children) [4].
- Papillary CPs tend to be more solid circumscribed masses that lack the typical calcification and "machinery oil" cyst content seen in adamantinomatous tumors.
- The tumors often involve or sit within the third ventricle.
- Histologically, the tumor consists of well-differentiated, squamous-lined papillae surrounding cores of fibrovascular stroma (Fig. 21.15).
- The squamous-like epithelium lacks true keratin formation and keratohyalin granules, thereby differing from epidermoid and dermoid cysts.
- Papillary tumors do not have the microcystic degeneration, keratinous nodules, and cholesterol clefts that are so characteristic of the adamantinomatous variant.

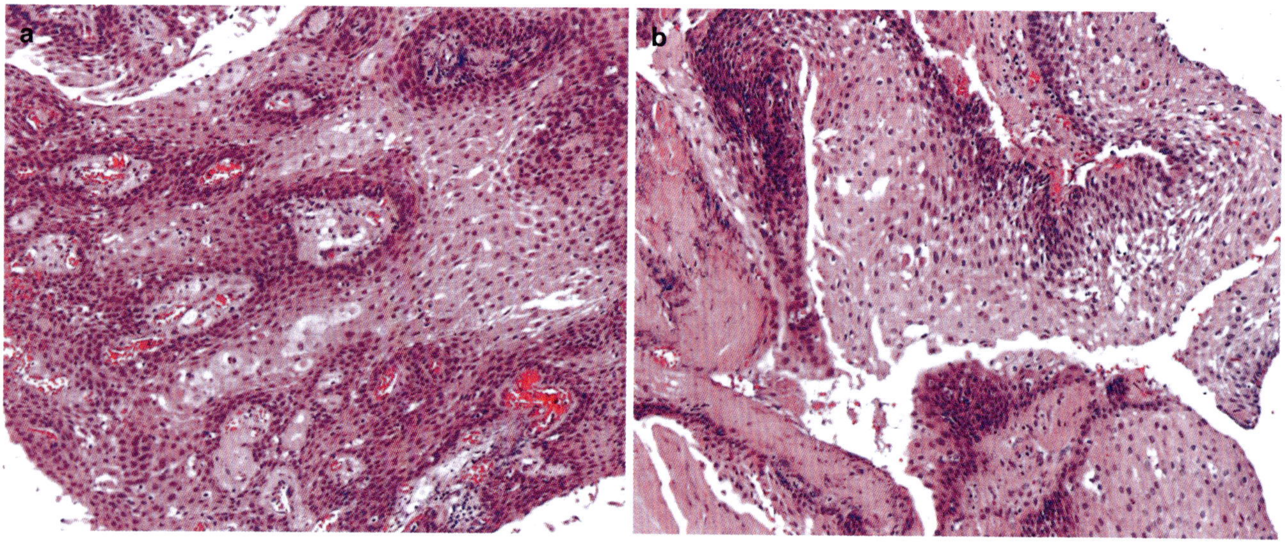

Fig. 21.15 Papillary craniopharyngioma. Papillary CP shows papillary formations composed of pseudostratified epithelium and may have a moderate degree of lymphocytic infiltrates in the fibrous vascular cores (H&E) (**a**). The pseudostratified epithelium shows no superficial maturation or keratin formation (**b**)

21.4 Clinical Management

Clinical management of CPs often requires multimodality treatment consisting of surgery, radiation-based intervention, and sometimes local chemotherapy. Recurrence and disease progression are frequent.

21.5 Surgical Management

- Common surgical approaches for resection of CPs include transcortical-intraventricular, interhemispheric-transcallosal, pterional-transsylvian, subfrontal, and extended transsphenoidal approaches [13, 15, 29–32].
- In recent years, extended endoscopic endonasal approaches have been utilized for CPs, with good results [31, 33–37].
- Gross total resection often may be challenging because of adherence to surrounding structures, especially in cases of reoperation [19].
- Preservation of the pituitary stalk should always be attempted unless complete panhypopituitarism and diabetes insipidus already exist and there is potential for total resection along with the infundibulum.
- Conservative resection is warranted for tumors demonstrating invasion of the hypothalamus, in order to maintain a high quality of life for the patient [38].
- Reported gross total resection rates vary from 45 to 90 %, depending on the approach and the reported tumor characteristics [13, 19].

21.5.1 Postoperative Management

- Vision may improve in up to 74–87 % of patients following surgery [13, 35].
- Some degree of hypopituitarism requiring hormonal replacement therapy is required in 65–90 % of patients following surgery [17].
- Panhypopituitarism occurs in up to 43 % of patients following surgery [17].
- Permanent diabetes insipidus develops in up to 60 % of patients following surgery [17].
- Long-term survival rates have been reported to be about 90 % at 10 years after surgery [19].
- Long-term recurrence-free survival rates have been reported to be about 38–100 % at 10 years after surgery; these rates depend mostly on the degree of surgical tumor resection [7, 19].
- There has been some debate as to whether adamantinomatous CPs demonstrate a higher potential for recurrence; recent analyses have reported similar or slightly higher rates than for their papillary counterparts [4, 18, 20].
- Radiation therapy or reoperation may be indicated in cases of residual disease or demonstrated recurrence and/or growth of tumor.
- Recurrence-free survival has been reported to be 74–81 % following gross total removal, 41–42 % following subtotal resection, and 83–90 % following subtotal resection with radiation therapy [1]. Selection bias is a major determinant of outcome in these studies.
- Stereotactic radiosurgery has provided limited benefits for CPs, with a wide range of tumor control rates reported, ranging from 36 to 100 % [39, 40].
- A typical marginal dose of 12 Gy is utilized for single-fraction radiosurgical treatment. Fractionated radiation therapy doses are up to 64 Gy.
- Stereotactic radiosurgery is more successful for solid tumors than for cystic or mixed lesions, with a long-term tumor control rate of up to 90 % [39].
- For recurrent cystic tumors, the use of intracystic bleomycin and carmustine wafers (Gliadel®; Eisai Inc., Woodcliff Lake, NJ) has been reported with limited efficacy [41, 42].
- Targeted molecular therapy is a promising avenve for treating *BRAF*$^+$ papillary CPs.

References

1. Karavitaki N, Cudlip S, Adams CB, Wass JA. Craniopharyngiomas. Endocr Rev. 2006;27:371–97.
2. Prabhu VC, Brown HG. The pathogenesis of craniopharyngiomas. Childs Nerv Syst. 2005;21:622–7.
3. Jane Jr JA, Laws ER. Craniopharyngioma. Pituitary. 2006;9: 323–6.
4. Crotty TB, Scheithauer BW, Young Jr WF, Davis DH, Shaw EG, Miller GM, Burger PC. Papillary craniopharyngioma: a clinicopathological study of 48 cases. J Neurosurg. 1995;83:206–14.
5. Iwasaki K, Kondo A, Takahashi JB, Yamanobe K. Intraventricular craniopharyngioma: report of two cases and review of the literature. Surg Neurol. 1992;38:294–301.
6. Brunel H, Raybaud C, Peretti-Viton P, Lena G, Girard N, Paz-Paredes A, et al. Craniopharyngioma in children: MRI study of 43 cases. Neurochirurgie. 2002;48:309–18.
7. Karavitaki N, Brufani C, Warner JT, Adams CB, Richards P, Ansorge O, et al. Craniopharyngiomas in children and adults: systematic analysis of 121 cases with long-term follow-up. Clin Endocrinol (Oxf). 2005;62:397–409.
8. Elliott RE, Wisoff JH. Successful surgical treatment of craniopharyngioma in very young children. J Neurosurg Pediatr. 2009;3: 397–406.
9. Jagannathan J, Dumont AS, Jane Jr JA, Laws Jr ER. Pediatric sellar tumors: diagnostic procedures and management. Neurosurg Focus. 2005;18, E6.
10. Bunin GR, Surawicz TS, Witman PA, Preston-Martin S, Davis F, Bruner JM. The descriptive epidemiology of craniopharyngioma. J Neurosurg. 1998;89:547–51.
11. Fatemi N, Dusick JR, de Paiva Neto MA, Kelly DF. The endonasal microscopic approach for pituitary adenomas and other parasellar tumors: a 10-year experience. Neurosurgery. 2008;63:244–56; discussion 256.
12. Saeger W, Ludecke DK, Buchfelder M, Fahlbusch R, Quabbe HJ, Petersenn S. Pathohistological classification of pituitary tumors: 10 years of experience with the German Pituitary Tumor Registry. Eur J Endocrinol. 2007;156:203–16.
13. Chakrabarti I, Amar AP, Couldwell W, Weiss MH. Long-term neurological, visual, and endocrine outcomes following transnasal resection of craniopharyngioma. J Neurosurg. 2005;102:650–7.
14. Laws ER. Craniopharyngiomas in children and young adults. Prog Exp Tumor Res. 1987;30:335–40.
15. Zada G, Laws ER. Surgical management of craniopharyngiomas in the pediatric population. Horm Res Paediatr. 2010;74:62–6.
16. Honegger J, Barocka A, Sadri B, Fahlbusch R. Neuropsychological results of craniopharyngioma surgery in adults: a prospective study. Surg Neurol. 1998;50:19–28; discussion 28–9.
17. Honegger J, Buchfelder M, Fahlbusch R. Surgical treatment of craniopharyngiomas: endocrinological results. J Neurosurg. 1999;90: 251–7.
18. Adamson TE, Wiestler OD, Kleihues P, Yasargil MG. Correlation of clinical and pathological features in surgically treated craniopharyngiomas. J Neurosurg. 1990;73:12–7.
19. Fahlbusch R, Honegger J, Paulus W, Huk W, Buchfelder M. Surgical treatment of craniopharyngiomas: experience with 168 patients. J Neurosurg. 1999;90:237–50.
20. Weiner HL, Wisoff JH, Rosenberg ME, Kupersmith MJ, Cohen H, Zagzag D, et al. Craniopharyngiomas: a clinicopathological analysis of factors predictive of recurrence and functional outcome. Neurosurgery. 1994;35:1001–10; discussion 1010–1.
21. Zada G, Lin N, Ojerholm E, Ramkissoon S, Laws ER. Craniopharyngioma and other cystic epithelial lesions of the sellar region: a review of clinical, imaging, and histopathological relationships. Neurosurg Focus. 2010;28:E4.
22. Van Effenterre R, Boch AL. Craniopharyngioma in adults and children: a study of 122 surgical cases. J Neurosurg. 2002;97:3–11.
23. Sartoretti-Schefer S, Wichmann W, Aguzzi A, Valavanis A. MR differentiation of adamantinous and squamous-papillary craniopharyngiomas. AJNR Am J Neuroradiol. 1997;18:77–87.
24. Choi SH, Kwon BJ, Na DG, Kim JH, Han MH, Chang KH. Pituitary adenoma, craniopharyngioma, and Rathke cleft cyst involving both intrasellar and suprasellar regions: differentiation using MRI. Clin Radiol. 2007;62:453–62.
25. Harrison MJ, Morgello S, Post KD. Epithelial cystic lesions of the sellar and parasellar region: a continuum of ectodermal derivatives? J Neurosurg. 1994;80:1018–25.
26. Goodrich JT, Post KD, Duffy P. Ciliated craniopharyngioma. Surg Neurol. 1985;24:105–11.
27. Eldevik OP, Blaivas M, Gabrielsen TO, Hald JK, Chandler WF. Craniopharyngioma: radiologic and histologic findings and recurrence. AJNR Am J Neuroradiol. 1996;17:1427–39.
28. Brastianos PK, Taylor-Weiner A, Manley PE, Jones RT, Dias-Santagata D, Thorner AR, et al. Exome sequencing identifies *BRAF* mutations in papillary craniopharyngiomas. Nat Genet. 2014;46:161–5.
29. Komotar RJ, Roguski M, Bruce JN. Surgical management of craniopharyngiomas. J Neurooncol. 2009;92:283–96.
30. Laws Jr ER. Transsphenoidal removal of craniopharyngioma. Pediatr Neurosurg. 1994;21 Suppl 1:57–63.
31. Laws ER. Endoscopic surgery for cystic lesions of the pituitary region. Nat Clin Pract Endocrinol Metab. 2008;4:662–3.
32. Laws Jr ER. Transsphenoidal microsurgery in the management of craniopharyngioma. J Neurosurg. 1980;52:661–6.
33. Cavallo LM, Prevedello D, Esposito F, Laws Jr ER, Dusick JR, Messina A, et al. The role of the endoscope in the transsphenoidal management of cystic lesions of the sellar region. Neurosurg Rev. 2008;31:55–64; discussion 64.
34. Cavallo LM, Prevedello DM, Solari D, Gardner PA, Esposito F, Snyderman CH, et al. Extended endoscopic endonasal transsphenoidal approach for residual or recurrent craniopharyngiomas. J Neurosurg. 2009;111:578–89.
35. Leng LZ, Greenfield JP, Souweidane MM, Anand VK, Schwartz TH. Endoscopic, endonasal resection of craniopharyngiomas: analysis of outcome including extent of resection, cerebrospinal fluid leak, return to preoperative productivity, and body mass index. Neurosurgery. 2012;70:110–23; discussion 123–4.
36. Kaptain GJ, Vincent DA, Sheehan JP, Laws Jr ER. Transsphenoidal approaches for the extracapsular resection of midline suprasellar and anterior cranial base lesions. Neurosurgery. 2001;49:94–100; discussion 100–1.
37. Couldwell WT, Weiss MH, Rabb C, Liu JK, Apfelbaum RI, Fukushima T. Variations on the standard transsphenoidal approach to the sellar region, with emphasis on the extended approaches and parasellar approaches: surgical experience in 105 cases. Neurosurgery. 2004;55:539–47; discussion 547–50.
38. Zada G, Cappabianca P. Transsphenoidal surgery for craniopharyngiomas: the lessons of experience, timing, and restraint. World Neurosurg. 2010;74:256–8.
39. Gopalan R, Dassoulas K, Rainey J, Sherman JH, Sheehan JP. Evaluation of the role of Gamma Knife surgery in the treatment of craniopharyngiomas. Neurosurg Focus. 2008;24:E5.
40. Laws Jr ER, Vance ML. Radiosurgery for pituitary tumors and craniopharyngiomas. Neurosurg Clin N Am. 1999;10:327–36.
41. Laws Jr ER, Morris AM, Maartens N. Gliadel for pituitary adenomas and craniopharyngiomas. Neurosurgery. 2003;53:255–69; discussion 259–60.
42. Caceres A. Intracavitary therapeutic options in the management of cystic craniopharyngioma. Childs Nerv Syst. 2005;21:705–18.

Rathke Cleft Cysts

22

Gabriel Zada, M. Beatriz S. Lopes, Srinivasan Mukundan Jr., and Edward R. Laws Jr.

22.1 Epidemiology and Clinical Presentation

- Rathke cleft cysts (RCCs) are benign, cystic remnants of the craniopharyngeal duct that are typically located in the sellar and suprasellar region [1, 2].
- RCCs are often discovered incidentally; they have been identified in up to 22 % of the population according to routine autopsy specimens [3].
- Despite their relatively high prevalence, they produce clinical symptoms in a minority of patients, comprising only 2–9 % of all sellar lesions undergoing surgical resection [4–9].
- They show a slight female preponderance.
- The typical age at the time of clinical presentation is generally between 40 and 50 years [6, 7, 10].
- Typical symptoms associated with RCCs include headache, endocrine dysfunction, and vision loss [6, 11, 12].
- Diabetes insipidus and hyperprolactinemia are relatively common endocrine findings.
- RCCs rarely present with chemical meningitis, abscess, inflammatory hypophysitis, or intracystic hemorrhage and apoplexy [7, 13].
- Uncommonly, RCCs can cause symptoms in children, potentially resulting in somatic and/or sexual retardation as well as the more common symptoms related to mass effect [14].

G. Zada (✉)
Deptartment of Neurosurgery, University of Southern California, Los Angeles, CA, USA
e-mail: gzada@usc.edu

M.B.S. Lopes
Deptartment of Pathology, University of Virginia, Charlottesville, VA, USA

S. Mukundan Jr.,
Department of Radiology, Brigham and Women's Hospital, Boston, MA, USA

E.R. Laws Jr.,
Deptartment of Neurosurgery, Brigham and Women's Hospital, Boston, MA, USA

22.2 Imaging Features

- On MRI, RCCs often appear as well-circumscribed, centrally located spherical or ovoid lesions of the sellar region (Figs. 22.1, 22.2, 22.3, 22.4, 22.5, 22.6, 22.7, 22.8, 22.9, 22.10, 22.11, 22.12, 22.13, 22.14, 22.15, 22.16, 22.17, 22.18, 22.19, 22.20, and 22.21).
- Most of these smooth contoured cysts are unilobar, with a diameter ranging between 5 and 40 mm (mean about 17 mm) [7, 15, 16].
- They are often identified as having an epicenter located between the anterior and posterior pituitary gland in the region of the pars intermedia.
- The majority of lesions are intrasellar or intrasellar and suprasellar, with reports of purely suprasellar lesions occurring in a minority of patients [17, 18].
- The normal pituitary gland may be displaced in any direction by an RCC, including circumferentially if the cyst arises in and remains encased within the gland [19, 20].
- In most cases, administration of gadolinium contrast demonstrates little or no enhancement of the cyst wall or contents on MRI [10, 21, 22].
- A thin peripheral rim of enhancement has been attributed to inflammation or squamous metaplasia of the cyst wall, or to a circumferential rim of displaced pituitary gland [7, 19].
- The signal intensity of the cyst contents on MRI demonstrates high variability on T1 and T2 sequences, and has been reported to correlate with the nature of the cystic contents [23–25].
- Although most RCCs display a homogeneous signal intensity, up to 40 % contain a waxy intracystic nodule composed of protein and cellular debris, which typically fails to enhance following contrast administration [19, 21, 22].
- "Atypical" RCCs, or those with squamous metaplasia, inflammation, and/or multiple recurrences, may demonstrate a thickened, contrast-enhancing wall [12].
- RCCs tend to develop attachment to the pituitary stalk, which plays a major role in the development of postoperative diabetes insipidus and pituitary insufficiency following complete cyst removal [2, 26, 27].

G. Zada et al. (eds.), *Atlas of Sellar and Parasellar Lesions: Clinical, Radiologic, and Pathologic Correlations*,
DOI 10.1007/978-3-319-22855-6_22

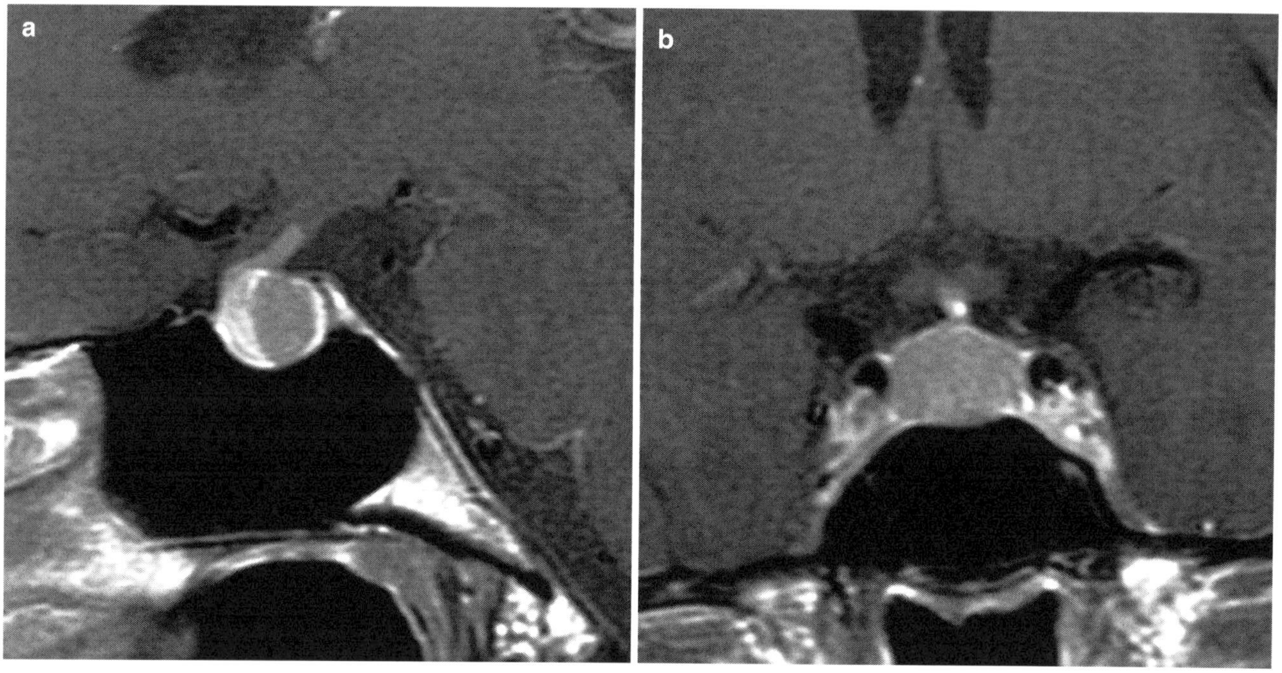

Fig. 22.1 Rathke cleft cyst. (**a**) Sagittal T1-weighted post-gadolinium image. (**b**) Coronal T1-weighted post-gadolinium image. A homogeneous, nonenhancing lesion is seen in the posterior sella, displacing the pituitary gland anteriorly. The pituitary stalk mildly deviates to the left

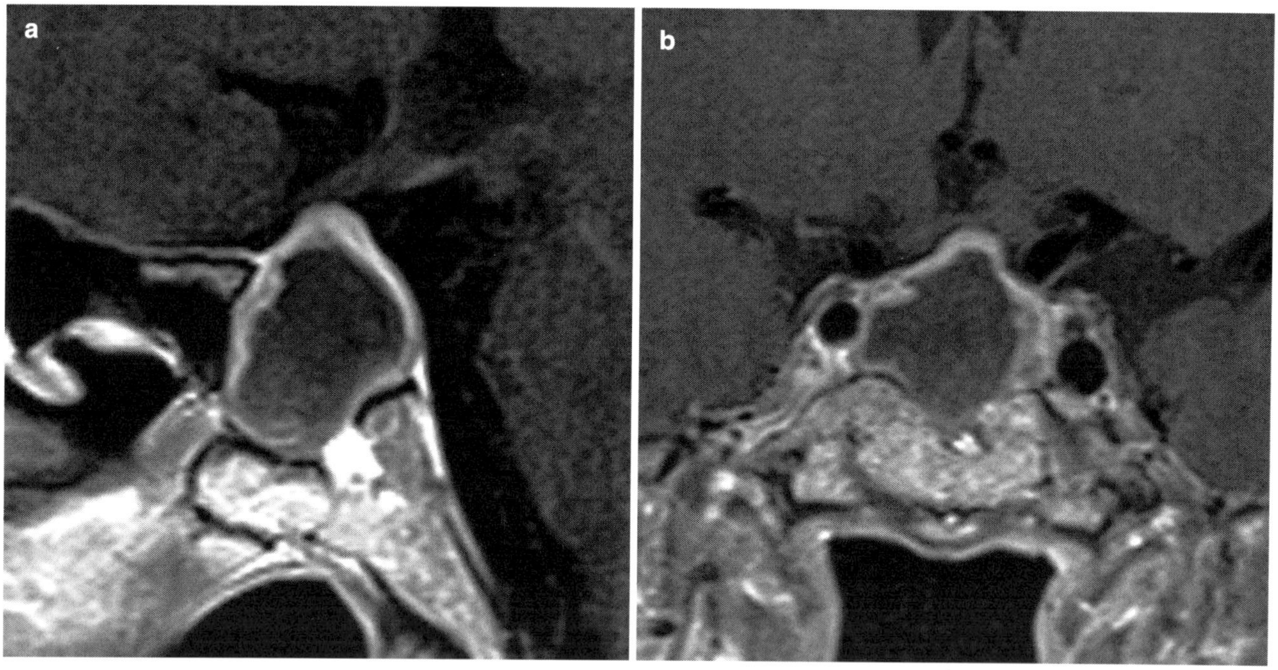

Fig. 22.2 Rathke cleft cyst. (**a**) Sagittal T1-weighted post-gadolinium image. (**b**) Coronal T1-weighted post-gadolinium image. There is a cystic lesion with peripheral enhancement in the sella, with erosion of the sellar floor and extension to the suprasellar cistern, displacing the optic chiasm

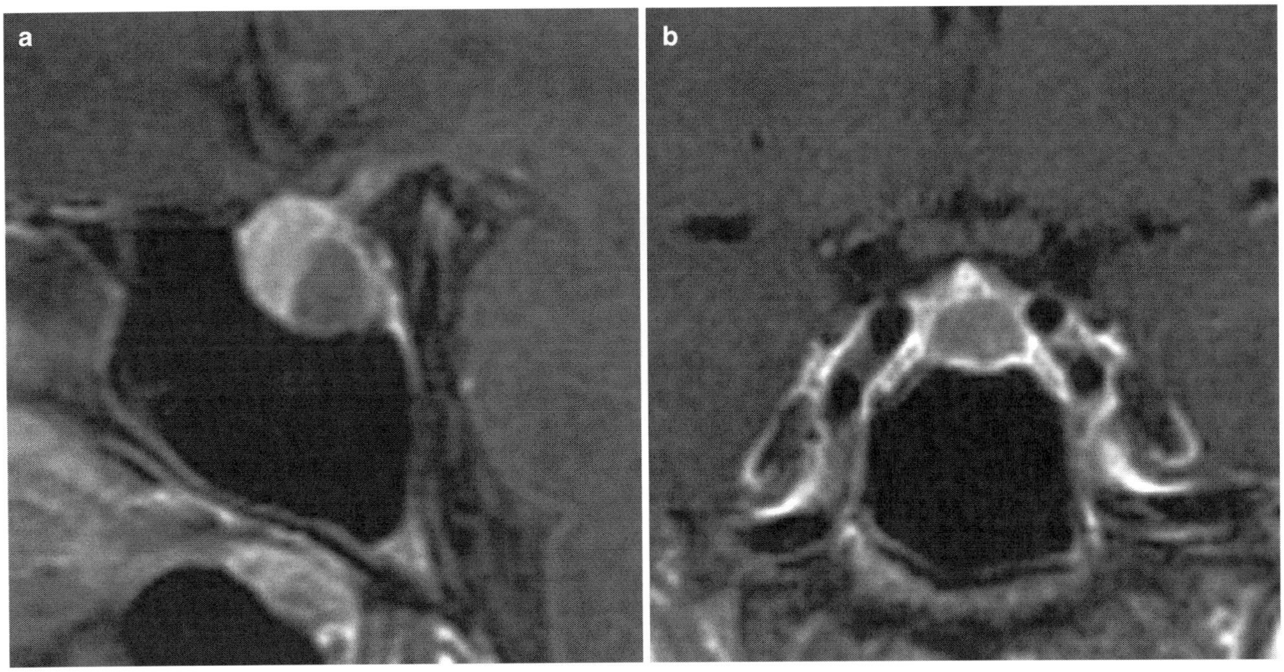

Fig. 22.3 Rathke cleft cyst. (**a**) Sagittal T1-weighted post-gadolinium image. (**b**) Coronal T1-weighted post-gadolinium image. A cystic lesion is centered in the posterior sella, displacing the pituitary gland anteriorly and superiorly

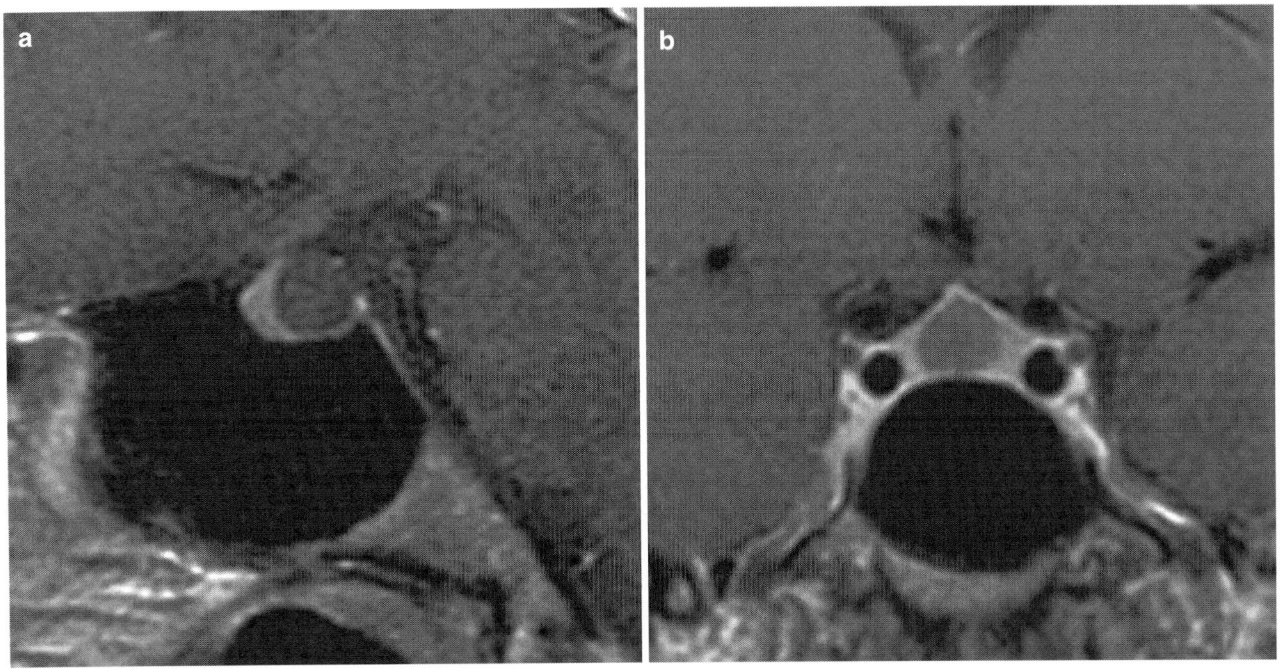

Fig. 22.4 Rathke cleft cyst. (**a**) Sagittal T1-weighted post-gadolinium image. (**b**) Coronal T1-weighted post-gadolinium image. A cystic lesion is located in the posterior sella, displacing the pituitary gland anteriorly

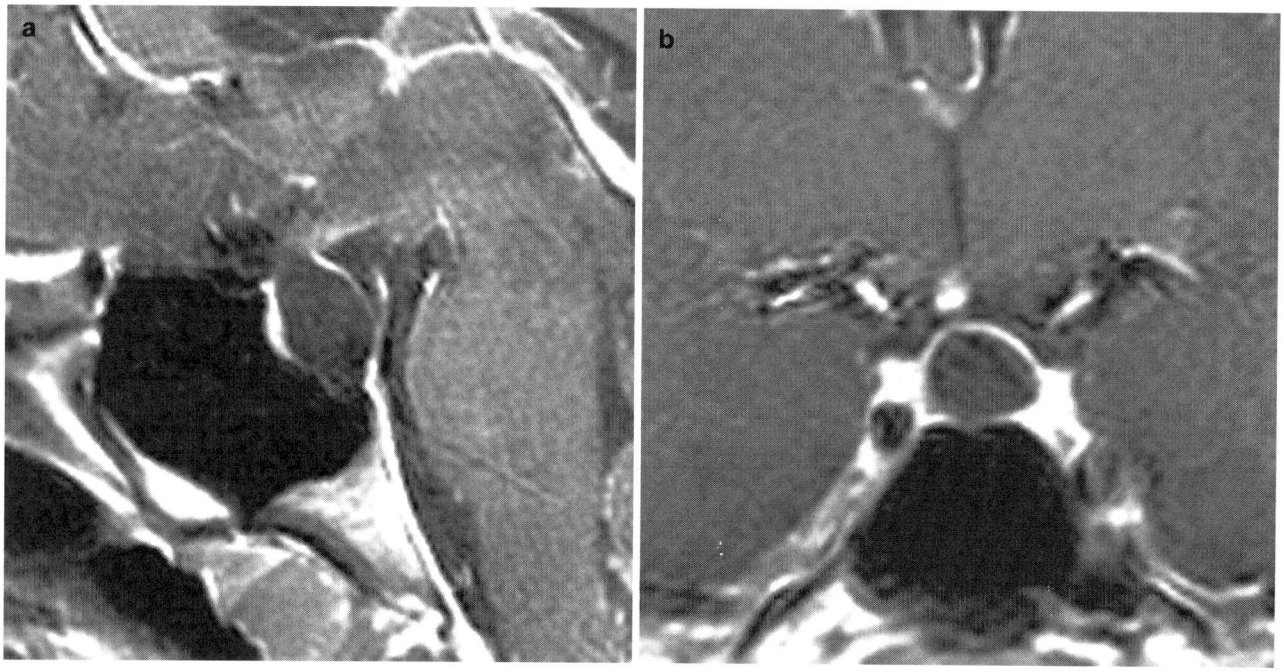

Fig. 22.5 Rathke cleft cyst. (**a**) Sagittal T1-weighted post-gadolinium image. (**b**) Coronal T1-weighted post-gadolinium image. There is a cystic lesion in the posterior sella, displacing the pituitary gland anteriorly. There is remodeling of the sellar floor

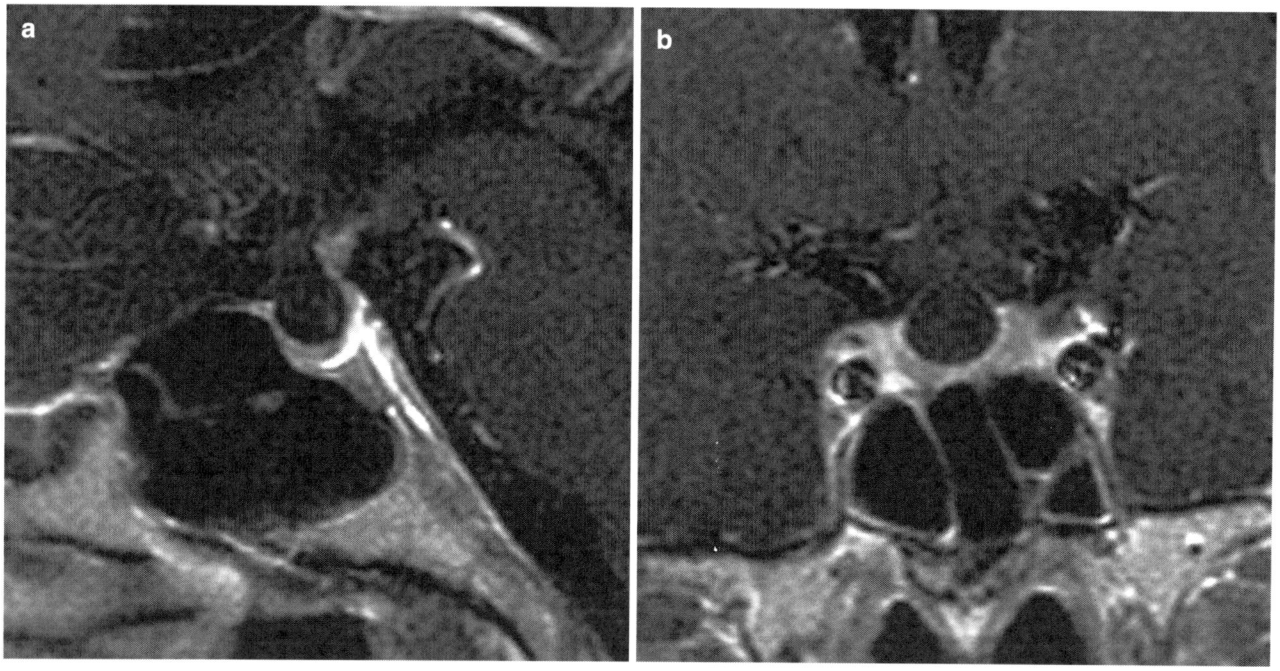

Fig. 22.6 Rathke cleft cyst. (**a**) Sagittal T1-weighted post-gadolinium image. (**b**) Coronal T1-weighted post-gadolinium image. A cystic sellar lesion displaces the pituitary gland inferiorly and the stalk posteriorly

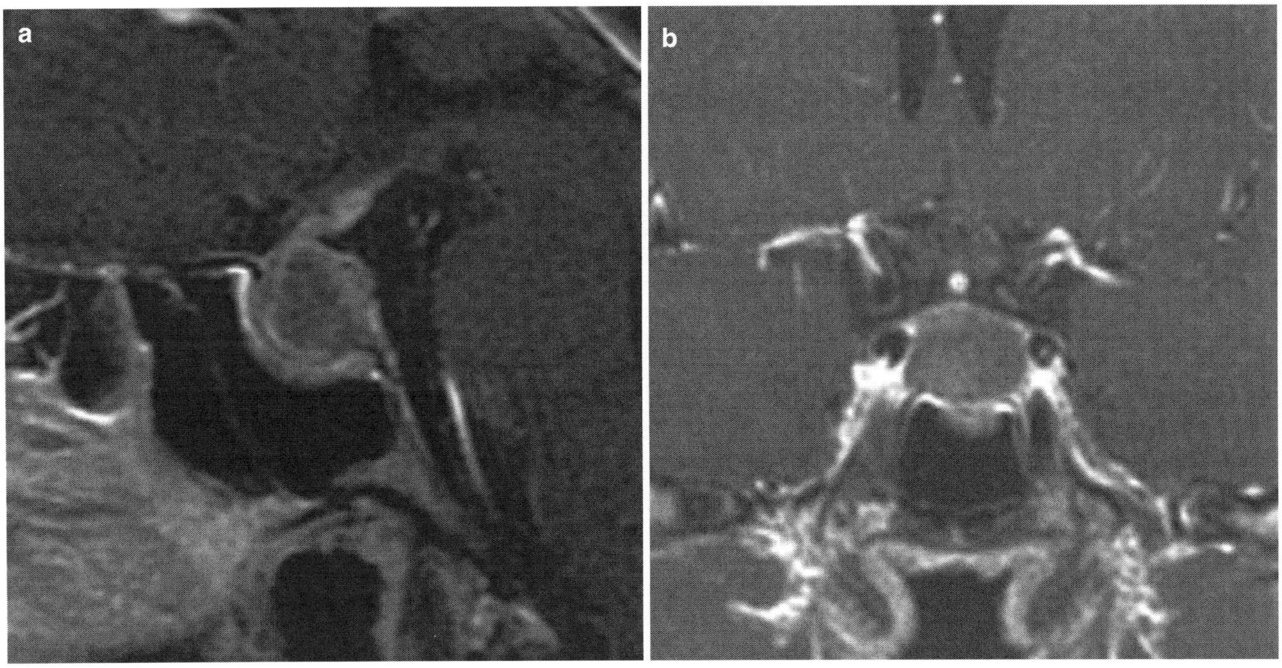

Fig. 22.7 Rathke cleft cyst. (**a**) Sagittal T1-weighted post-gadolinium image. (**b**) Coronal T1-weighted post-gadolinium image. There is a cystic lesion in the posterior sella displacing the pituitary gland and stalk anteriorly. There is remodeling of the sellar floor

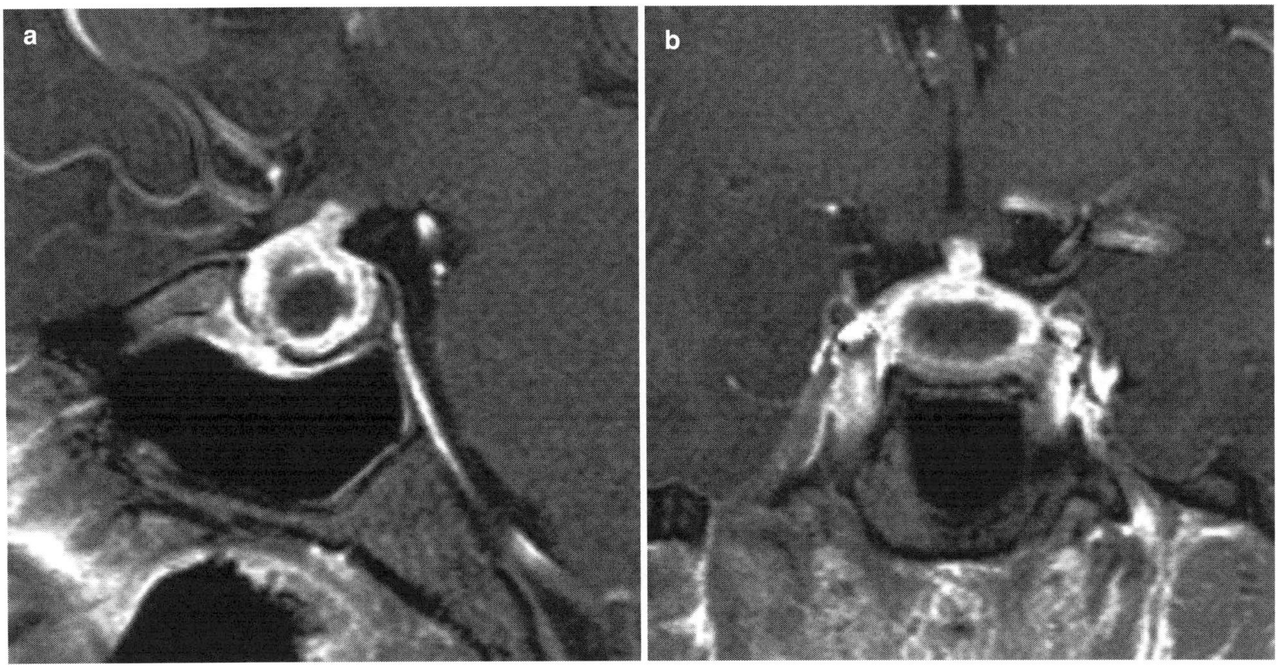

Fig. 22.8 Rathke cleft cyst. (**a**) Sagittal T1-weighted post-gadolinium image. (**b**) Coronal T1-weighted post-gadolinium image. A cystic lesion within the sella displaces the stalk anteriorly. There is remodeling of the sellar floor

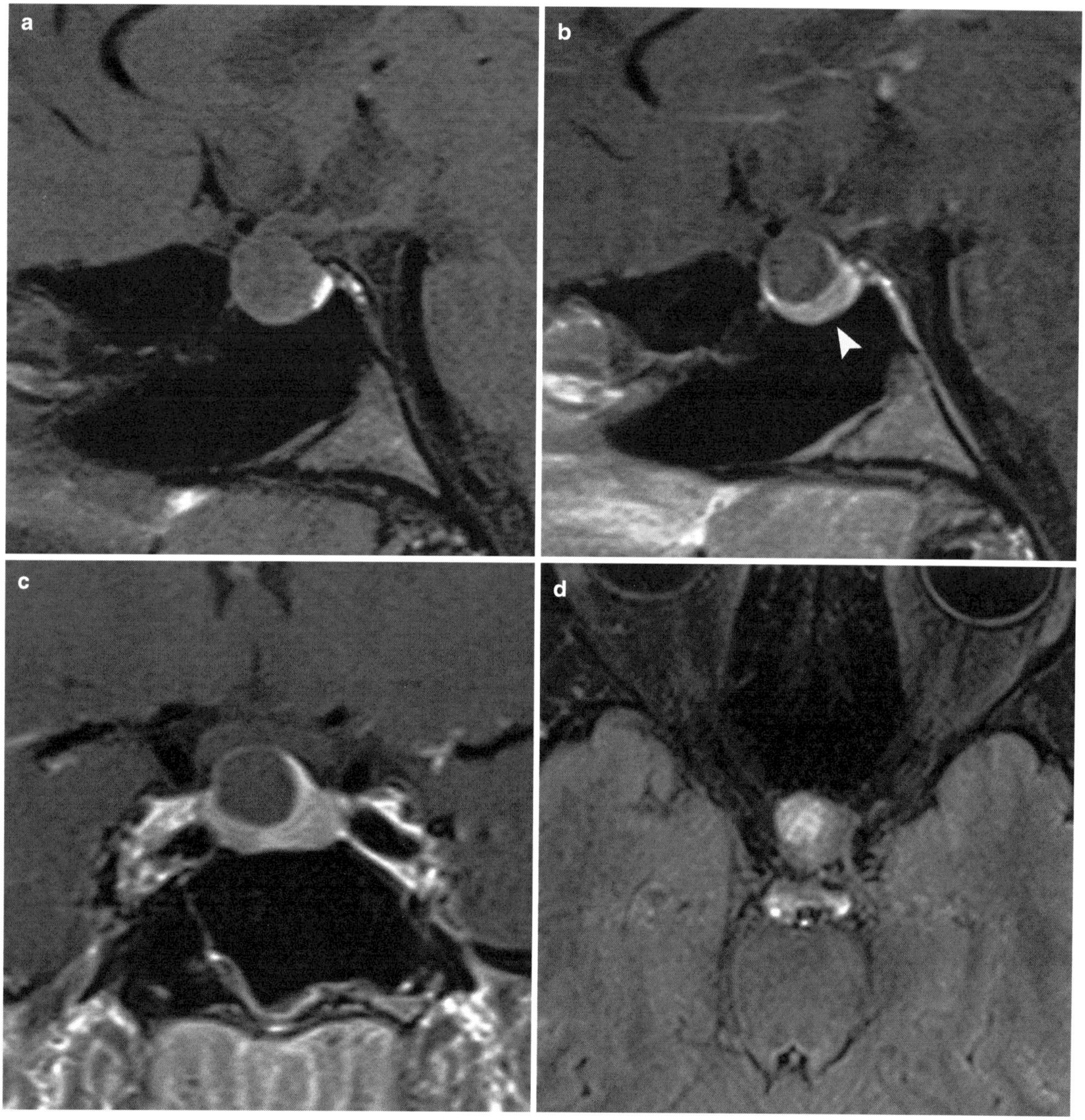

Fig. 22.9 Rathke cleft cyst. (**a**) Sagittal T1-weighted pre-gadolinium image. (**b**) Sagittal T1-weighted post-gadolinium image white arrow points to normal pituitary. (**c**) Coronal T1-weighted post-gadolinium image. (**d**) Axial FLuid Attenuated Inversion Recovery (FLAIR) image. There is a cystic lesion in the sella, displacing the pituitary stalk anteriorly. There is remodeling of the sellar floor. The optic chiasm is mildly elevated

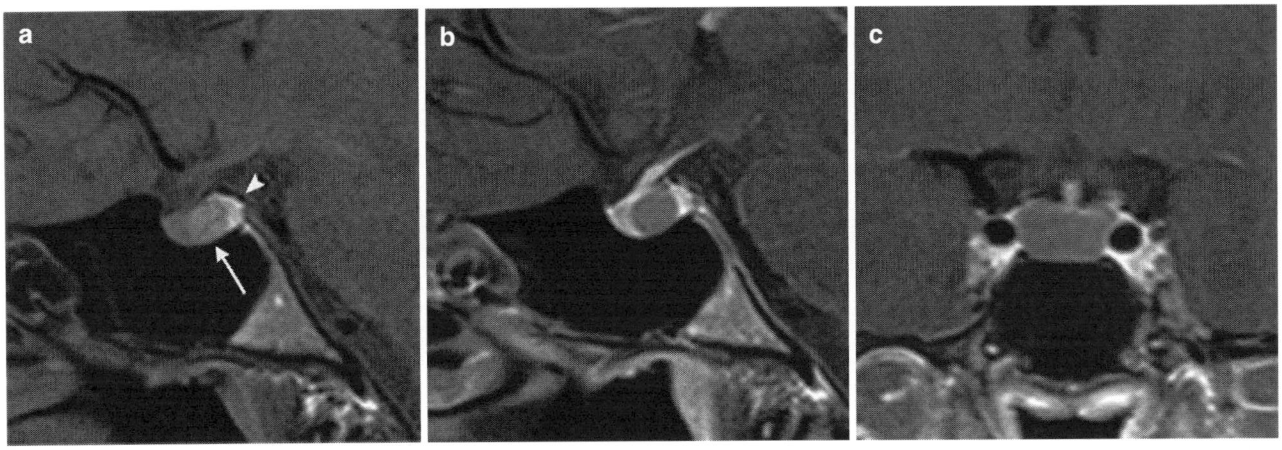

Fig. 22.10 Rathke cleft cyst. (**a**) Sagittal T1-weighted pre-gadolinium image. (**b**) Sagittal T1-weighted post-gadolinium image. (**c**) Coronal T1-weighted post-gadolinium image. A homogeneous, cystic lesion (*arrow*) contains T1 hyperintense material between the adenohypophysis and neurohypophysis (*arrowhead*)

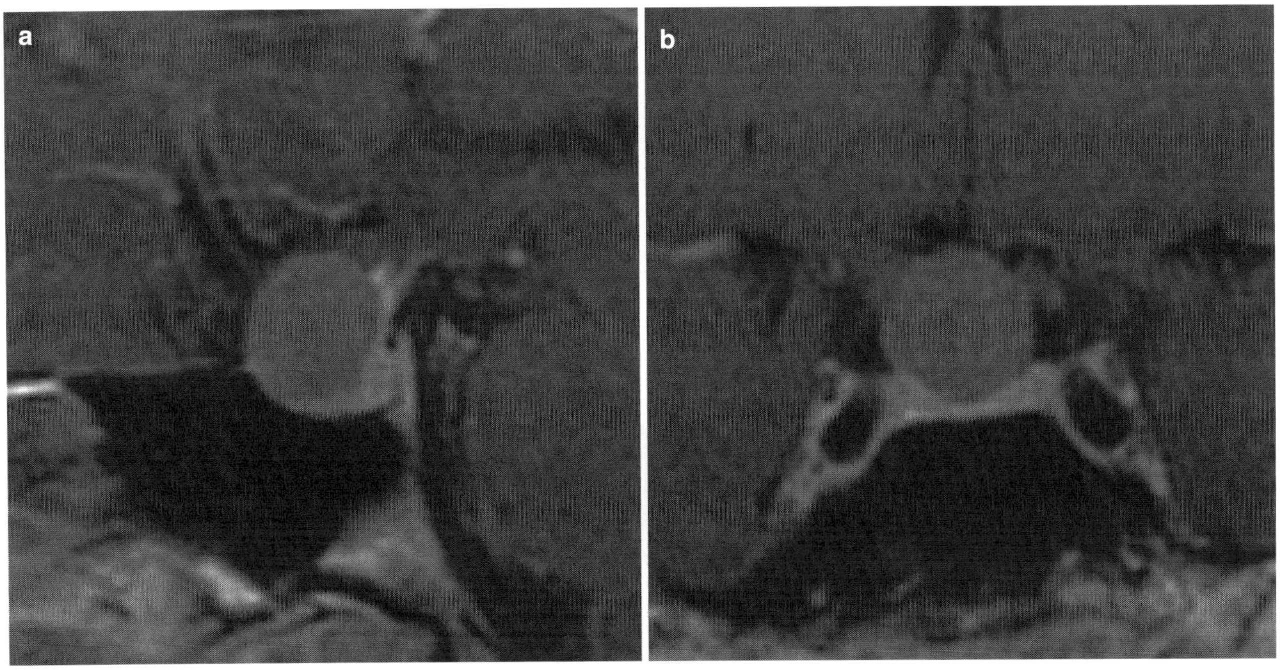

Fig. 22.11 Rathke cleft cyst. (**a**) Sagittal T1-weighted post-gadolinium image. (**b**) Coronal T1-weighted post-gadolinium image. There is a cystic lesion in the anterior sella, displacing the pituitary gland inferiorly and the pituitary stalk posteriorly

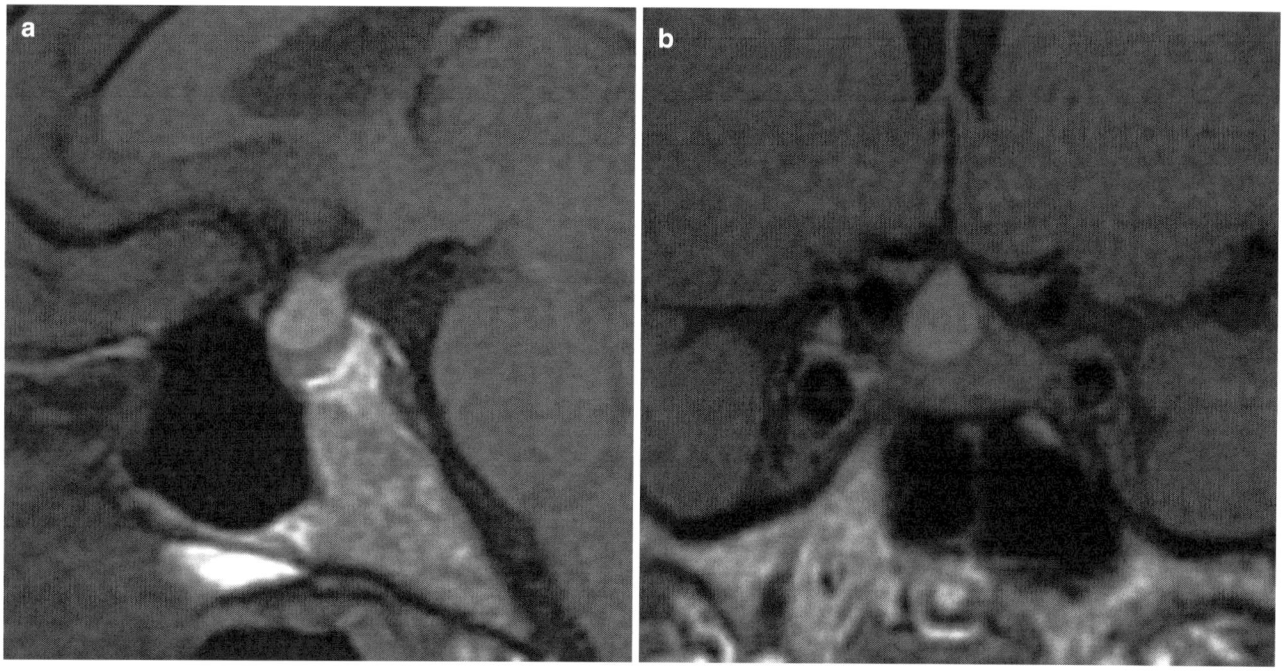

Fig. 22.12 Rathke cleft cyst. (**a**) Sagittal T1-weighted pre-gadolinium image. (**b**) Coronal T1-weighted pre-gadolinium image. A cystic lesion contains T1 hyperintense material in the anterior sella, displacing the pituitary gland inferiorly

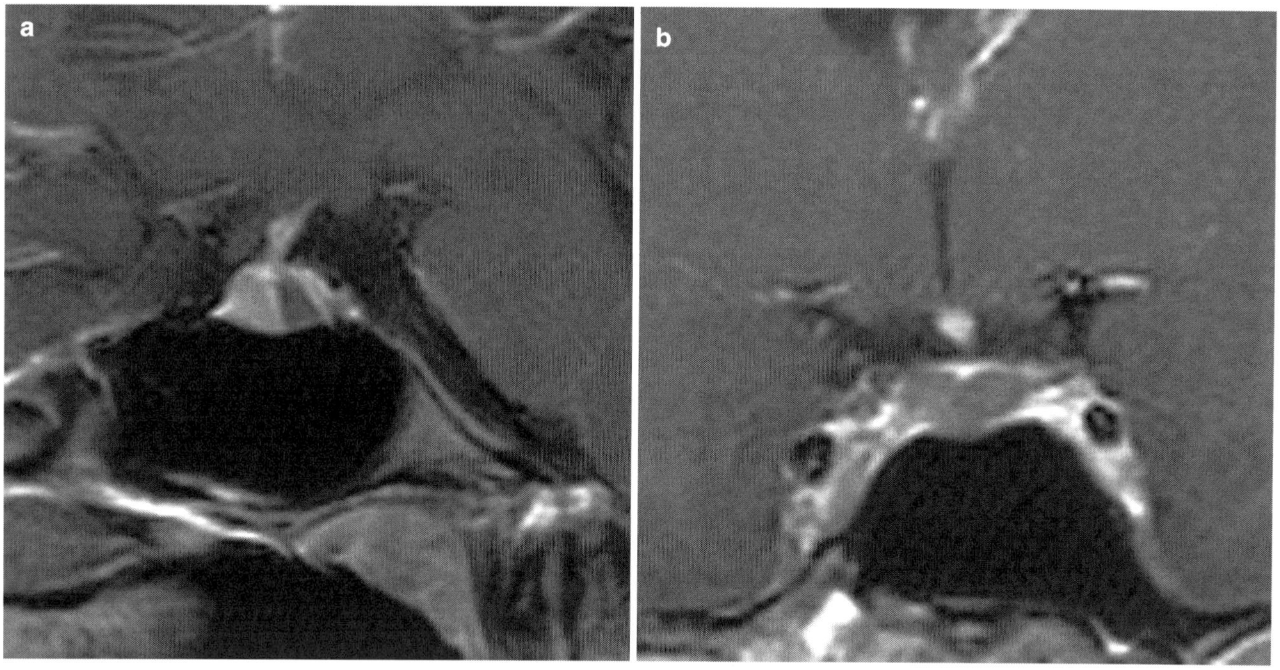

Fig. 22.13 Rathke cleft cyst. (**a**) Sagittal T1-weighted post-gadolinium image. (**b**) Coronal T1-weighted post-gadolinium image. A homogeneous, nonenhancing lesion is located between the adenohypophysis and neurohypophysis

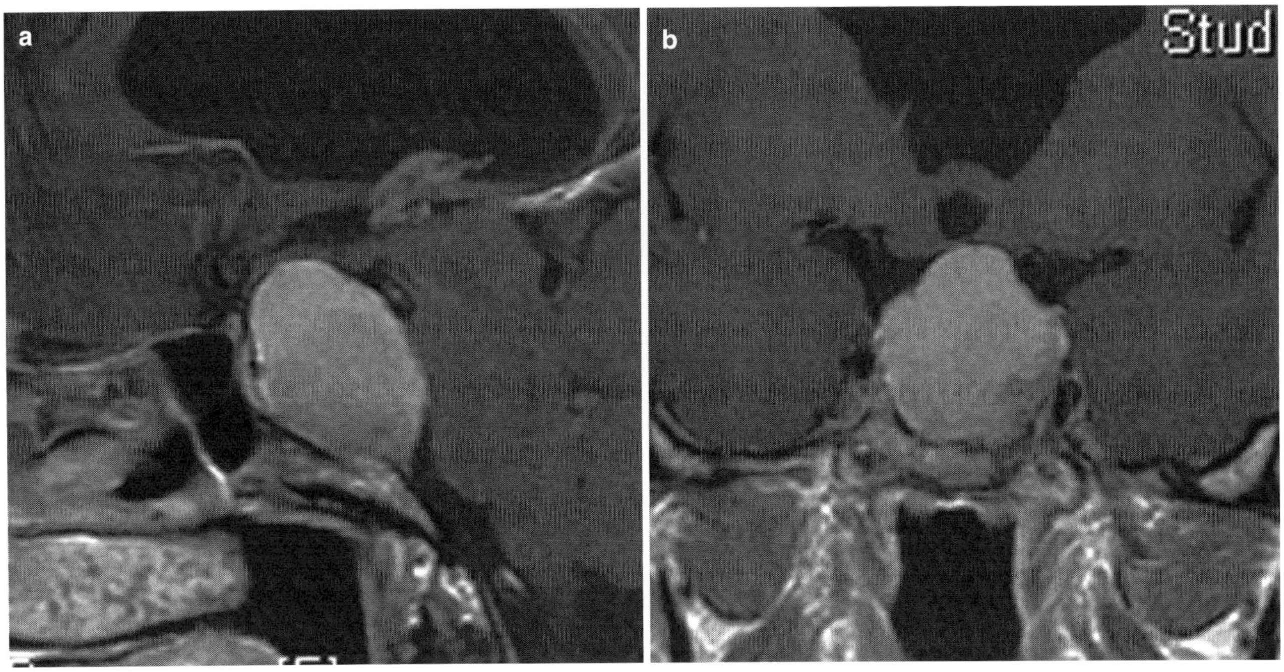

Fig. 22.14 Rathke cleft cyst. (**a**) Sagittal T1-weighted post-gadolinium image. (**b**) Coronal T1-weighted post-gadolinium image. There is a large, T1 hyperintense lesion eroding the sellar floor and extending to the suprasellar cistern, mildly elevating the optic chiasm. The mass extends posteriorly, abutting the pons

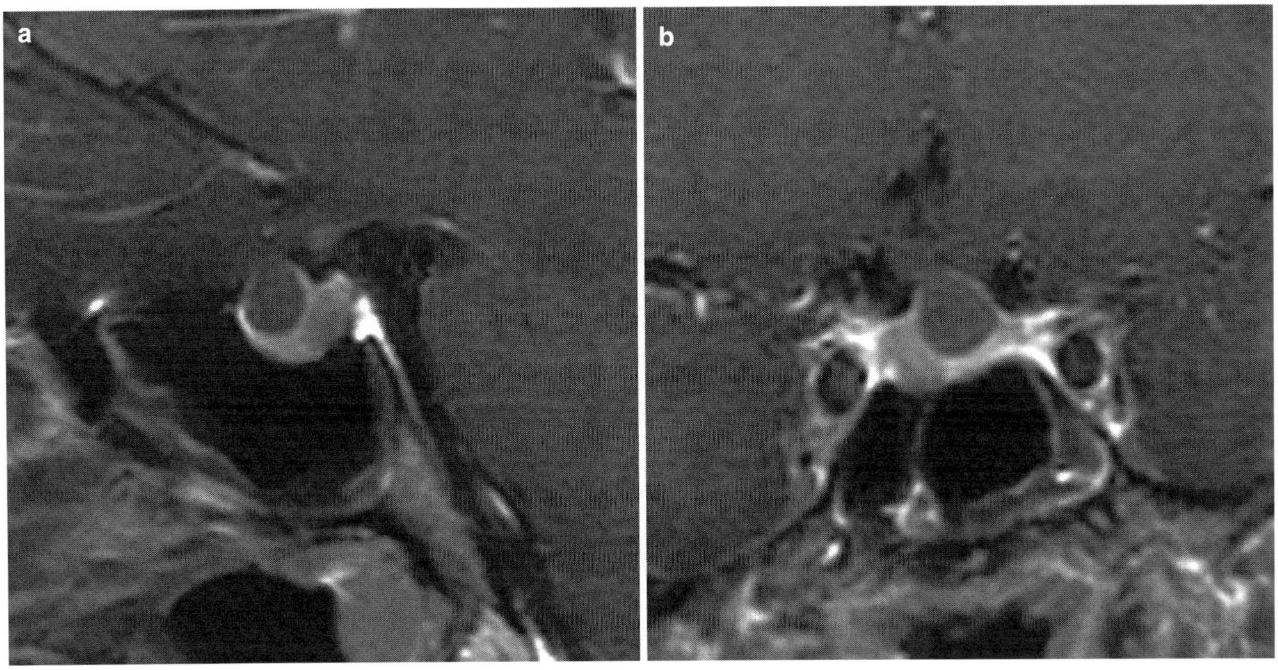

Fig. 22.15 Rathke cleft cyst. (**a**) Sagittal T1-weighted post-gadolinium image. (**b**) Coronal T1-weighted post-gadolinium image. There is a cystic lesion in the anterior sella, displacing the pituitary gland inferiorly. In addition, there is a hypoenhancing mass in the right aspect of the sella, likely to represent an incidental pituitary adenoma

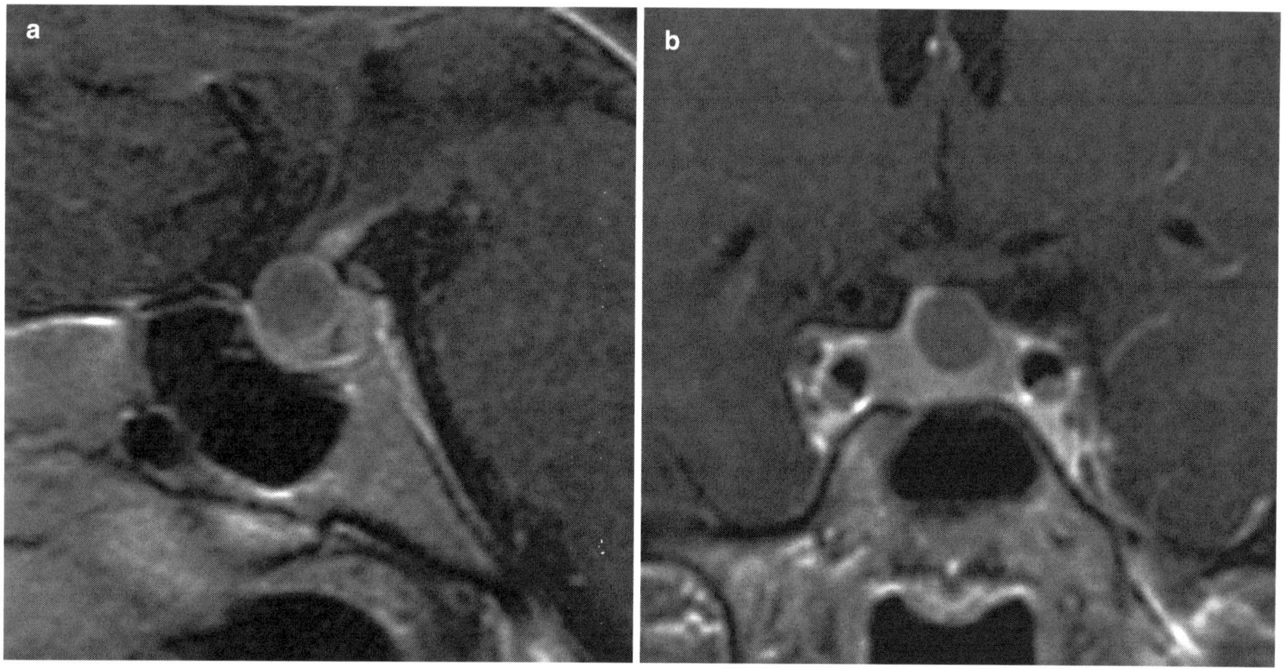

Fig. 22.16 Rathke cleft cyst. (**a**) Sagittal T1-weighted post-gadolinium image. (**b**) Coronal T1-weighted post-gadolinium image. A cystic lesion is present in the anterior sella, displacing the pituitary gland inferiorly. The pituitary stalk is deviated to the right

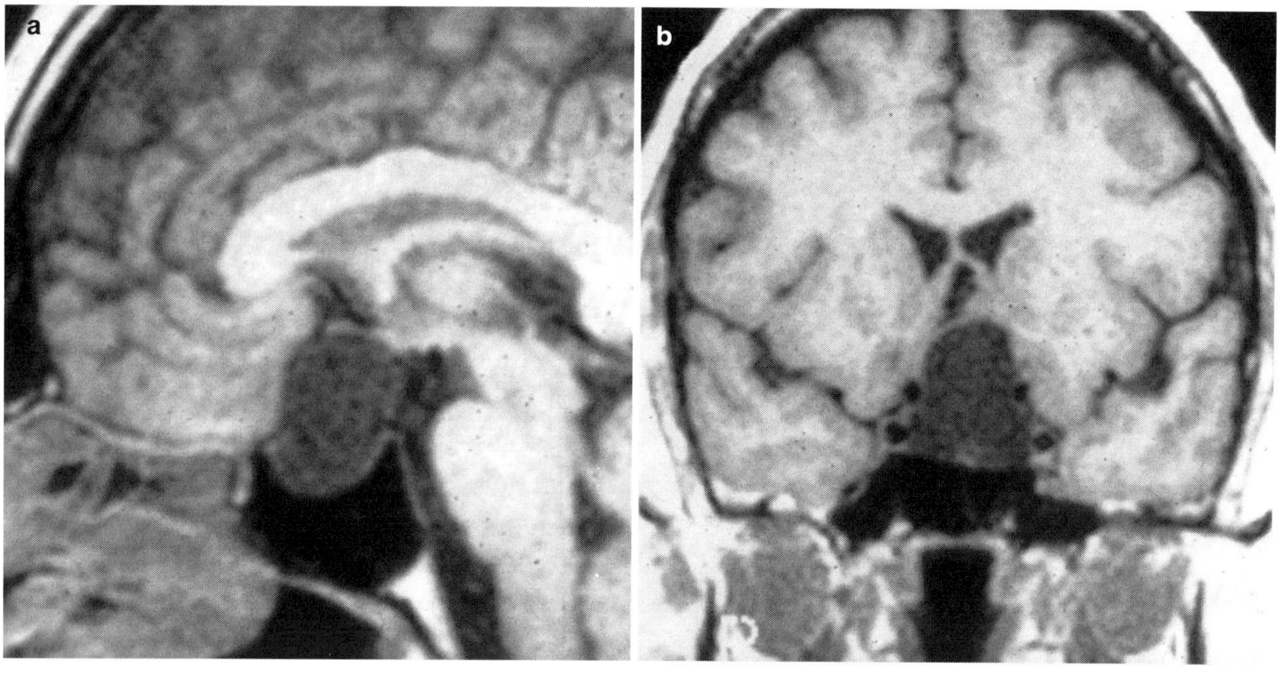

Fig. 22.17 Rathke cleft cyst. (**a**) Sagittal T1-weighted pre-gadolinium image. (**b**) Coronal T1-weighted pre-gadolinium image. A cystic sellar/suprasellar lesion elevates the left hypothalamus

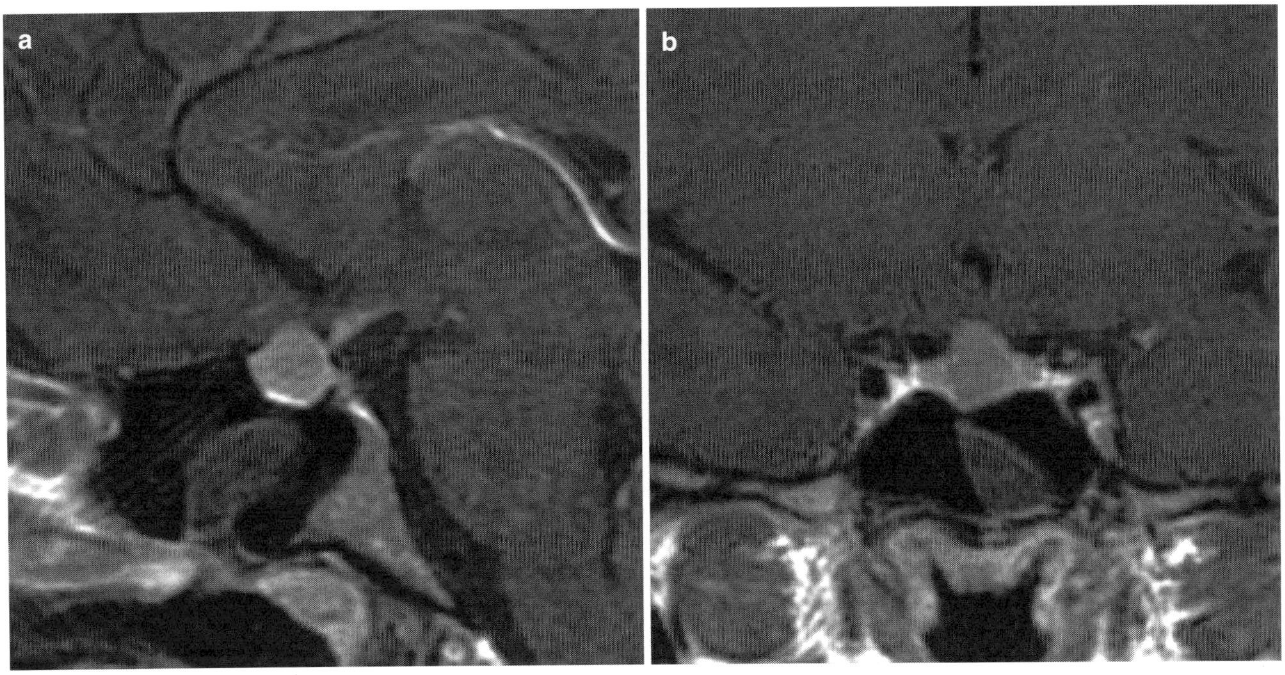

Fig. 22.18 Rathke cleft cyst. (**a**) Sagittal T1-weighted pre-gadolinium image. (**b**) Coronal T1-weighted pre-gadolinium image. There is a nonenhancing, T1 hyperintense sellar lesion with mild suprasellar extension

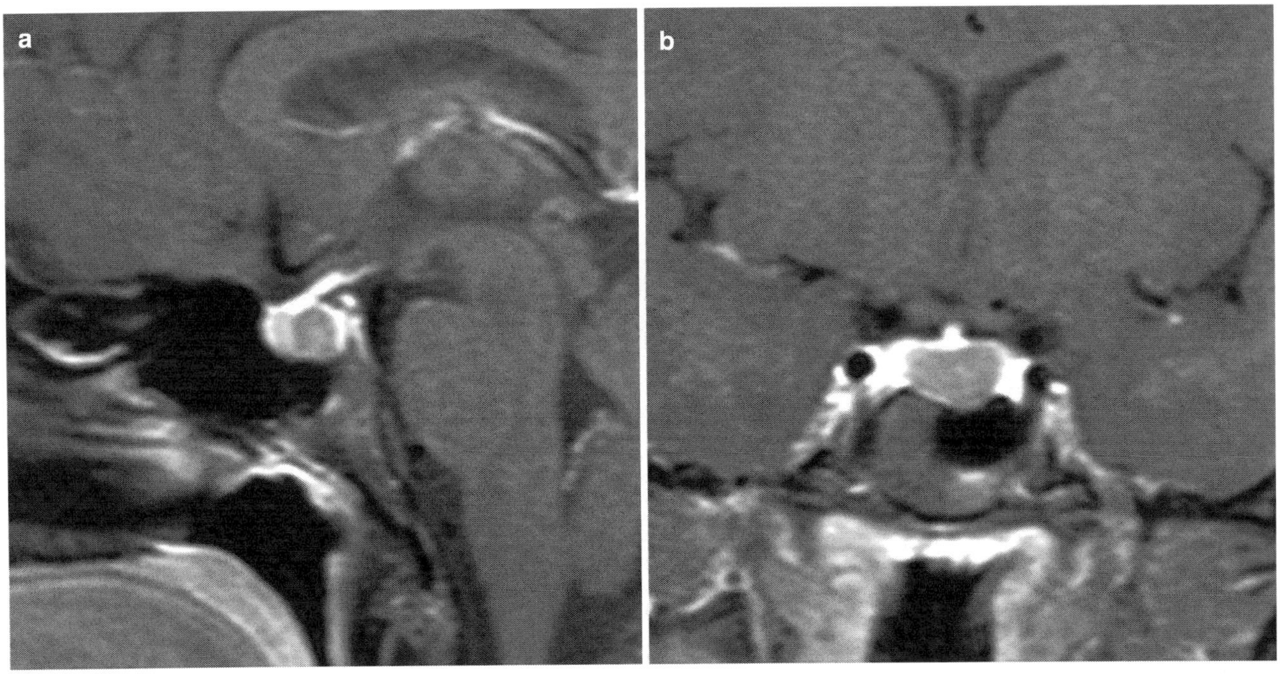

Fig. 22.19 Rathke cleft cyst. (**a**) Sagittal T1-weighted post-gadolinium image. (**b**) Coronal T1-weighted post-gadolinium image white arrow. A cystic lesion is centered between the adenohypophysis and neurohypophysis. The lesion is posterior and inferior to the pituitary stalk

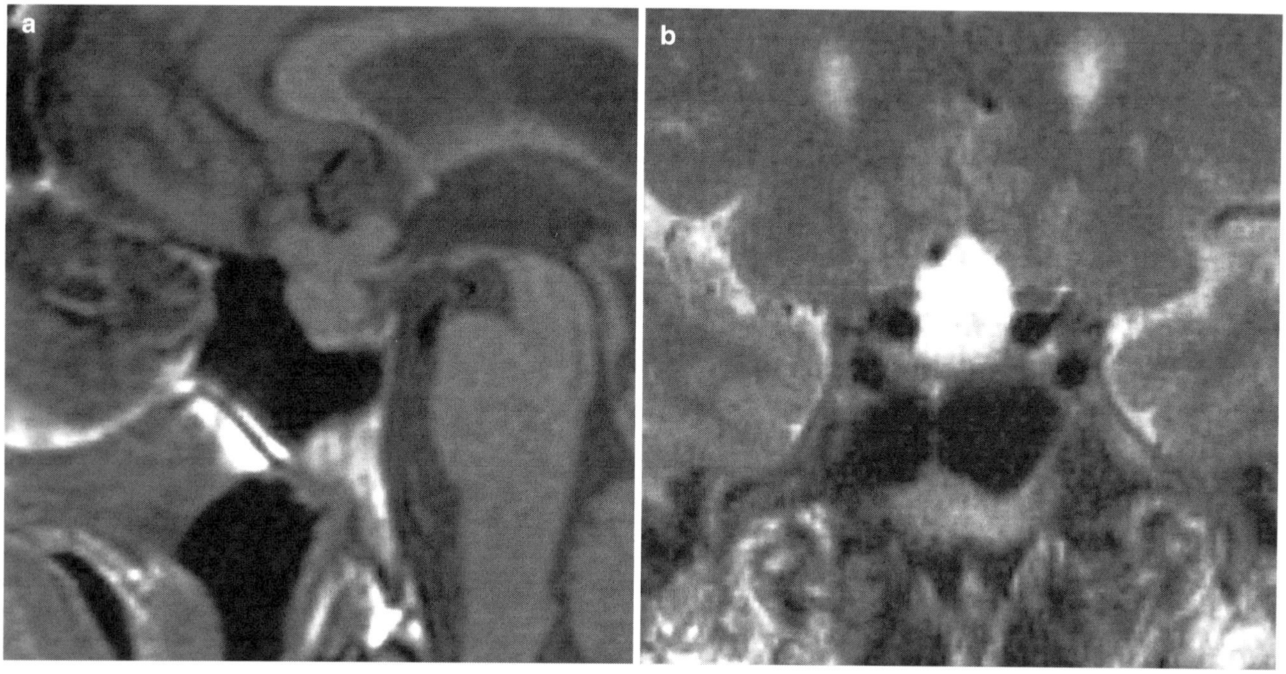

Fig. 22.20 Rathke cleft cyst. (**a**) Sagittal T1-weighted pre-gadolinium image. (**b**) Coronal T2-weighted image. There is a cystic lesion in the sella with superior extension to the anterior interhemispheric fissure

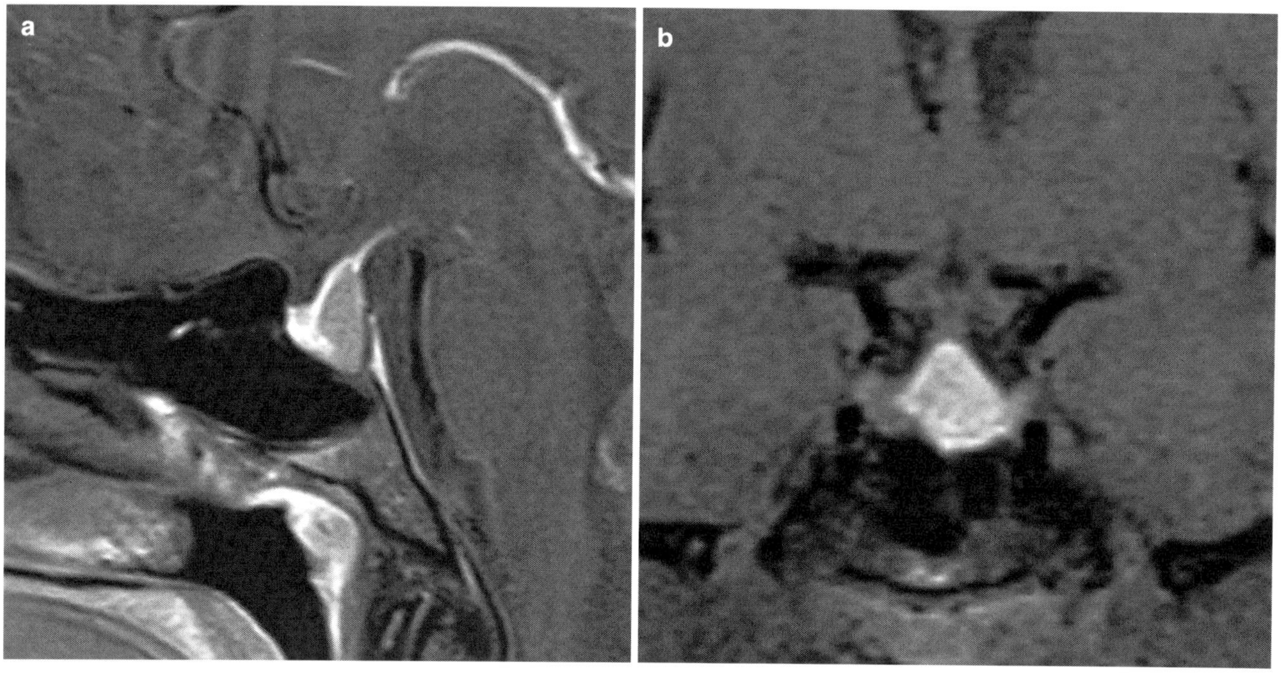

Fig. 22.21 Rathke cleft cyst. (a) Sagittal T1-weighted post-gadolinium image. (**b**) Coronal T1-weighted pre-gadolinium image. A cystic lesion in the posterior sella contains T1 hyperintense material displacing the pituitary gland anteriorly

22.3 Histopathology

- RCCs typically demonstrate simple columnar or cuboidal epithelium, often with ciliated or mucinous goblet cells. Pseudostratified columnar cells are also commonly observed in specimens of RCCs (Fig. 22.22).
- Occasional adenohypophyseal cells also may be observed in the epithelium lining.
- It is not unusual to see RCCs with squamous metaplasia and xanthomatous changes, particularly when there is also evidence of old hemorrhage and inflammatory infiltration. Squamous metaplasia of RCCs has been noted to occur in 9–39 % of patients and is associated with higher rates of cyst recurrence [6, 7, 28].
- It is essential to differentiate between an RCC with squamous metaplasia, an epidermoid cyst, and craniopharyngioma, for better surveillance of possible recurrence and other complications.

22.4 Clinical Management

- Most patients with RCCs remain asymptomatic, do not require surgical management, and can be monitored with serial imaging studies.
- Endoscopic transsphenoidal operations are now widely used to fenestrate and drain RCCs.
- Complete resection of the cyst wall is not typically recommended, as it is associated with a higher incidence of postoperative diabetes insipidus [10].
- Intracystic alcohol administration following surgical fenestration has not been shown to reduce the risk of RCC recurrence and is not routinely recommended [29].
- Sellar floor reconstruction is not recommended if no CSF leak is identified, in order to promote continuous drainage of the cyst following the operation.
- Previous studies have demonstrated high rates (>90 %) of complete resolution of the cyst following surgical drainage [6, 10, 30].
- Headache and visual symptoms frequently improve, but hypopituitarism is less likely to improve following drainage [12].
- Overall long-term recurrence rates following fenestration or resection of RCCs have varied from 3 to 33 % and have been reported to correlate with several factors, including the radiologic enhancement pattern of the cyst wall, the presence of squamous metaplasia or stratified epithelium, the aggressiveness of cyst wall resection, and the placement of an abdominal fat graft [6, 7, 10, 31, 32].
- Serial imaging is recommended on a yearly basis following surgery.

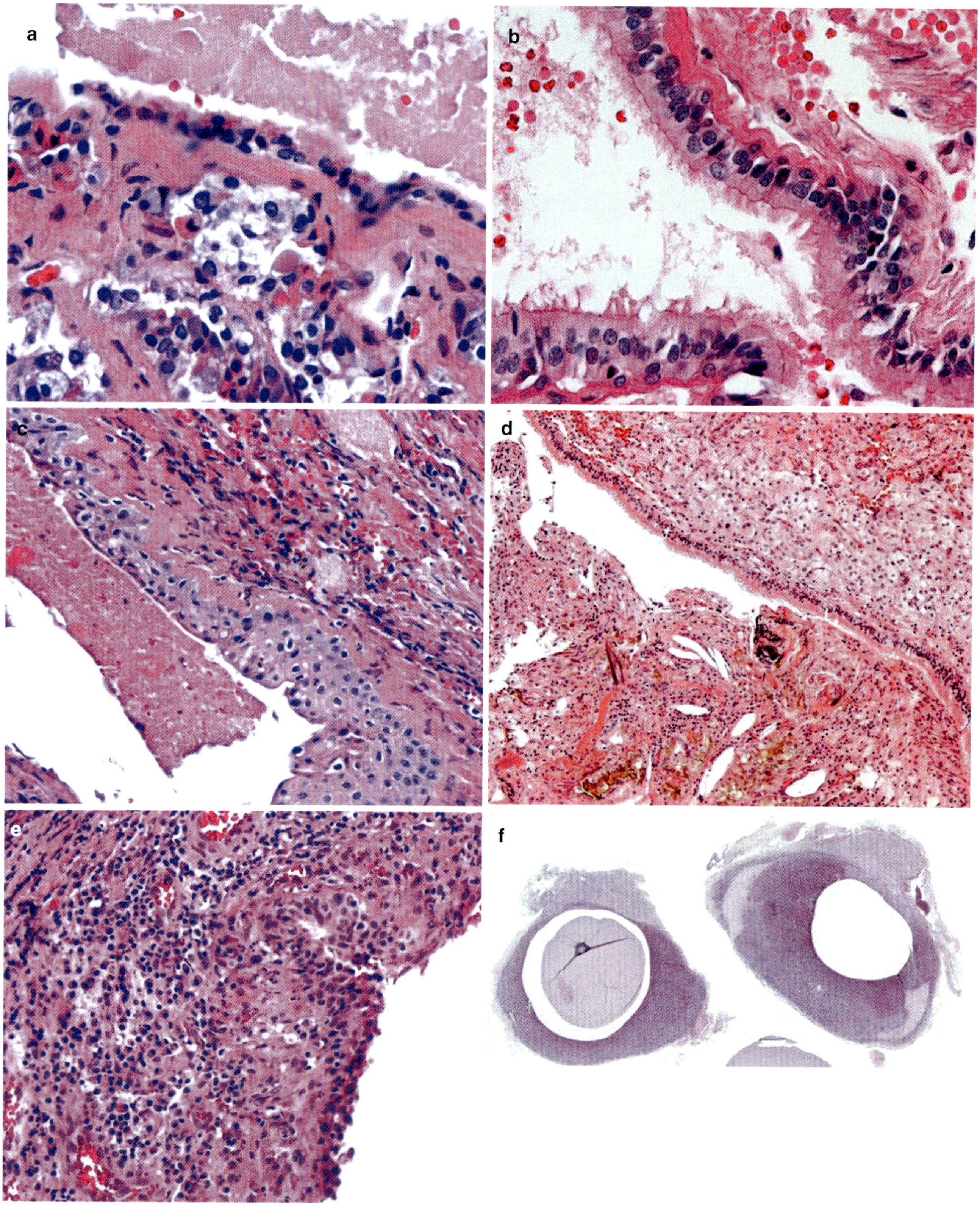

Fig. 22.22 Rathke cleft cyst (H&E). (**a**) The normal Rathke cleft is composed of a single cuboidal epithelium resting adjacent to the pituitary gland. (**b**) Rathke cleft cysts (RCCs) show similar epithelial lining, composed of cuboidal to columnar cells with ciliated borders. (**c**) Squamous metaplasia is not an uncommon finding in these cysts. (**d**) Xanthomatous inflammatory changes arising from an RCC. (**e**) Secondary hypophysitis may be present as a result of inflammation triggered by subclinical rupture of the cyst. (**f**) An autopsy specimen with an incidental, nonsymptomatic RCC

References

1. Couldwell WT, Weiss MH. Nonadenomatous lesions of the pituitary. In: Krisht A, Tindall GT, editors. Pituitary disorders: comprehensive management. Baltimore: Lippincott Williams & Wilkins; 1999.
2. Kanter AS, Sansur CA, Jane Jr JA, Laws Jr ER. Rathke's cleft cysts. Front Horm Res. 2006;34:127–57.
3. Teramoto A, Hirakawa K, Sanno N, Osamura Y. Incidental pituitary lesions in 1,000 unselected autopsy specimens. Radiology. 1994;193:161–4.
4. Zada G, Liu CY, Fishback D, Singer PA, Weiss MH. Recognition and management of delayed hyponatremia following transsphenoidal pituitary surgery. J Neurosurg. 2007;106:66–71.
5. Zada G, Kelly DF, Cohan P, Wang C, Swerdloff R. Endonasal transsphenoidal approach for pituitary adenomas and other sellar lesions: an assessment of efficacy, safety, and patient impressions. J Neurosurg. 2003;98:350–8.
6. Aho CJ, Liu C, Zelman V, Couldwell WT, Weiss MH. Surgical outcomes in 118 patients with Rathke cleft cysts. J Neurosurg. 2005;102:189–93.
7. Kim JE, Kim JH, Kim OL, Paek SH, Kim DG, Chi JG, Jung HW. Surgical treatment of symptomatic Rathke cleft cysts: clinical features and results with special attention to recurrence. J Neurosurg. 2004;100:33–40.
8. Voelker JL, Campbell RL, Muller J. Clinical, radiographic, and pathological features of symptomatic Rathke's cleft cysts. J Neurosurg. 1991;74:535–44.
9. Saeger W, Ludecke DK, Buchfelder M, Fahlbusch R, Quabbe HJ, Petersenn S. Pathohistological classification of pituitary tumors: 10 years of experience with the German Pituitary Tumor Registry. Eur J Endocrinol. 2007;156:203–16.
10. Benveniste RJ, King WA, Walsh J, Lee JS, Naidich TP, Post KD. Surgery for Rathke cleft cysts: technical considerations and outcomes. J Neurosurg. 2004;101:577–84.
11. Isono M, Kamida T, Kobayashi H, Shimomura T, Matsuyama J. Clinical features of symptomatic Rathke's cleft cyst. Clin Neurol Neurosurg. 2001;103:96–100.
12. Zada G. Rathke cleft cysts: a review of clinical and surgical management. Neurosurg Focus. 2011;31, E1. doi:10.3171/2011.5.FOCUS1183.
13. Shimoji T, Shinohara A, Shimizu A, Sato K, Ishii S. Rathke cleft cysts. Surg Neurol. 1984;21:295–310.
14. Zada G, Ditty B, McNatt SA, McComb JG, Krieger MD. Surgical treatment of Rathke cleft cysts in children. Neurosurgery. 2009;64:1132–7; author reply 1037–8.
15. Nishioka H, Haraoka J, Izawa H, Ikeda Y. Magnetic resonance imaging, clinical manifestations, and management of Rathke's cleft cyst. Clin Endocrinol (Oxf). 2006;64:184–8.
16. Shin JL, Asa SL, Woodhouse LJ, Smyth HS, Ezzat S. Cystic lesions of the pituitary: clinicopathological features distinguishing craniopharyngioma, Rathke's cleft cyst, and arachnoid cyst. J Clin Endocrinol Metab. 1999;84:3972–82.
17. Barrow DL, Spector RH, Takei Y, Tindall GT. Symptomatic Rathke's cleft cysts located entirely in the suprasellar region: review of diagnosis, management, and pathogenesis. Neurosurgery. 1985;16:766–72.
18. Wenger M, Simko M, Markwalder R, Taub E. An entirely suprasellar Rathke's cleft cyst: case report and review of the literature. J Clin Neurosci. 2001;8:564–7.
19. Brassier G, Morandi X, Tayiar E, Riffaud L, Chabert E, Heresbach N, et al. Rathke's cleft cysts: surgical-MRI correlation in 16 symptomatic cases. J Neuroradiol. 1999;26:162–71.
20. Ross DA, Norman D, Wilson CB. Radiologic characteristics and results of surgical management of Rathke's cysts in 43 patients. Neurosurgery. 1992;30:173–8; discussion 178–9.
21. Byun WM, Kim OL, Kim D. MR imaging findings of Rathke's cleft cysts: significance of intracystic nodules. AJNR Am J Neuroradiol. 2000;21:485–8.
22. Binning MJ, Gottfried ON, Osborn AG, Couldwell WT. Rathke cleft cyst intracystic nodule: a characteristic magnetic resonance imaging finding. J Neurosurg. 2005;103:837–40.
23. Asari S, Ito T, Tsuchida S, Tsutsui T. MR appearance and cyst content of Rathke cleft cysts. J Comput Assist Tomogr. 1990;14:532–5.
24. Hayashi Y, Tachibana O, Muramatsu N, Tsuchiya H, Tada M, Arakawa Y, et al. Rathke cleft cyst: MR and biomedical analysis of cyst content. J Comput Assist Tomogr. 1999;23:34–8.
25. Tominaga JY, Higano S, Takahashi S. Characteristics of Rathke's cleft cyst in MR imaging. Magn Reson Med Sci. 2003;2:1–8.
26. Laws ER, Kanter AS. Rathke cleft cysts. J Neurosurg. 2004;101:571–2; discussion 572.
27. Nemergut EC, Zuo Z, Jane Jr JA, Laws Jr ER. Predictors of diabetes insipidus after transsphenoidal surgery: a review of 881 patients. J Neurosurg. 2005;103:448–54.
28. Le BH, Towfighi J, Kapadia SB, Lopes MB. Comparative immunohistochemical assessment of craniopharyngioma and related lesions. Endocr Pathol. 2007;18:23–30.
29. Lillehei KO, Widdel L, Astete CA, Wierman ME, Kleinschmidt-DeMasters BK, Kerr JM. Transsphenoidal resection of 82 Rathke cleft cysts: limited value of alcohol cauterization in reducing recurrence rates. J Neurosurg. 2011;114:310–7.
30. El-Mahdy W, Powell M. Transsphenoidal management of 28 symptomatic Rathke's cleft cysts, with special reference to visual and hormonal recovery. Neurosurgery. 1998;42:7–16; discussion 16–7.
31. Mukherjee JJ, Islam N, Kaltsas G, Lowe DG, Charlesworth M, Afshar F, et al. Clinical, radiological and pathological features of patients with Rathke's cleft cysts: tumors that may recur. J Clin Endocrinol Metab. 1997;82:2357–62.
32. Kasperbauer JL, Orvidas LJ, Atkinson JL, Abboud CF. Rathke cleft cyst: diagnostic and therapeutic considerations. Laryngoscope. 2002;112:1836–9.

23 Xanthogranuloma of the Sellar Region

Gabriel Zada, M. Beatriz S. Lopes, Srinivasan Mukundan Jr., and Edward Laws Jr.

23.1 Epidemiology and Clinical Presentation

- This lesion is also called a "cholesterol granuloma." (*See also* the next Chap. 24.)
- They have been reported to comprise a subset of lesions (up to 34 %) initially thought to be adamantinomatous craniopharyngiomas or Rathke's cleft cysts [1].
- They are likely to originate from Rathke's cleft cysts or pituitary adenomas with internal hemorrhage, inflammation, or both [2].
- They tend to occur in younger adult patients (mean, 27 years).
- In some patients, the lesion may be part of the Erdheim-Chester disease [3].
- They belong to a spectrum of disease that includes xanthogranulomas, xanthomatous hypophysitis, and xanthogranulomatous hypophysitis [4, 5]. (*See* "Inflammatory Hypophysitis" in Chap. 56.)
- Patients have a relatively high incidence of hypopituitarism and diabetes insipidus.

23.2 Imaging Features

- MRI shows a cystic sellar and suprasellar lesion with a thickened capsule [6].
- T2-weighted MRI shows a hypointense or mixed-intensity mass with an inhomogeneous contrast enhancement pattern [6, 7].
- Cholesterol clefts typically show high signal intensity on T1 images and low signal intensity on T2 images [2].
- Xanthogranulomas are smaller in diameter than craniopharyngiomas, and they tend to remain primarily intrasellar [1].
- Xanthogranulomas may extend to or invade the cavernous sinuses, an inflammatory process similar to the Tolosa-Hunt syndrome.

G. Zada, MD, MS (✉)
Department of Neurological Surgery, Keck School of Medicine, University of Southern California,
1200 N State Street, #3300, Los Angeles, CA 90033, USA
e-mail: gzada@usc.edu

M.B.S. Lopes, MD, PhD
Department of Pathology (Neuropathology), University of Virginia School of Medicine,
1215 Lee Street, Room 3060–HEP, Charlottesville, VA 22908, USA
e-mail: msl2e@virginia.edu

S. MukundanJr., PhD, MD
Department of Radiology, Brigham and Women's Hospital,
75 Francis Street, Boston, MA 02115, USA
e-mail: smukundan@partners.org

E. LawsJr., MD
Department of Neurosurgery, Brigham and Women's Hospital,
15 Francis Street, Boston, MA 02115, USA
e-mail: elaws@partners.org

G. Zada et al. (eds.), *Atlas of Sellar and Parasellar Lesions: Clinical, Radiologic, and Pathologic Correlations*,
DOI 10.1007/978-3-319-22855-6_23

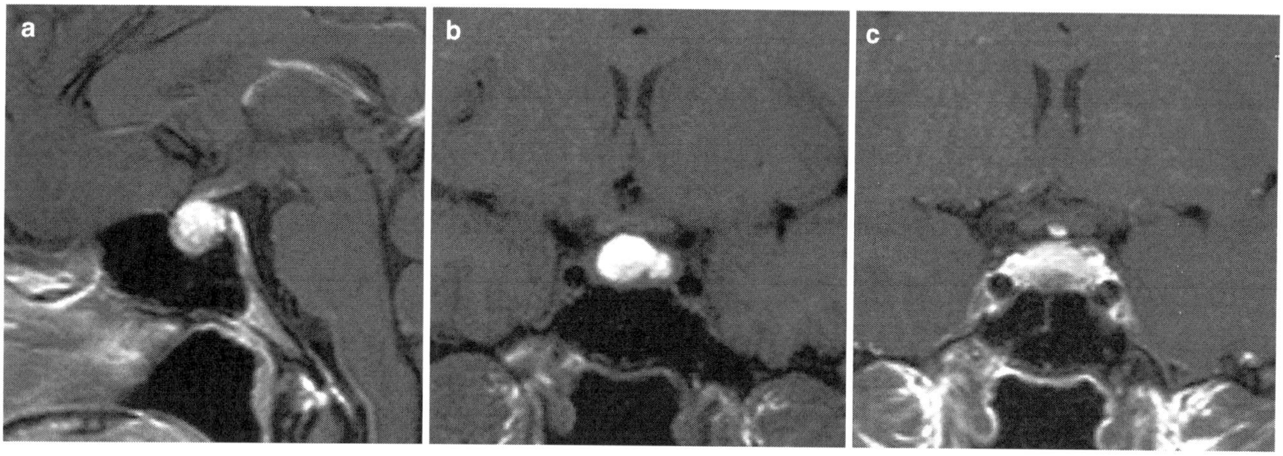

Fig. 23.1 (**a**) Sagittal T1-weighted post-gadolinium image. (**b**) Coronal T1-weighted pre-gadolinium image. (**c**) Coronal T1-weighted post-gadolinium image. There is a lobulated cystic lesion in the sella containing T1 hyperintense material. The pituitary stalk is displaced anteriorly

23.3 Histopathology

- Extensive inflammation with no readily identifiable epithelium is seen in the majority of cases [1, 8].
- Frequent histopathological findings include cholesterol clefts, macrophages, chronic inflammatory infiltrates, necrotic debris, foamy histiocytes, and hemosiderin deposits [4].
- Because these lesions may not have an epithelial lining, immunohistochemistry for cytokeratins is negative [8].
- Although they have been reported to comprise a distinct entity, it remains unknown whether they are derived from RCCs, craniopharyngiomas, and/or other lesions.
- Features of xanthogranuloma have been reported to be more consistent with RCCs than with craniopharyngiomas; they have demonstrated a high association with squamous metaplasia of these lesions [8], as seen in Fig. 22.22d.

23.4 Clinical Management

- Surgical management is the preferred primary treatment for symptomatic xanthogranulomas. Complete resection may be warranted if initial attempts at fenestration and drainage are unsuccessful.

References

1. Paulus W, Honegger J, Keyvani K, Fahlbusch R. Xanthogranuloma of the sellar region: a clinicopathological entity different from adamantinomatous craniopharyngioma. Acta Neuropathol. 1999;97:377–82.
2. Nishioka H, Shibuya M, Ohtsuka K, Ikeda Y, Haraoka J. Endocrinological and MRI features of pituitary adenomas with marked xanthogranulomatous reaction. Neuroradiology. 2010;52:997–1002.
3. Reithmeier T, Trost HA, Wolf S, Stolzle A, Feiden W, Lumenta CB. Xanthogranuloma of the Erdheim-Chester type within the sellar region: case report. Clin Neuropathol. 2002;21:24–8.
4. Burt MG, Morey AL, Turner JJ, Pell M, Sheehy JP, Ho KK. Xanthomatous pituitary lesions: a report of two cases and review of the literature. Pituitary. 2003;6:161–8.
5. Folkerth RD, Price Jr DL, Schwartz M, Black PM, De Girolami U. Xanthomatous hypophysitis. Am J Surg Pathol. 1998;22:736–41.
6. Sugata S, Hirano H, Yatsushiro K, Yunoue S, Nakamura K, Arita K. Xanthogranuloma in the suprasellar region. Neurol Med Chir (Tokyo). 2009;49:124–7.
7. Jung CS, Schanzer A, Hattingen E, Plate KH, Seifert V. Xanthogranuloma of the sellar region. Acta Neurochir (Wien). 2006;148:473–7.
8. Le BH, Towfighi J, Kapadia SB, Lopes MB. Comparative immunohistochemical assessment of craniopharyngioma and related lesions. Endocr Pathol. 2007;18:23–30.

Petrous Apex Cholesterol Granuloma

24

Gabriel Zada, M. Beatriz S. Lopes, Srinivasan Mukundan Jr., and Edward Laws Jr.

24.1 Epidemiology and Clinical Presentation

- The previous section covered xanthogranulomas of the sella.
- Cholesterol granulomas of the petrous apex may be caused by obstruction of the normal aeration of the petrous air cells (i.e., Eustachian tube obstruction), resulting in chronic accumulation of cholesterol deposits and remodeling of the skull base (obstruction-vacuum theory) [1].
- Another theory is that hyperplastic mucosa invades exposed bone marrow, resulting in chronic hemorrhage and inflammation of the petrous apex (exposed marrow theory) [2].
- Cholesterol granulomas of the petrous apex often present with any of the following symptoms: headache, visual dysfunction, hearing loss, serous otitis media, dizziness, tinnitus, facial pain, or hemifacial spasm [3].
- Patients are typically in the fourth to fifth decade of life [4].

24.2 Imaging Features

- Cholesterol granulomas of the petrous apex typically demonstrate increased signal intensity on both T1- and T2-weighted MR images and are nonenhancing (Figs. 24.1 and 24.2) [5, 6].
- Because blood products are present within the lesion, the lesion may appear markedly hypointense on susceptibility-sensitive sequences, and variable signal characteristics may be seen on diffusion-weighted imaging.
- MRI is the preferred modality for assessing the relationship of the granuloma to surrounding structures, differentiating granulomas from other cystic lesions of the petrous apex (such as arachnoid cysts, and epidermoid cysts), and demonstrating the degree of postoperative drainage.
- CT imaging typically demonstrates variable degrees of bony erosion [7], but the bony margins should be indicative of smooth remodeling rather than aggressive destruction.
- The average diameter of symptomatic petrous apex cholesterol granulomas is 3 cm [8].
- Erosion of the clivus and extension into the sphenoid sinus are commonly noted.
- MRI is better than CT scans for postsurgical follow-up. Recurrent cholesterol granuloma will show a new area of T1 shortening within the preexisting cavity. Fat-saturated sequences may be necessary to distinguish a recurrent lesion from fat-packing material.

G. Zada, MD, MS (✉)
Department of Neurological Surgery, Keck School of Medicine, University of Southern California, 1200 N State Street, #3300, Los Angeles, CA 90033, USA
e-mail: gzada@usc.edu

M.B.S. Lopes, MD, PhD
Department of Pathology (Neuropathology), University of Virginia School of Medicine, 1215 Lee Street, Room 3060–HEP, Charlottesville, VA 22908, USA
e-mail: msl2e@virginia.edu

S. Mukundan Jr., PhD, MD
Department of Radiology, Brigham and Women's Hospital, 75 Francis Street, Boston, MA 02115, USA
e-mail: smukundan@partners.org

E. Laws Jr., MD
Department of Neurosurgery, Brigham and Women's Hospital, 15 Francis Street, Boston, MA 02115, USA
e-mail: elaws@partners.org

G. Zada et al. (eds.), *Atlas of Sellar and Parasellar Lesions: Clinical, Radiologic, and Pathologic Correlations*, DOI 10.1007/978-3-319-22855-6_24

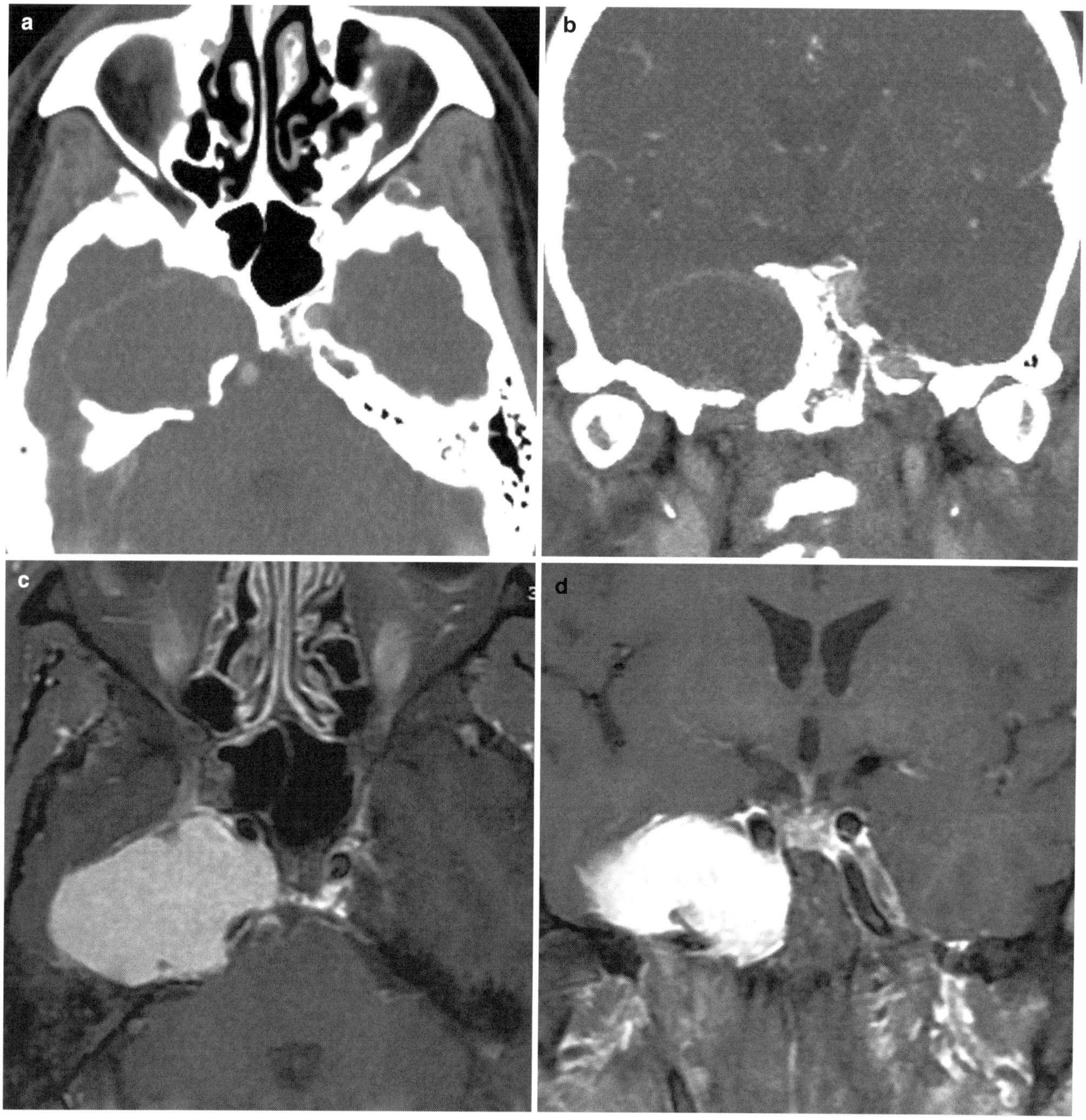

Fig. 24.1 Petrous apex cholesterol granuloma. (**a**) Axial CT image with contrast enhancement. (**b**) Coronal CT image with contrast enhancement. (**c**) Axial T1-weighted gadolinium-enhanced image. (**d**) Coronal T1-weighted gadolinium-enhanced image. There is an ovoid cystic lesion in the right petrous apex, containing predominantly T1-hyperintense material. The right internal carotid artery is displaced anteriorly

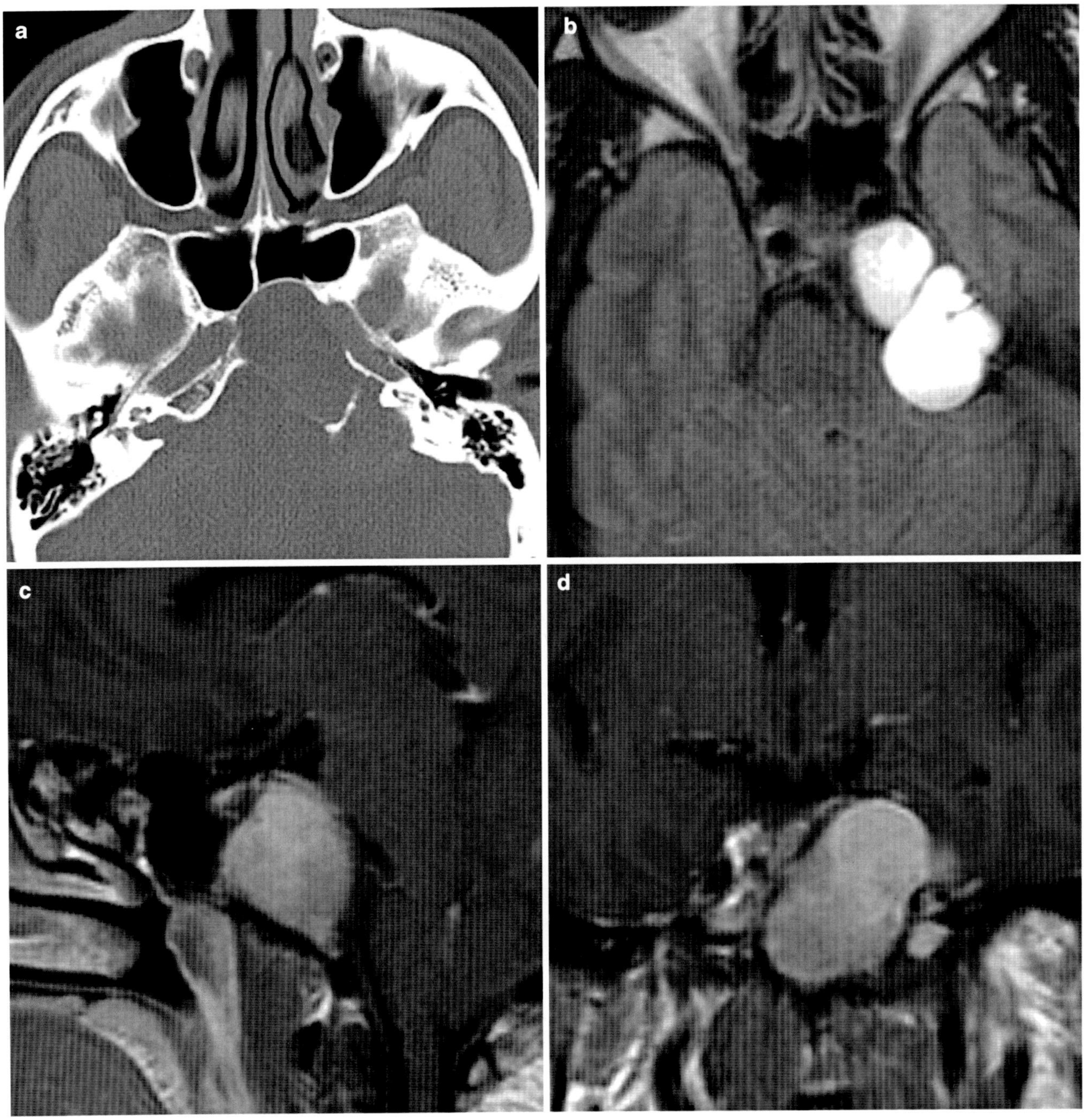

Fig. 24.2 Petrous apex cholesterol granuloma. (**a**) Axial CT image with contrast enhancement. (**b**) Axial FLAIR image. (**c**) Sagittal T1-weighted gadolinium-enhanced image. (**d**) Coronal T1-weighted gadolinium-enhanced image. There is an expansile cystic lesion in the left petrous apex containing T1-hyperintense material. The cyst expanded to the clivus body with anterior displacement of the left cavernous internal carotid artery. Posteriorly, the cyst indents the brainstem

24.3 Histopathology

- Chocolate-colored fluid contents are often grossly observed.
- Petrous apex cholesterol granulomas are characterized by cholesterol clefts surrounded by histiocytes, lymphocytes, plasma cells, and multinucleated foreign-body giant cells [9].
- Areas of old hemorrhage and inflammation with hemosiderin-laden macrophages are typically observed (Fig. 24.3) [10].

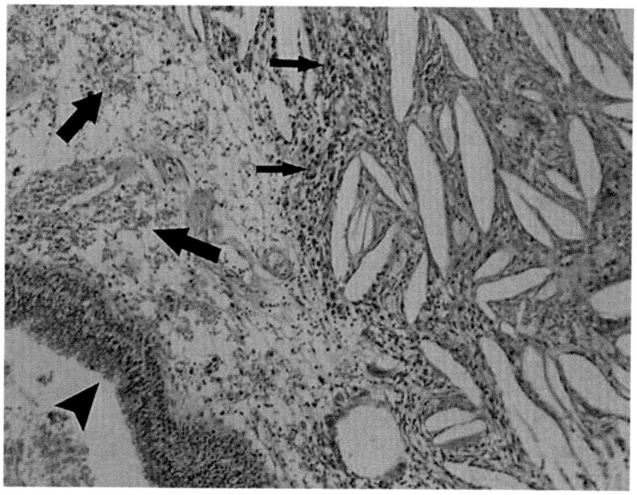

Fig. 24.3 In a petrous apex cholesterol granuloma, a large number of submucosal spindle-shaped, empty clefts surrounded by inflammatory cells are shown. The intact respiratory epithelium is noted (*arrowhead*). Focal hemorrhage (*large arrows*) and hemosiderin-laden macrophages (*small arrows*) are also shown (H&E stain, ×100) (Adapted from Chao [10]; with permission)

24.4 Clinical Management

- Surgical management is the preferred primary treatment for symptomatic petrous apex cholesterol granulomas.
- Open surgical approaches such as a middle cranial fossa or infracochlear approach have been traditionally used [11].
- Endoscopic endonasal approaches for selected cholesterol granulomas offer the potential for effective and safe marsupialization and drainage [12].
- Symptomatic improvement, including resolution of cranial nerve deficits, has been reported in 80–100 % of patients [12, 13].
- A primary surgical goal is to establish a long-standing drainage route, such as into the sphenoid sinus.
- Some authors have advocated insertion of a Silastic stent to maintain patency of the drainage route [8, 12].
- Maximal safe resection of the cyst wall may reduce the risk for recurrence [1, 4].
- Symptomatic recurrence has been reported in 15–35 % of patients; this rate may be higher in patients who have undergone simple fenestration without the use of a stent [8].

References

1. Eisenberg MB, Haddad G, Al-Mefty O. Petrous apex cholesterol granulomas: evolution and management. J Neurosurg. 1997;86:822–9.
2. Jackler RK, Cho M. A new theory to explain the genesis of petrous apex cholesterol granuloma. Otol Neurotol. 2003;24:96–106; discussion 106.
3. Brodkey JA, Robertson JH, Shea 3rd JJ, Gardner G. Cholesterol granulomas of the petrous apex: combined neurosurgical and otological management. J Neurosurg. 1996;85:625–33.
4. Terao T, Onoue H, Hashimoto T, Ishibashi T, Kogure T, Abe T. Cholesterol granuloma in the petrous apex: case report and review. Acta Neurochir (Wien). 2001;143:947–52.
5. Greenberg JJ, Oot RF, Wismer GL, Davis KR, Goodman ML, Weber AE, Montgomery WW. Cholesterol granuloma of the petrous apex: MR and CT evaluation. AJNR Am J Neuroradiol. 1988;9:1205–14.
6. Martin N, Sterkers O, Mompoint D, Julien N, Nahum H. Cholesterol granulomas of the middle ear cavities: MR imaging. Radiology. 1989;172:521–5.
7. Durgam A, Batra PS. Paranasal sinus cholesterol granuloma: systematic review of diagnostic and management aspects. Int Forum Allergy Rhinol. 2013;3:242–7.
8. Hoa M, House JW, Linthicum Jr FH. Petrous apex cholesterol granuloma: maintenance of drainage pathway, the histopathology of surgical management and histopathologic evidence for the exposed marrow theory. Otol Neurotol. 2012;33:1059–65.
9. Leon ME, Chavez C, Fyfe B, Nagorsky MJ, Garcia FU. Cholesterol granuloma of the maxillary sinus. Arch Pathol Lab Med. 2002;126:217–9.
10. Chao TK. Cholesterol granuloma of the maxillary sinus. Eur Arch Otorhinolaryngol. 2006;263:592–7.
11. Scopel TF, Fernandez-Miranda JC, Pinheiro-Neto CD, Peris-Celda M, Paluzzi A, Gardner PA, et al. Petrous apex cholesterol granulomas: endonasal versus infracochlear approach. Laryngoscope. 2012;122:751–61.
12. Paluzzi A, Gardner P, Fernandez-Miranda JC, Pinheiro-Neto CD, Scopel TF, Koutourousiou M, Snyderman CH. Endoscopic endonasal approach to cholesterol granulomas of the petrous apex: a series of 17 patients: clinical article. J Neurosurg. 2012; 116:792–8.
13. Brackmann DE, Toh EH. Surgical management of petrous apex cholesterol granulomas. Otol Neurotol. 2002;23:529–33.

Sellar Region Arachnoid Cysts

25

Gabriel Zada, M. Beatriz S. Lopes, Srinivasan Mukundan Jr., and Edward Laws Jr.

25.1 Epidemiology and Clinical Presentation

- Arachnoid cysts are developmental anomalies that can originate anywhere in the CNS.
- They are often discovered as an incidental finding, remain asymptomatic, and can be monitored with serial imaging.
- They rarely cause symptoms requiring surgical intervention.
- Among major series of transsphenoidal operations, arachnoid cysts comprise 0.22–0.8 % of lesions [1–3].
- The mean age of patients at the time of clinical diagnosis is 47 years [1].
- The clinical presentation typically includes headache, amenorrhea or galactorrhea, anterior pituitary insufficiency, and/or visual dysfunction [1, 4–6].
- Hyperprolactinemia due to stalk effect is a common laboratory finding [1, 4].

25.2 Imaging Features

- On MR imaging, arachnoid cysts in this region typically appear as ovoid cystic lesions with sellar and suprasellar components.
- Compared with CSF, cyst contents are typically isointense or hyperintense on T1-weighted MR imaging (Figs. 25.1, 25.2, 25.3, 25.4, 25.5, and 25.6) [1].
- Expansion of the sella turcica is commonly observed.
- The mean cyst diameter of surgically treated cases is 20–24 mm [6].
- These cysts can often be differentiated from other cystic lesions of the sellar region with the use of MR diffusion-weighted imaging (DWI). The apparent diffusion coefficient (ADC) of arachnoid is similar to that of stationary water [7].

G. Zada, MD, MS (✉)
Department of Neurological Surgery, Keck School of Medicine, University of Southern California, 1200 N State Street, #3300, Los Angeles, CA 90033, USA
e-mail: gzada@usc.edu

M.B.S. Lopes, MD, PhD
Department of Pathology (Neuropathology), University of Virginia School of Medicine, 1215 Lee Street, Room 3060–HEP, Charlottesville, VA 22908, USA
e-mail: msl2e@virginia.edu

S. Mukundan Jr., PhD, MD
Department of Radiology, Brigham and Women's Hospital, 75 Francis Street, Boston, MA 02115, USA
e-mail: smukundan@partners.org

E. Laws Jr., MD
Department of Neurosurgery, Brigham and Women's Hospital, 15 Francis Street, Boston, MA 02115, USA
e-mail: elaws@partners.org

G. Zada et al. (eds.), *Atlas of Sellar and Parasellar Lesions: Clinical, Radiologic, and Pathologic Correlations*,
DOI 10.1007/978-3-319-22855-6_25

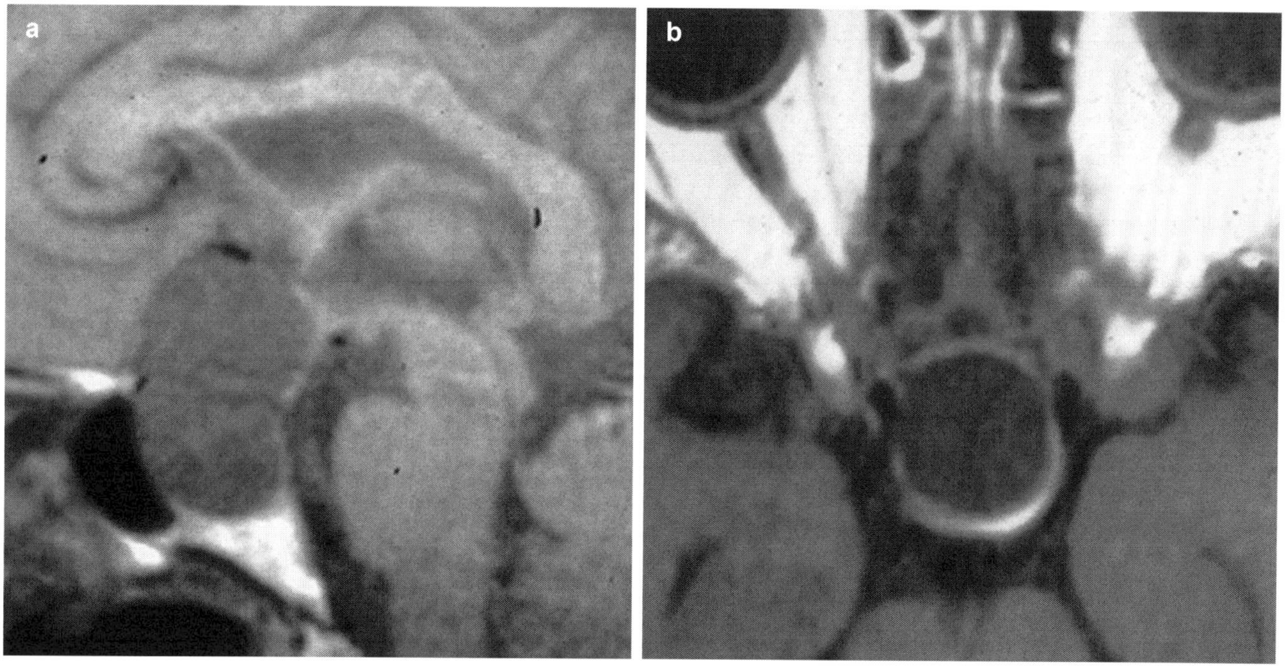

Fig. 25.1 Arachnoid cyst. (**a**) Sagittal T1-weighted post-gadolinium image. (**b**) Coronal T1-weighted post-gadolinium image. A nonenhancing lesion is located in the sella with suprasellar extension. The signal intensity of the lesion is similar to the cerebrospinal fluid (CSF). There is remodeling of the sellar floor. The optic chiasm is elevated by the mass

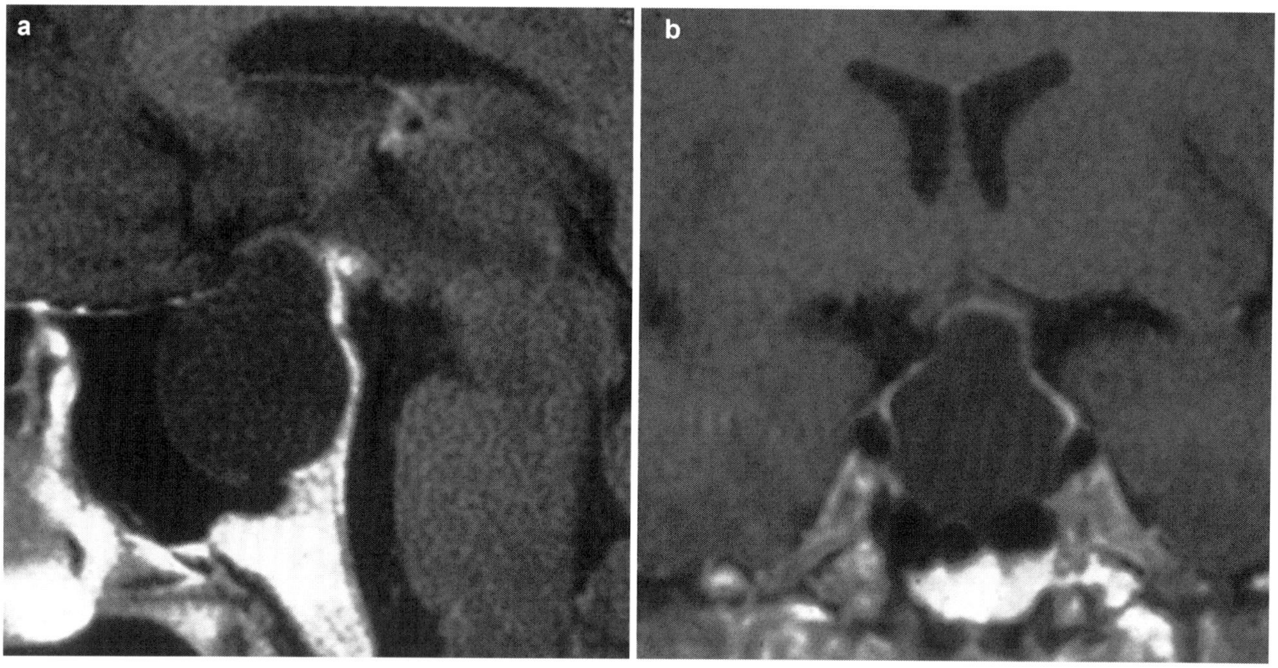

Fig. 25.2 Arachnoid cyst. (**a**) Sagittal T1-weighted post-gadolinium image. (**b**) Coronal T1-weighted post-gadolinium image. A nonenhancing lesion in the sella is present with suprasellar extension and remodeling of the sellar floor. The signal intensity of the lesion is similar to the CSF. The optic chiasm is mildly elevated by the mass

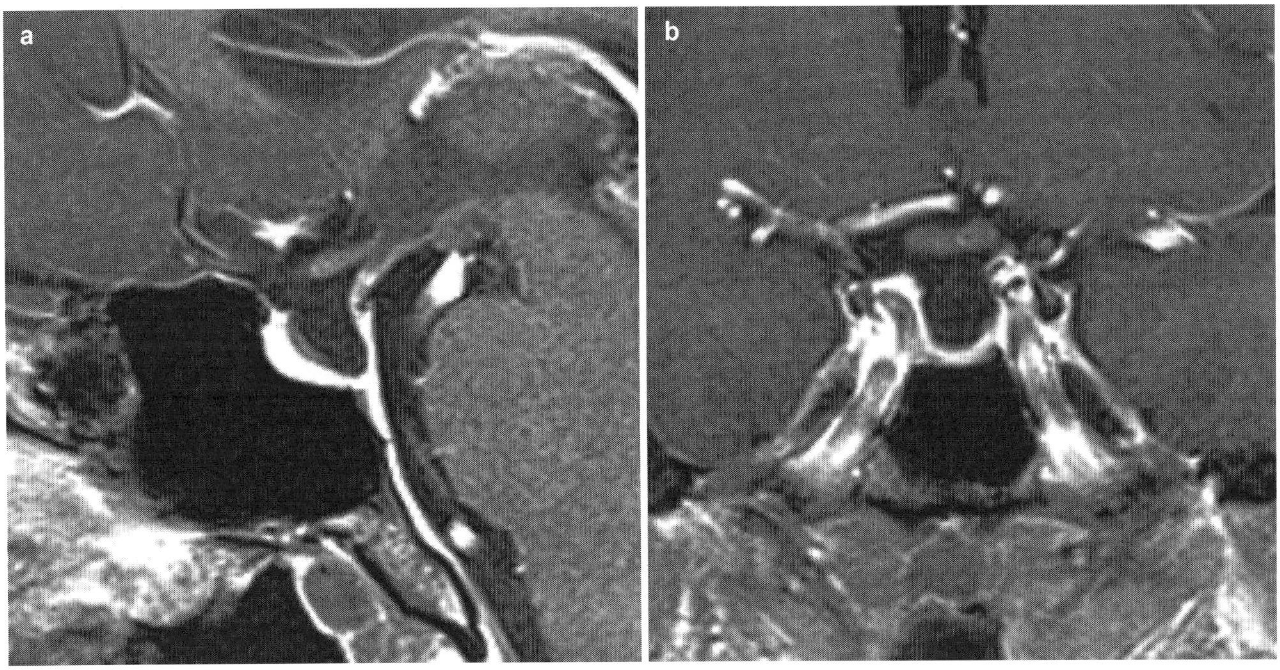

Fig. 25.3 Arachnoid cyst. (**a**) Sagittal T1-weighted post-gadolinium image. (**b**) Coronal T1-weighted post-gadolinium image. There is posterior displacement of the pituitary stalk; the depressed appearance of the pituitary gland suggests the presence of a collection with signal intensity similar to that of the CSF. The wall of the cystic collection is not visualized on these images

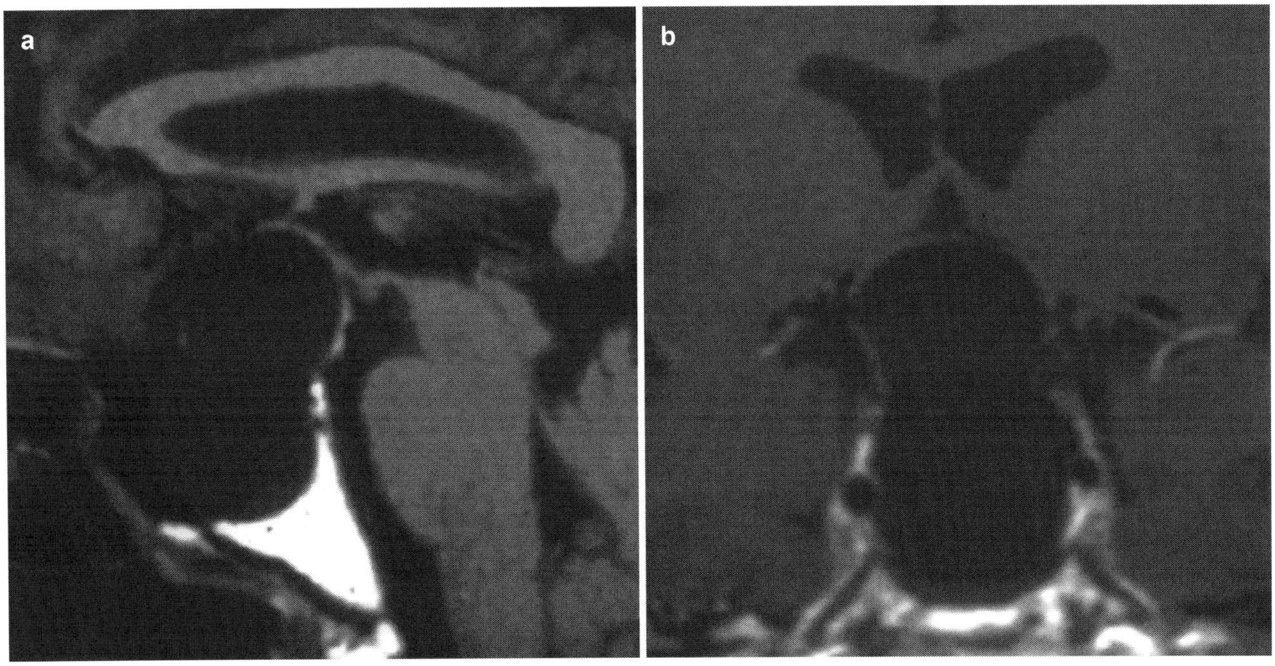

Fig. 25.4 Arachnoid cyst. (**a**) Sagittal T1-weighted post-gadolinium image. (**b**) Coronal T1-weighted post-gadolinium image. There is a nonenhancing lesion in the sella, with suprasellar extension and remodeling of the sellar floor. The signal intensity of the lesion is similar to the CSF. The optic chiasm is elevated by the mass

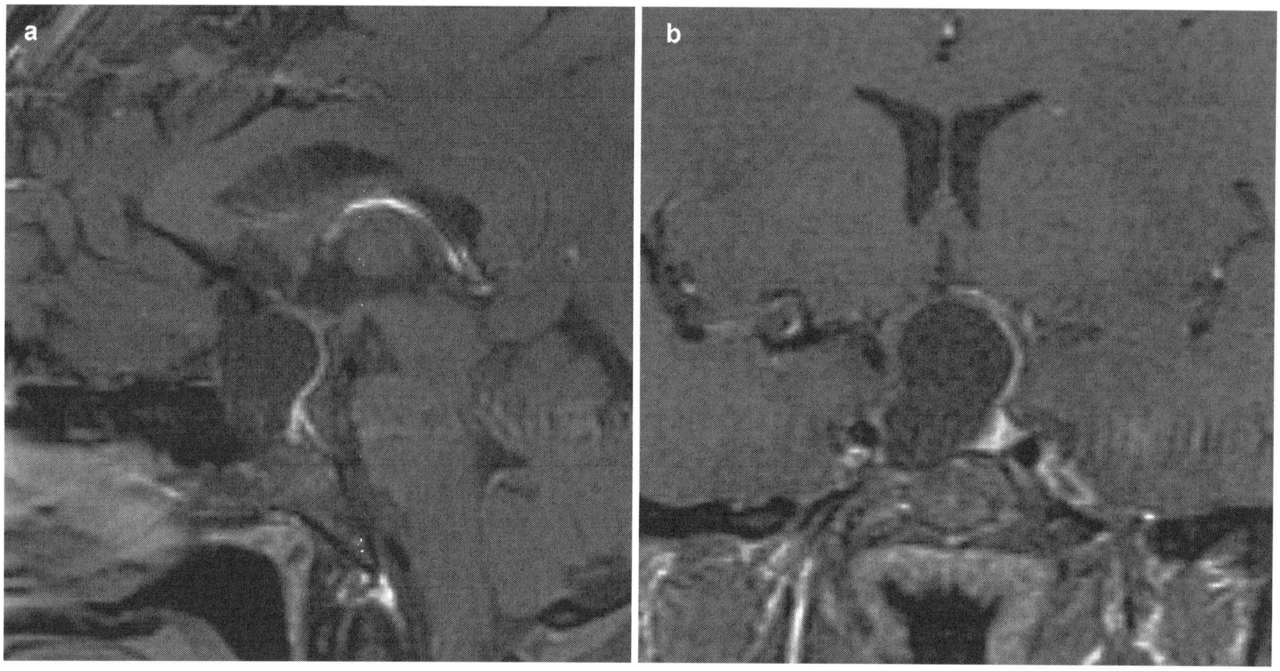

Fig. 25.5 Arachnoid cyst. (**a**) Sagittal T1-weighted post-gadolinium image. (**b**) Coronal T1-weighted post-gadolinium image. A nonenhancing lesion is located in the right aspect of the sella, with suprasellar extension and remodeling of the sellar floor. The signal intensity of the lesion is similar to the CSF. The optic chiasm is elevated by the mass

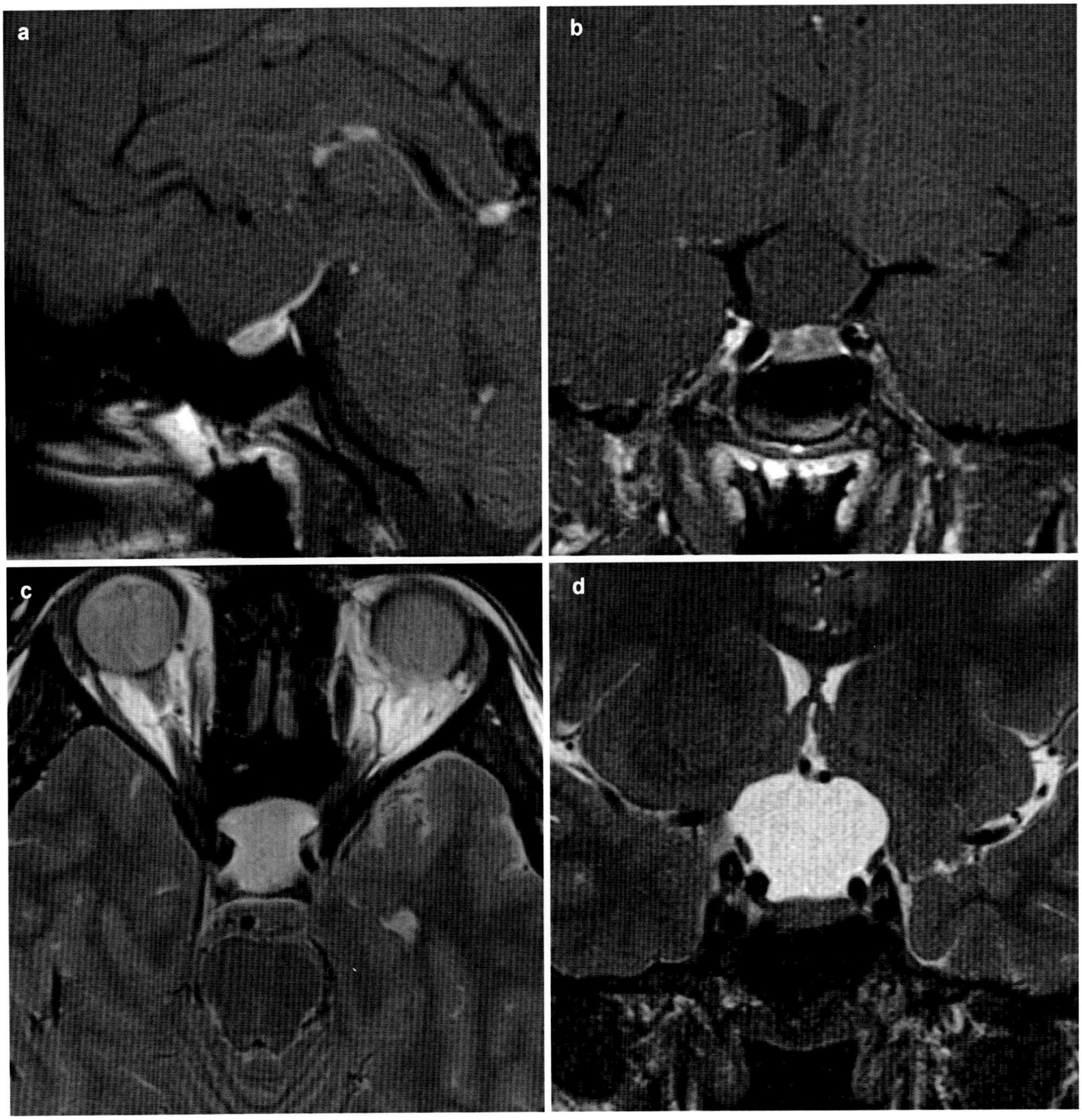

Fig. 25.6 Arachnoid cyst. (**a**) Sagittal T1-weighted precontrast image. (**b**) Coronal T1-weighted precontrast image. (**c**) Axial T2-weighted image. (**d**) Coronal T2-weighted image. A nonenhancing suprasellar collection displays signal intensity similar to that of the CSF. There is downward effacement of the sellar contents by the collection. The A1 segments of both anterior cerebral arteries are elevated by the collection

25.3 Histopathology

- *Pathophysiology*: Normally, no arachnoid layer is located below the level of the diaphragma sellae. Arachnoid cysts are thought to develop in this region secondary to a congenitally wide aperture in the diaphragma sellae, allowing arachnoid and cerebrospinal fluid (CSF) to enter the sella turcica via a ball-valve effect. Ultimately, the arachnoid membrane apposes and the CSF space no longer communicates, forming a sequestered (noncommunicating) cyst with an arachnoid lining, as opposed to an empty sella condition. (*See* "Empty Sella Syndrome" in Chap. 66.)
- The structure of an arachnoid cyst wall is similar to that of normal arachnoid membrane.
- The inner surface of the cyst wall is composed of arachnoid cells with slender processes and large amounts of extracellular space; microvilli are not found (Fig. 25.7) [8].
- Immunostaining of the cyst wall can be used to differentiate arachnoid cysts from epithelial cysts, because the arachnoid cysts demonstrate negative immunoreactivity for glial fibrillary acidic protein (GFAP), S-100 protein, prealbumin, and carcinoembryonic antigen (CEA) [9].
- The protein concentration of arachnoid cysts has been measured to range between 300 and 25,500 mg/L [1].

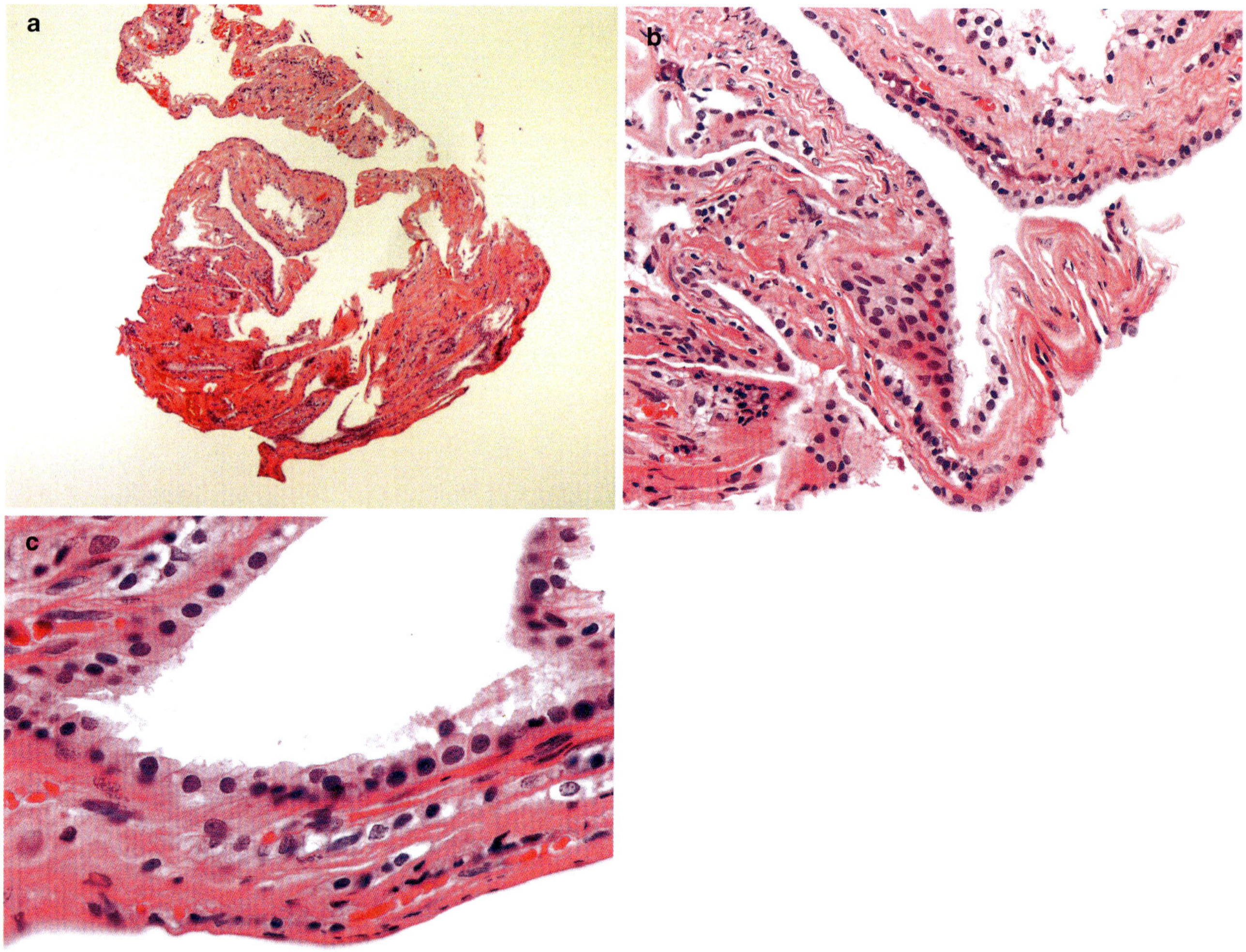

Fig. 25.7 Arachnoid cyst. (**a**) Arachnoid cysts are composed of a single layer of flat to cuboidal cells lying in a delicate, fibrovascular stroma. (**b**, **c**) Unlike a Rathke cleft cyst, the cells are devoid of cilia and other epithelial-like properties

25.4 Clinical Management

- Surgical intervention may be required for patients with symptomatic sellar region arachnoid cysts.
- In patients with symptoms referable to an arachnoid cyst, a transsphenoidal approach with fenestration of the cyst and partial versus complete cyst wall resection is the standard approach [4, 7].
- Endoscopic transsphenoidal fenestration of intrasellar and suprasellar arachnoid cysts has become the preferred approach in many major institutions [10, 11].
- Other authors have reported successful obliteration of the cyst using autologous fat, without enlarging the communication with the suprasellar cistern [6].
- Craniotomy with fenestration into the parasellar CSF cisterns has been advocated for larger or recurrent arachnoid cysts with extrasellar extension [12, 13].
- In rare cases, a CSF-diverting shunt may be required for additional management of refractory cysts [12, 13].
- Visual loss and hyperprolactinemia are likely to improve following surgical drainage; improvement of anterior pituitary insufficiency is less likely [4, 12].
- Rates of intraoperative and postoperative CSF leaks are higher than in patients undergoing transsphenoidal surgery for other sellar lesions, especially if communication with subarachnoid cisterns is created [1].
- Prolapse of the optic chiasm may occur following treatment of this condition.
- Recurrence has been reported in 20–50 % of patients [1, 5, 6]. Close monitoring for recurrence is recommended.

References

1. Dubuisson AS, Stevenaert A, Martin DH, Flandroy PP. Intrasellar arachnoid cysts. Neurosurgery. 2007;61:505–13; discussion 513.
2. Fatemi N, Dusick JR, de Paiva Neto MA, Kelly DF. The endonasal microscopic approach for pituitary adenomas and other parasellar tumors: a 10-year experience. Neurosurgery. 2008;63:244–56; discussion 256.
3. Saeger W, Ludecke DK, Buchfelder M, Fahlbusch R, Quabbe HJ, Petersenn S. Pathohistological classification of pituitary tumors: 10 years of experience with the German Pituitary Tumor Registry. Eur J Endocrinol. 2007;156:203–16.
4. Meyer FB, Carpenter SM, Laws Jr ER. Intrasellar arachnoid cysts. Surg Neurol. 1987;28:105–10.
5. Shin JL, Asa SL, Woodhouse LJ, Smyth HS, Ezzat S. Cystic lesions of the pituitary: clinicopathological features distinguishing craniopharyngioma, Rathke's cleft cyst, and arachnoid cyst. J Clin Endocrinol Metab. 1999;84:3972–82.
6. McLaughlin N, Vandergrift A, Ditzel Filho LF, Shahlaie K, Eisenberg AA, Carrau RL, et al. Endonasal management of sellar arachnoid cysts: simple cyst obliteration technique. J Neurosurg. 2012;116:728–40.
7. Tsuruda JS, Chew WM, Moseley ME, Norman D. Diffusion-weighted MR imaging of the brain: value of differentiating between extraaxial cysts and epidermoid tumors. AJR Am J Roentgenol. 1990;155:1059–65; discussion 1066–8.
8. Miyagami M, Tsubokawa T. Histological and ultrastructural findings of benign intracranial cysts. Noshuyo Byori. 1993;10:151–60.
9. Inoue T, Matsushima T, Fukui M, Iwaki T, Takeshita I, Kuromatsu C. Immunohistochemical study of intracranial cysts. Neurosurgery. 1988;23:576–81.
10. Cavallo LM, Prevedello D, Esposito F, Laws Jr ER, Dusick JR, Messina A, et al. The role of the endoscope in the transsphenoidal management of cystic lesions of the sellar region. Neurosurg Rev. 2008;31:55–64; discussion 64.
11. Laws ER. Endoscopic surgery for cystic lesions of the pituitary region. Nat Clin Pract Endocrinol Metab. 2008;4:662–3.
12. Pierre-Kahn A, Capelle L, Brauner R, Sainte-Rose C, Renier D, Rappaport R, Hirsch JF. Presentation and management of suprasellar arachnoid cysts. Review of 20 cases. J Neurosurg. 1990;73:355–9.
13. Rappaport ZH. Suprasellar arachnoid cysts: options in operative management. Acta Neurochir (Wien). 1993;122:71–5.

Sellar Region Epidermoid and Dermoid Cysts

26

Gabriel Zada, M. Beatriz S. Lopes, Srinivasan Mukundan Jr., and Edward Laws Jr.

26.1 Epidemiology and Clinical Presentation

- Epidermoid and dermoid cysts are developmental anomalies that can occur anywhere in the cranial cavity [1].
- Epidermoid cysts often arise in a paramedian location, most commonly in the region of the cerebellopontine angle (CPA) [2, 3].
- Dermoid lesions typically arise in the midline [4]. The most common location is also in the posterior fossa, where they are often associated with Klippel-Feil syndrome or other craniocervical anomalies. They also may occur in the nasal cavity, with extension through the skull base [5, 6].
- These cysts may occasionally present as suprasellar or parasellar lesions [7].
- Rarely, they may present as isolated intrasellar lesions (limited primarily to case reports).
- These lesions make up 0.2–0.7 % of major transsphenoidal series [8, 9].
- Sellar region epidermoid and dermoid tumors typically present in middle-aged patients with symptoms of mass effect, including headache, visual loss, and endocrine dysfunction [10–12].
- Some reports have also described a clinical presentation mimicking pituitary apoplexy [2, 13].
- The cyst contents can be caustic to the surrounding tissue, and in some cases the cyst presents with acute rupture causing chemical meningitis, hemorrhage, seizure, neurological deficits, and/or psychosis [14–19].

26.2 Imaging Features

- CT imaging typically demonstrates a midline, hypodense mass in the suprasellar region, with signal intensity similar to that of the CSF.
- MRI frequently demonstrates hypointense T1 signal intensity and heterogeneous T2 hyperintensity that has been reported to correlate with cyst contents (Figs. 26.1, 26.2, 26.3, 26.4, and 26.5) [19].
- Demonstration of restricted diffusion on diffusion-weighted imaging (DWI) has been shown to be useful in differentiating dermoid and epidermoid lesions from other types of cystic pathology, particularly arachnoid cysts [20]. DWI is also highly sensitive for the presence of residual cyst and the detection of recurrence.
- In cases of ruptured dermoid tumors, multiple regions of hypodensity on CT scans and T1 shortening on MRI consistent with disseminated fat droplets may be seen throughout the subarachnoid space or within the ventricular system [19, 21]. Because the fat droplets have lower density than CSF, they tend to layer in antigravity positions within the ventricular system.

G. Zada, MD, MS (✉)
Department of Neurological Surgery, Keck School of Medicine, University of Southern California, 1200 N State Street, #3300, Los Angeles, CA 90033, USA
e-mail: gzada@usc.edu

M.B.S. Lopes, MD, PhD
Department of Pathology (Neuropathology), University of Virginia School of Medicine, 1215 Lee Street, Room 3060–HEP, Charlottesville, VA 22908, USA
e-mail: msl2e@virginia.edu

S. Mukundan Jr., PhD, MD
Department of Radiology, Brigham and Women's Hospital, 75 Francis Street, Boston, MA 02115, USA
e-mail: smukundan@partners.org

E. Laws Jr., MD
Department of Neurosurgery, Brigham and Women's Hospital, 15 Francis Street, Boston, MA 02115, USA
e-mail: elaws@partners.org

G. Zada et al. (eds.), *Atlas of Sellar and Parasellar Lesions: Clinical, Radiologic, and Pathologic Correlations*,
DOI 10.1007/978-3-319-22855-6_26

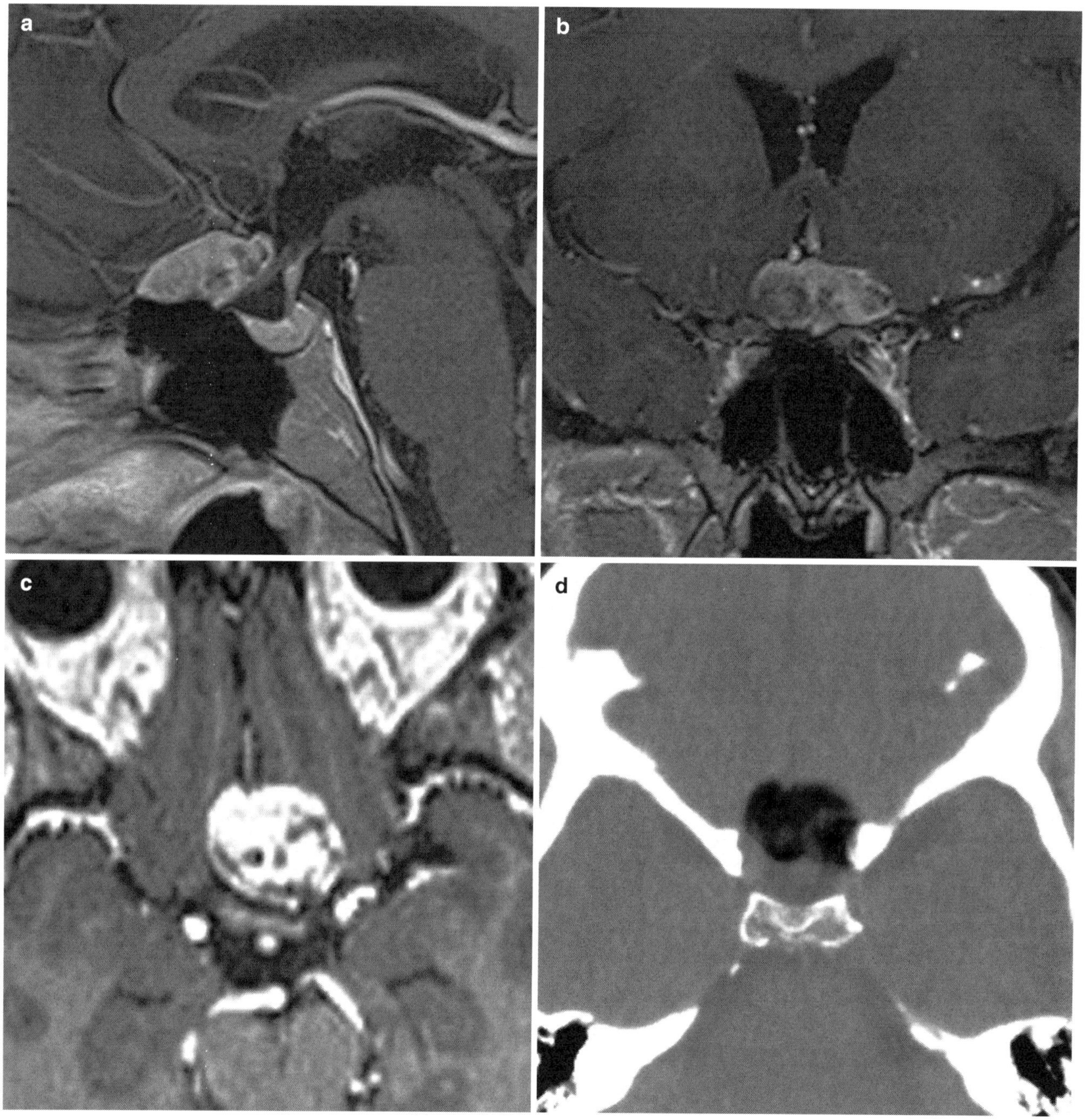

Fig. 26.1 Dermoid cyst. (**a**) Sagittal T1-weighted post-gadolinium image. (**b**) Coronal T1-weighted post-gadolinium image. (**c**) Axial CT image. A lobulated mass is located above the planum sphenoidale anterior to the pituitary stalk. (**d**) On a CT scan, the lesion has areas of low attenuation indicating the presence of fat. The anterior cerebral arteries are posterior to the lesion

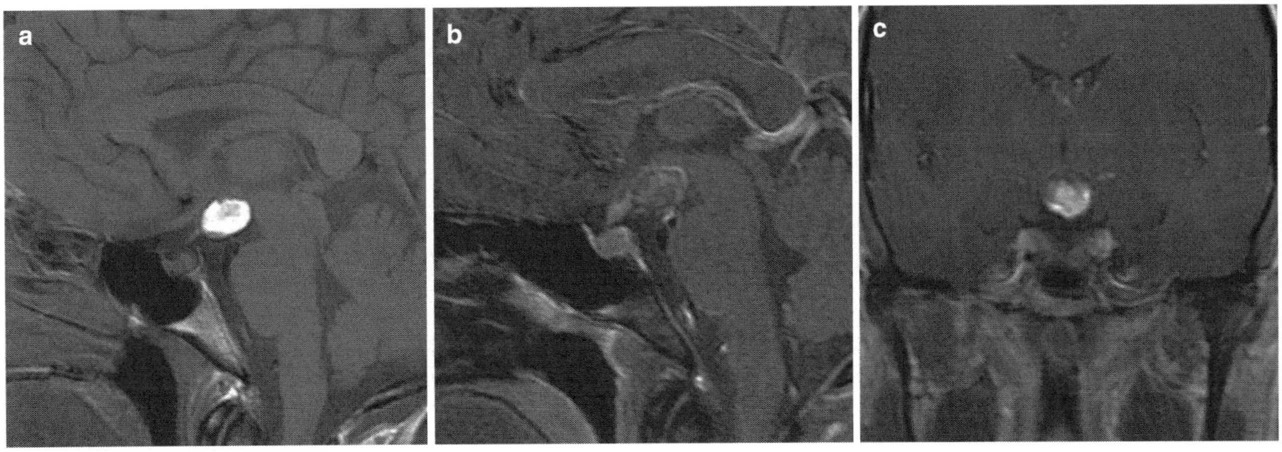

Fig. 26.2 Dermoid cyst. (**a**) Sagittal T1-weighted noncontrast image. (**b**) Sagittal T1-weighted post-gadolinium enhanced image. (**c**) Coronal T1-weighted noncontrast image. Showing a T1 hyperintense heterogeneous and minimally enhancing dermoid cyst of the interpeduncular cisterns posterior to the infundibulum

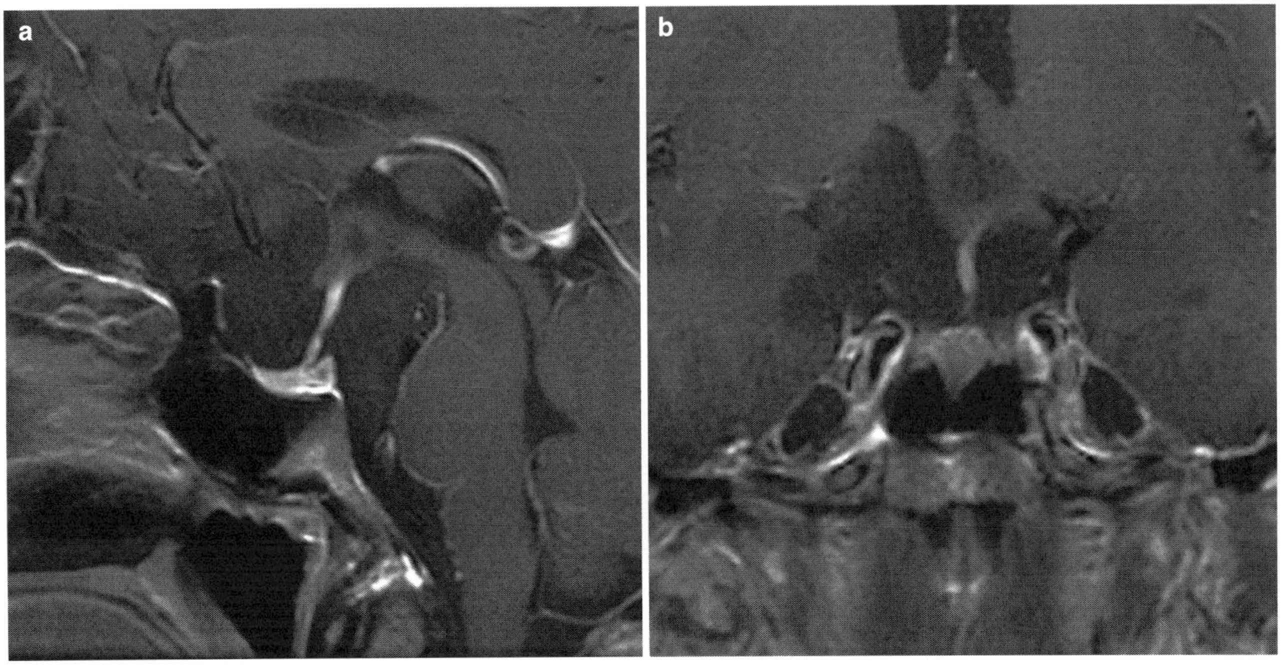

Fig. 26.3 Epidermoid cyst. (**a**) Sagittal T1-weighted post-gadolinium image. (**b**) Coronal T1-weighted post-gadolinium image. There is a cystic lesion in the suprasellar region surrounding the pituitary stalk. The lesion elevates the hypothalami

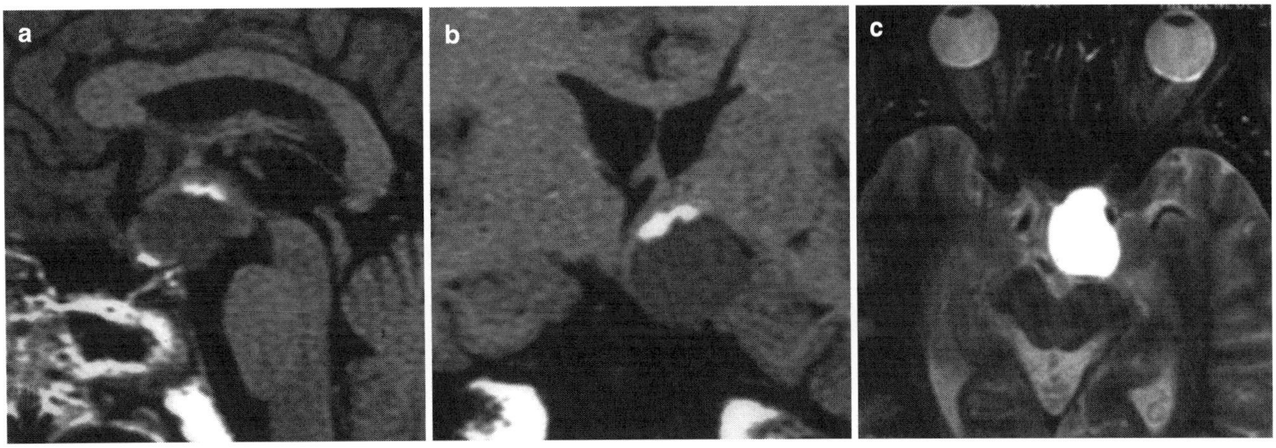

Fig. 26.4 (**a**) Sagittal T1-weighted pre-gadolinium image. (**b**) Coronal T1-weighted pre-gadolinium image. (**c**) Axial T2-weighted image. A cystic suprasellar lesion contains regions of T1 hyperintensity, possibly representing fat or proteinaceous material. The lesion elevates the left hypothalamus

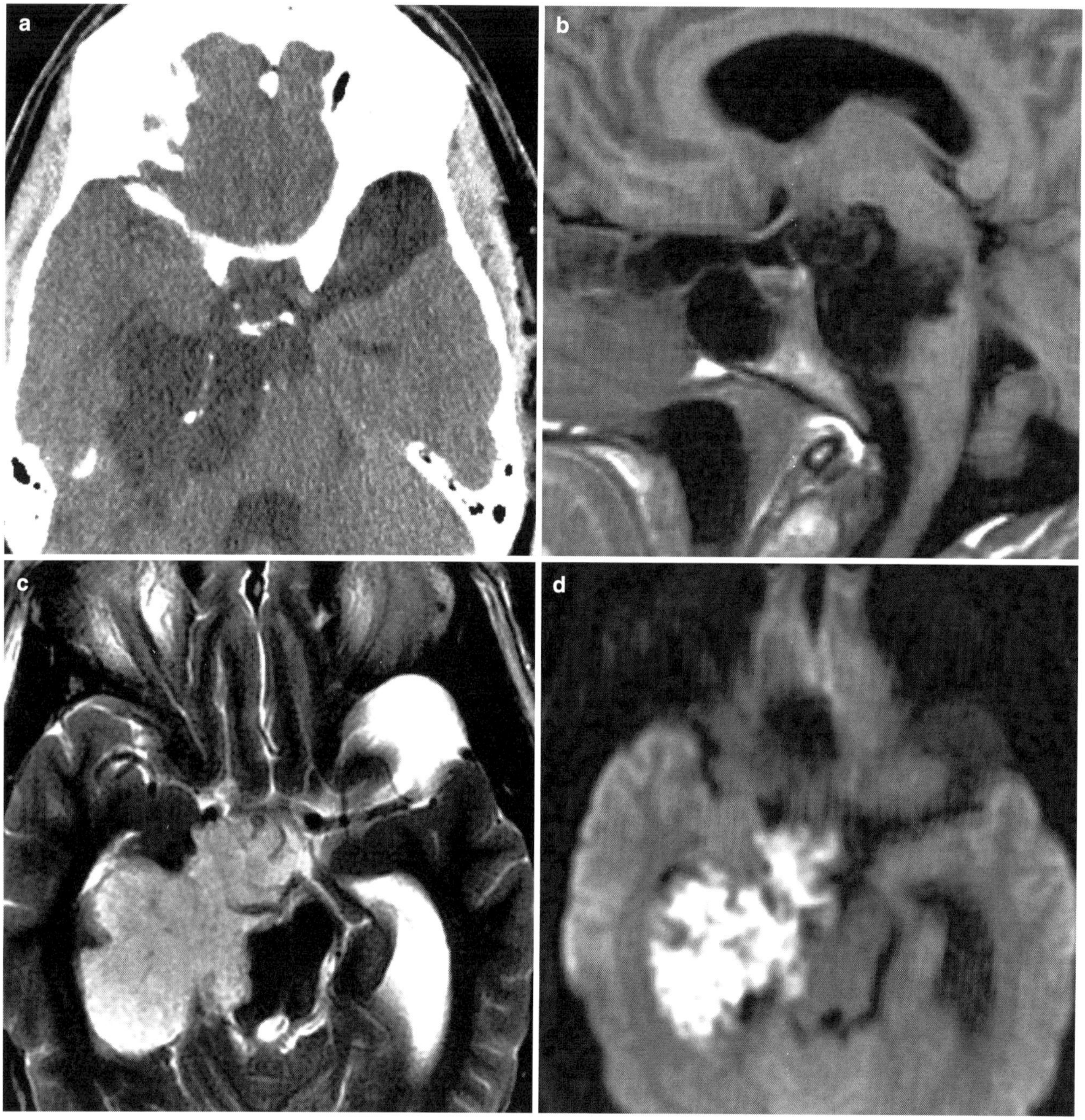

Fig. 26.5 (**a**) Axial CT scan. (**b**) Sagittal T1-weighted pre-gadolinium image. (**c**) Axial T2-weighted image. (**d**) Axial diffusion-weighted image (DWI). There is a cystic lesion in the suprasellar region, extending to the right ambient cistern and choroidal fissure. There are punctate calcifications along the septated part of the lesion. On DWI, there is increased signal intensity

26.3 Histopathology

- Epidermoid cysts typically exhibit a thin layer of squamous epithelium with a keratohyaline granular layer and a "flaky" keratin formation resting in a fibrocollagenous stroma (Fig. 26.6a, b).
- In addition to squamous epithelium, dermoid cysts contain adnexal structures such as hair follicles and glandular elements (Fig. 26.6c, d).
- Both cystic sellar lesions (particularly epidermoid cysts) may rupture to cause an exuberant inflammatory reaction in the surrounding parenchyma, resulting in secondary hypophysitis and meningitis.

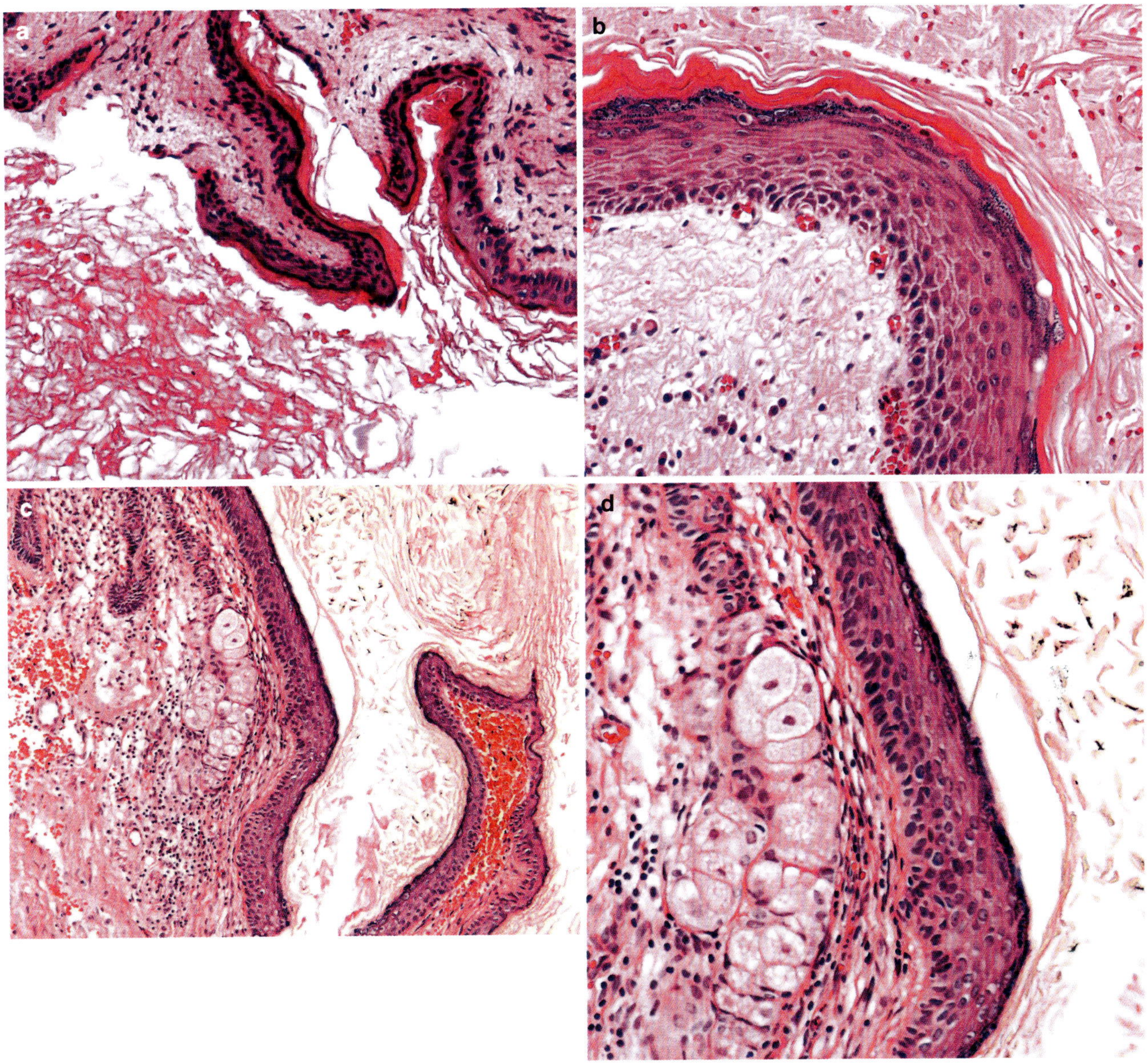

Fig. 26.6 Epidermoid and dermoid cysts. (**a**) Low-magnification view of an epidermoid cyst displays the squamous, stratified epithelium lining resting in a fibrous stroma. (**b**) The epithelium lining shows squamous epithelium with a keratohyaline granular layer and formation of flaky (acellular) keratin. (**c, d**) Dermoid cysts, on the other hand, show (in addition to the squamous, keratinizing epithelium) adnexal structures beneath the epithelium, including sebaceous glands

26.4 Clinical Management

- Surgical resection remains the most effective modality; no adjunctive measures have been proven to be of significant benefit in the management of these lesions.
- Extended endonasal microscopic and endoscopic skull base approaches have been utilized for resection of intrasellar and suprasellar dermoid and epidermoid cysts [6, 8, 11, 22–26].
- Endoscopy-assisted keyhole approaches may be ideally suited for these lesions because of the ability to look around surgical corners and resect additional cyst contents with the assistance of angled endoscopes [27, 28].
- Open cranial approaches are often required for larger or more invasive tumors [1, 29].
- Intraoperatively, dermoid and epidermoid cysts often can prove to be adhesive lesions that are not safely amenable to a gross total resection. The cyst capsule and contents cannot consistently be dissected off key vascular and nervous structures to achieve an acceptable outcome with minimal morbidity. In such cases, conservative resection is recommended.
- Steroids are recommended for up to 1 week following rupture or surgery, to reduce the risk of complications from chemical meningitis.
- A long-term recurrence rate of 26 % has been reported for all epidermoid and dermoid cysts, mandating serial monitoring of these patients [1].

References

1. Gormley WB, Tomecek FJ, Qureshi N, Malik GM. Craniocerebral epidermoid and dermoid tumours: a review of 32 cases. Acta Neurochir (Wien). 1994;128:115–21.
2. Sani S, Smith A, Leppla DC, Ilangovan S, Glick R. Epidermoid cyst of the sphenoid sinus with extension into the sella turcica presenting as pituitary apoplexy: case report. Surg Neurol. 2005;63:394–7; discussion 397.
3. Zhou LF. Intracranial epidermoid tumours: thirty-seven years of diagnosis and treatment. Br J Neurosurg. 1990;4:211–6.
4. Caldarelli M, Massimi L, Kondageski C, Di Rocco C. Intracranial midline dermoid and epidermoid cysts in children. J Neurosurg. 2004;100:473–80.
5. Uglietta JP, Boyko OB, Rippe DJ, Fuller GN, Schiff SJ, Heinz ER. Intracerebral extension of nasal dermoid cyst: CT appearance. J Comput Assist Tomogr. 1989;13:1061–4.
6. Weiss DD, Robson CD, Mulliken JB. Transnasal endoscopic excision of midline nasal dermoid from the anterior cranial base. Plast Reconstr Surg. 1998;102:2119–23.
7. Akdemir G, Daglioglu E, Ergungor MF. Dermoid lesion of the cavernous sinus: case report and review of the literature. Neurosurg Rev. 2004;27:294–8.
8. Fatemi N, Dusick JR, de Paiva Neto MA, Kelly DF. The endonasal microscopic approach for pituitary adenomas and other parasellar tumors: a 10-year experience. Neurosurgery. 2008;63:244–56; discussion 256.
9. Saeger W, Ludecke DK, Buchfelder M, Fahlbusch R, Quabbe HJ, Petersenn S. Pathohistological classification of pituitary tumors: 10 years of experience with the German Pituitary Tumor Registry. Eur J Endocrinol. 2007;156:203–16.
10. Boggan JE, Davis RL, Zorman G, Wilson CB. Intrasellar epidermoid cyst. Case report. J Neurosurg. 1983;58:411–5.
11. Oge K, Ozgen T. Transsphenoidal removal of an intra- and suprasellar epidermoid cyst. Neurochirurgia (Stuttg). 1991;34: 94–6.
12. Lin CJ, Jou JR, Woung LC, Tu YK, Jeng YM, Chang HC. Suprasellar dermoid cyst presenting as acquired exotropia. J Pediatr Ophthalmol Strabismus. 2003;40:47–50.
13. Tuna H, Torun F, Torun AN, Erdogan A. Intrasellar epidermoid cyst presenting as pituitary apoplexy. J Clin Neurosci. 2008;15: 1154–6.
14. Mamata H, Matsumae M, Yanagimachi N, Matsuyama S, Takamiya Y, Tsugane R. Parasellar dermoid tumor with intra-tumoral hemorrhage. Eur Radiol. 1998;8:1594–7.
15. Takeuchi H, Kubota T, Kabuto M, Izaki K. Ruptured suprasellar dermoid cyst presenting olfactory delusion (Eigengeruchs erlebnis). Neurosurgery. 1993;33:97–9.
16. Venkatesh SK, Phadke RV, Trivedi P, Bannerji D. Asymptomatic spontaneous rupture of suprasellar dermoid cyst: a case report. Neurol India. 2002;50:480–3.
17. Cohen JE, Abdallah JA, Garrote M. Massive rupture of suprasellar dermoid cyst into ventricles. Case illustration. J Neurosurg. 1997;87:963.
18. Ahmad I, Tominaga T, Ogawa A, Yoshimoto T. Ruptured suprasellar dermoid associated with middle cerebral artery aneurysm: case report. Surg Neurol. 1992;38:341–6.
19. Smith AS, Benson JE, Blaser SI, Mizushima A, Tarr RW, Bellon EM. Diagnosis of ruptured intracranial dermoid cyst: value MR over CT. AJNR Am J Neuroradiol. 1991;12:175–80.
20. Tsuruda JS, Chew WM, Moseley ME, Norman D. Diffusion-weighted MR imaging of the brain: value of differentiating between extraaxial cysts and epidermoid tumors. AJR Am J Roentgenol. 1990;155:1059–65; discussion 1066–8.
21. Liu JK, Gottfried ON, Salzman KL, Schmidt RH, Couldwell WT. Ruptured intracranial dermoid cysts: clinical, radiographic, and surgical features. Neurosurgery. 2008;62:377–84; discussion 384.
22. Duz B, Secer HI, Tosun F, Gonul E. Endoscopic endonasal resection of a midline intradural frontobasal dermoid tumour. Minim Invasive Neurosurg. 2007;50:363–6.
23. Baskin DS, Wilson CB. Transsphenoidal treatment of non-neoplastic intrasellar cysts. A report of 38 cases. J Neurosurg. 1984;60:8–13.
24. Esposito F, Becker DP, Villablanca JP, Kelly DF. Endonasal transsphenoidal transclival removal of prepontine epidermoid tumors: technical note. Neurosurgery. 2005;56:E443; discussion E443.
25. Dusick JR, Esposito F, Kelly DF, Cohan P, DeSalles A, Becker DP, Martin NA. The extended direct endonasal transsphenoidal approach for nonadenomatous suprasellar tumors. J Neurosurg. 2005;102:832–41.
26. McCoul ED, Chow S, Lee DL, Anand VK, Schwartz TH. Endoscopic endonasal approach for resection of ventral skull base keratinaceous cysts. Int Forum Allergy Rhinol. 2012;2:258–63.
27. Watanabe T, Ito E, Sato T, Ichikawa M, Oda K, Ando H, et al. Combined microsurgical and endoscopic removal of extensive suprasellar and prepontine epidermoid tumors. Neurol Med Chir (Tokyo). 2011;51:684–8.
28. Truchman A. Endoscopic-assisted resection of intracranial epidermoid tumors. World Neurosurg 2014;(3–4):450–4.
29. Yasargil MG, Abernathey CD, Sarioglu AC. Microneurosurgical treatment of intracranial dermoid and epidermoid tumors. Neurosurgery. 1989;24:561–7.

Colloid Cysts of the Sellar Region

27

Gabriel Zada, M. Beatriz S. Lopes, Srinivasan Mukundan Jr., and Edward Laws Jr.

27.1 Epidemiology and Clinical Presentation

- Colloid cysts are benign growths typically (99 %) arising in the third ventricle near the foramen of Monro.
- In rare cases, they can arise in the sellar or suprasellar region; they comprise less than 0.5 % of surgically treated sellar lesions [1, 2].
- They often arise in the region of the pars intermedia, located between the anterior and posterior pituitary gland, and may be challenging to differentiate from Rathke's cleft cysts (RCCs).
- They can present clinically with signs of local mass effect, including headache, visual loss, or hypopituitarism [3, 4].

27.2 Imaging Features

- On CT imaging, most colloid cysts are hyperdense and typically ovoid or rounded in shape.
- On MRI, colloid cysts may produce a variety of signal intensity. In the pituitary region, they are typically located in the pars intermedia and may be difficult to differentiate from RCCs. Most are hyperintense on T1-weighted imaging, with variable T2-weighted imaging characteristics [5]. Mild enhancement of the cyst capsule can be noted (Figs. 27.1, 27.2, and 27.3). Many colloid cysts will demonstrate restricted diffusion on diffusion-weighted imaging (DWI) sequences [2].

G. Zada, MD, MS (✉)
Department of Neurological Surgery, Keck School of Medicine, University of Southern California, 1200 N State Street, #3300, Los Angeles, CA 90033, USA
e-mail: gzada@usc.edu

M.B.S. Lopes, MD, PhD
Department of Pathology (Neuropathology), University of Virginia School of Medicine, 1215 Lee Street, Room 3060–HEP, Charlottesville, VA 22908, USA
e-mail: msl2e@virginia.edu

S. MukundanJr., PhD, MD
Department of Radiology, Brigham and Women's Hospital, 75 Francis Street, Boston, MA 02115, USA
e-mail: smukundan@partners.org

E. LawsJr., MD
Department of Neurosurgery, Brigham and Women's Hospital, 15 Francis Street, Boston, MA 02115, USA
e-mail: elaws@partners.org

G. Zada et al. (eds.), *Atlas of Sellar and Parasellar Lesions: Clinical, Radiologic, and Pathologic Correlations*,
DOI 10.1007/978-3-319-22855-6_27

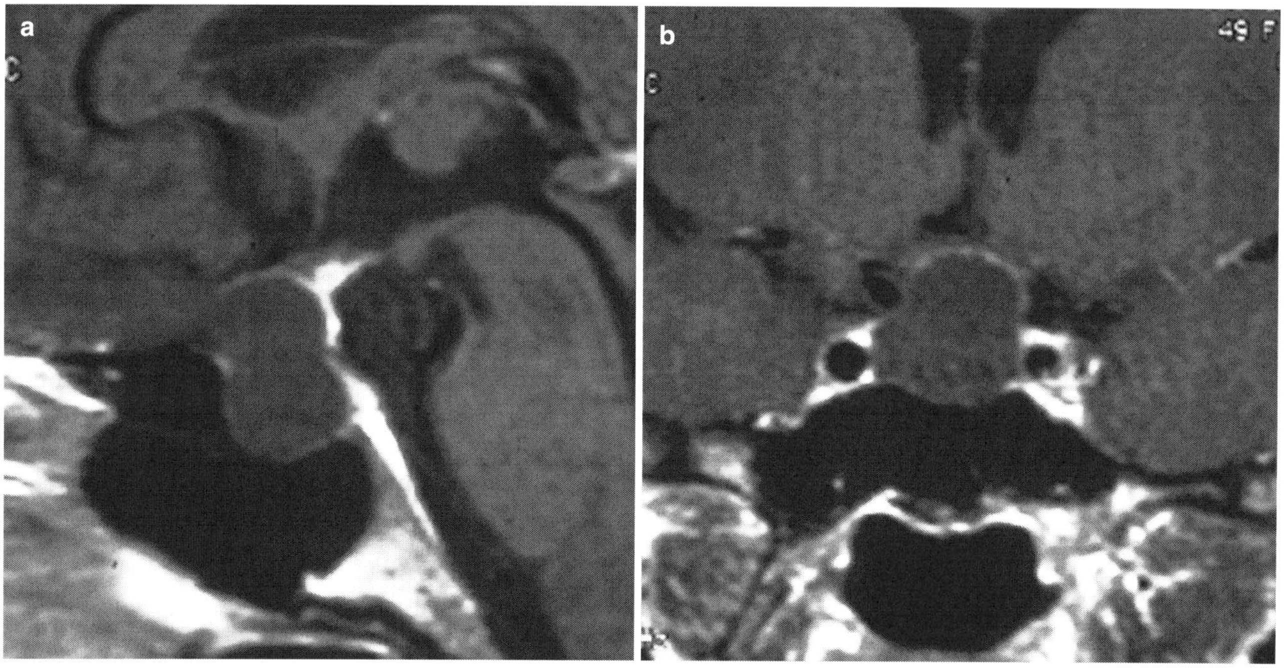

Fig. 27.1 Colloid cyst. (**a**) Sagittal T1-weighted post-gadolinium image. (**b**) Coronal T1-weighted post-gadolinium image. A lobular cyst with a thin rim of enhancement is centered in the sella, with suprasellar extension. The sellar floor is remodeled. The optic chiasm appears to be elevated by the cyst

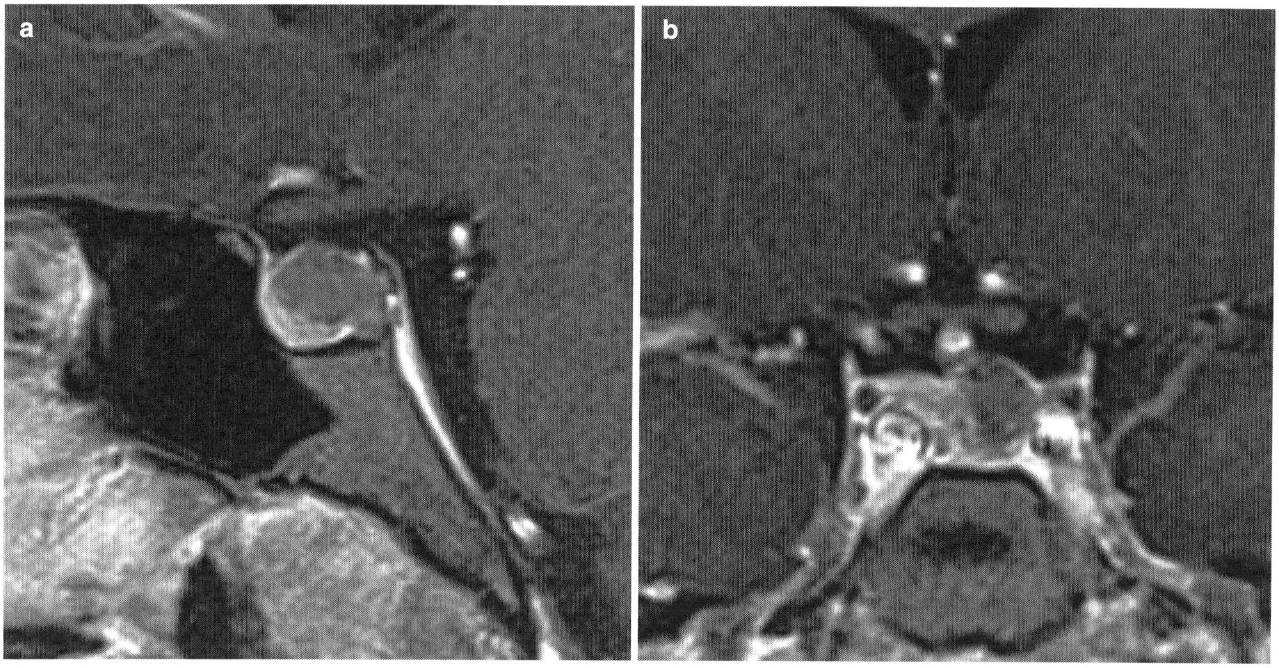

Fig. 27.2 Colloid cyst. (**a**) Sagittal T1-weighted post-gadolinium image. (**b**) Coronal T1-weighted post-gadolinium image. A slightly hyperintense cyst is centered in the left sella, displacing the normal pituitary tissue to the left. The sellar floor is expanded

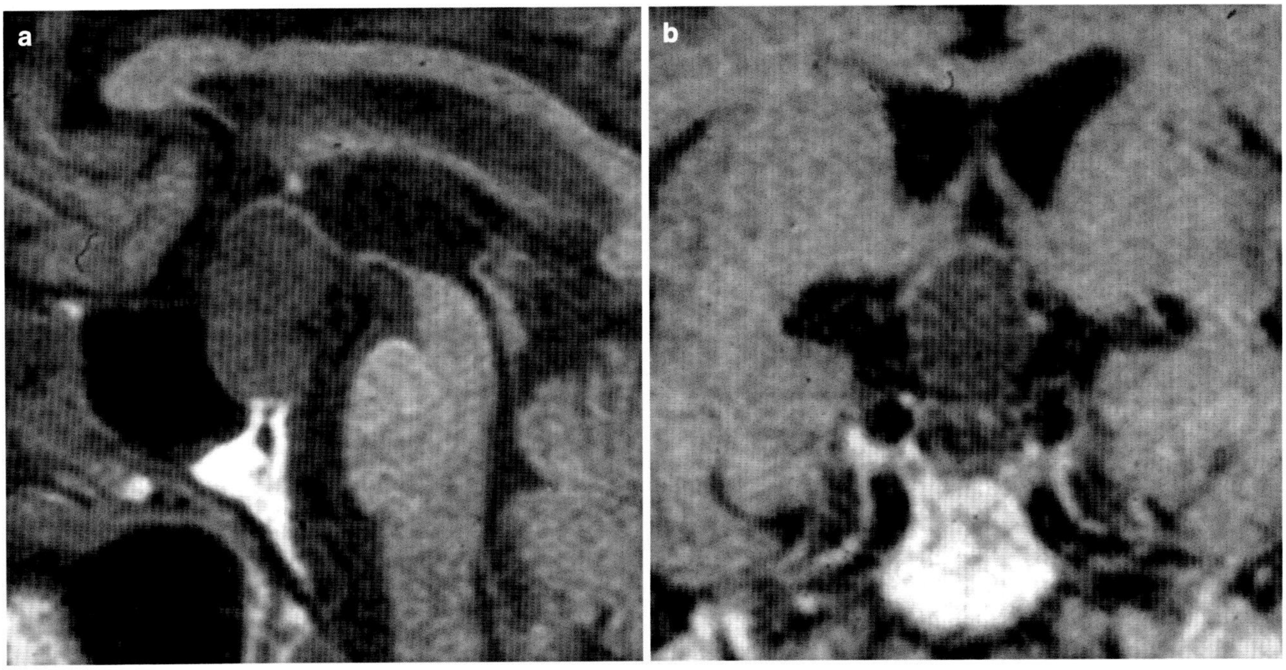

Fig. 27.3 Colloid cyst. (**a**) Sagittal T1-weighted nonenhanced image. (**b**) Coronal T1-weighted nonenhanced image. A lobular cyst with a thin rim of enhancement is centered in the sella, with suprasellar extension. The sellar floor is remodeled. The optic chiasm appears to be elevated by the cyst

27.3 Histopathology

- Colloid cysts are typically filled with a whitish or yellowish, relatively thick, colloid (mucopolysaccharide) substance. Areas of old hemorrhage and cholesterol accumulation may give the contents of the cyst a denser consistency.
- There may be a dense, calcified component within the cyst.
- Histologically, colloid cysts are lined by a single layer of cuboidal or columnar epithelium with interspersed ciliated and goblet cells (Fig. 27.4).
- Colloid cysts are often indistinguishable from RCCs; many consider them the same entity [6].

27.4 Clinical Management

- Transsphenoidal surgical resection is recommended for symptomatic colloid cysts of the pituitary region.
- Improvement in headaches, visual dysfunction, and reversal of pituitary axis deficiencies have been reported in most patients following resection [4].

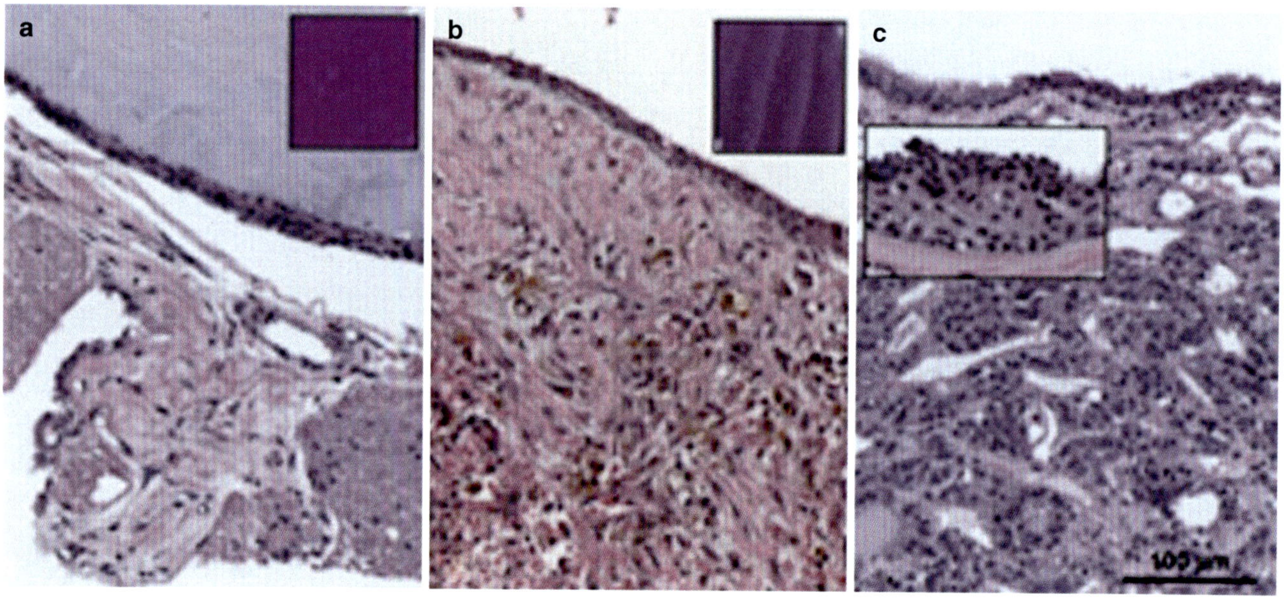

Fig. 27.4 Histology of colloid cysts and Rathke's cleft cyst (RCC). (**a**) Cyst wall of a colloid cyst of the third ventricle. (**b**) Cyst wall of a colloid cyst with partially ciliated cells and numerous siderophages in the cyst wall. (**c**) RCC with numerous ciliated cells. *Insets* show colloidal cyst contents (**a**, **b**) and focal squamous metaplasia (**c**) (original magnification ×200; insets ×400. H&E staining; insets *A* and *B* show periodic acid–Schiff staining) (Adapted from Bender et al. [5], with permission)

References

1. Saeger W, Ludecke DK, Buchfelder M, Fahlbusch R, Quabbe HJ, Petersenn S. Pathohistological classification of pituitary tumors: 10 years of experience with the German Pituitary Tumor Registry. Eur J Endocrinol. 2007;156:203–16.
2. Bladowska J, Bednarek-Tupikowska G, Biel A, Sasiadek M. Colloid cyst of the pituitary gland: case report and literature review. Pol J Radiol. 2010;75:88–93.
3. Clarke PR, Rowbotham GF. Colloid cyst of the pituitary gland causing chiasmal compression. Br J Surg. 1956;44:107–8.
4. Nomikos P, Buchfelder M, Fahlbusch R. Intra- and suprasellar colloid cysts. Pituitary. 1999;2:123–6.
5. Bender B, Honegger JB, Beschorner R, Ernemann U, Horger M. MR imaging findings in colloid cysts of the sellar region: comparison with colloid cysts of the third ventricle and Rathke's cleft cysts. Acad Radiol. 2013;20:1457–65.
6. Lach B, Scheithauer BW, Gregor A, Wick MR. Colloid cyst of the third ventricle. A comparative immunohistochemical study of neuraxis cysts and choroid plexus epithelium. J Neurosurg. 1993;78:101–11.

Part VI

Other Neoplasms of the Anterior Skull Base, Sellar, and Parasellar Regions

Meningioma of the Sellar and Parasellar Region

28

Gabriel Zada, M. Beatriz S. Lopes,
Srinivasan Mukundan Jr., and Edward Laws Jr.

28.1 Epidemiology and Clinical Presentation

- Meningiomas are commonly occurring extra-axial lesions originating from the arachnoid cap cells of the dura.
- They are typically benign, slow-growing lesions that present secondary to mass effect on surrounding structures.
- Meningiomas in the sellar and parasellar region may arise from any point along the dural skull base, including the tuberculum sellae, planum sphenoidale, anterior or clinoid processes, sphenoid wing, cavernous sinuses, petroclival region, diaphragma sellae, or clivus.
- Meningiomas typically comprise 1–3 % of sellar lesions resected in major transsphenoidal series [1, 2]. Purely intrasellar meningiomas are quite uncommon and may present with hypopituitarism, headache, and visual loss [3, 4]. Most purely intrasellar meningiomas arise from inferior leaves of the diaphragma sellae [5, 6].
- Meningiomas of the sellar region may present with headache, visual loss, hypopituitarism, cranial nerve paresis, proptosis, hydrocephalus, or any combination of these conditions.
- Tuberculum sellae meningiomas frequently present with visual loss, causing a bilateral superior quadrantanopsia that gradually evolves into a full bitemporal hemianopsia.
- Presentation of intrasellar meningioma mimicking pituitary apoplexy has been reported [7, 8].

28.2 Imaging Features

- Meningiomas are dural-based, often homogenously enhancing lesions that are noted to arise from the skull base (Figs. 28.1, 28.2, 28.3, 28.4, 28.5, 28.6, 28.7, 28.8, 28.9, 28.10, and 28.11).
- They may demonstrate varying patterns of intensity on T2-weighted imaging, based on the protein and water content of the tumor.
- Diaphragma sellae or tuberculum sellae meningiomas often mimic imaging features of a pituitary macroadenoma [5, 9, 10].
- Several features may help differentiate sellar meningioma from pituitary macroadenoma [5]:
  - Bright, homogeneous enhancement seen with meningioma.
  - A suprasellar rather than intrasellar tumor epicenter.
  - A dural tail sign seen with meningiomas.
  - Distinct pituitary gland with variable enhancement seen inferior to the tumor and diaphragma sellae in some cases.
  - Meningiomas may cause stenosis of the cavernous internal carotid artery, whereas pituitary adenomas rarely do so.

G. Zada, MD, MS (✉)
Department of Neurological Surgery, Keck School of Medicine, University of Southern California, 1200 N State Street, #3300, Los Angeles, CA 90033, USA
e-mail: gzada@usc.edu

M.B.S. Lopes, MD, PhD
Department of Pathology (Neuropathology), University of Virginia School of Medicine, 1215 Lee Street, Room 3060–HEP, Charlottesville, VA 22908, USA
e-mail: msl2e@virginia.edu

S. Mukundan Jr., PhD, MD
Department of Radiology, Brigham and Women's Hospital, 75 Francis Street, Boston, MA 02115, USA
e-mail: smukundan@partners.org

E. Laws Jr., MD
Department of Neurosurgery, Brigham and Women's Hospital, 15 Francis Street, Boston, MA 02115, USA
e-mail: elaws@partners.org

G. Zada et al. (eds.), *Atlas of Sellar and Parasellar Lesions: Clinical, Radiologic, and Pathologic Correlations*, DOI 10.1007/978-3-319-22855-6_28

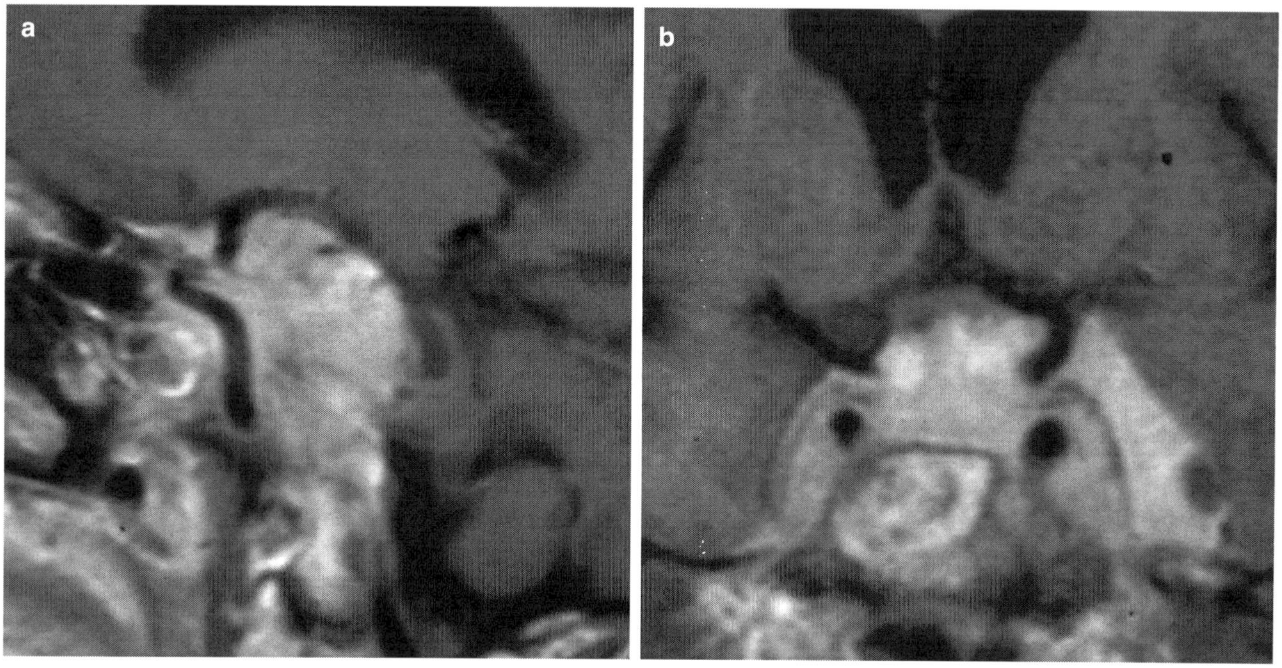

Fig. 28.1 Meningioma. (**a**) Sagittal T1-weighted gadolinium-enhanced image. (**b**) Coronal T1-weighted gadolinium-enhanced image. A large, enhancing mass is centered in the left parasellar region, with involvement of the sella. The pituitary gland is not visualized

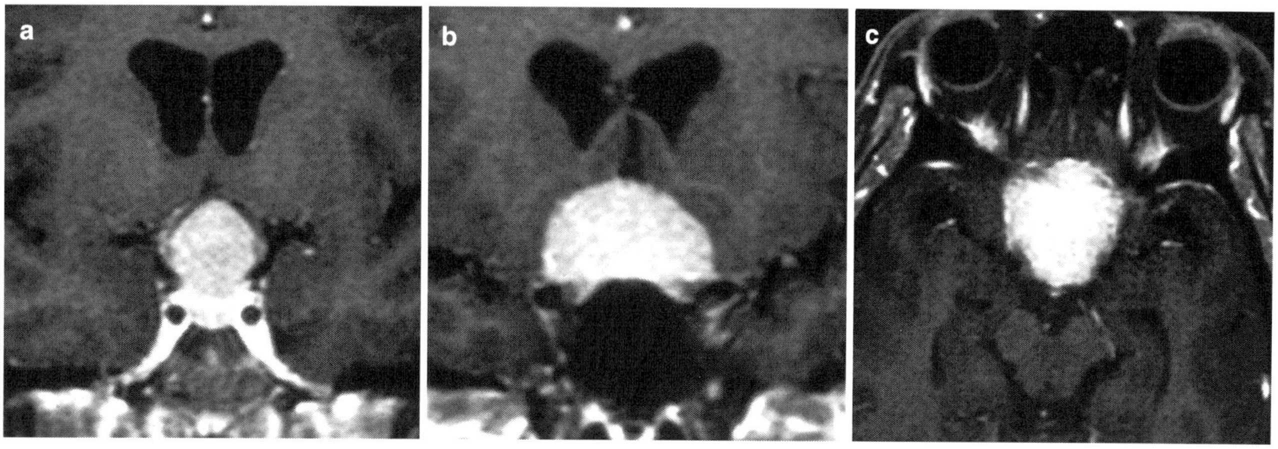

Fig. 28.2 Meningioma. (**a**, **b**) Coronal T1-weighted gadolinium-enhanced images. (**c**) Axial T1-weighted gadolinium-enhanced image. There is an enhancing mass centered in the planum sphenoidale extending to the anterior sella

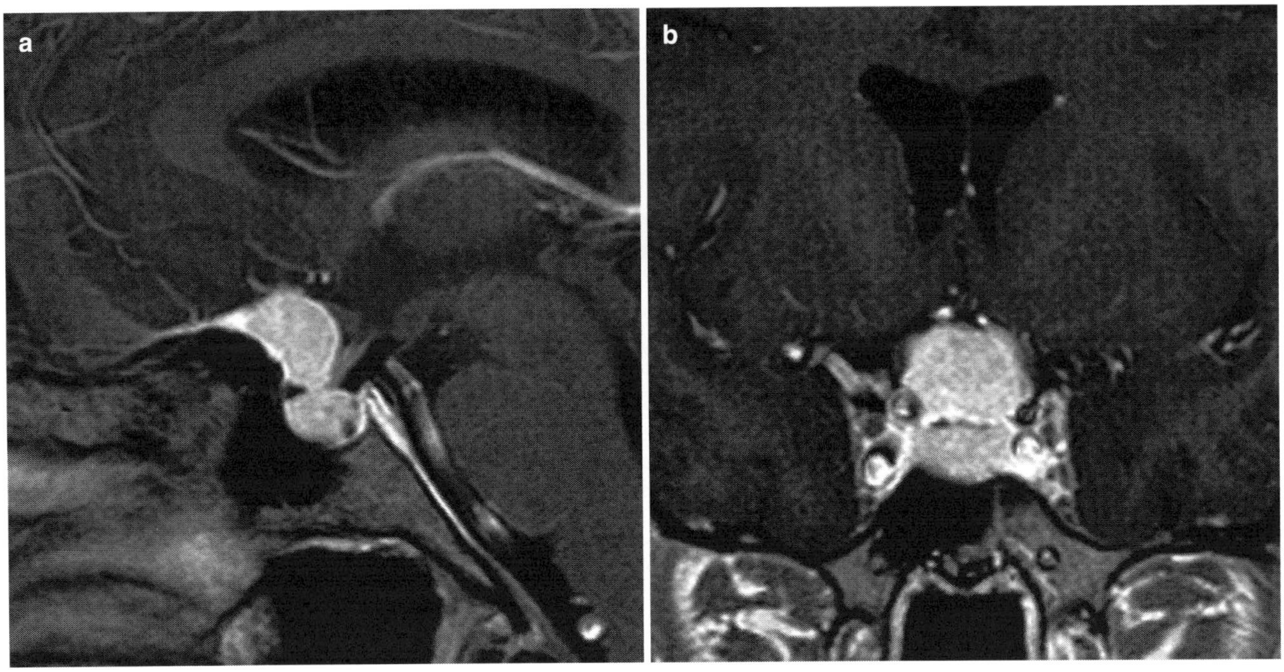

Fig. 28.3 Tuberculum sellae meningioma. (**a**) Sagittal T1-weighted gadolinium-enhanced image. (**b**) Coronal T1-weighted gadolinium-enhanced image. A dural-based enhancing mass is centered in the planum sphenoidale, extending to the anterior sella. The mass is above the pituitary gland and anterior to the pituitary stalk. The mass abuts bilateral cavernous internal carotid arteries without encasement

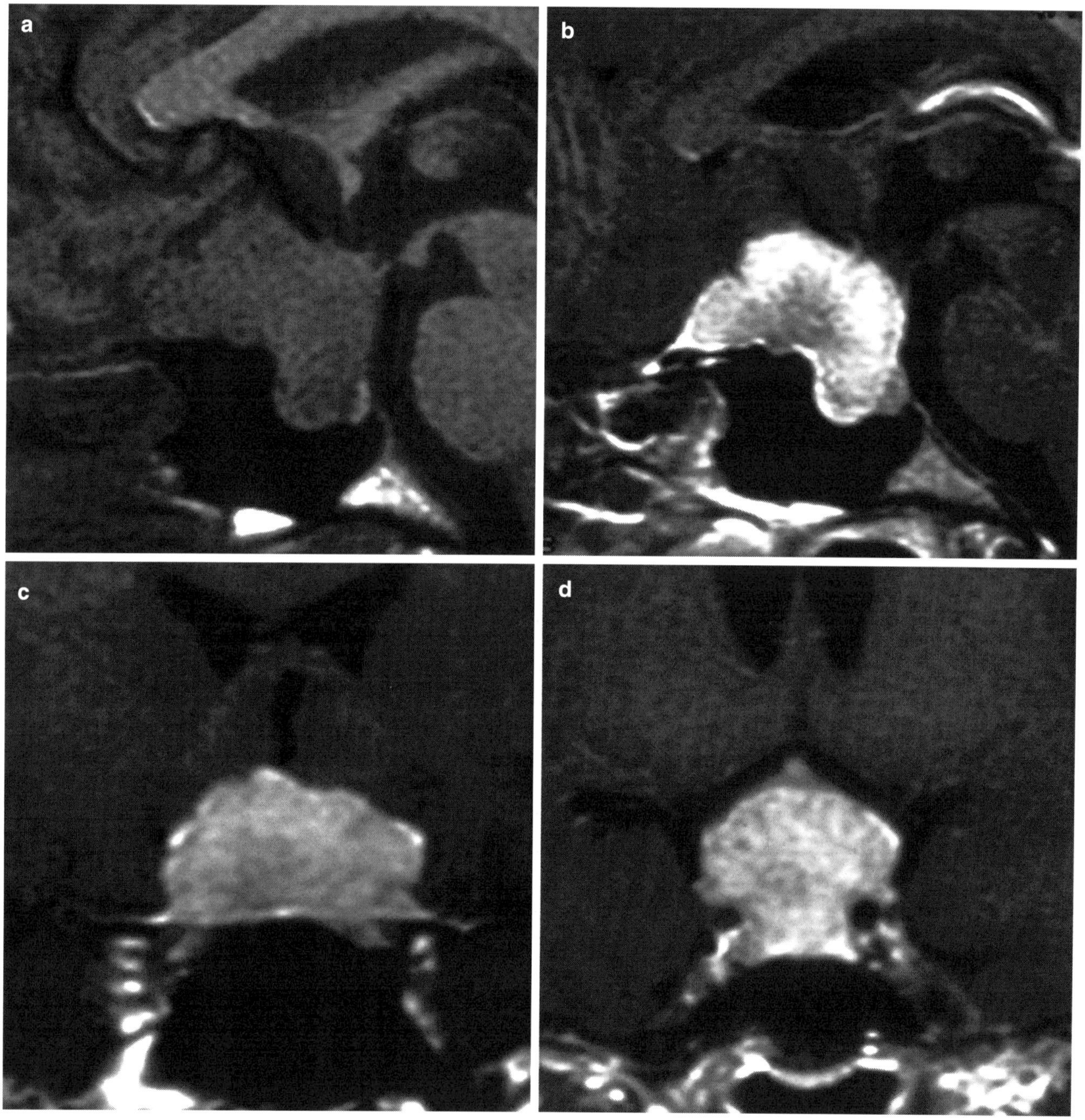

Fig. 28.4 Meningioma. (**a**) Sagittal T1-weighted precontrast image. (**b**) Sagittal T1-weighted gadolinium-enhanced image. (**c, d**) Coronal T1-weighted gadolinium-enhanced images. A dural-based enhancing mass is centered in the planum sphenoidale, extending to the anterior sella. The mass is above the pituitary gland, which is flattened against the sellar floor. The mass surrounds bilateral cavernous internal carotid arteries

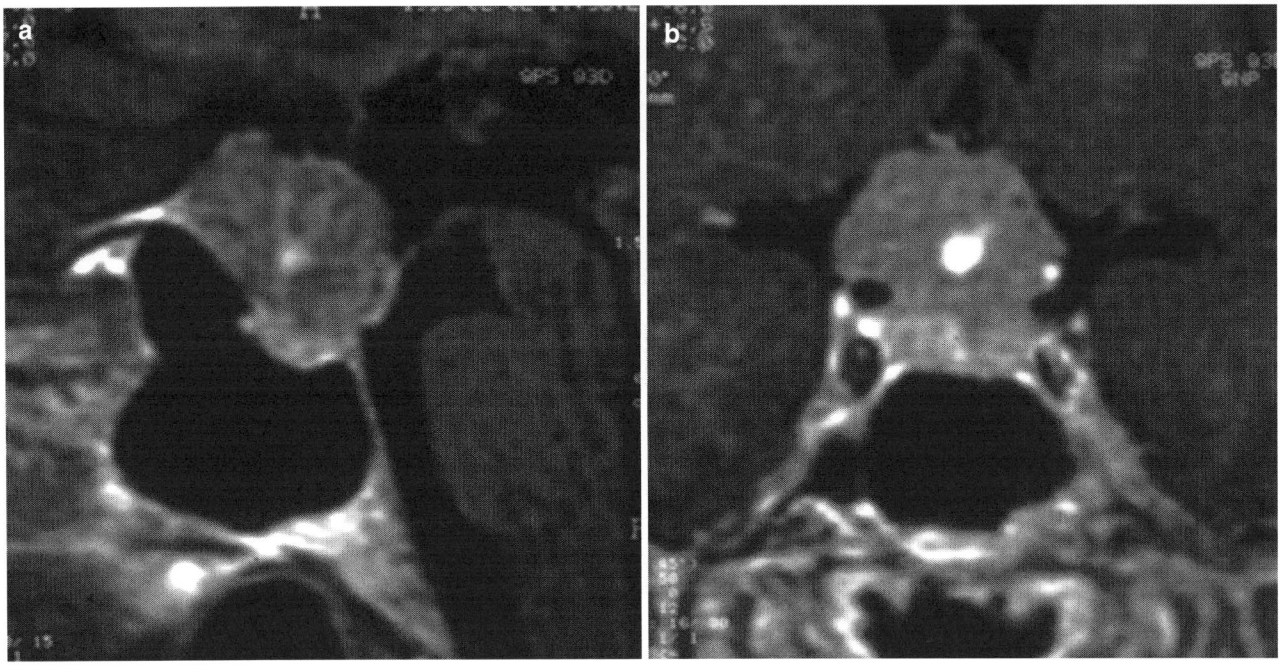

Fig. 28.5 Meningioma. (**a**) Sagittal T1-weighted gadolinium-enhanced image. (**b**) Coronal T1-weighted gadolinium-enhanced image. A heterogeneously enhancing mass is located in the suprasellar region, with a dural tail in the planum sphenoidale. The mass is above the pituitary gland. The mass surrounds the right cavernous internal carotid artery

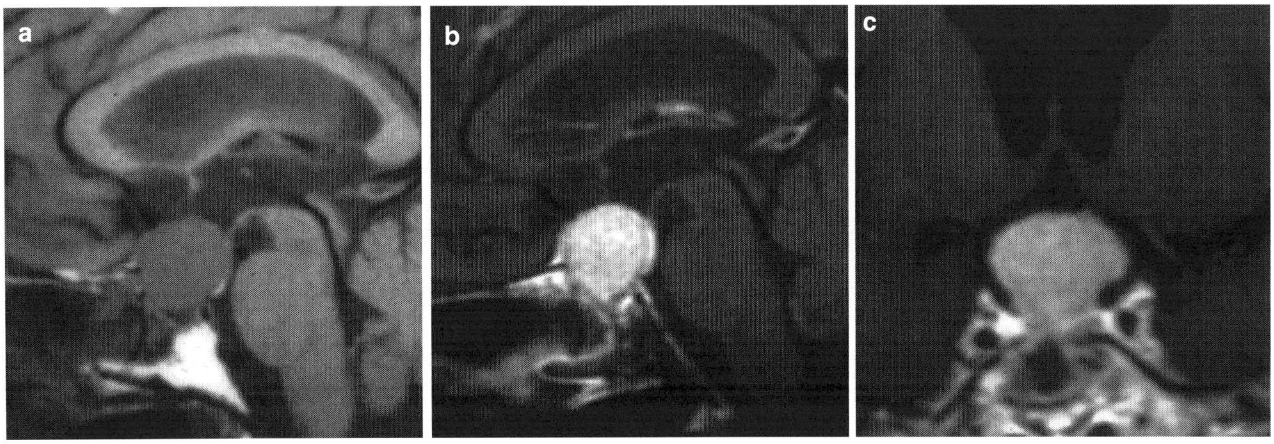

Fig. 28.6 Meningioma. (**a**) Sagittal T1-weighted precontrast image. (**b**) Sagittal T1-weighted gadolinium-enhanced image. (**c**) Coronal T1-weighted gadolinium-enhanced image. There is an enhancing mass centered in the suprasellar region, with a dural tail in the planum sphenoidale. The pituitary gland is not well visualized. The mass abuts the cavernous internal carotid arteries bilaterally

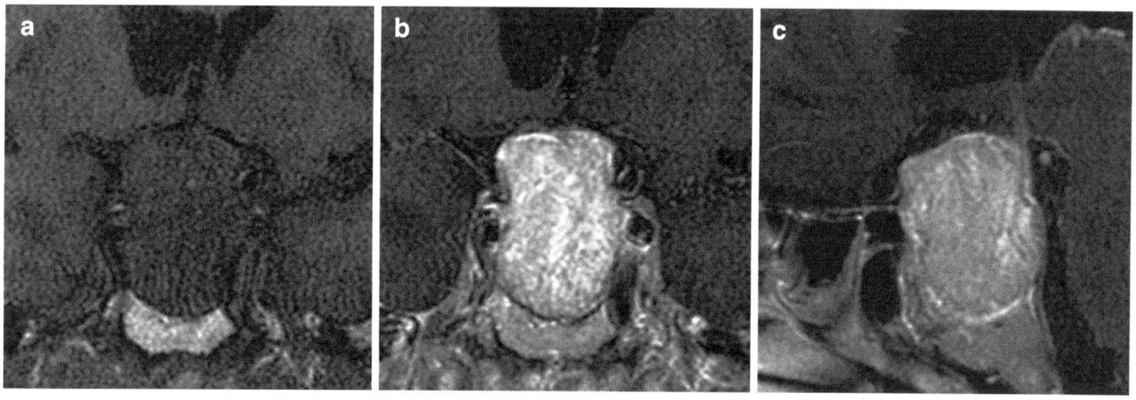

Fig. 28.7 Meningioma. (**a**) Coronal T1-weighted precontrast image. (**b**) Coronal T1-weighted gadolinium-enhanced image. (**c**) Sagittal T1-weighted gadolinium-enhanced image. A heterogeneously enhancing mass is centered in the sella and the suprasellar regions. The pituitary gland is not well visualized, and the sellar floor appears eroded. Superiorly, the mass elevates the optic chiasm

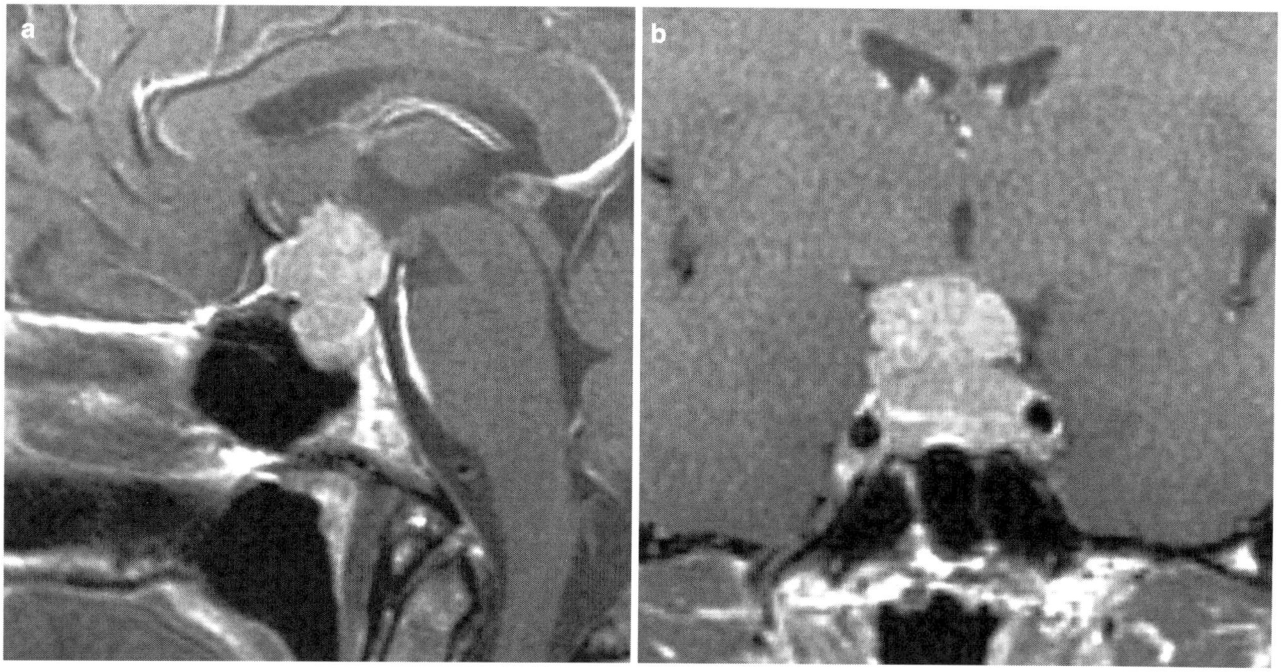

Fig. 28.8 Diaphragma of sellae meningioma. (**a**) Sagittal T1-weighted gadolinium-enhanced image. (**b**) Coronal T1-weighted gadolinium-enhanced image. An enhancing mass is centered in the sella/suprasellar region. There is a small dural attachment at the planum sphenoidale. The pituitary gland is not well visualized. The mass surrounds the right cavernous internal carotid artery

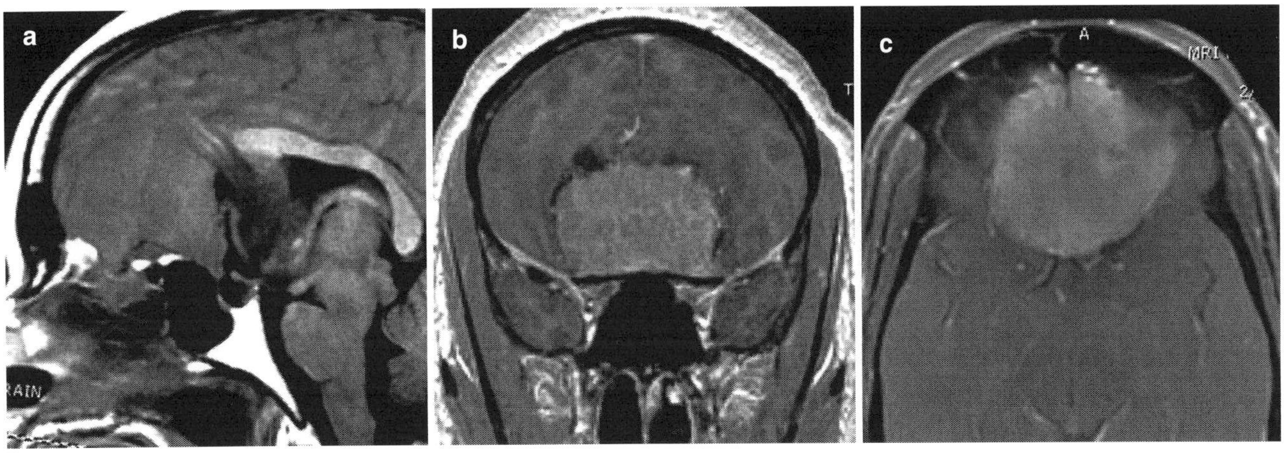

Fig. 28.9 Meningioma. (**a**) Sagittal T1-weighted precontrast image. (**b**) Coronal T1-weighted gadolinium-enhanced image. (**c**) Axial T1-weighted gadolinium-enhanced image. There is a large, enhancing mass arising from the olfactory groove and planum sphenoidale, compressing the frontal lobes. The pituitary gland is separate from the mass

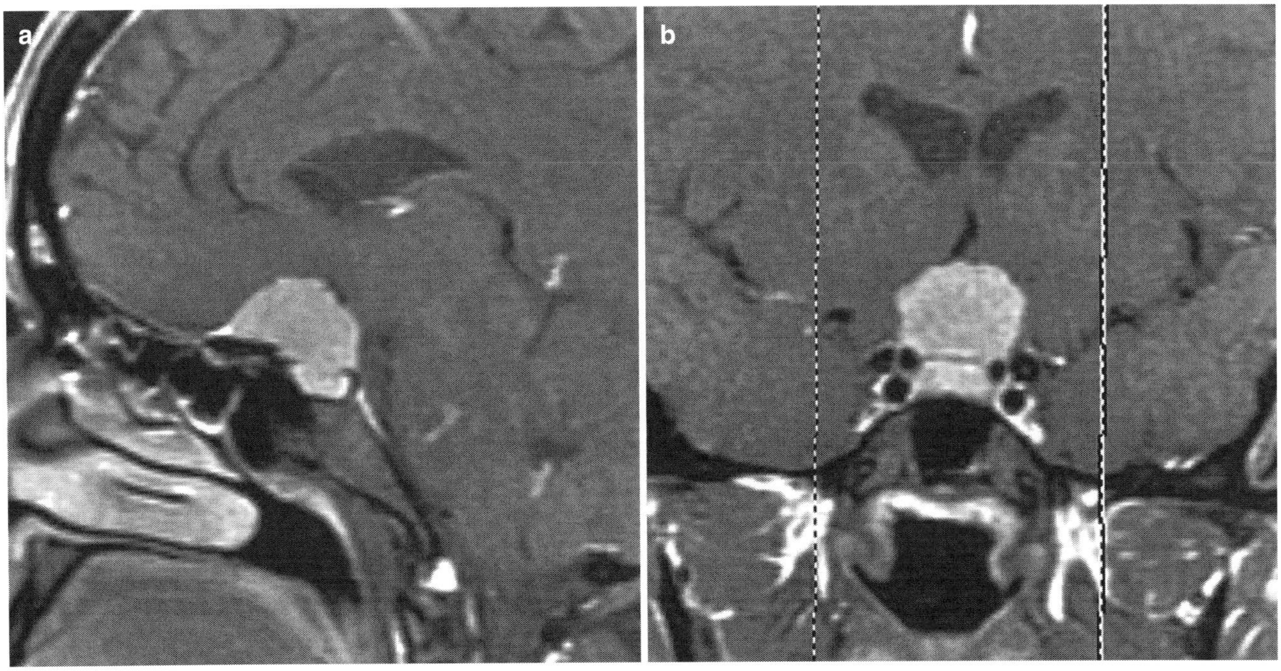

Fig. 28.10 Meningioma. (**a**) Sagittal T1-weighted gadolinium-enhanced image. (**b**) Coronal T1-weighted gadolinium-enhanced image. An enhancing mass in the planum sphenoidale extends to the anterior sella. The pituitary gland is seen in the inferior aspect of the sella, immediately inferior to the mass

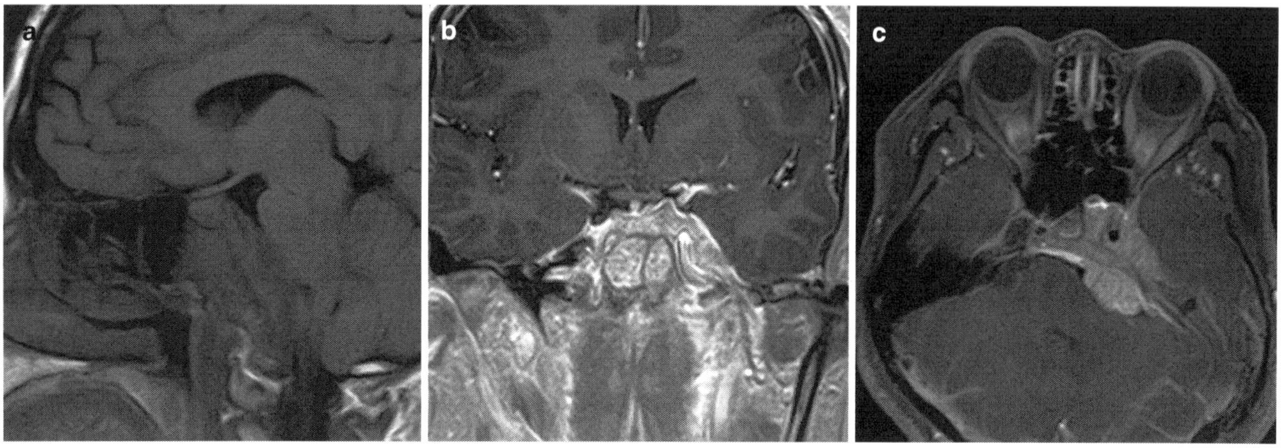

Fig. 28.11 Meningioma. (**a**) Sagittal T1-weighted precontrast image. (**b**) Coronal T1-weighted gadolinium-enhanced image. (**c**) Axial T1-weighted gadolinium-enhanced image with fat saturation. An enhancing mass is seen in the left sphenoid-clival ligament, with components in both left middle cranial fossae involving the cavernous sinus, as well as in the prepontine region, mildly effacing the pons. The mass likely encases the left cavernous internal carotid artery, but flow void (**c**) indicates that it remains patent

28.3 Histopathology

- Meningiomas are typically benign lesions with meningothelial, fibroblastic, or mixed components. Meningothelial whorls and psammoma bodies are common (Fig. 28.12).
- The World Health Organization (WHO) classifies meningiomas as benign (WHO I), atypical (WHO II), or anaplastic/malignant (WHO III). Atypical and anaplastic meningiomas are aggressive subtypes with a higher MIB-1 labeling index, mitotic features, and nuclear pleomorphism.
- WHO Grade II meningiomas are characterized by any of these parameters:
  - A mitotic index of 4 or more per 10 high-power field
  - At least three of the five following parameters:
    - Sheeting architecture (loss of whorling and/or fascicles)
    - Small cell formation (high nucleus-to-cytoplasm ratio)
    - Macronucleoli
    - Hypercellularity
    - Spontaneous necrosis (i.e., not induced by embolization or radiation)
  - Brain invasion
- WHO Grade III meningiomas are characterized by a mitotic index of 20 or more per high-power field and/or frank anaplasia (sarcoma-, carcinoma-, or melanoma-like histology).

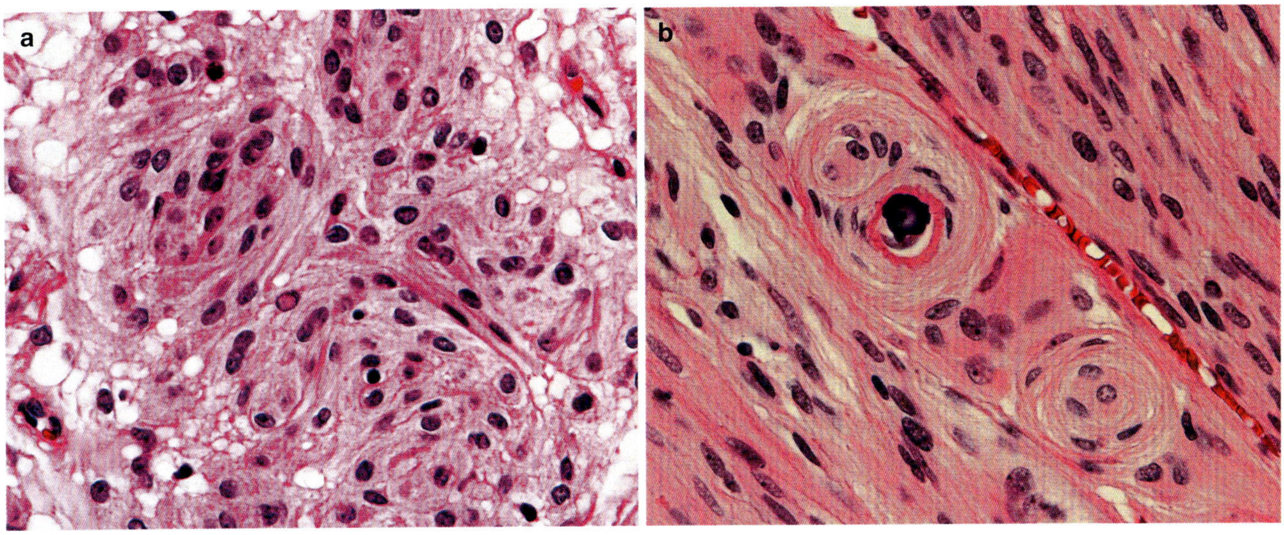

Fig. 28.12 Meningioma. Similar to meningiomas arising in any portion of the CNS, sellar tumors may exhibit a variety of meningioma subtypes. (**a**) A meningothelial meningioma shows well-differentiated cells with prominent syncytial arrangements; note the characteristic intranuclear pseudoinclusion. (**b**) A transitional meningioma is composed of elongated spindle cells arranged in fascicles side-by-side with well-formed meningothelial whorls and psammoma bodies

28.4 Clinical and Surgical Management

- The surgical approach is frequently dictated by the relationship of the tumor to the neurovascular structures of the sellar and parasellar region, particularly the optic nerves and chiasm, carotid arteries, and pituitary gland and stalk. The position of the optic chiasm relative to the tuberculum sellae (pre-fixed or post-fixed optic chiasm) often plays a major role in the selection of the approach [11].
- Microscopic analysis has shown that meningiomas frequently demonstrate evidence of microinvasion of the cranial nerves and carotid artery wall, making a gross total resection unsafe (if not impossible) in some cases [12, 13].
- The main goals of surgery are complete tumor resection (when possible), surgical cytoreduction, preservation of visual function, and preservation of pituitary function.
- Meningiomas are frequently firm and vascular lesions. Preoperative arterial embolization of tumor feeders may be warranted if the diagnosis is established ahead of time [3].
- Optimal patient selection remains paramount in dictating the preferred surgical approach and improving patient outcomes [14, 15].
- Open craniotomy remains the gold-standard approach for many sellar-region meningiomas [14, 16, 17]. Transcranial approaches such as a pterional, orbitozygomatic, or supraorbital/subfrontal approaches have typically been used to access the sellar region and anterior skull base.
- Over the past several decades, extended transsphenoidal approaches have been utilized with good results for the resection of selected skull base meningiomas, especially for intrasellar meningiomas [1, 18–21].
- Extended endoscopic skull base approaches have been reported with acceptable outcomes over the past decade, but extensive skull base reconstruction may be required following tumor removal [22–24].
- For large or giant meningiomas, optimal tumor debulking may require a combination of surgical approaches to achieve a safe and maximal resection [3].
- Preoperative tumor embolization may be beneficial in selected patients and may reduce operative blood loss and the requirement for blood transfusions. The complication rate associated with preoperative embolization is 3–4 % [25].

28.4.1 Radiotherapy and Radiosurgery

- Surgical debulking with postoperative stereotactic radiosurgery has become a widely accepted paradigm of management for many skull base meningiomas, especially those with cavernous sinus invasion.
- Single-fraction radiosurgery offers excellent rates (>90 %) of long-term tumor control for residual skull base meningiomas with minimal complications, but it is generally limited to lesions that are more than 3–5 mm from the optic apparatus [26–28].
- The dose depends on the tumor volume and proximity to the optic apparatus and pituitary gland; typical doses for single-fraction radiosurgery are 14–16 Gy delivered to the 50 % isodose line.
- Fractionated stereotactic radiosurgery has been used to treat perioptic lesions that are closer to the optic nerve and chiasm, with excellent rates of tumor control and a very low incidence of visual loss [29].

28.4.2 Clinical Follow-up and Further Treatment

- Recurrences may occur more than a decade after surgery with adjunctive radiation, mandating long-term radiological surveillance.
- Refractory or multiply recurrent meningiomas not amenable to further resection or radiation-based interventions (especially atypical or anaplastic meningiomas) have been treated with somatostatin analogs, hydroxyurea, temozolomide, or interferon-α, with varying and usually disappointing results [30, 31, 32].

References

1. Fatemi N, Dusick JR, de Paiva Neto MA, Kelly DF. The endonasal microscopic approach for pituitary adenomas and other parasellar tumors: a 10-year experience. Neurosurgery. 2008;63:244–56; discussion 256.
2. Saeger W, Ludecke DK, Buchfelder M, Fahlbusch R, Quabbe HJ, Petersenn S. Pathohistological classification of pituitary tumors: 10 years of experience with the German Pituitary Tumor Registry. Eur J Endocrinol. 2007;156:203–16.
3. Nozaki K, Nagata I, Yoshida K, Kikuchi H. Intrasellar meningioma: case report and review of the literature. Surg Neurol. 1997;47:447–52; discussion 452–4.
4. Grisoli F, Vincentelli F, Raybaud C, Harter M, Guibout M, Baldini M. Intrasellar meningioma. Surg Neurol. 1983;20:36–41.
5. Taylor SL, Barakos JA, Harsh GR, Wilson CB. Magnetic resonance imaging of tuberculum sellae meningiomas: preventing preoperative misdiagnosis as pituitary macroadenoma. Neurosurgery. 1992;31:621–7; discussion 627.
6. Kinjo T, Al-Mefty O, Ciric I. Diaphragma sellae meningiomas. Neurosurgery. 1995;36:1082–92.
7. Orakdogeny M, Karadereler S, Berkman Z, Ersahin M, Ozdogan C, Aker F. Intra-suprasellar meningioma mimicking pituitary apoplexy. Acta Neurochir (Wien). 2004;146:511–5.
8. Kudo H, Takaishi Y, Minami H, Takamoto T, Kitazawa S, Maeda S, Tamaki N. Intrasellar meningioma mimicking pituitary apoplexy: case report. Surg Neurol. 1997;48:374–81.
9. Michael AS, Paige ML. MR imaging of intrasellar meningiomas simulating pituitary adenomas. J Comput Assist Tomogr. 1988;12:944–6.
10. Abe T, Matsumoto K, Homma H, Kawamura N, Iwata T, Nemoto S. Dorsum sellae meningioma mimicking pituitary macroadenoma: case report. Surg Neurol. 1999;51:543–6; discussion 546–7.

11. Rhoton Jr AL. The sellar region. Neurosurgery. 2002;51:S335–74.
12. Larson JJ, van Loveren HR, Balko MG, Tew Jr JM. Evidence of meningioma infiltration into cranial nerves: clinical implications for cavernous sinus meningiomas. J Neurosurg. 1995;83:596–9.
13. Sen C, Hague K. Meningiomas involving the cavernous sinus: histological factors affecting the degree of resection. J Neurosurg. 1997;87:535–43.
14. de Divitiis E, Esposito F, Cappabianca P, Cavallo LM, de Divitiis O. Tuberculum sellae meningiomas: high route or low route? A series of 51 consecutive cases. Neurosurgery. 2008;62:556–63.
15. Zada G, Du R, Laws Jr ER. Defining the "edge of the envelope": patient selection in treating complex sellar-based neoplasms via transsphenoidal versus open craniotomy. J Neurosurg. 2011;114:286–300.
16. Mathiesen T, Kihlstrom L. Visual outcome of tuberculum sellae meningiomas after extradural optic nerve decompression. Neurosurgery. 2006;59:570–6.
17. Fahlbusch R, Schott W. Pterional surgery of meningiomas of the tuberculum sellae and planum sphenoidale: surgical results with special consideration of ophthalmological and endocrinological outcomes. J Neurosurg. 2002;96:235–43.
18. Couldwell WT, Weiss MH, Rabb C, Liu JK, Apfelbaum RI, Fukushima T. Variations on the standard transsphenoidal approach to the sellar region, with emphasis on the extended approaches and parasellar approaches: surgical experience in 105 cases. Neurosurgery. 2004;55:539–47; discussion 547–50.
19. Honegger J, Fahlbusch R, Buchfelder M, Huk WJ, Thierauf P. The role of transsphenoidal microsurgery in the management of sellar and parasellar meningioma. Surg Neurol. 1993;39:18–24.
20. Kitano M, Taneda M, Nakao Y. Postoperative improvement in visual function in patients with tuberculum sellae meningiomas: results of the extended transsphenoidal and transcranial approaches. J Neurosurg. 2007;107:337–46.
21. Kaptain GJ, Vincent DA, Sheehan JP, Laws Jr ER. Transsphenoidal approaches for the extracapsular resection of midline suprasellar and anterior cranial base lesions. Neurosurgery. 2001;49:94–100; discussion 100–1.
22. Schwartz TH, Fraser JF, Brown S, Tabaee A, Kacker A, Anand VK. Endoscopic cranial base surgery: classification of operative approaches. Neurosurgery. 2008;62:991–1002; discussion 1002–5.
23. Gardner PA, Kassam AB, Thomas A, Snyderman CH, Carrau RL, Mintz AH, Prevedello DM. Endoscopic endonasal resection of anterior cranial base meningiomas. Neurosurgery. 2008;63:36–52; discussion 52–4.
24. de Divitiis E, Cavallo LM, Esposito F, Stella L, Messina A. Extended endoscopic transsphenoidal approach for tuberculum sellae meningiomas. Neurosurgery. 2008;62:1192–201.
25. Borg A, Ekanayake J, Mair R, Smedley T, Brew S, Kitchen N, et al. Preoperative particle and glue embolization of meningiomas: indications, results and lessons learned from 117 consecutive patients. Neurosurgery. 2013;73:ons244–51; discussion ons252.
26. Hasegawa T, Kida Y, Yoshimoto M, Koike J, Iizuka H, Ishii D. Long-term outcomes of Gamma Knife surgery for cavernous sinus meningioma. J Neurosurg. 2007;107:745–51.
27. Kuo JS, Chen JC, Yu C, Zelman V, Giannotta SL, Petrovich Z, et al. Gamma knife radiosurgery for benign cavernous sinus tumors: quantitative analysis of treatment outcomes. Neurosurgery. 2004;54:1385–93; discussion 1393–4.
28. Zada G, Pagnini PG, Yu C, Erickson KT, Hirschbein J, Zelman V, Apuzzo ML. Long-term outcomes and patterns of tumor progression after gamma knife radiosurgery for benign meningiomas. Neurosurgery. 2010;67:322–8; discussion 328–9.
29. Pham CJ, Chang SD, Gibbs IC, Jones P, Heilbrun MP, Adler Jr JR. Preliminary visual field preservation after staged CyberKnife radiosurgery for perioptic lesions. Neurosurgery. 2004;54:799–810; discussion 810–2.
30. Chamberlain MC. The role of chemotherapy and targeted therapy in the treatment of intracranial meningioma. Curr Opin Oncol. 2012;24:666–71.
31. Chamberlain MC, Tsao-Wei DD, Groshen S. Temozolomide for treatment-resistant recurrent meningioma. Neurology. 2004;62:1210–2.
32. Muazzam A. Recent developments in chemotherapy for meningiomas: A Review. Neurosurg Focus 2013;35(6):E18.

Hemangiopericytoma

29

Gabriel Zada, M. Beatriz S. Lopes, Srinivasan Mukundan Jr., and Edward Laws Jr.

29.1 Epidemiology and Clinical Presentation

- Hemangiopericytoma (HPC) is a relatively uncommon tumor of the anterior skull base and paranasal sinuses; very rarely, it arises in the sellar region [1].
- In the sellar region, HPC typically presents with symptoms and signs of local mass effect, including headaches, visual loss, and/or hypopituitarism, often mimicking a pituitary adenoma.
- More commonly, HPC may arise as a primary sinonasal tumor (5 % of HPC cases). Also known as glomangiopericytomas, these are a distinct entity but are related to HPCs. These tumors are likely to present with nasal obstruction or epistaxis [2].
- HPC typically arises in the sixth or seventh decade of life [3].

29.2 Imaging Features

- HPC of the sellar region may closely resemble pituitary adenoma on standard MR imaging [4].
- Most HPCs are larger than 4 cm in maximal diameter at the time of diagnosis.
- On CT, HPCs are typically hyperdense with heterogeneous contrast enhancement; they often show bony erosion (Fig. 29.1).
- On MR imaging, they are typically isointense to brain matter and demonstrate heterogeneous contrast enhancement. A dural tail is present in approximately half of cases [5].

G. Zada, MD, MS (✉)
Department of Neurological Surgery, Keck School of Medicine, University of Southern California, 1200 N State Street, #3300, Los Angeles, CA 90033, USA
e-mail: gzada@usc.edu

M.B.S. Lopes, MD, PhD
Department of Pathology (Neuropathology), University of Virginia School of Medicine, 1215 Lee Street, Room 3060–HEP, Charlottesville, VA 22908, USA
e-mail: msl2e@virginia.edu

S. Mukundan Jr., PhD, MD
Department of Radiology, Brigham and Women's Hospital, 75 Francis Street, Boston, MA 02115, USA
e-mail: smukundan@partners.org

E. Laws Jr., MD
Department of Neurosurgery, Brigham and Women's Hospital, 15 Francis Street, Boston, MA 02115, USA
e-mail: elaws@partners.org

G. Zada et al. (eds.), *Atlas of Sellar and Parasellar Lesions: Clinical, Radiologic, and Pathologic Correlations*, DOI 10.1007/978-3-319-22855-6_29

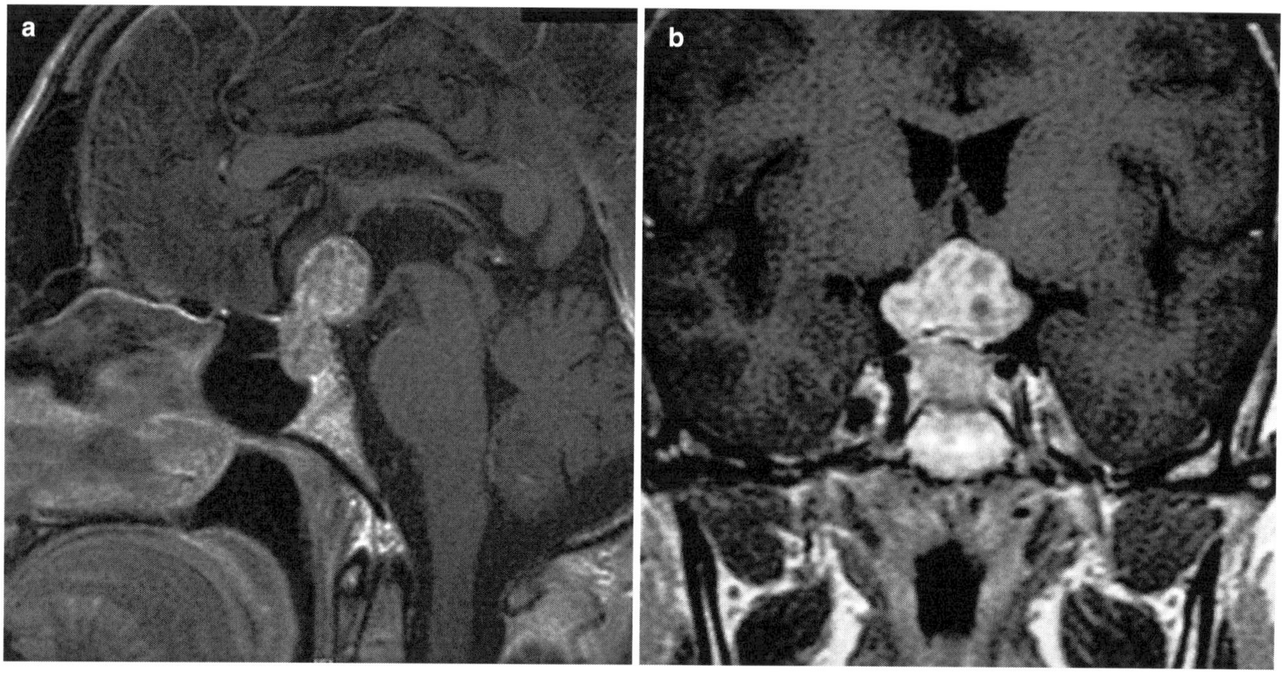

Fig. 29.1 Hemangiopericytoma. (**a**) Sagittal T1-weighted gadolinium-enhanced image. (**b**) Coronal T1-weighted gadolinium-enhanced image. An enhancing mass is seen in the sellar and suprasellar region, arising from the region of the diaphragma sellae, with compression of the optic apparatus. The pituitary gland cannot be distinguished from the mass (Adapted with permission from Jalali R et al., Acta Neurochir (Wien) (2008) 150:67–71)

29.3 Histopathology

- HPC is a mesenchymal, non-meningothelial tumor, closed related to the solitary fibrous tumor of the soft tissues [6, 7].
- HPC is histologically characterized by high cellularity, closed apposed cells with round to ovoid nuclei arranged in a haphazard pattern, and intermixed by a rich network of thin-walled branching vessels (Fig. 29.2). Limited fibrous stroma is present.
- In rare cases, malignant HPC can arise in the sellar region [8].
- Sinonasal HPC is a distinct entity characterized by a diffuse, subepithelial proliferation of bland, uniform, closely packed spindle cells. A unique vascular network composed of variably sized, staghorn-appearing vascular channels, often with perivascular hyalinization, is often observed. Most cases are immunopositive for vimentin and smooth muscle actin staining [3, 9].

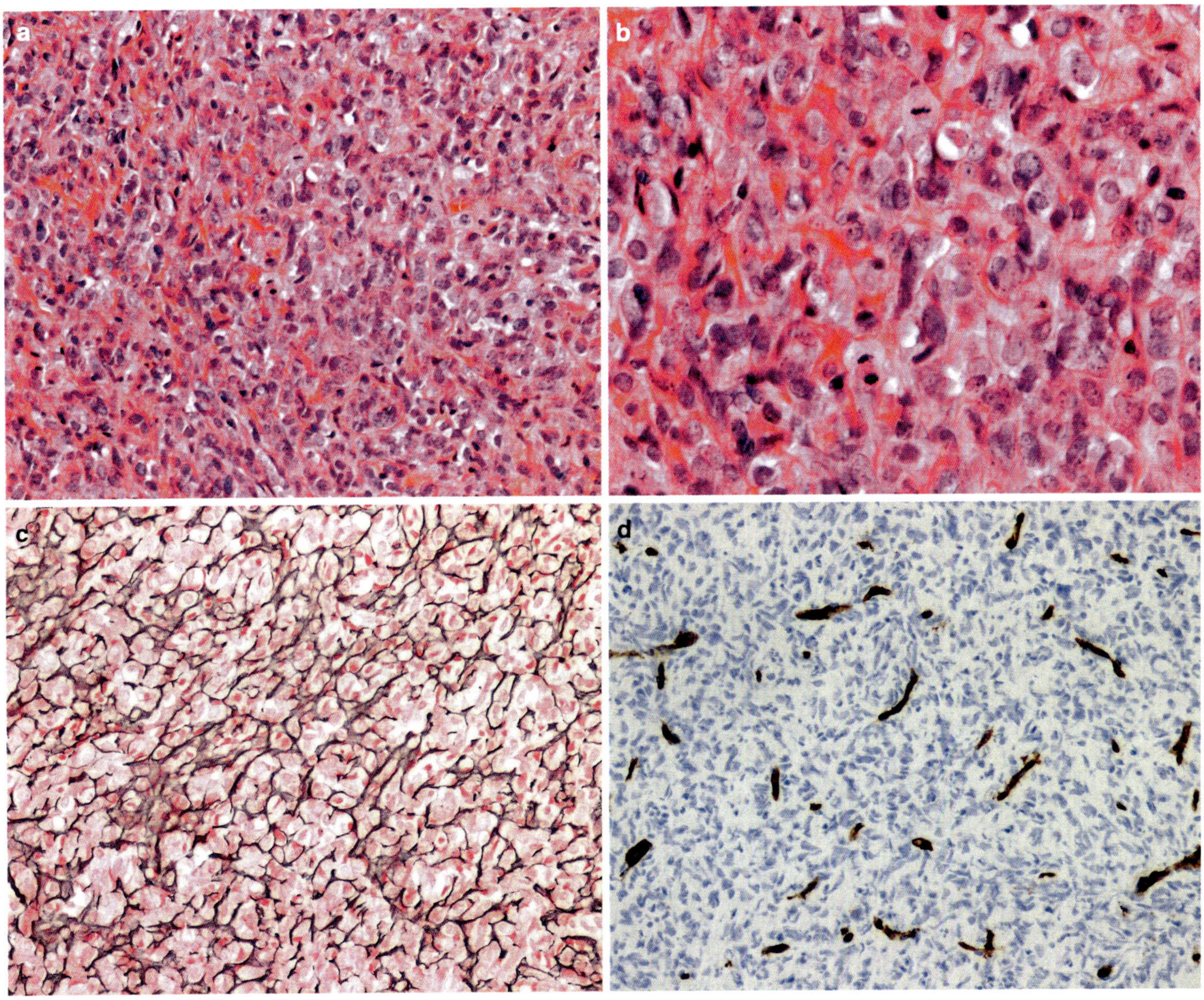

Fig. 29.2 Hemangiopericytoma. Hemangiopericytomas are hypercellular neoplasms composed of sheets of oval to spindle-shaped tumor cells with well-delineated cytoplasmic borders and oval and elongated nuclei (**a**, **b**). Mitotic activity may be obvious (**b**). A prominent network of delicate vascular clefts is seen (**a**), which is accentuated by immunoreactivity for reticulin (**c**) or endothelial cell immunomarkers like CD31 (**d**)

29.4 Clinical and Surgical Management

- The primary treatment of skull base HPC is surgical resection, followed by radiation-based treatment for any residual disease. Endoscopic endonasal resection is the preferred approach for most sinonasal and sellar region HPCs [10].
- HPC is an extremely vascular tumor. A priori knowledge of the diagnosis may offer an opportunity for preoperative embolization in selected cases.
- Recurrence is noted in up to 92 % of patients following surgical excision. Complete excision is recommended whenever possible and is known to correlate with a lower recurrence rate [3, 11, 12].
- Metastatic HPC has been reported in up to 20 % of cases.
- Stereotactic radiosurgery has demonstrated a long-term tumor control rate of 47 % [13].
- HPC is characterized by a high rate of recurrence and disease progression, mandating vigilant postoperative monitoring.

References

1. Juco J, Horvath E, Smyth H, Rotondo F, Kovacs K. Hemangiopericytoma of the sella mimicking pituitary adenoma: case report and review of the literature. Clin Neuropathol. 2007;26:288–93.
2. Hofmann V, Holzhausen HJ, Koesling S, Knipping S. Sinonasal hemangiopericytoma. Rev Laryngol Otol Rhinol (Bord). 2010;131:313–5.
3. Thompson LD, Miettinen M, Wenig BM. Sinonasal-type hemangiopericytoma: a clinicopathologic and immunophenotypic analysis of 104 cases showing perivascular myoid differentiation. Am J Surg Pathol. 2003;27:737–49.
4. Kanda Y, Mase M, Aihara N, Yamada K, Sugino F, Tateyama H. Sellar hemangiopericytoma mimicking pituitary adenoma. Surg Neurol. 2001;55:113–5.
5. Chiechi MV, Smirniotopoulos JG, Mena H. Intracranial hemangiopericytomas: MR and CT features. AJNR Am J Neuroradiol. 1996;17:1365–71.
6. Morrison DA, Bibby K. Sellar and suprasellar hemangiopericytoma mimicking pituitary adenoma. Arch Ophthalmol. 1997;115:1201–3.
7. Schirmer CM, Heilman CB. Hemangiopericytomas of the skull base. Neurosurg Focus. 2011;30, E10.
8. Das P, Haresh KP, Suri V, Sharma MC, Sharma BS, Sarkar C. Malignant hemangiopericytoma of pituitary fossa. Indian J Pathol Microbiol. 2010;53:109–11.
9. Eichhorn JH, Dickersin GR, Bhan AK, Goodman ML. Sinonasal hemangiopericytoma. A reassessment with electron microscopy, immunohistochemistry, and long-term follow-up. Am J Surg Pathol. 1990;14:856–66.
10. Tessema B, Eloy JA, Folbe AJ, Anstead AS, Mirani NM, Jourdy DN, et al. Endoscopic management of sinonasal hemangiopericytoma. Otolaryngol Head Neck Surg. 2012;146:483–6.
11. Duval M, Hwang E, Kilty SJ. Systematic review of treatment and prognosis of sinonasal hemangiopericytoma. Head Neck. 2013;35:1205–10.
12. Thiringer JK, Costantino PD, Houston G. Sinonasal hemangiopericytoma: case report and literature review. Skull Base Surg. 1995;5:185–90.
13. Olson C, Yen CP, Schlesinger D, Sheehan J. Radiosurgery for intracranial hemangiopericytomas: outcomes after initial and repeat Gamma Knife surgery. J Neurosurg. 2010;112:133–9.

Schwannomas of the Sellar and Parasellar Region

30

Gabriel Zada, M. Beatriz S. Lopes, Srinivasan Mukundan Jr., and Edward Laws Jr.

30.1 Epidemiology and Clinical Presentation

- Schwannomas are typically benign neoplasms arising from the Schwann cells of peripheral and cranial nerves. The most common intracranial nerves of origin are the eighth, fifth, and seventh cranial nerves, followed by the other cranial nerves [1].
- Intrasellar and parasellar schwannomas are relatively rare but have been reported.
- These tumors may present with signs of local mass effect (headache, visual loss, hypopituitarism) or dysfunction of the nerve of origin.
- Intrasellar schwannomas are potentially thought to arise from perivascular or ectopic Schwann cells, lateral nerve plexi within the cavernous sinus, or Schwann cells from dural nerve twigs [2]. These tumors make up less than 1 % of major transsphenoidal series for sellar pathology [3].
- In the parasellar region, schwannomas may arise from any of the cranial nerves coursing through the cavernous sinus (especially the trigeminal nerve), the skull base foramina or fissures, or more distal paranasal locations (e.g., the pterygopalatine fossa), thereby presenting as primary cavernous sinus, skull base, or paranasal sinus masses [4].
- Primary sinonasal schwannomas may arise from the pterygopalatine fossa, sinonasal tract, nasal septum, or ethmoidal region. These tumors may present with nasal obstruction, epistaxis, pain, and/or anosmia.

30.2 Imaging Features

- Primary intrasellar schwannoma may be difficult to distinguish from pituitary adenoma.
- On MRI, schwannomas are typically isointense to brain on both T1- and T2-weighted MR images, with mild contrast enhancement and occasional cystic or hemorrhagic features (Figs. 30.1, 30.2, 30.3, and 30.4) [5].
- On CT imaging, bony erosion and remodeling of the skull base and paranasal sinuses are common features (Fig. 30.4). Smooth widening of the skull base foramina is a reliable imaging sign of schwannomas.

G. Zada, MD, MS (✉)
Department of Neurological Surgery, Keck School of Medicine, University of Southern California, 1200 N State Street, #3300, Los Angeles, CA 90033, USA
e-mail: gzada@usc.edu

M.B.S. Lopes, MD, PhD
Department of Pathology (Neuropathology), University of Virginia School of Medicine, 1215 Lee Street, Room 3060–HEP, Charlottesville, VA 22908, USA
e-mail: msl2e@virginia.edu

S. Mukundan Jr., PhD, MD
Department of Radiology, Brigham and Women's Hospital, 75 Francis Street, Boston, MA 02115, USA
e-mail: smukundan@partners.org

E. Laws Jr., MD
Department of Neurosurgery, Brigham and Women's Hospital, 15 Francis Street, Boston, MA 02115, USA
e-mail: elaws@partners.org

G. Zada et al. (eds.), *Atlas of Sellar and Parasellar Lesions: Clinical, Radiologic, and Pathologic Correlations*,
DOI 10.1007/978-3-319-22855-6_30

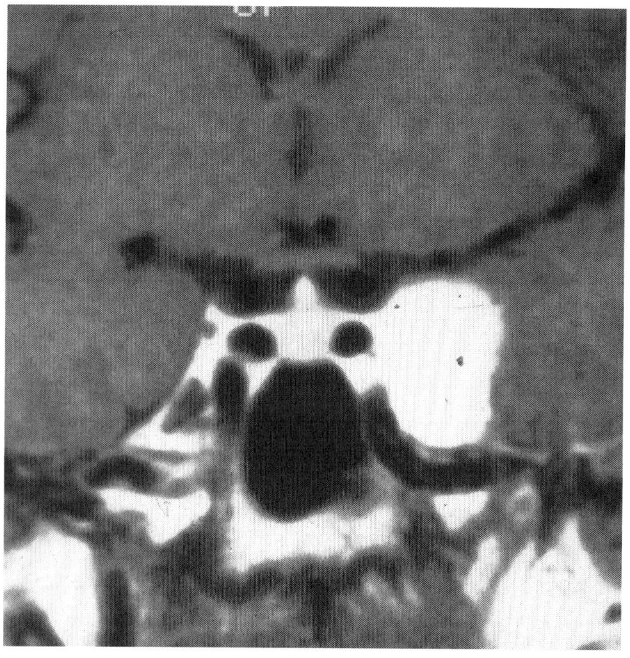

Fig. 30.1 Schwannoma of the trigeminal nerve. Coronal T1-weighted gadolinium-enhanced MR image. A large enhancing mass is centered in the left parasellar region

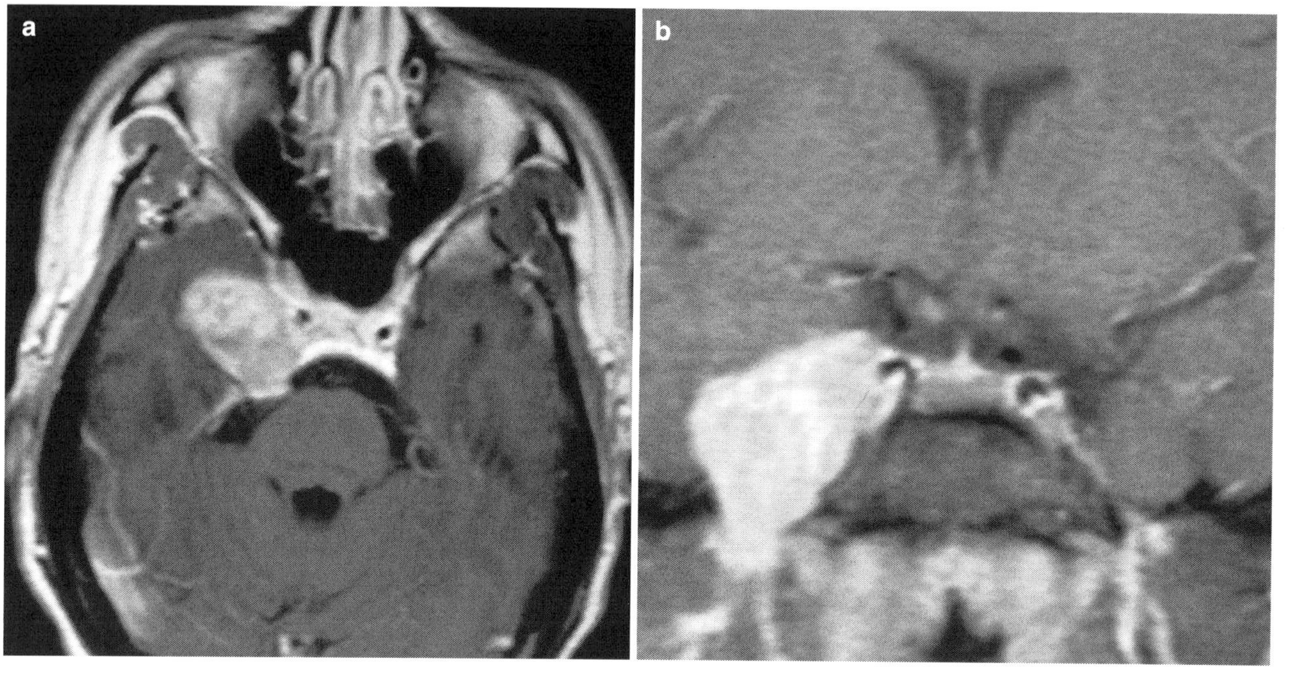

Fig. 30.2 Trigeminal schwannoma. (**a**) Axial T1-weighted gadolinium-enhanced image. (**b**) Coronal T1-weighted gadolinium-enhanced image. There is a large right parasellar, enhancing mass centered in the right Meckel's cave, extending through the right foramen ovale

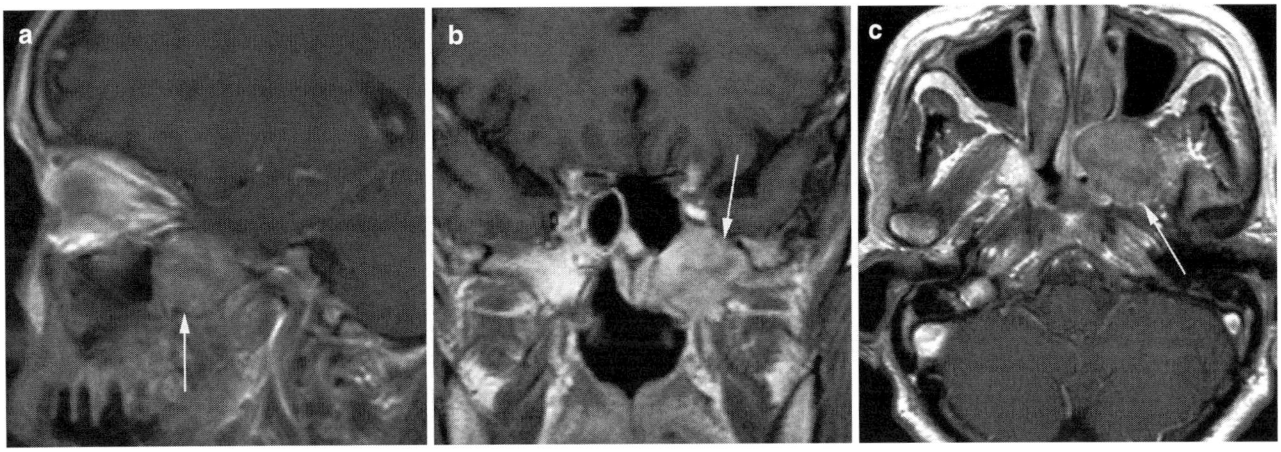

Fig. 30.3 Maxillary nerve schwannoma. (**a**) Sagittal T1-weighted gadolinium-enhanced image. (**b**) Coronal T1-weighted gadolinium-enhanced image. (**c**) Axial T1-weighted gadolinium-enhanced image. There is a heterogeneously enhancing mass (*arrows*) centered immediately below the left foramen ovale, extending anteriorly to the left pterygopalatine fossa

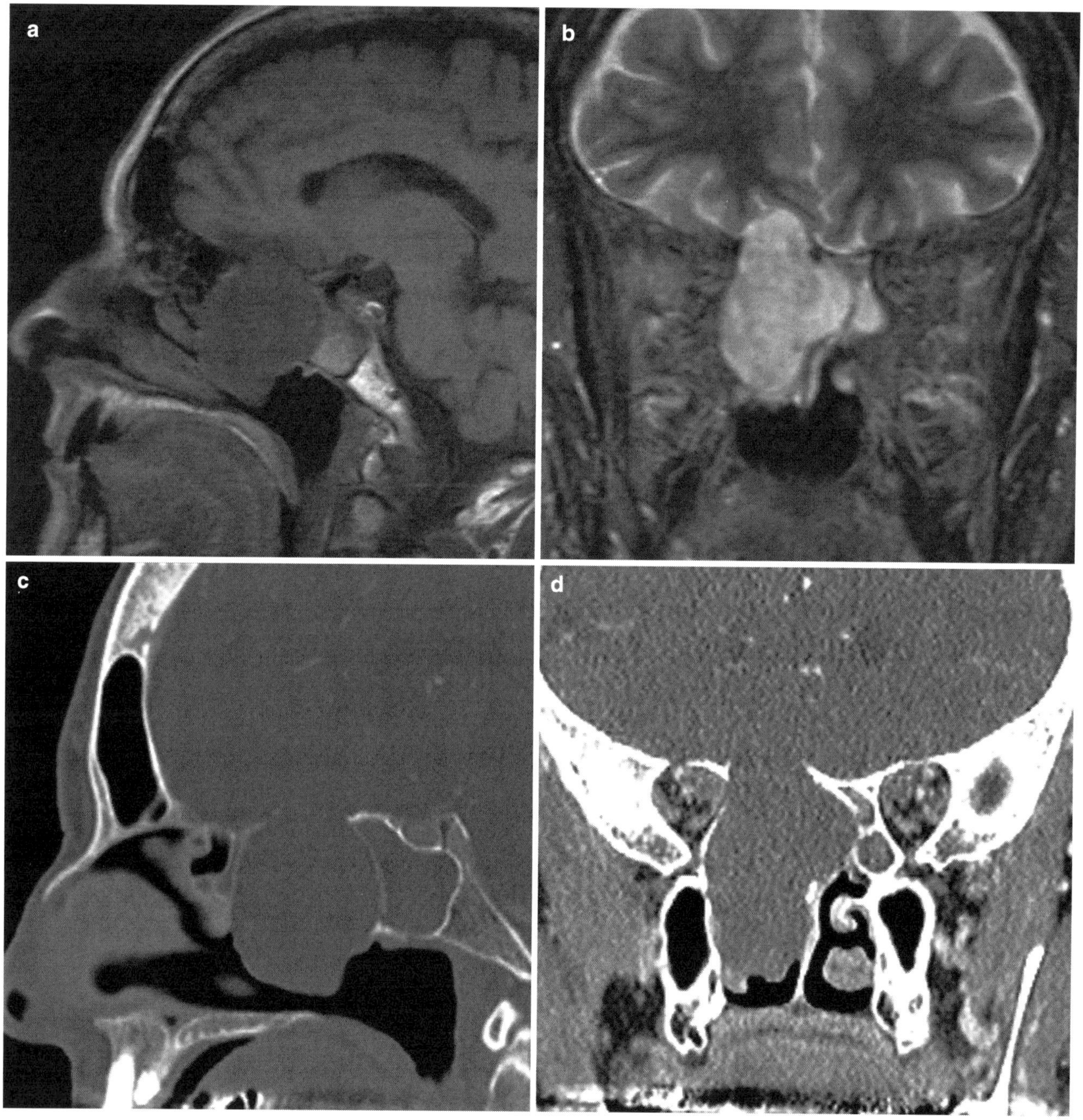

Fig. 30.4 Schwannoma. (**a**) Sagittal T1-weighted non-enhanced image. (**b**) Coronal T2-weighted image. (**c**) Sagittal CT image in bone algorithm. (**d**) Coronal CT image in soft tissue algorithm. A heterogeneously enhancing mass is centered in the right posterior ethmoid, with marked bony remodeling superiorly, medially, and inferiorly. Superiorly, the mass expands into the right anterior cranial fossa abutting the frontal lobe. Medially, the mass displaces the bony septum and narrows the sphenoid sinuses. Inferiorly, the mass expands into the nasal cavity. The sphenoid sinuses are completely obstructed

30.3 Histopathology

- Typical histopathological features of parasellar and sinonasal schwannoma include spindle cell proliferation with low mitotic activity and a low MIB-1 labeling index.
- Diffuse immunoreactivity for S100 is typically noted, with negative staining of CD34 and epithelial membrane antigen (EMA) [6].
- Classic features of schwannoma—cellular Antoni A and loose Antoni B areas, Verocay bodies, and hyalinized, thickened vessels—are typically observed but not always found in parasellar and sinonasal schwannoma (Fig. 30.5) [7, 8].
- Rare, malignant schwannomas with rhabdomyoblastic differentiation (Triton tumors) of the parasellar or sinonasal region have been reported; these tumors require multimodality treatment with radiation and chemotherapy [9].

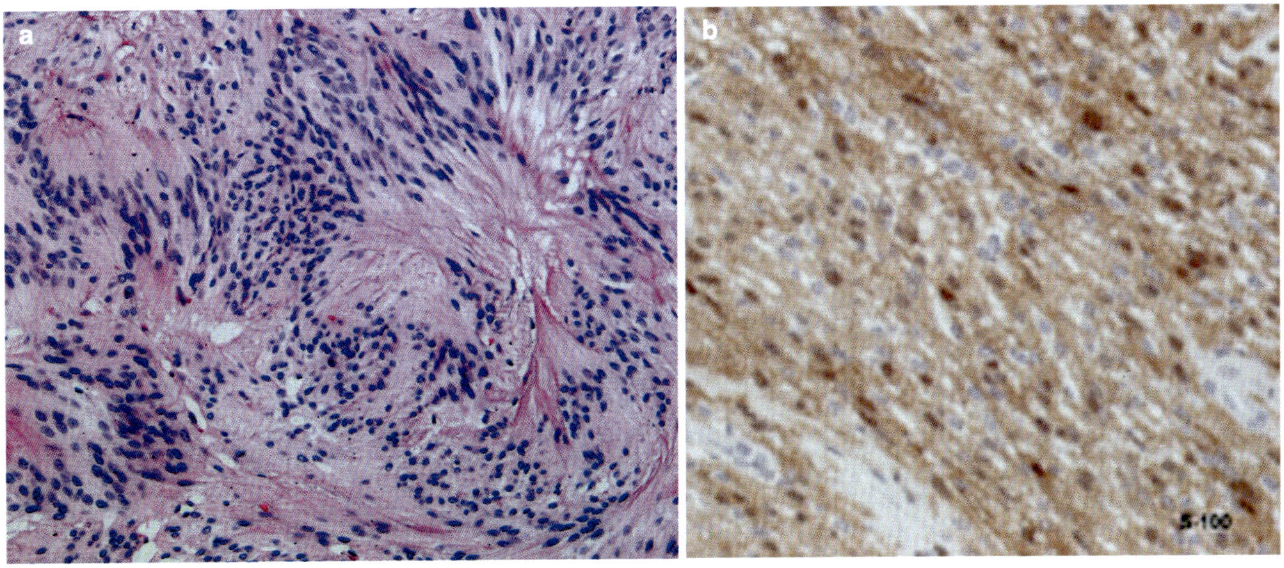

Fig. 30.5 Schwannoma. (**a**) A schwannoma consisting of dense fascicles in an Antoni A arrangement and nuclear palisading (H&E, Å ~20), and (**b**) Differentiated Schwann cells expressing S-100 protein (Adapted with permission from Rallis et al. [8])

30.4 Clinical and Surgical Management

- Successful transsphenoidal resection of intrasellar and suprasellar schwannoma has been reported numerous times, typically with improvement in visual function [10, 11].
- Endonasal endoscopic approaches may be useful for resection of schwannomas arising in the sinonasal region and more laterally or anteriorly in the skull base, such as the cribriform region, sinonasal tract, or pterygopalatine fossa [12–14].
- Schwannomas of the skull base are often characterized by a rich blood supply, making the tumors quite vascular.
- For primary cavernous sinus (i.e., trigeminal) schwannomas, open craniotomy with an extradural temporopolar or similar approach may be utilized with excellent surgical results. Facial hypoesthesia is the major adverse outcome associated with this approach [15–17].
- Following gross resection of benign parasellar and sinonasal schwannomas, the recurrence rate has been reported to be extremely low (<10 %) [6, 14].

30.4.1 Radiotherapy and Radiosurgery

- Stereotactic radiosurgery (fractionated or unfractionated) has been reported to achieve successful long-term control of parasellar schwannomas in over 90 % of cases [18–20].

30.4.2 Clinical Follow-up and Further Treatment

- Vigilant serial monitoring for tumor recurrence or progression is recommended following surgical resection and/or radiation.
- Patients with malignant schwannoma or Triton tumors require aggressive multimodality therapy consisting of surgical resection, radiation, and chemotherapy.

References

1. Sarma S, Sekhar LN, Schessel DA. Nonvestibular schwannomas of the brain: a 7-year experience. Neurosurgery. 2002;50:437–48; discussion 448–9.
2. Honegger J, Koerbel A, Psaras T, Petrick M, Mueller K. Primary intrasellar schwannoma: clinical, aetiopathological and surgical considerations. Br J Neurosurg. 2005;19:432–8.
3. Saeger W, Ludecke DK, Buchfelder M, Fahlbusch R, Quabbe HJ, Petersenn S. Pathohistological classification of pituitary tumors: 10 years of experience with the German Pituitary Tumor Registry. Eur J Endocrinol. 2007;156:203–16.
4. Prabhu SS, Bruner JM. Large oculomotor schwannoma presenting as a parasellar mass: a case report and literature review. Surg Neurol Int. 2010;1:15.
5. Kim YS, Kim HJ, Kim CH, Kim J. CT and MR imaging findings of sinonasal schwannoma: a review of 12 cases. AJNR Am J Neuroradiol. 2013;34:628–33.
6. Buob D, Wacrenier A, Chevalier D, Aubert S, Quinchon JF, Gosselin B, Leroy X. Schwannoma of the sinonasal tract: a clinicopathologic and immunohistochemical study of 5 cases. Arch Pathol Lab Med. 2003;127:1196–9.
7. Perez MT, Farkas J, Padron S, Changus JE, Webster EL. Intrasellar and parasellar cellular schwannoma. Ann Diagn Pathol. 2004;8:142–50.
8. Rallis G, Stathopoulos P, Mezitis M, Sakellaridis N, Machera H, Zachariades N. Combined craniofacial approach for the removal of a large trigeminal schwannoma invading the infratemporal fossa. Oral Maxillofac Surg. 2012;16:211–6.
9. Heffner DK, Gnepp DR. Sinonasal fibrosarcomas, malignant schwannomas, and "Triton" tumors. A clinicopathologic study of 67 cases. Cancer. 1992;70:1089–101.
10. Esposito F, Cappabianca P, Del Basso De Caro M, Cavallo LM, Rinaldi C, De Divitiis E. Endoscopic endonasal transsphenoidal removal of an intra-suprasellar schwannoma mimicking a pituitary adenoma. Minim Invasive Neurosurg. 2004;47:230–4.
11. Maartens NF, Ellegala DB, Vance ML, Lopes MB, Laws Jr ER. Intrasellar schwannomas: report of two cases. Neurosurgery. 2003;52:1200–5; discussion 1205–6.
12. Pasquini E, Sciarretta V, Farneti G, Ippolito A, Mazzatenta D, Frank G. Endoscopic endonasal approach for the treatment of benign schwannoma of the sinonasal tract and pterygopalatine fossa. Am J Rhinol. 2002;16:113–8.
13. Liu JK, Eloy JA. Expanded endoscopic endonasal transcribriform approach for resection of anterior skull base olfactory schwannoma. J Neurosurg. 2012;32:E3.
14. Shin SS, Gardner PA, Stefko ST, Madhok R, Fernandez-Miranda JC, Snyderman CH. Endoscopic endonasal approach for nonvestibular schwannomas. Neurosurgery. 2011;69:1046–57; discussion 1057.
15. Zada G, Day JD, Giannotta SL. The extradural temporopolar approach: a review of indications and operative technique. Neurosurg Focus. 2008;25:E3.
16. Wanibuchi M, Fukushima T, Zomordi AR, Nonaka Y, Friedman AH. Trigeminal schwannomas: skull base approaches and operative results in 105 patients. Neurosurgery. 2012;70:132–43; discussion 143–4.
17. Al-Mefty O, Ayoubi S, Gaber E. Trigeminal schwannomas: removal of dumbbell-shaped tumors through the expanded Meckel cave and outcomes of cranial nerve function. J Neurosurg. 2002; 96:453–63.
18. Choi CY, Soltys SG, Gibbs IC, Harsh GR, Sakamoto GT, Patel DA, et al. Stereotactic radiosurgery of cranial nonvestibular schwannomas: results of single- and multisession radiosurgery. Neurosurgery. 2011;68:1200–8; discussion 1208.
19. Hayashi M, Chernov M, Tamura N, Yomo S, Ochiai T, Nagai M, et al. Gamma Knife surgery for abducent nerve schwannoma. Report of 4 cases. J Neurosurg. 2010;113:136–43.
20. Phi JH, Paek SH, Chung HT, Jeong SS, Park CK, Jung HW, Kim DG. Gamma Knife surgery and trigeminal schwannoma: is it possible to preserve cranial nerve function? J Neurosurg. 2007;107: 727–32.

Chordoma and Chondrosarcoma

31

Gabriel Zada, M. Beatriz S. Lopes,
Srinivasan Mukundan Jr., and Edward Laws Jr.

31.1 Epidemiology and Clinical Presentation

31.1.1 Chordoma

- Chordomas are locally aggressive tumors originating from notochord remnants along the neural axis, especially at the rostral and caudal extents (clivus and sacrum).
- Typically, these invasive, expansile lesions present secondary to mass effect on surrounding structures.
- The median age at presentation is 38–46 years; the age for chondrosarcoma may be slightly higher [1–3].
- Overall, chordomas occur more frequently in men, but intracranial chordomas demonstrate an even predilection for both sexes.
- Chordomas occur most frequently in the sacral region (50 %), followed by the clivus (35 %) and additional spinal regions (10–15 %).
- Less commonly, they present primarily as intrasellar, retrosellar, nasopharyngeal, or foramen magnum region lesions [4–6].
- Chordomas comprise 0.5–2 % of sellar lesions in major transsphenoidal series [7, 8].
- Diplopia caused by abducens nerve paresis is the most common presenting sign of a clival chordoma [9]. The abducens nerve enters Dorello's canal in the clivus and ascends until it enters the cavernous sinus, thus making it susceptible to injury by the tumor or during surgical resection of chordomas.
- Other commonly associated symptoms and signs are headache, visual loss, hypopituitarism, weakness, and dysequilibrium [2, 9].

31.1.2 Chondrosarcoma

- Chondrosarcomas are rare lesions originating from cartilage; they typically arise in the long bones and pelvis.
- Less than 10 % occur intracranially or in the neck [10].
- Chondrosarcomas are distinct pathological entities that are reported to portend better long-term outcomes [9, 11].
- They comprise 0.17 % of surgically resected lesions in major transsphenoidal series [7].

G. Zada, MD, MS (✉)
Department of Neurological Surgery, Keck School of Medicine, University of Southern California, 1200 N State Street, #3300, Los Angeles, CA 90033, USA
e-mail: gzada@usc.edu

M.B.S. Lopes, MD, PhD
Department of Pathology (Neuropathology), University of Virginia School of Medicine, 1215 Lee Street, Room 3060–HEP, Charlottesville, VA 22908, USA
e-mail: msl2e@virginia.edu

S. Mukundan Jr., PhD, MD
Department of Radiology, Brigham and Women's Hospital, 75 Francis Street, Boston, MA 02115, USA
e-mail: smukundan@partners.org

E. Laws Jr., MD
Department of Neurosurgery, Brigham and Women's Hospital, 15 Francis Street, Boston, MA 02115, USA
e-mail: elaws@partners.org

G. Zada et al. (eds.), *Atlas of Sellar and Parasellar Lesions: Clinical, Radiologic, and Pathologic Correlations*, DOI 10.1007/978-3-319-22855-6_31

31.2 Imaging Features

- Chordomas can originate anywhere along the clivus and are typically centered on the midline. In many cases, they remain extradural, but they may invade the dura and neurovascular structures of the posterior fossa, interpeduncular cistern, and prepontine cistern [9].
- Retrosellar, retroclival, and/or petroclival extension is often found and may result in compression of the brainstem.
- Cavernous sinus invasion has been reported in 37–75 % of cases (Fig. 31.1) [1].
- CT imaging demonstrates lytic bony erosion of the clivus, often with intratumoral calcification [12, 13].

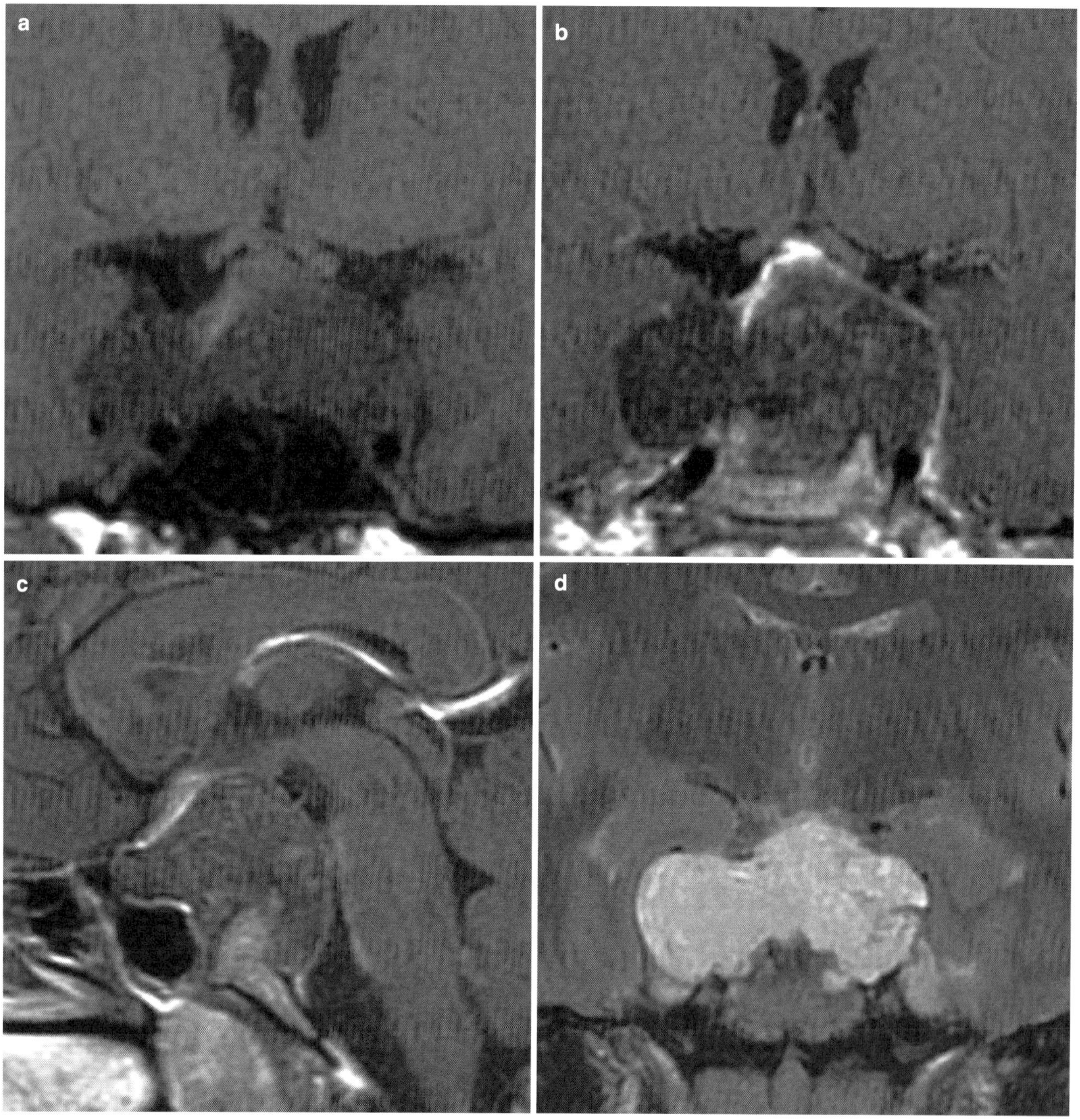

Fig. 31.1 Chordoma. (**a**) Coronal T1-weighted pre-gadolinium image. (**b**) Coronal T1-weighted post-gadolinium image. (**c**) Sagittal T1-weighted post-gadolinium image. (**d**) Coronal T2-weighted image. A large, lobular, heterogeneously enhancing mass is centered in the sella, eroding the clivus and displacing the pituitary gland superiorly. The mass is predominantly hyperintense on the T2-weighted image (**d**). There is invasion of the cavernous sinus bilaterally. A prepontine component is seen abutting the pons

- The lesions are typically hypointense or isointense on T1 imaging and hyperintense on T2 imaging owing to a relatively high fluid content (Figs. 31.2, 31.3, and 31.4) [13, 14].
- Heterogeneous contrast enhancement is often seen [13].
- A chondroid variant of chordoma occurs, with features of both chordoma and chondrosarcoma.
- MRI usually cannot differentiate chondrosarcoma from chordoma. Chondrosarcomas are typically paramedian in origin, arising near the petroclival fissure (Fig. 31.5), however, whereas chordomas are typically centered on the midline [3, 12].

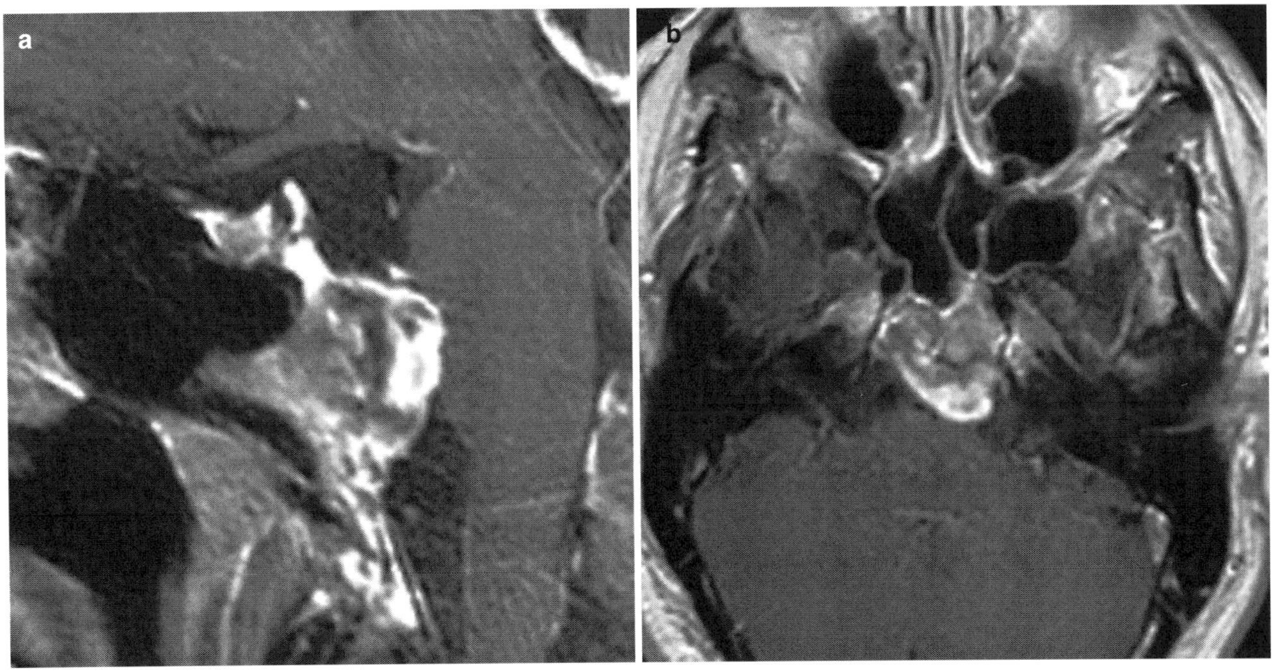

Fig. 31.2 Chordoma. (**a**) Sagittal T1-weighted post-gadolinium image. (**b**) Axial T1-weighted post-gadolinium image. There is a lobular, heterogeneously enhancing mass centered in the upper clivus, with an exophytic component extending to the prepontine cistern abutting the pons. The mass appears separate from the sella

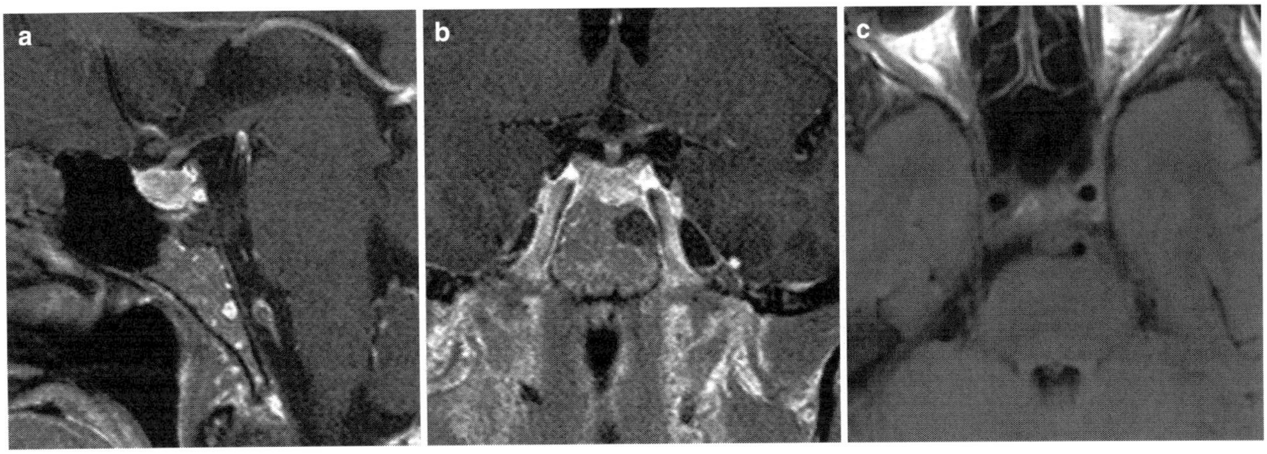

Fig. 31.3 Chordoma. (**a**) Sagittal T1-weighted post-gadolinium image. (**b**) Coronal T1-weighted post-gadolinium image. (**c**) Axial fluid attenuated inversion recovery (FLAIR) image. A small, hypoenhancing mass is located in the left posterior upper clivus, extending to the prepontine cistern. The mass appears separate from the sella

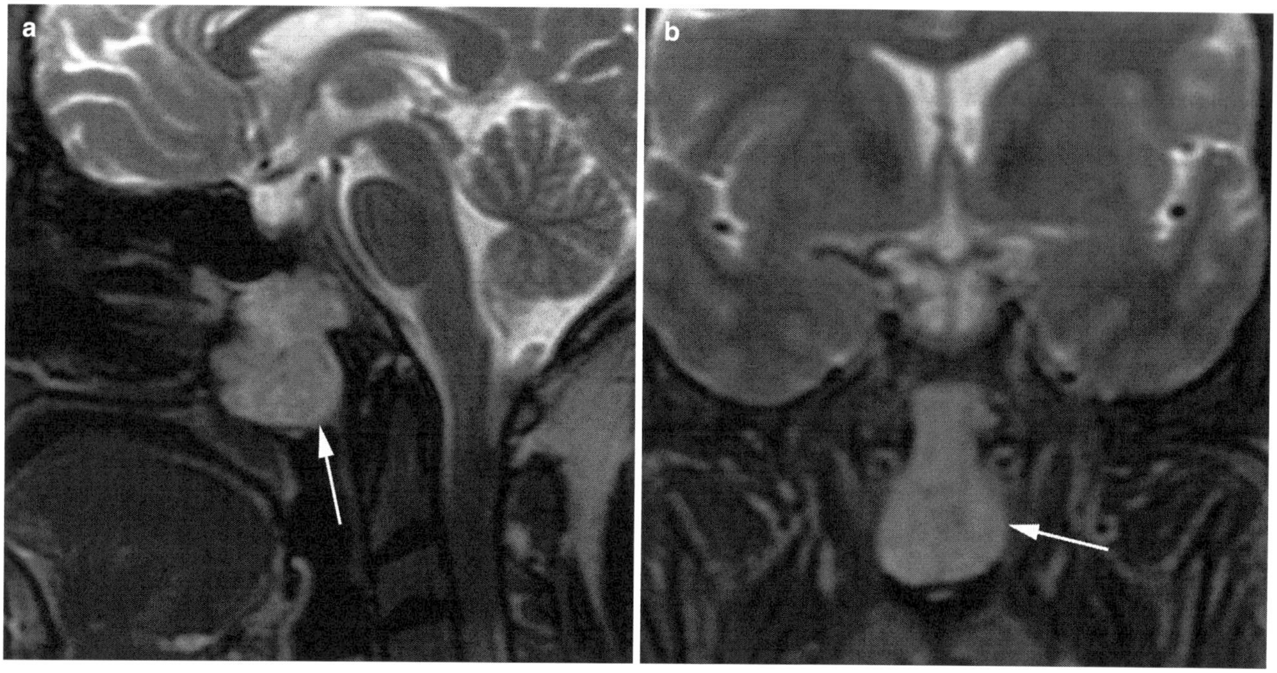

Fig. 31.4 Chordoma. (**a**) Sagittal T2-weighted image. (**b**) Coronal T2-weighted image. A lobular, slightly T2 hyperintense mass (*arrows*) arises from the anterior clivus and extends to the roof of the nasopharynx

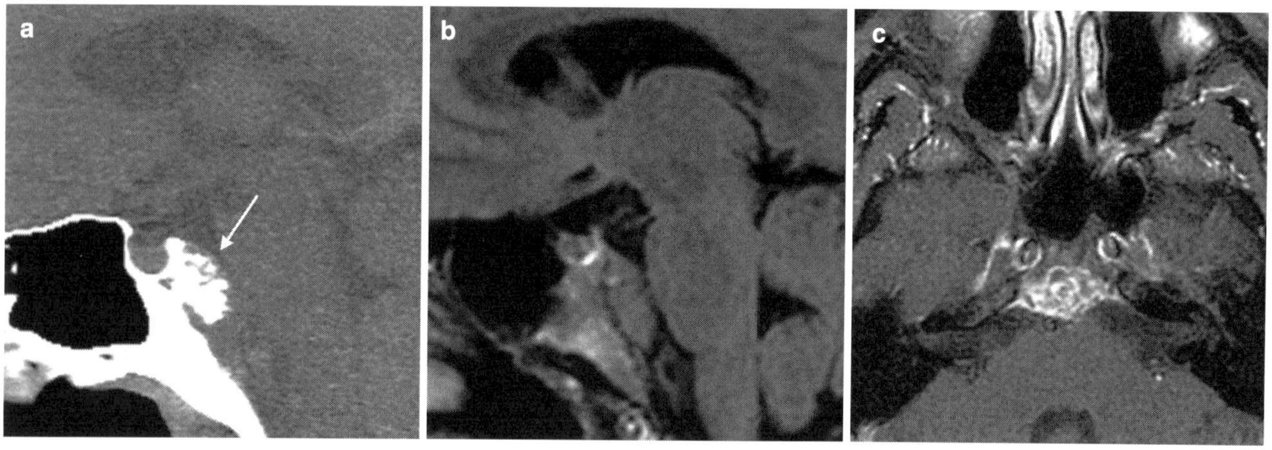

Fig. 31.5 Chondrosarcoma. (**a**) Sagittal CT image. (**b**) Sagittal FLAIR image. (**c**) Axial T1-weighted, fat-saturated post-gadolinium image. A calcified, exophytic mass is centered in the upper posterior clivus (*arrow*), appearing separate from the sella

31.3 Pathology

- Chordomas are low-grade malignant neoplasms derived from the notochord.
- Small polygonal cells with eosinophilic cytoplasm and eccentric nuclei are immersed in a mucoid matrix [4]. Vacuolated ("bubble-bearing"), physaliphorous cells are the hallmark finding on histopathological analysis.
- The tumor cells are arranged in lobules and can form cords or small nests.
- Chordomas typically demonstrate immunoreactivity for S100, vimentin, and epithelial-like markers such as EMA and cytokeratin (Fig. 31.6) [9].
- Brachyury is commonly overexpressed in chordomas and can be used to differentiate chordoma from chondrosarcoma and other tumors.
- The chondroid subtype of chordoma is characterized by hyalinization and does not appear to be associated with worsened patient outcomes [3, 15].
- Microscopic metastatic lesions may be found in up to 40 % of patients on autopsy studies but are grossly identified in 10–20 % [4].
- Chondrosarcomas are sarcomatous neoplasms with various degrees of cartilaginous differentiation.
- Most chondrosarcomas occur in long bones, but involvement of the base of the skull and sacrum is common.
- Chondrosarcomas are characterized by epithelioid-like or spindle cells immersed in a myxoid or cartilaginous matrix similar to that seen in chordomas.
- Chondrosarcomas demonstrate mesenchymal markers including vimentin and S100 protein, but these tumors do not demonstrate immunoreactivity for epithelial markers including EMA and cytokeratin, which are typically positive in chordoma and chondroid chordomas (Fig. 31.7) [3, 4, 9].

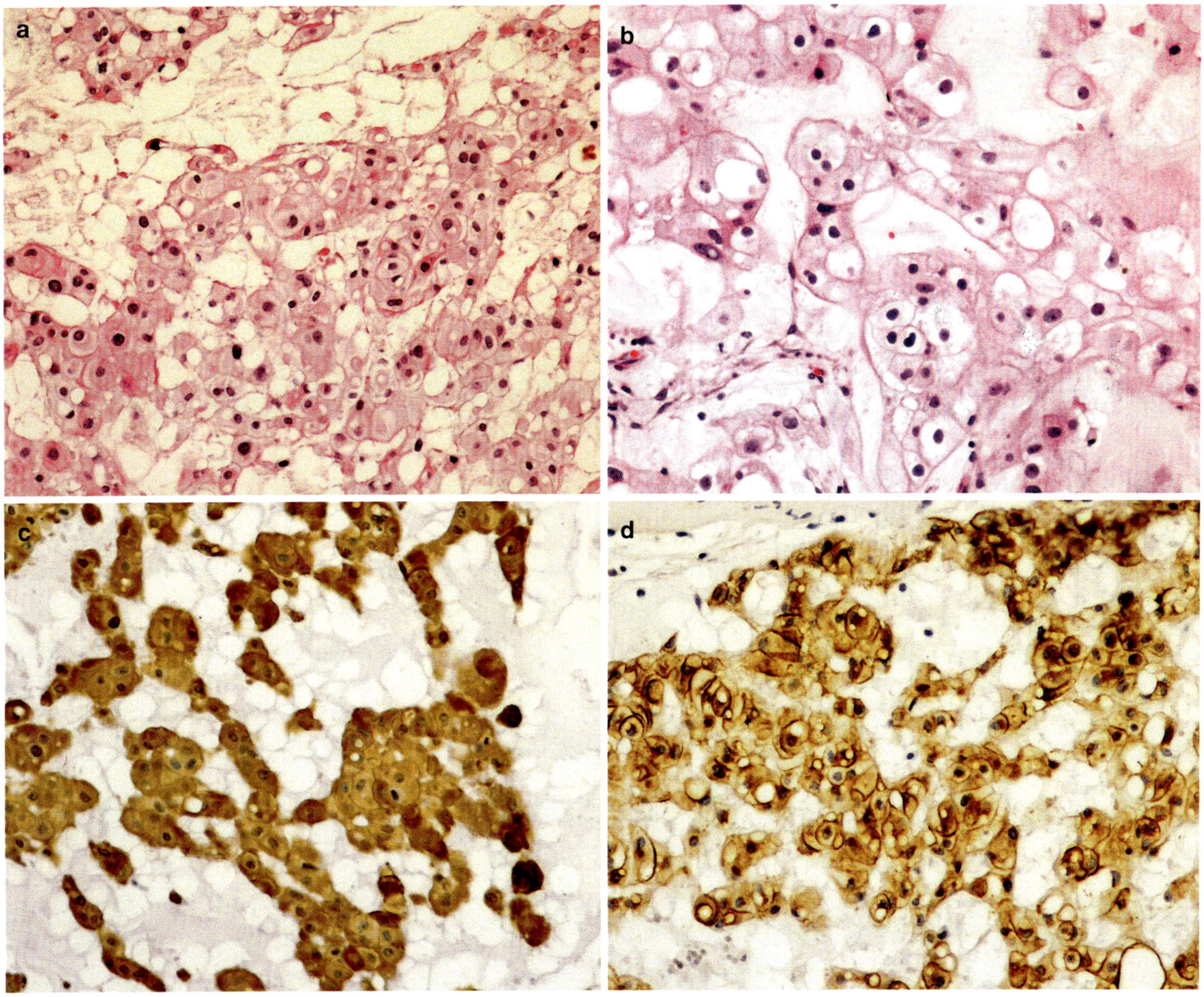

Fig. 31.6 Chordoma. Chordomas are characteristically composed of physaliphorous cells with pale to clear, foamy, or bubbling cytoplasm arranged in cords and trabecules and immersed in a myxoid stroma (**a**, **b**). As a derivative of the notochord, chordomas express mesenchymal markers including vimentin and S100 (**c**), as well epithelial markers like epithelial membrane antigen (EMA) (**d**) and cytokeratin

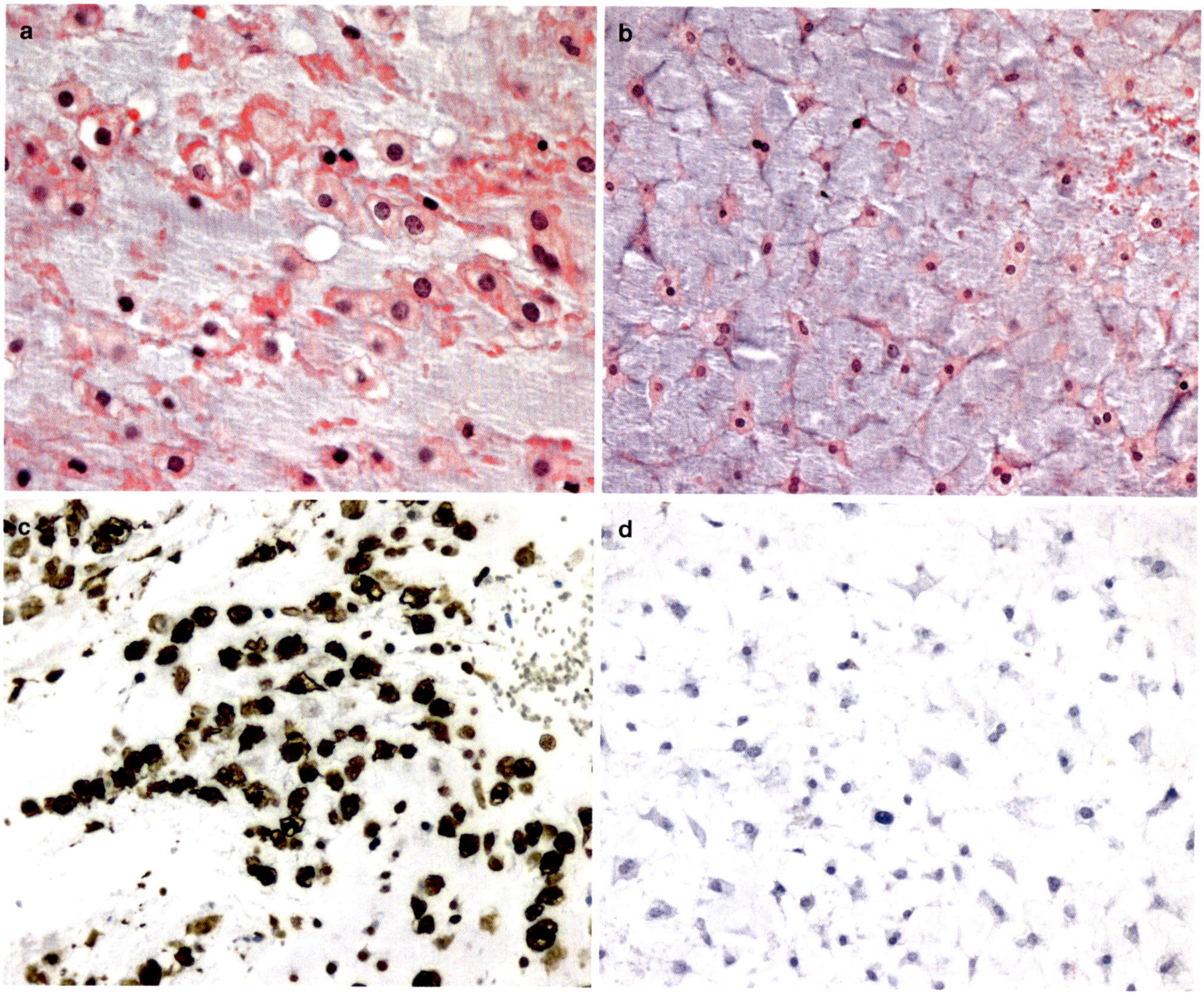

Fig. 31.7 Chondrosarcoma. Chondrosarcoma demonstrates epithelioid cells (**a**) or stellate-like cells (**b**) immersed in a cartilaginous stroma, which may be similar to those seen in chordomas. Although chondrosarcomas are immunopositive for S100 protein (**c**), unlike chordomas, they do not express epithelial markers, including EMA (**d**)

31.4 Clinical and Surgical Management

- Aggressive (if possible, gross total) surgical resection has been advocated for clival chordomas, but resection is frequently limited by extension and invasion of critical neurovascular structures [4, 16].
- Chordomas are typically extradural lesions and should therefore be resected via extradural approaches, when feasible [1].
- The surgical approach is often dictated by the location and boundaries of the lesion. An extended or combined skull base approach may be preferred to achieve as radical a resection as possible. Far lateral or combined transpetrosal approaches often are indicated to achieve maximal resection of these lesions. In the past, a variety of skull base approaches, including subfrontal, extradural temporopolar, transbasal, transoral, and lateral transcondylar approaches, have been used [1, 11, 17].
- Staged procedures are frequently necessary to achieve optimal tumor debulking [11].
- Extended transsphenoidal approaches have been used to approach selected chordomas of the clivus [8, 18–20].
- In recent years, extended endoscopic techniques have been used to resect selected clival chordomas that do not demonstrate a significant degree of lateral extension or encasement of the vertebrobasilar system [21, 22].
- More complex paramedian skull base approaches have been described for resecting the lateral components of these tumors, including the transpterygoid and transmaxillary approaches. The risk of internal carotid artery exposure and injury is increased with these techniques [23].
- Extensive skull base reconstruction techniques, such as vascularized, pedicle-based nasoseptal flaps, have been effective in reducing the risk of postoperative cerebrospinal fluid (CSF) leaks [23].
- Gross total or radical resection rates of 33–83 % have been reported [3, 9, 11, 23, 24].
- Postoperative neurological complications have been reported in 20–60 % of patients, with cranial nerve paresis being the most common [9, 11].

31.4.1 Radiotherapy and Radiosurgery

- Various modalities of stereotactic radiosurgery have been implemented for residual or recurrent chordomas, with limited results.
- Fractionated proton beam therapy has offered some success in long-term tumor control of chordomas, with reported 5-year survival rates of 79 %. Improved patient outcomes have been reported following proton beam radiosurgery, compared with surgery alone [3, 25].
- Unfractionated stereotactic radiosurgery (e.g., Gamma Knife) has demonstrated limited results for chordomas, with recent studies reporting long-term tumor control rates of 50 % [26].
- Interstitial brachytherapy using iodine isotopes for recurrent chordoma has been attempted with limited success [27].

31.4.2 Clinical Follow-up

- Five-year progression-free survival has been reported to be 65–79 % [11, 25].
- Five-year overall survival rates of 51–79 % have been reported, depending significantly on the age at diagnosis [2, 28].
- Better outcomes have been reported in patients presenting with cranial nerve paresis, either because they present earlier in the course of the disease or because the tumor growth patterns are more favorable in this condition.
- Survival rates drop significantly for progressive and recurrent tumors following multimodal management, with a reported 5-year patient survival of 5 % [29].
- Patients with chondrosarcoma have significantly better long-term progression-free and overall survival outcomes [3].

References

1. Al-Mefty O, Borba LA. Skull base chordomas: a management challenge. J Neurosurg. 1997;86:182–9.
2. Forsyth PA, Cascino TL, Shaw EG, Scheithauer BW, O'Fallon JR, Dozier JC, Piepgras DG. Intracranial chordomas: a clinicopathological and prognostic study of 51 cases. J Neurosurg. 1993;78:741–7.
3. Almefty K, Pravdenkova S, Colli BO, Al-Mefty O, Gokden M. Chordoma and chondrosarcoma: similar, but quite different, skull base tumors. Cancer. 2007;110:2457–67.
4. Lanzino G, Dumont AS, Lopes MB, Laws Jr ER. Skull base chordomas: overview of disease, management options, and outcome. Neurosurg Focus. 2001;10(3):E12.
5. Thodou E, Kontogeorgos G, Scheithauer BW, Lekka I, Tzanis S, Mariatos P, Laws Jr ER. Intrasellar chordomas mimicking pituitary adenoma. J Neurosurg. 2000;92:976–82.
6. Campbell WM, McDonald TJ, Unni KK, Laws Jr ER. Nasal and paranasal presentations of chordomas. Laryngoscope. 1980;90:612–8.
7. Saeger W, Ludecke DK, Buchfelder M, Fahlbusch R, Quabbe HJ, Petersenn S. Pathohistological classification of pituitary tumors: 10 years of experience with the German Pituitary Tumor Registry. Eur J Endocrinol. 2007;156:203–16.
8. Fatemi N, Dusick JR, de Paiva Neto MA, Kelly DF. The endonasal microscopic approach for pituitary adenomas and other parasellar tumors: a 10-year experience. Neurosurgery. 2008;63:244–56; discussion 256.
9. Colli BO, Al-Mefty O. Chordomas of the skull base: follow-up review and prognostic factors. Neurosurg Focus. 2001;10(3):E1.
10. Gadwal SR, Fanburg-Smith JC, Gannon FH, Thompson LD. Primary chondrosarcoma of the head and neck in pediatric patients: a clinicopathologic study of 14 cases with a review of the literature. Cancer. 2000;88:2181–8.

11. Gay E, Sekhar LN, Rubinstein E, Wright DC, Sen C, Janecka IP, Snyderman CH. Chordomas and chondrosarcomas of the cranial base: results and follow-up of 60 patients. Neurosurgery. 1995;36:887–96; discussion 896–7.
12. Weber AL, Liebsch NJ, Sanchez R, Sweriduk Jr ST. Chordomas of the skull base. Radiologic and clinical evaluation. Neuroimaging Clin N Am. 1994;4:515–27.
13. Erdem E, Angtuaco EC, Van Hemert R, Park JS, Al-Mefty O. Comprehensive review of intracranial chordoma. Radiographics. 2003;23:995–1009.
14. Larson 3rd TC, Houser OW, Laws Jr ER. Imaging of cranial chordomas. Mayo Clin Proc. 1987;62:886–93.
15. Wold LE, Laws Jr ER. Cranial chordomas in children and young adults. J Neurosurg. 1983;59:1043–7.
16. Harsh GR, editor. Chordomas and chondrosarcomas of the skull base and spine. New York: Thieme; 2003.
17. Zada G, Day JD, Giannotta SL. The extradural temporopolar approach: a review of indications and operative technique. Neurosurg Focus. 2008;25(6):E3.
18. Maira G, Pallini R, Anile C, Fernandez E, Salvinelli F, La Rocca LM, Rossi GF. Surgical treatment of clival chordomas: the transsphenoidal approach revisited. J Neurosurg. 1996;85:784–92.
19. Couldwell WT, Weiss MH, Rabb C, Liu JK, Apfelbaum RI, Fukushima T. Variations on the standard transsphenoidal approach to the sellar region, with emphasis on the extended approaches and parasellar approaches: surgical experience in 105 cases. Neurosurgery. 2004;55:539–47; discussion 547–50.
20. Laws Jr ER. Transsphenoidal surgery for tumors of the clivus. Otolaryngol Head Neck Surg. 1984;92:100–1.
21. Carrabba G, Dehdashti AR, Gentili F. Surgery for clival lesions: open resection versus the expanded endoscopic endonasal approach. Neurosurg Focus. 2008;25(6):E7.
22. Fraser JF, Nyquist GG, Moore N, Anand VK, Schwartz TH. Endoscopic endonasal transclival resection of chordomas: operative technique, clinical outcome, and review of the literature. J Neurosurg. 2010;112:1061–9.
23. Stippler M, Gardner PA, Snyderman CH, Carrau RL, Prevedello DM, Kassam AB. Endoscopic endonasal approach for clival chordomas. Neurosurgery. 2009;64:268–77; discussion 277–8.
24. Menezes AH, Gantz BJ, Traynelis VC, McCulloch TM. Cranial base chordomas. Clin Neurosurg. 1997;44:491–509.
25. Hug EB, Loredo LN, Slater JD, DeVries A, Grove RI, Schaefer RA, et al. Proton radiation therapy for chordomas and chondrosarcomas of the skull base. J Neurosurg. 1999;91:432–9.
26. Dassoulas K, Schlesinger D, Yen CP, Sheehan J. The role of Gamma Knife surgery in the treatment of skull base chordomas. J Neurooncol. 2009;94:243–8.
27. Gutin PH, Leibel SA, Hosobuchi Y, Crumley RL, Edwards MS, Wilson CB, et al. Brachytherapy of recurrent tumors of the skull base and spine with iodine-125 sources. Neurosurgery. 1987;20:938–45.
28. Hug EB. Review of skull base chordomas: prognostic factors and long-term results of proton-beam radiotherapy. Neurosurg Focus. 2001;10(3):E11.
29. Fagundes MA, Hug EB, Liebsch NJ, Daly W, Efird J, Munzenrider JE. Radiation therapy for chordomas of the base of skull and cervical spine: patterns of failure and outcome after relapse. Int J Radiat Oncol Biol Phys. 1995;33:579–84.

Hemangioblastomas of the Sellar and Suprasellar Region

32

Gabriel Zada, M. Beatriz S. Lopes, Srinivasan Mukundan Jr., and Edward Laws Jr.

32.1 Epidemiology and Clinical Presentation

- Hemangioblastoma of the pituitary and parasellar region is a rare diagnosis. Within the central nervous system, they are typically confined to the cerebellum and spinal cord.
- They can occur sporadically or as part of the von Hippel-Lindau (VHL) syndrome [1].
- The prevalence of infundibular hemangioblastoma in patients with VHL is 3 %, making this the most common site for supratentorial hemangioblastoma [2].
- In the sellar region, they usually arise in the region of the pituitary stalk (infundibulum), yet they typically remain asymptomatic, without evidence of hypopituitarism [3].
- In rare cases, sellar or suprasellar hemangioblatomas can present with hypopituitarism and/or visual loss [4–8].
- In rare cases, they may hemorrhage and present with pituitary apoplexy (Fig. 32.1) [9].

G. Zada, MD, MS (✉)
Department of Neurological Surgery, Keck School of Medicine, University of Southern California, 1200 N State Street, #3300, Los Angeles, CA 90033, USA
e-mail: gzada@usc.edu

M.B.S. Lopes, MD, PhD
Department of Pathology (Neuropathology), University of Virginia School of Medicine, 1215 Lee Street, Room 3060–HEP, Charlottesville, VA 22908, USA
e-mail: msl2e@virginia.edu

S. Mukundan Jr., PhD, MD
Department of Radiology, Brigham and Women's Hospital, 75 Francis Street, Boston, MA 02115, USA
e-mail: smukundan@partners.org

E. Laws Jr., MD
Department of Neurosurgery, Brigham and Women's Hospital, 15 Francis Street, Boston, MA 02115, USA
e-mail: elaws@partners.org

G. Zada et al. (eds.), *Atlas of Sellar and Parasellar Lesions: Clinical, Radiologic, and Pathologic Correlations*,
DOI 10.1007/978-3-319-22855-6_32

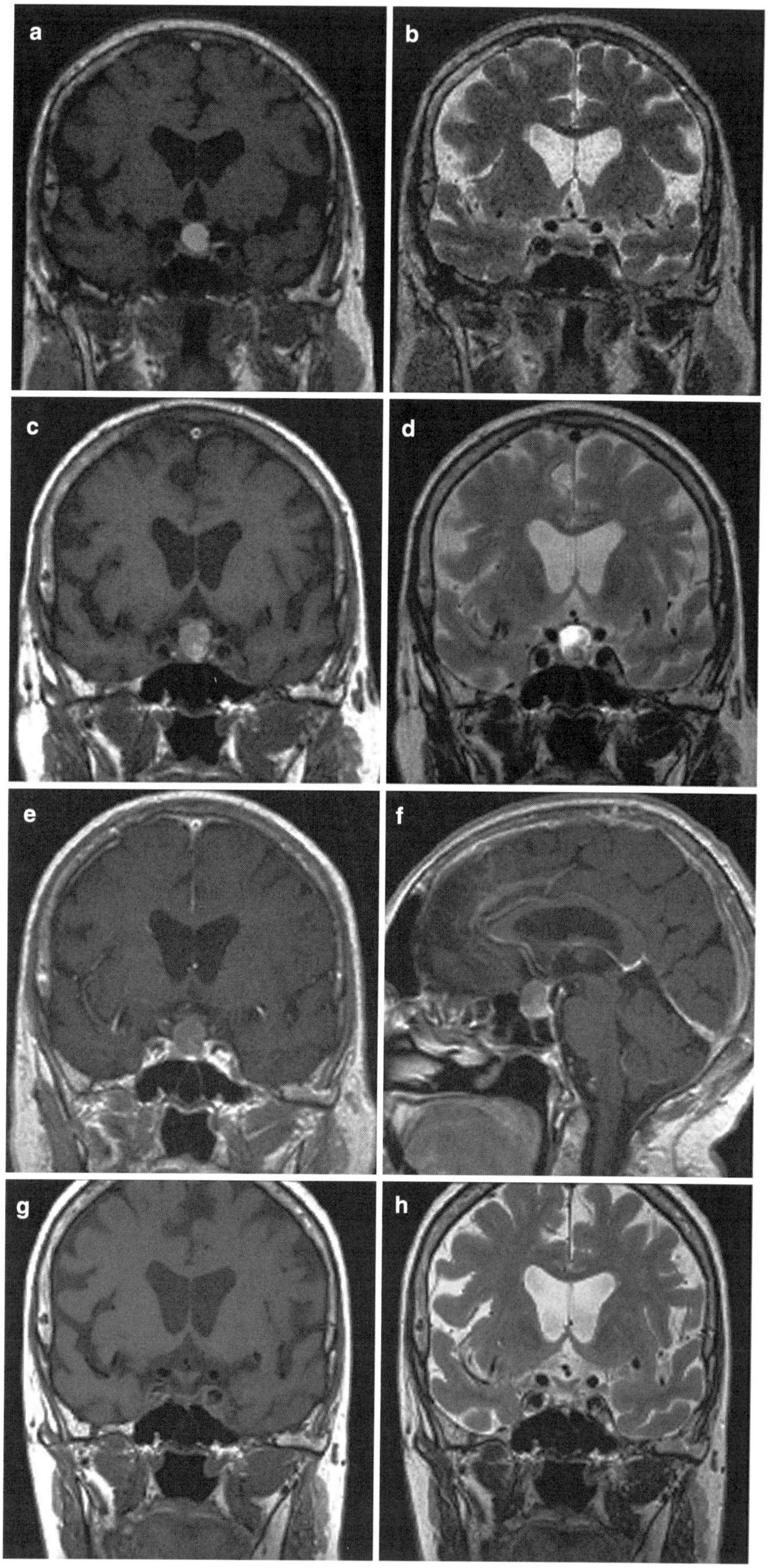

Fig. 32.1 Hemangioblastoma. (**a**, **b**) T1- and T2-weighted MRI scans taken 2 years prior to presentation. (**c**) This T1-weighted MRI scan reveals a partly vesicular, hyperintense, and slightly increased (vs **a** and **b**) intrasellar and suprasellar mass of 16 mm in diameter, with progressive compression of the prechiasmatic portions of the optic nerves bilaterally. (**d**) T2-weighted MRI scan showing the vesicular portion as hypointense; normal pituitary tissue could not be clearly delineated. (**e**, **f**) No enhancement is evident on T1-weighted imaging after intravenous administration of gadolinium. (**g**, **h**) An MRI scan taken 16 months postoperatively showed regular display of the remaining pituitary gland with good chiasmatic decompression and no signs of tumor recurrence (Adapted from Schar et al. [9]; with permission)

32.2 Imaging Features

- Infundibular hemangioblastomas are typically less than 1 cm in diameter and are avidly and homogeneously enhancing solid masses [2]. Supratentorial hemangioblastomas arising in other regions may be solid or cystic and solid, often with an enhancing mural nodule [10].
- In the sellar region and anterior skull base, larger hemangioblastomas are often characterized by large intratumoral flow voids and the absence of a dural tail. They are typically isointense to brain on T1-weighted images and hyperintense on T2-weighted images, with avid contrast enhancement [6, 7].
- On CT images, the solid portion is typically hyperdense.
- The solid portion often can be visualized with angiographic imaging.

32.3 Histopathology

- Hemangioblastoma is characterized by vascular proliferation of capillaries of variable size, along with a variable degree of stromal cells containing pink to clear foamy and lipid-laden cytoplasm (Fig. 32.2). Cystic change is commonly observed, yet necrosis is uncommon.
- Histologically, hemangioblastoma may be difficult to differentiate from renal cell carcinoma or meningioma. Renal cell carcinoma and meningioma are typically immunopositive for EMA, however, whereas hemangioblastoma is not.
- More specific and useful markers include podoplanin (D2-40) and inhibin A that are positive in hemangioblastomas but negative in renal cell carcinomas.

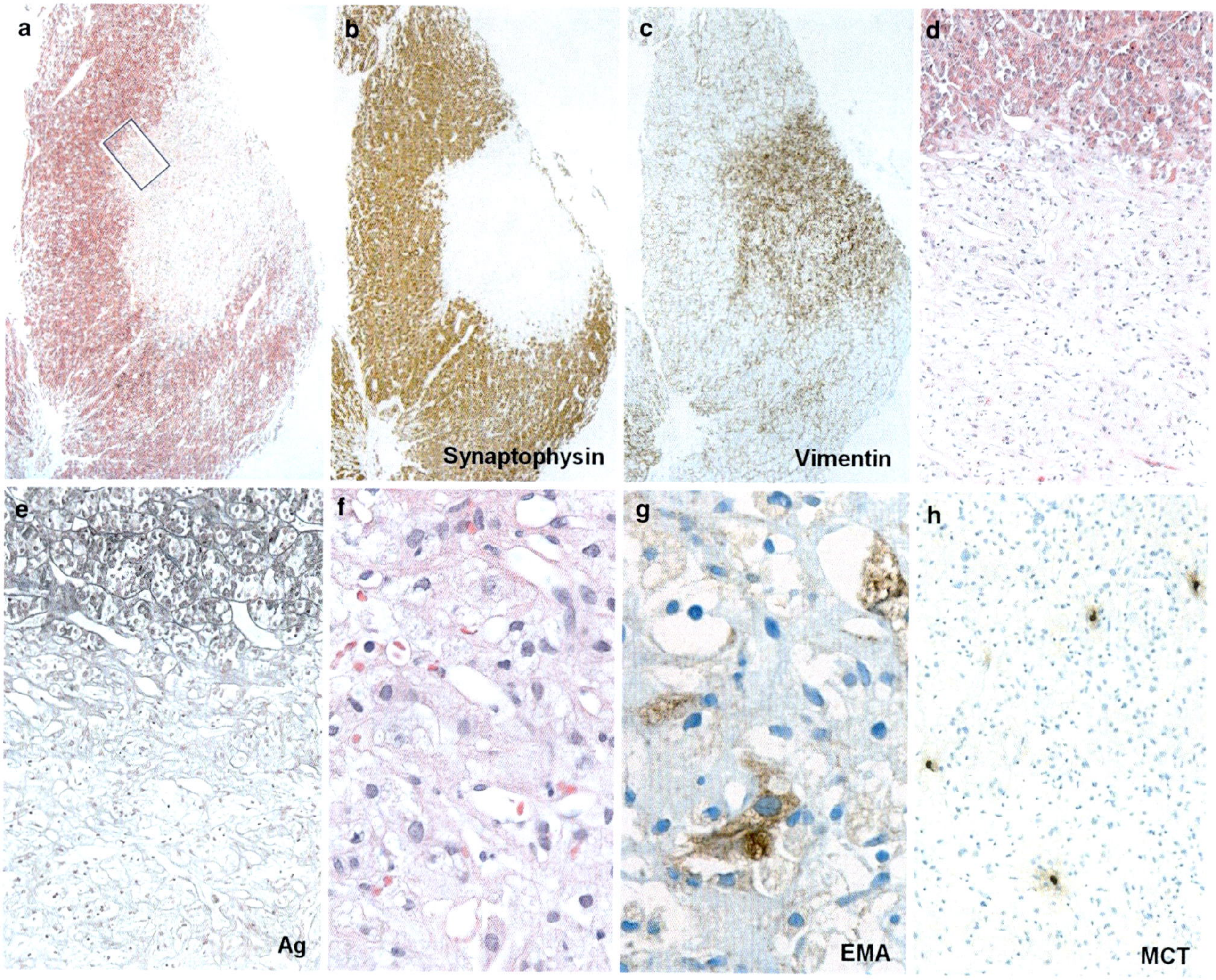

Fig. 32.2 Well-circumscribed hemangioblastoma (HBL) nodule partly surrounded by a crescent-shaped mantle of peritumoral pituitary parenchyma. (**a**) Optical contrast between the faint eosinophilic hue of the HBL nidus and the bright red granular quality of adjacent somatotrophs. (**b**, **c**) Adjacent section planes treated with immunohistochemistry, showing segregation of adenohypophyseal neuroendocrine cells (**b**) and mesenchymal-like immunophenotype (**c**) of the HBL nodule. (**d**) Detail view of boxed area in panel (**a**) shows the HBL comprise an irregular, reticular meshwork of tortuous, thin-walled capillaries that tend to be interspersed with pale stromal cells. (**e**) Gomori's reticulin stain highlighting the brisk transition from the acinar outline of native adenohypophyseal follicles (*upper third*) to the vascular-dominated basement membrane pattern of HBL. (**f**) High-power view of HBL showing polygonal contours and cytoplasmic vacuolation of stromal cells encased by capillaries. Some nuclear pleomorphism, as also evident in this microscopic field, is of no prognostic significance. (**g**) A minority of stromal cells were stained for EMA. (**h**) Scattered mast cells are a characteristic complement of HBL. If not labeled otherwise, microphotographs have been made using H&E stain. Original magnifications: **a**–**c**, ×30; **d**, **e**, and **h**, ×100; **f** and **g**, ×400 (Adapted from Schar et al. [9]; with permission)

32.4 Clinical and Surgical Management

- A majority of sellar and suprasellar region hemangioblastomas will remain asymptomatic without any evidence of hypopituitarism, so they can be serially monitored without need for surgical intervention [2].
- If symptomatic, these lesions can be resected via a transsphenoidal or open skull base craniotomy [3, 8, 9].
- Various modalities of radiation and stereotactic radiosurgery have been successfully implemented for hemangioblastomas not amenable to further surgical resection [8, 11, 12].
- Various pharmacologic agents, such as thalidomide and sunitinib, have been used for refractory cases of hemangioblastoma occurring within the CNS [13, 14].
- Patients with newly diagnosed hemangioblastoma should be screened for VHL, with complete ophthalmologic imaging and screening for renal or hepatic lesions.

References

1. Goto T, Nishi T, Kunitoku N, Yamamoto K, Kitamura I, Takeshima H, et al. Suprasellar hemangioblastoma in a patient with von Hippel-Lindau disease confirmed by germline mutation study: case report and review of the literature. Surg Neurol. 2001;56:22–6.
2. Lonser RR, Butman JA, Kiringoda R, Song D, Oldfield EH. Pituitary stalk hemangioblastomas in von Hippel-Lindau disease. J Neurosurg. 2009;110:350–3. doi:10.3171/2008.4.17532.
3. Fomekong E, Hernalsteen D, Godfraind C, D'Haens J, Raftopoulos C. Pituitary stalk hemangioblastoma: the fourth case report and review of the literature. Clin Neurol Neurosurg. 2007;109:292–8.
4. Barton JC, Goncalves E, Santani A, Chandra-Sekar B, Morris EC, Carter BB, Stolle CA. Hypogonadotrophic hypogonadism due to intrasellar hemangioblastoma in von Hippel-Lindau syndrome. Am J Med Genet A. 2009;149A:549–51.
5. Dan NG, Smith DE. Pituitary hemangioblastoma in a patient with von Hippel-Lindau disease. Case report. J Neurosurg. 1975;42:232–5.
6. Prabhu K, Daniel RT, Chacko G, Chacko AG. Optic nerve haemangioblastoma mimicking a planum sphenoidale meningioma. Br J Neurosurg. 2009;23:561–3.
7. Rumboldt Z, Gnjidic Z, Talan-Hranilovic J, Vrkljan M. Intrasellar hemangioblastoma: characteristic prominent vessels on MR imaging. AJR Am J Roentgenol. 2003;180:1480–1.
8. Sawin PD, Follett KA, Wen BC, Laws Jr ER. Symptomatic intrasellar hemangioblastoma in a child treated with subtotal resection and adjuvant radiosurgery. Case report. J Neurosurg. 1996;84:1046–50.
9. Schär RT, Vajtai I, Sahli R, Seiler RW. Manifestation of a sellar hemangioblastoma due to pituitary apoplexy: a case report. J Med Case Rep. 2011;5:496.
10. Peyre M, David P, Van Effenterre R, Francois P, Thys M, Emery E, et al. Natural history of supratentorial hemangioblastomas in von Hippel-Lindau disease. Neurosurgery. 2010;67:577–87; discussion 587.
11. Patrice SJ, Sneed PK, Flickinger JC, Shrieve DC, Pollock BE, Alexander 3rd E, et al. Radiosurgery for hemangioblastoma: results of a multiinstitutional experience. Int J Radiat Oncol Biol Phys. 1996;35:493–9.
12. Asthagiri AR, Mehta GU, Zach L, Li X, Butman JA, Camphausen KA, Lonser RR. Prospective evaluation of radiosurgery for hemangioblastomas in von Hippel-Lindau disease. Neuro Oncol. 2010;12:80–6.
13. Piribauer M, Czech T, Dieckmann K, Birner P, Hainfellner JA, Prayer D, et al. Stabilization of a progressive hemangioblastoma under treatment with thalidomide. J Neurooncol. 2004;66:295–9.
14. Reyes-Botero G, Gallego Perez-Larraya J, Sanson M. Sporadic CNS hemangioblastomatosis, response to sunitinib and secondary polycythemia. J Neurooncol. 2012;107:439–40.

Cavernous Sinus Cavernous Hemangiomas

33

Gabriel Zada, M. Beatriz S. Lopes, Srinivasan Mukundan Jr., and Edward Laws Jr.

33.1 Epidemiology and Clinical Presentation

- Cavernous sinus cavernous hemangiomas (CSCHs) are distinct from cavernous malformations (angiomas) [1].
- CSCHs are benign vascular tumors, not true vascular malformations; they frequently present with headaches and cranial nerve paresis [1, 2].
- Cavernous angiomas, on the other hand, are true vascular malformations that may be located anywhere in the brain. (*See* Chap. 61.)
- CSCHs comprise 2–3 % of cavernous sinus tumors.
- The mean age of patients with CSCHs is 43 years; there is female predilection [3].
- CSCHs occasionally may extend medially into the sella turcica and mimic pituitary adenomas [4–9].
- CSCHs represent 0.07 % of lesions treated in major transsphenoidal series [10].
- In rare cases, cavernous hemangiomas may arise in the sphenoid sinus, potentially resulting in visual deficits and headaches [11].

33.2 Imaging Features

- On MRI, CSCHs often show hypointensity or isointensity on T1-weighted imaging and hyperintensity on T2-weighted imaging (Fig. 33.1). Avid contrast enhancement is common in CSCHs [12, 13].
- On dynamic-enhancement MRI, CSCHs typically demonstrate heterogeneous contrast enhancement with initial enhancement [3].
- In angiographic studies, one third of CSCHs are occult; a blush in the cavernous sinus can be seen for the other two thirds [1].

G. Zada, MD, MS (✉)
Department of Neurological Surgery, Keck School of Medicine, University of Southern California, 1200 N State Street, #3300, Los Angeles, CA 90033, USA
e-mail: gzada@usc.edu

M.B.S. Lopes, MD, PhD
Department of Pathology (Neuropathology), University of Virginia School of Medicine, 1215 Lee Street, Room 3060–HEP, Charlottesville, VA 22908, USA
e-mail: msl2e@virginia.edu

S. Mukundan Jr., PhD, MD
Department of Radiology, Brigham and Women's Hospital, 75 Francis Street, Boston, MA 02115, USA
e-mail: smukundan@partners.org

E. Laws Jr., MD
Department of Neurosurgery, Brigham and Women's Hospital, 15 Francis Street, Boston, MA 02115, USA
e-mail: elaws@partners.org

G. Zada et al. (eds.), *Atlas of Sellar and Parasellar Lesions: Clinical, Radiologic, and Pathologic Correlations*, DOI 10.1007/978-3-319-22855-6_33

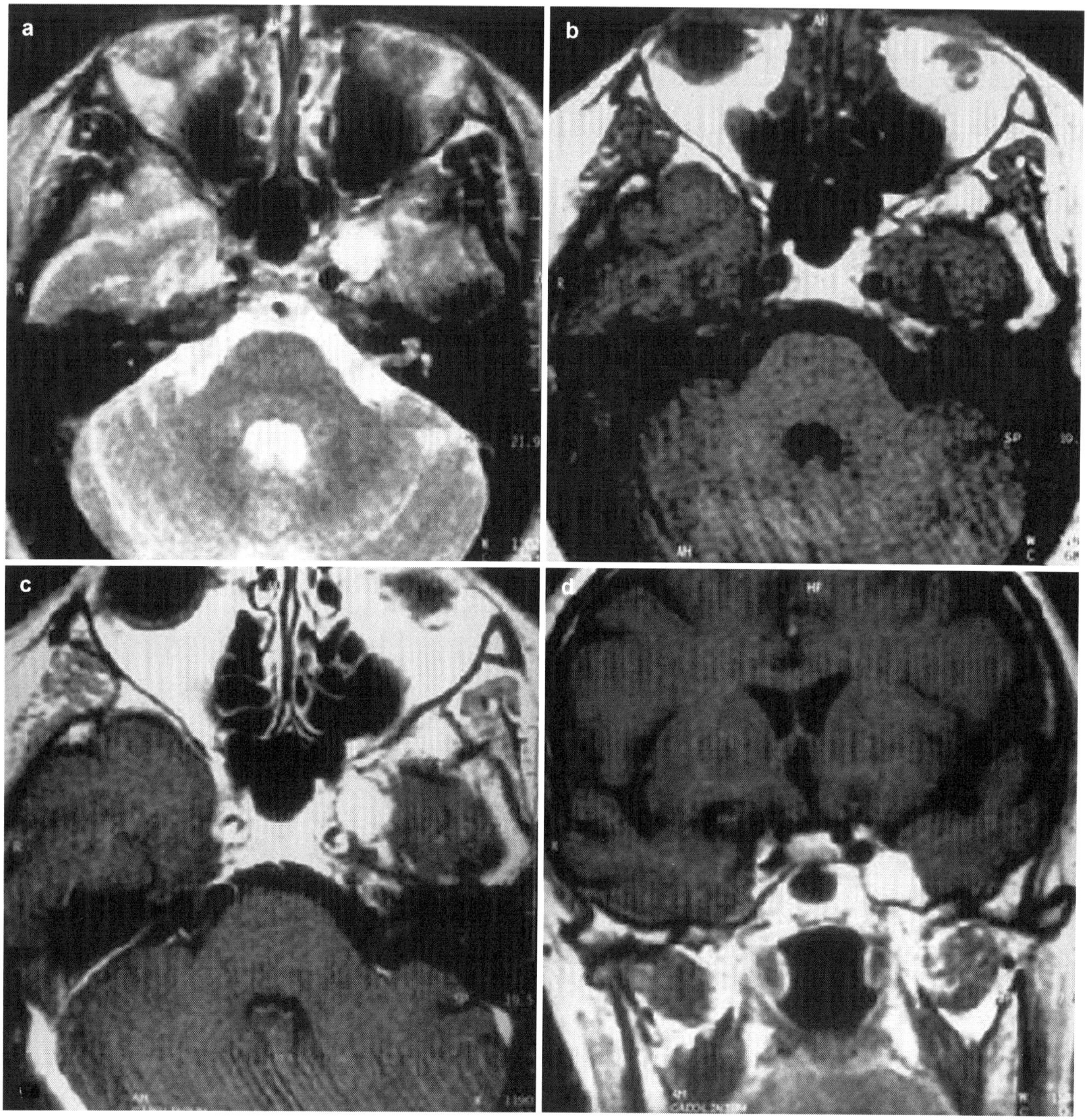

Fig. 33.1 Cavernous sinus cavernous hemangioma. (**a**) Axial T2-weighted MRI showing a rounded, hyperintense lesion in the left parasellar region and cavernous sinus. (**b**) Axial T1-weighted MRI shows the same lesion that is isointense to gray matter. (**c**, **d**) Axial and coronal contrast-enhanced T1-weighted MRI shows avid contrast enhancement of the left cavernous sinus hemangioma (adapted from Tannouri et al with permission, Neuroradiology. 2001;43:317–320)

33.3 Histopathology

- CSCHs are frequently lined by a pseudocapsule. Vascular channels are commonly seen, with intratumoral hemorrhage and calcification being rare findings in CSCHs (Fig. 33.2).
- CSCHs can be classified as one of two subtypes [14]:
  - Type A CSCHs are characterized by adjacent thin-walled, sinusoidal vessels with little intervening connective tissue. These CSCHs are associated with a high degree of intraoperative bleeding.
  - Type B CSCHs are characterized by more interconnective tissue and fewer sinusoidal vessels. These CSCHs are easier to resect surgically because they are associated with less bleeding.

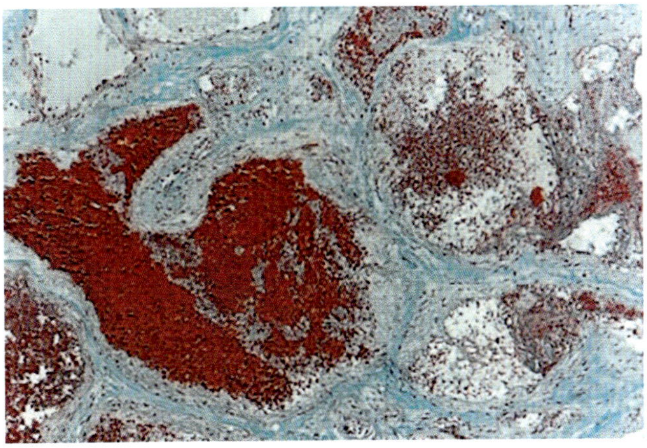

Fig. 33.2 Masson trichrome stain showing a cavernous hemangioma with compact, sclerotic vessels and little interstitium (adapted from Tannouri et al with permission, Neuroradiology. 2001;43:317–320)

33.4 Clinical and Surgical Management

- When necessary, surgical resection of a symptomatic cavernous sinus cavernous hemangioma may be performed via an endonasal endoscopic approach or craniotomy [4].
- The extradural temporopolar approach to the cavernous sinus is often utilized when open craniotomy is recommended [15].
- Injection of fibrin glue has been successfully used to control intraoperative bleeding during resection of CSCHs [16].
- Although recurrence rates are low following surgical resection via craniotomy, the incidence of cranial nerve paresis is rather high [2].
- As a less invasive alternative, stereotactic radiosurgery has been successfully and safely used to treat CSCHs. Tumor volume is decreased in up to 80 % of cases. The typical treatment dose is 13–14 Gy [12, 17, 18].

References

1. Gonzalez LF, Lekovic GP, Eschbacher J, Coons S, Porter RW, Spetzler RF. Are cavernous sinus hemangiomas and cavernous malformations different entities? Neurosurg Focus. 2006;21(1), e6.
2. Goel A, Muzumdar D, Sharma P. Extradural approach for cavernous hemangioma of the cavernous sinus: experience with 13 cases. Neurol Med Chir (Tokyo). 2003;43:112–8; discussion 119.
3. Jinhu Y, Jianping D, Xin L, Yuanli Z. Dynamic enhancement features of cavernous sinus cavernous hemangiomas on conventional contrast-enhanced MR imaging. AJNR Am J Neuroradiol. 2008; 29:577–81.
4. Fraser JF, Mass AY, Brown S, Anand VK, Schwartz TH. Transnasal endoscopic resection of a cavernous sinus hemangioma: technical note and review of the literature. Skull Base. 2008;18:309–15.
5. Hori S, Hayashi N, Nomoto K, Sato H, Hayashi T, Nagai S, et al. Cavernous sinus cavernous hemangioma largely extending into the sella turcica and mimicking pituitary adenoma: case report. Neurol Med Chir (Tokyo). 2010;50:330–2.
6. Chuang CC, Jung SM, Yang JT, Chang CN, Pai PC. Intrasellar cavernous hemangioma. J Clin Neurosci. 2006;13:672–5.
7. Cobbs CS, Wilson CB. Intrasellar cavernous hemangioma. Case report. J Neurosurg. 2001;94:520–2.
8. Lombardi D, Giovanelli M, de Tribolet N. Sellar and parasellar extra-axial cavernous hemangiomas. Acta Neurochir (Wien). 1994;130:47–54.
9. Buonaguidi R, Canapicci R, Mimassi N, Ferdeghini M. Intrasellar cavernous hemangioma. Neurosurgery. 1984;14:732–4.
10. Saeger W, Ludecke DK, Buchfelder M, Fahlbusch R, Quabbe HJ, Petersenn S. Pathohistological classification of pituitary tumors: 10 years of experience with the German Pituitary Tumor Registry. Eur J Endocrinol. 2007;156:203–16.
11. Dufour H, Fesselet J, Métellus P, Figarella-Branger D, Grisoli F. Cavernous hemangioma of the sphenoid sinus: case report and review of the literature. Surg Neurol. 2001;55:169–73; discussion 173.
12. Kida Y, Kobayashi T, Mori Y. Radiosurgery of cavernous hemangiomas in the cavernous sinus. Surg Neurol. 2001;56:117–22; discussion 122–3.
13. Sohn CH, Kim SP, Kim IM, Lee JH, Lee HK. Characteristic MR imaging findings of cavernous hemangiomas in the cavernous sinus. AJNR Am J Neuroradiol. 2003;24:1148–51.
14. Shi J, Hang C, Pan Y, Liu C, Zhang Z. Cavernous hemangiomas in the cavernous sinus. Neurosurgery. 1999;45:1308–13; discussion 1313–4.
15. Zada G, Day JD, Giannotta SL. The extradural temporopolar approach: a review of indications and operative technique. Neurosurg Focus. 2008;25(6), E3.
16. Kim IM, Yim MB, Lee CY, Son EI, Kim DW, Kim SP, Sohn CH. Merits of intralesional fibrin glue injection in surgery for cavernous sinus cavernous hemangiomas. Technical note. J Neurosurg. 2002;97:718–21.
17. Chou CW, Wu HM, Huang CI, Chung WY, Guo WY, Shih YH, et al. Gamma knife surgery for cavernous hemangiomas in the cavernous sinus. Neurosurgery. 2010;67:611–6; discussion 616.
18. Li P, Ren H, Zhang S, Wang W. Clinical results of Gamma Knife surgery for cavernous sinus hemangiomas. J Neurosurg. 2012; 117:89–95.

Optic Pathway (Opticochiasmatic) and Hypothalamic Gliomas

34

Gabriel Zada, M. Beatriz S. Lopes,
Srinivasan Mukundan Jr., and Edward Laws Jr.

34.1 Epidemiology and Clinical Presentation

- Optic pathway gliomas (OPGs) are typically low-grade neoplasms presenting in pediatric patients, often with a history of neurofibromatosis-1 (NF-1).
- OPGs typically arise during the first decade of life. The mean age at diagnosis is 4–5 years.
- Clinical symptoms of OPGs often include visual loss, proptosis, hydrocephalus, precocious puberty, or hypopituitarism [1].
- The prevalence of NF-1 in children with OPGs is 60 % [2]. Conversely, nearly 20 % of patients with NF-1 develop OPGs [3].
- In rare cases, an OPG can present as a sellar mass [4].

34.2 Imaging Features

- OPGs associated with NF-1 are more commonly located along the anterior optic pathways and are likely to involve both optic nerves (Figs. 34.1 and 34.2). On the other hand, sporadic cases of OPG are more likely to involve the central optic chiasm and hypothalamus [5, 6]. Contrast enhancement can be used to evaluate posterior invasion of the optic tracts [3].
- On MRI, the average tumor diameter and volume in NF-1 patients are typically smaller than in non-NF patients. Similarly, OPGs in non-NF patients are more likely to demonstrate vessel encasement, cystic components, and the presence of hydrocephalus [6].
- Most OPGs are hypointense to isointense to the brain on T1-weighted MR imaging and hyperintense on T2-weighted imaging [7], and homogeneous contrast enhancement of OPGs is seen in 60–70 % of patients [6].

G. Zada, MD, MS (✉)
Department of Neurological Surgery, Keck School of Medicine, University of Southern California, 1200 N State Street, #3300, Los Angeles, CA 90033, USA
e-mail: gzada@usc.edu

M.B.S. Lopes, MD, PhD
Department of Pathology (Neuropathology), University of Virginia School of Medicine, 1215 Lee Street, Room 3060–HEP, Charlottesville, VA 22908, USA
e-mail: msl2e@virginia.edu

S. Mukundan Jr., PhD, MD
Department of Radiology, Brigham and Women's Hospital, 75 Francis Street, Boston, MA 02115, USA
e-mail: smukundan@partners.org

E. Laws Jr., MD
Department of Neurosurgery, Brigham and Women's Hospital, 15 Francis Street, Boston, MA 02115, USA
e-mail: elaws@partners.org

G. Zada et al. (eds.), *Atlas of Sellar and Parasellar Lesions: Clinical, Radiologic, and Pathologic Correlations*,
DOI 10.1007/978-3-319-22855-6_34

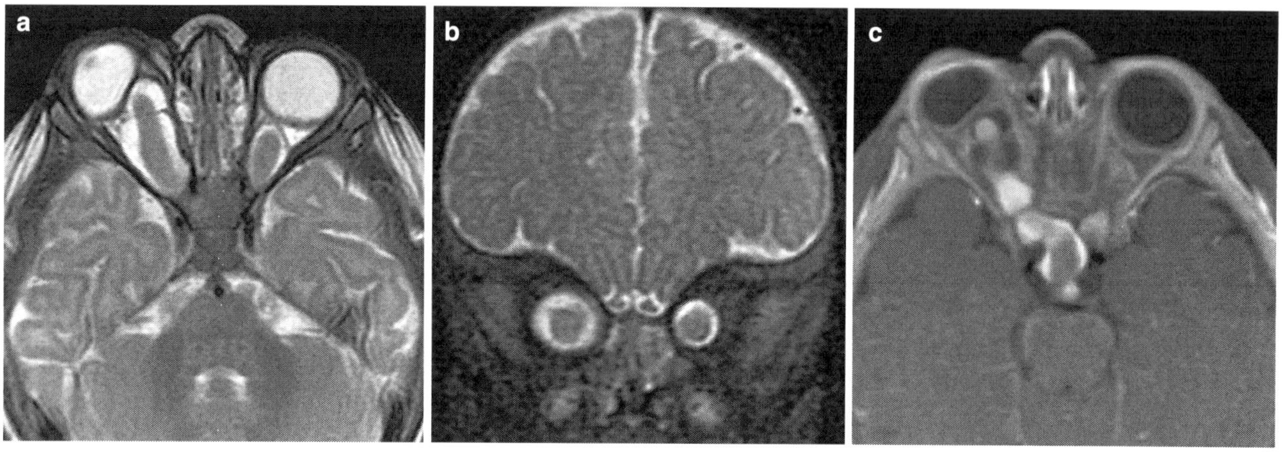

Fig. 34.1 Optic glioma. (**a**) Axial T2-weighted image. (**b**) Coronal T2 inversion-recovery (IR) image. (**c**) Axial T1-weighted gadolinium-enhanced image. The optic nerves are diffusely enlarged bilaterally, with enhancement extending to the optic chiasm. There is dilatation of the optic sheaths, and the right globe is displaced anterolaterally

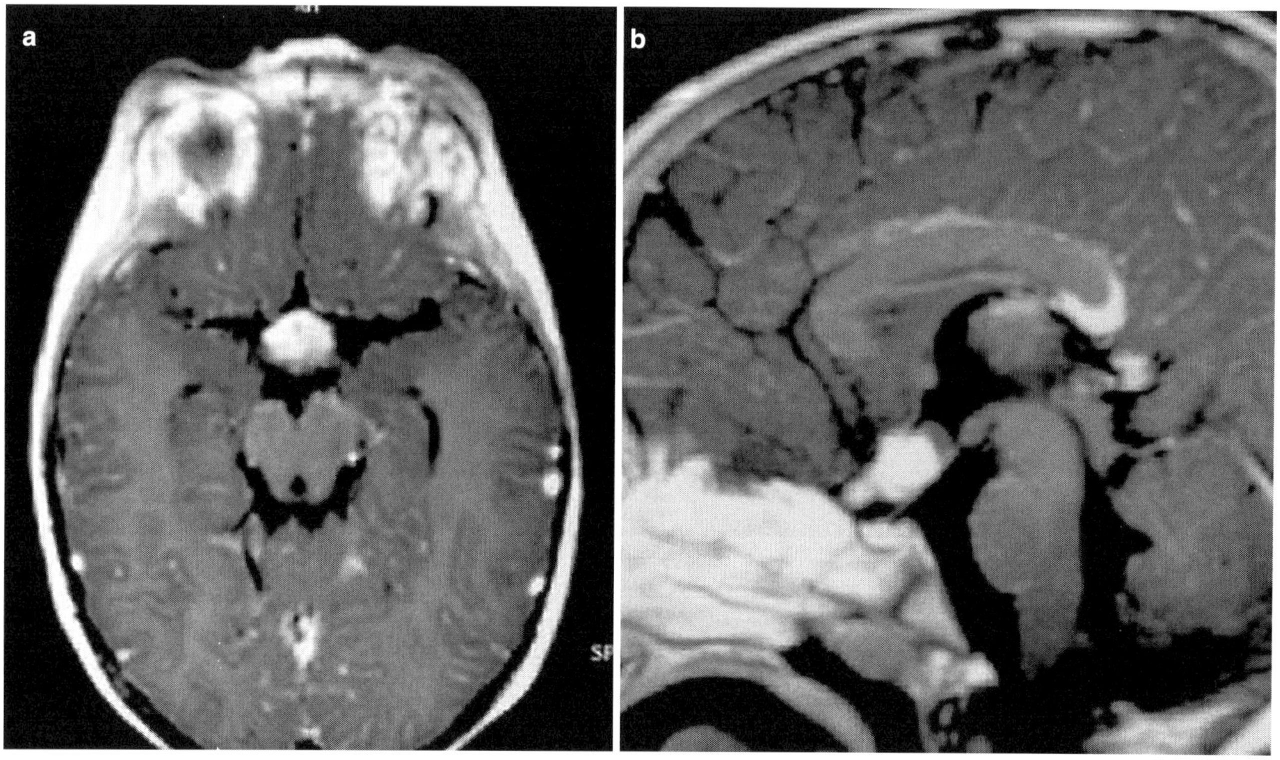

Fig. 34.2 Optic chiasm glioma in a 2-year-old patient with neurofibromatosis type 1. Axial (**a**) and sagittal (**b**) T1-weighted MR images after gadolinium administration show a homogeneously enhancing chiasmal tumor (Adapted with permission from Piccirilli et al. [15])

34.3 Histopathology

- OPGs are comprised of various histopathological glioma subsets, including pilocytic astrocytoma, diffuse infiltrating astrocytoma, and pilomyxoid astrocytoma.
- A majority of OPGs are pilocytic (WHO Grade I) astrocytomas, characterized by hypocellularity, glial fibrillary acidic protein (GFAP) immunoreactivity, and Rosenthal fibers (Figs. 34.3 and 34.4) [7]. Although mitoses are rare, microcystic degeneration is common.
- A minority of OPGs are diffuse (WHO II) astrocytomas or pilomyxoid astrocytomas. The latter are characterized by myxoid vascular and perivascular cellular arrangements without Rosenthal fibers [8].
- Although they are typically low-grade, indolent tumors, malignant transformation has been reported in 4–5 % of OPGs [9].

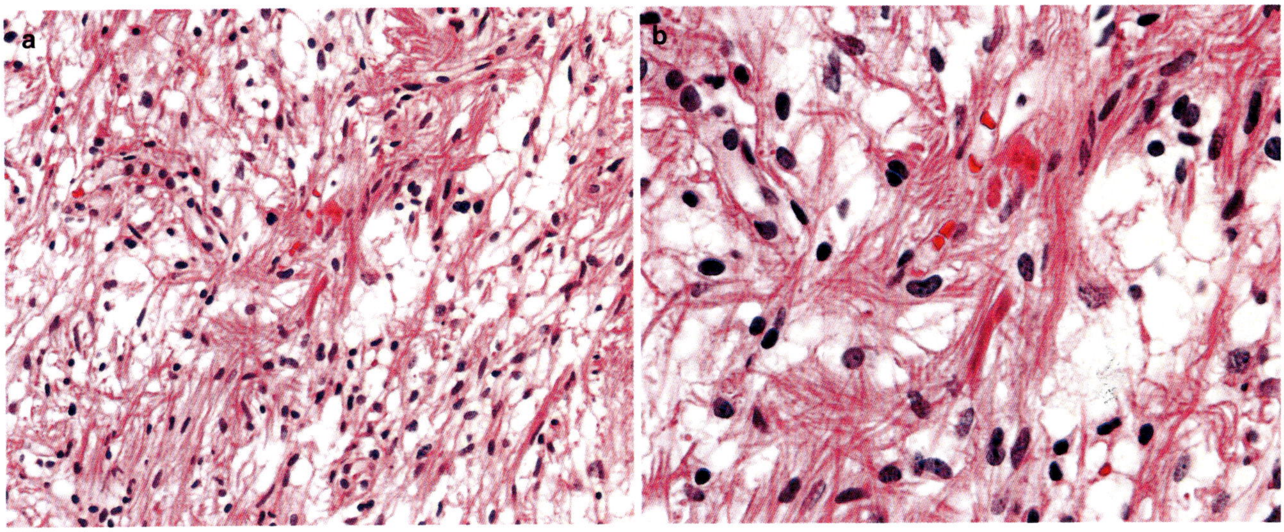

Fig. 34.3 Hypothalamic pilocytic astrocytoma. (**a**) Typical biphasic arrangement of compact, fibrillary pattern admixed with hypocellular and microcystic areas. (**b**) Numerous Rosenthal fibers are intermixed with the piloid cells

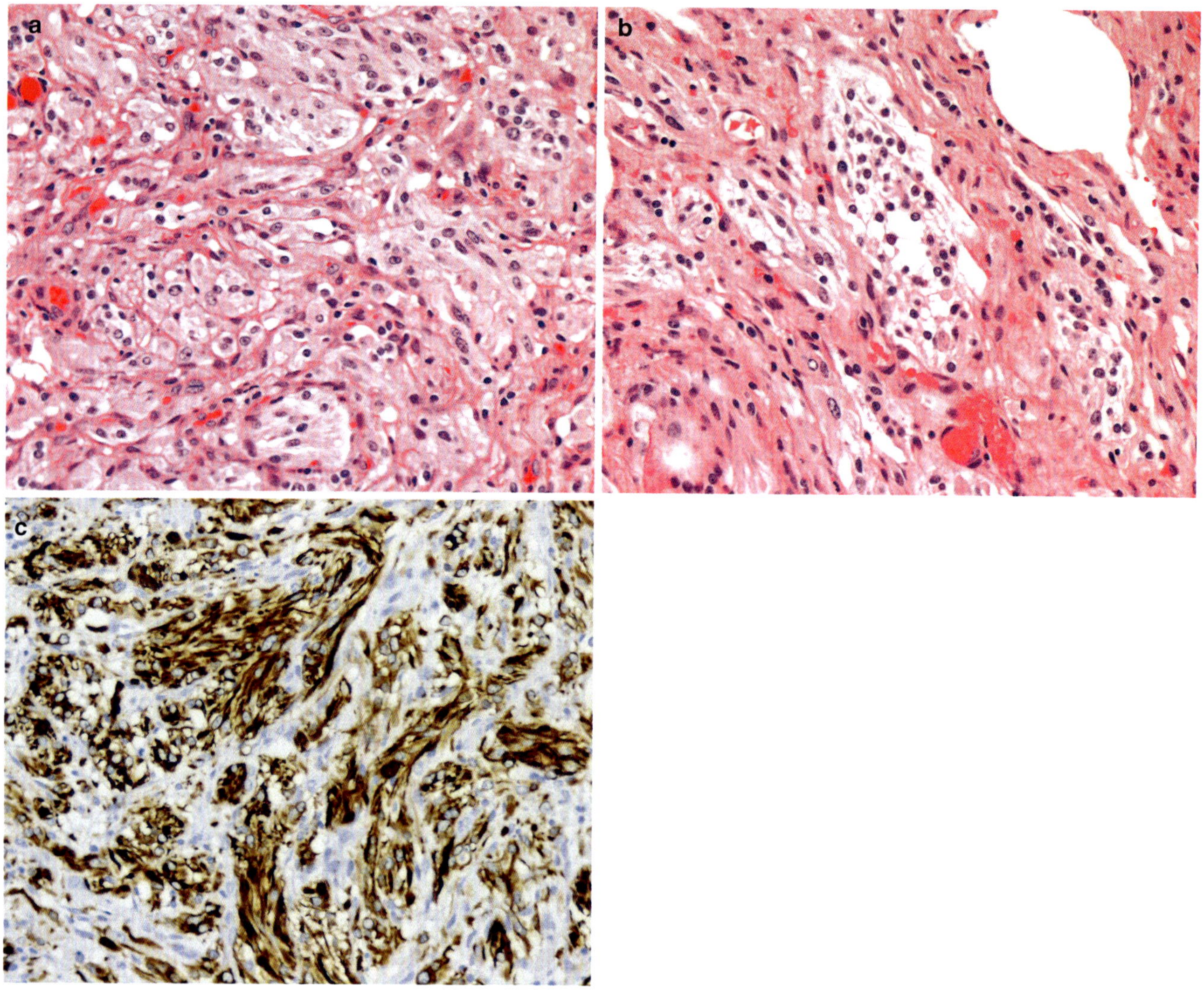

Fig. 34.4 Optic nerve pilocytic astrocytoma. Representative sections from a cystic tumor arising from the optic chiasm and involving the suprasellar region in a 13-month-old boy who presents with vomiting. The tumor shows spindle cells with coarse fibrillar processes and minimal nuclear pleomorphism arranged in fascicles (**a**). Rosenthal fibers are not prominent. A focal biphasic pattern is present (**b**). Immunohistochemical staining for glial fibrillary acidic protein (GFAP) is strongly positive (**c**)

34.4 Clinical and Surgical Management

- Multimodality algorithms for OPGs include surgical resection versus biopsy, chemotherapy, and radiation treatments. Many clinicians advocate the use of early chemotherapy, reserving radiation treatment for as late as possible in children [10, 11].
- Surgical treatment for OPGs is rarely curative and typically is limited to biopsies or minimal debulking. Many authors support empiric treatment with chemotherapy based on clinical and imaging diagnosis alone, with surgery reserved for refractory cases [12]. Early surgery may be indicated for large tumors causing hydrocephalus or for those with unilateral optic nerve involvement [7].
- Chemotherapeutic agents often used to treat OPGs include cisplatin and vincristine [13].
- Stereotactic radiosurgery (typically fractionated) has been used to treat OPGs [14].
- 10-year overall patient survival is greater than 90 %, but progression occurs in nearly half of patients [2].
- Ophthalmologic examinations should be performed every 3 months to monitor for disease progression [3].

References

1. Cnossen MH, Stam EN, Cooiman LC, Simonsz HJ, Stroink H, Oranje AP, et al. Endocrinologic disorders and optic pathway gliomas in children with neurofibromatosis type 1. Pediatrics. 1997;100:667–70.
2. Nicolin G, Parkin P, Mabbott D, Hargrave D, Bartels U, Tabori U, et al. Natural history and outcome of optic pathway gliomas in children. Pediatr Blood Cancer. 2009;53:1231–7.
3. Shamji MF, Benoit BG. Syndromic and sporadic pediatric optic pathway gliomas: review of clinical and histopathological differences and treatment implications. Neurosurg Focus. 2007; 23(5), E3.
4. Tekkok IH, Tahta K, Saglam S. Optic nerve glioma presenting as a huge intrasellar mass. Case report. J Neurosurg Sci. 1994;38:137–40.
5. Taylor T, Jaspan T, Milano G, Gregson R, Parker T, Ritzmann T, et al. Radiological classification of optic pathway gliomas: experience of a modified functional classification system. Br J Radiol. 2008;81:761–6.
6. Kornreich L, Blaser S, Schwarz M, Shuper A, Vishne TH, Cohen IJ, et al. Optic pathway glioma: correlation of imaging findings with the presence of neurofibromatosis. AJNR Am J Neuroradiol. 2001;22:1963–9.
7. Binning MJ, Liu JK, Kestle JR, Brockmeyer DL, Walker ML. Optic pathway gliomas: a review. Neurosurg Focus. 2007;23(5), E2.
8. Ceppa EP, Bouffet E, Griebel R, Robinson C, Tihan T. The pilomyxoid astrocytoma and its relationship to pilocytic astrocytoma: report of a case and a critical review of the entity. J Neurooncol. 2007;81:191–6.
9. Ater J, Tarbell N, Laws Jr E. Optic nerve, chiasmal, and hypothalamic tumors. In: Levin VA, editor. Cancer in the nervous system. 2nd ed. Oxford: Oxford University Press; 2002. p. 158–70.
10. Stieber VW. Radiation therapy for visual pathway tumors. J Neuroophthalmol. 2008;28:222–30.
11. Jahraus CD, Tarbell NJ. Optic pathway gliomas. Pediatr Blood Cancer. 2006;46:586–96.
12. Sawamura Y, Kamada K, Kamoshima Y, Yamaguchi S, Tajima T, Tsubaki J, Fujimaki T. Role of surgery for optic pathway/hypothalamic astrocytomas in children. Neuro Oncol. 2008;10:725–33.
13. Kato T, Sawamura Y, Tada M, Ikeda J, Ishii N, Abe H. Cisplatin/vincristine chemotherapy for hypothalamic/visual pathway astrocytomas in young children. J Neurooncol. 1998;37:263–70.
14. Combs SE, Schulz-Ertner D, Moschos D, Thilmann C, Huber PE, Debus J. Fractionated stereotactic radiotherapy of optic pathway gliomas: tolerance and long-term outcome. Int J Radiat Oncol Biol Phys. 2005;62:814–9.
15. Piccirilli M, Lenzi J, Delfinis C, Trasimeni G, Salvati M, Raco A. Spontaneous regression of optic pathways gliomas in three patients with neurofibromatosis type 1 and critical review of the literature. Childs Nerv Syst. 2006;22:1332–7.

Pituicytomas and Sellar Ependymomas

35

Gabriel Zada, M. Beatriz S. Lopes, Srinivasan Mukundan Jr., and Edward Laws Jr.

35.1 Epidemiology and Clinical Presentation

- Pituicytoma, a new pathological entity defined by the WHO in 2007, is a variant of a low-grade astrocytoma originating in the neurohypophysis [1, 2].
- In the past, pituicytoma has been referred to as infundibuloma, choristoma, granular cell tumor, or granular cell myoblastoma. (*See* the following section on Granular Cell Tumor.)
- Pituicytoma typically occurs in adults and frequently mimics a pituitary adenoma [2–4].
- Astrocytoma and pituicytoma collectively comprise 0.22–0.65 % of all lesions treated in major transsphenoidal series [5, 6].
- There is a slight male predilection of 1.6:1 [7].
- Pituicytoma can present with visual loss, headache, and/or hypopituitarism. Even though pituicytoma is a primary tumor of the neurohypophysis, diabetes insipidus is not a common finding at presentation [8, 9].
- Sellar ependymoma is a rare variant of pituicytoma, described in only four cases to date [10].

35.2 Imaging Features

- On MRI, pituicytoma often appears as a solid, discrete, sellar, and suprasellar mass that enhances avidly and homogeneously with contrast (Fig. 35.1) [4, 8, 11].
- It mimics the appearance of a meningioma or pituitary adenoma [12].
- Pituicytomas are typically isointense to gray matter on T1-weighted MR imaging and isointense or hyperintense on T2-weighted imaging [13].
- Approximately one quarter will appear separate from the anterior pituitary gland [8].

G. Zada, MD, MS (✉)
Department of Neurological Surgery, Keck School of Medicine, University of Southern California, 1200 N State Street, #3300, Los Angeles, CA 90033, USA
e-mail: gzada@usc.edu

M.B.S. Lopes, MD, PhD
Department of Pathology (Neuropathology), University of Virginia School of Medicine, 1215 Lee Street, Room 3060–HEP, Charlottesville, VA 22908, USA
e-mail: msl2e@virginia.edu

S. Mukundan Jr., PhD, MD
Department of Radiology, Brigham and Women's Hospital, 75 Francis Street, Boston, MA 02115, USA
e-mail: smukundan@partners.org

E. Laws Jr., MD
Department of Neurosurgery, Brigham and Women's Hospital, 15 Francis Street, Boston, MA 02115, USA
e-mail: elaws@partners.org

G. Zada et al. (eds.), *Atlas of Sellar and Parasellar Lesions: Clinical, Radiologic, and Pathologic Correlations*,
DOI 10.1007/978-3-319-22855-6_35

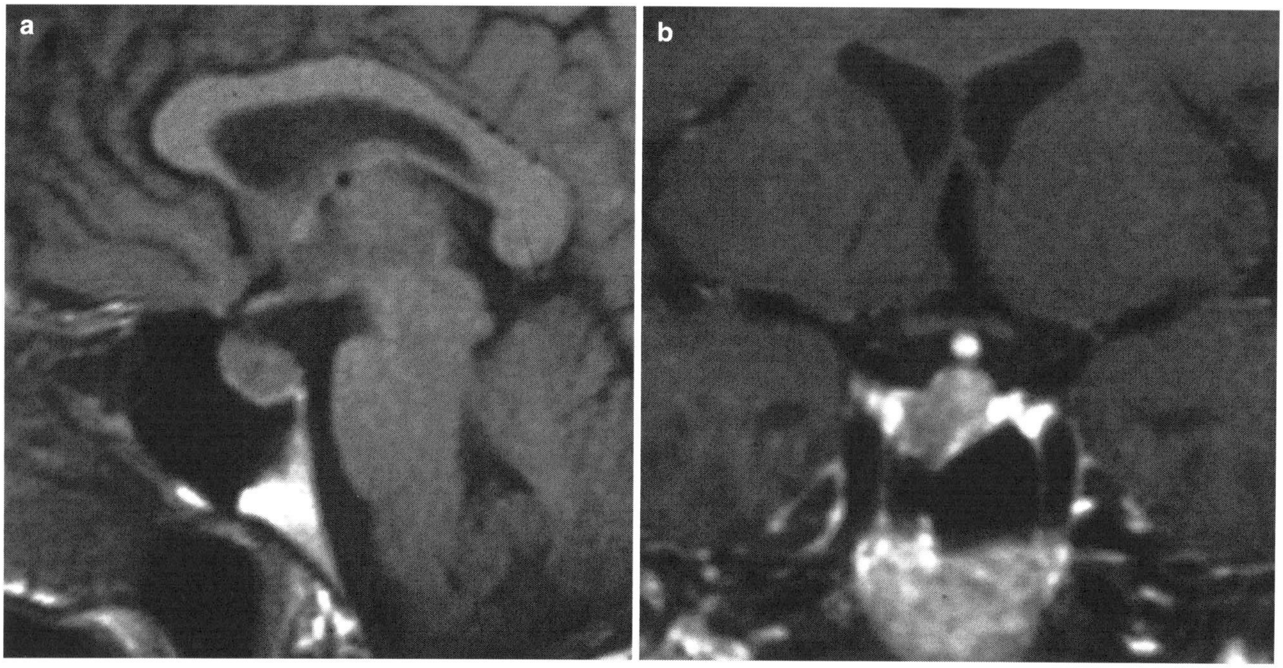

Fig. 35.1 Pituicytoma. (**a**) Sagittal T1-weighted precontrast image. (**b**) Coronal T1-weighted gadolinium-enhanced image. There is a hypoenhancing lesion in the right aspect of the sella, without suprasellar extension. Remodeling of the right sellar floor is also seen

35.3 Histopathology

- Pituicytoma is classified as a WHO Grade I spindle cell astrocytic tumor originating in the neurohypophysis or infundibulum.
- Pituicytoma consists of plump spindle cells with slightly pleomorphic nuclei, pinpoint nucleoli, and rare or absent mitoses [2].
- Specimens are generally positive for S100 and vimentin immunostaining and are nonreactive for synaptophysin and neurofilament protein [2]. GFAP staining may be focally or diffusely positive (Fig. 35.2).
- Most significantly, pituicytomas show strong nuclear TTF-1 immunoreacitivity (Fig. 35.2e).
- The MIB-1 labeling index is reported to be low (1–2 %) in most cases [14].
- Pituicytoma can be differentiated from normal neurohypophysis, which contains axons and Herring bodies [2].
- Pituicytomas also can be differentiated from pilocytic astrocytomas, which have Rosenthal fibers and granular bodies [15].
- Ultrastructural analysis shows absence of secretory granules in pituicytoma [16].
- Sellar ependymoma is a rare lesion with classic ependymal cell findings; it is thought to arise from ependymal pituicytes [10].

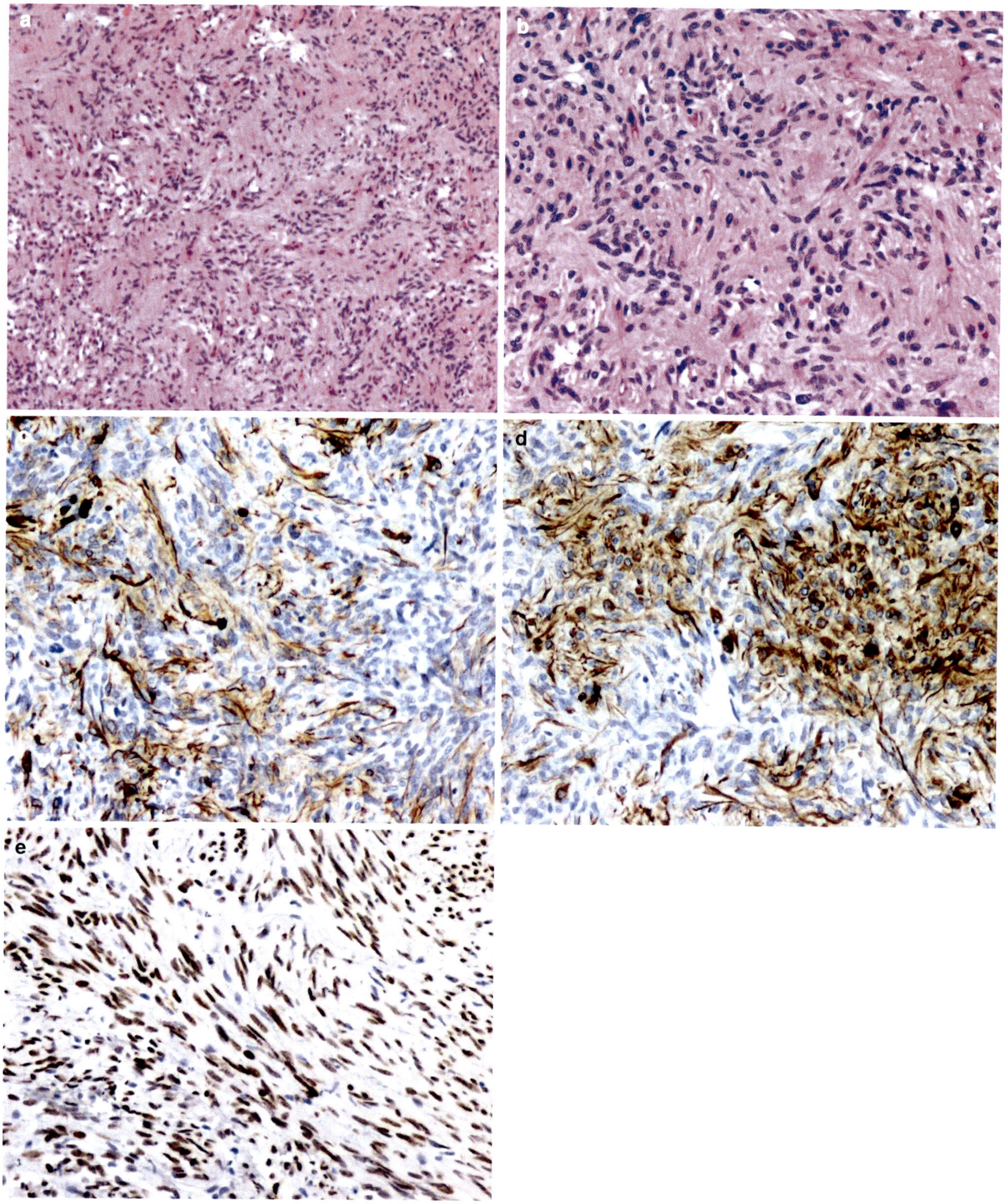

Fig. 35.2 Pituicytoma. Pituicytomas are characterized by elongated fibrillary cells arranged in a fascicular pattern. The cells have a piloid, fibrillary appearance similar to pilocytic astrocytomas (**a**, **b**, H&E stain). Tumor cells are strongly immunoreactive for GFAP (**c**) and vimentin (**d**). Thyroid transcription factor 1 (TTF-1) nuclear immunoreactivity is strongly positive in pituicytomas (**e**) and seems to confirm an origin from the intrinsic glial cell of the pituitary, the pituicyte

35.4 Clinical and Surgical Management

- Transsphenoidal surgery is typically an effective approach for intrasellar pituicytoma. For purely suprasellar pituicytoma, craniotomy may be preferred, as pituicytomas have been reported to be highly vascular, firm tumors that may result in considerable intraoperative bleeding [17].
- Aggressive surgical management is recommended when feasible, although a gross total resection often cannot be achieved safely.
- The vascular supply of pituicytomas has been shown to derive in part from the superior hypophyseal arteries, and selective embolization prior to surgery has been suggested if the diagnosis is known ahead of time [3, 17].
- Although no large series with long-term follow-up are available, gross total resection has been associated with long-term recurrence-free follow-up. Recurrence appears to be common following subtotal surgical resection, occurring in roughly 39 % of patients [9, 18].
- Adjunctive radiation therapy may have been beneficial in anecdotal cases, although no clear clinical benefit has been shown [9].
- Hormone replacement therapy for hypopituitarism is often required after treatment.

References

1. Louis DN, Ohgaki H, Wiestler OD, Cavenee WK, Burger PC, Jouvet A, et al. The 2007 WHO classification of tumours of the central nervous system. Acta Neuropathol. 2007;114:97–109.
2. Brat DJ, Scheithauer BW, Staugaitis SM, Holtzman RN, Morgello S, Burger PC. Pituicytoma: a distinctive low-grade glioma of the neurohypophysis. Am J Surg Pathol. 2000;24:362–8.
3. Gibbs WN, Monuki ES, Linskey ME, Hasso AN. Pituicytoma: diagnostic features on selective carotid angiography and MR imaging. AJNR Am J Neuroradiol. 2006;27:1639–42.
4. Hurley TR, D'Angelo CM, Clasen RA, Wilkinson SB, Passavoy RD. Magnetic resonance imaging and pathological analysis of a pituicytoma: case report. Neurosurgery. 1994;35:314–7; discussion 317.
5. Saeger W, Ludecke DK, Buchfelder M, Fahlbusch R, Quabbe HJ, Petersenn S. Pathohistological classification of pituitary tumors: 10 years of experience with the German Pituitary Tumor Registry. Eur J Endocrinol. 2007;156:203–16.
6. Furtado SV, Ghosal N, Venkatesh PK, Gupta K, Hegde AS. Diagnostic and clinical implications of pituicytoma. J Clin Neurosci. 2010;17:938–43.
7. Brat DJ, Scheithauer BW, Fuller GN, Tihan T. Newly codified glial neoplasms of the 2007 WHO Classification of Tumours of the Central Nervous System: angiocentric glioma, pilomyxoid astrocytoma and pituicytoma. Brain Pathol. 2007;17:319–24.
8. Covington MF, Chin SS, Osborn AG. Pituicytoma, spindle cell oncocytoma, and granular cell tumor: clarification and meta-analysis of the world literature since 1893. AJNR Am J Neuroradiol. 2011;32:2067–72.
9. Pirayesh Islamian A, Buslei R, Saeger W, Fahlbusch R. Pituicytoma: overview of treatment strategies and outcome. Pituitary. 2012; 15:227–36.
10. Scheithauer BW, Swearingen B, Whyte ET, Auluck PK, Stemmer-Rachamimov AO. Ependymoma of the sella turcica: a variant of pituicytoma. Hum Pathol. 2009;40:435–40.
11. Uesaka T, Miyazono M, Nishio S, Iwaki T. Astrocytoma of the pituitary gland (pituicytoma): case report. Neuroradiology. 2002;44:123–5.
12. Chakraborti S, Mahadevan A, Govindan A, Sridhar K, Mohan NV, Satish IR, et al. Pituicytoma: report of three cases with review of literature. Pathol Res Pract. 2013;209:52–8.
13. Hammoud DA, Munter FM, Brat DJ, Pomper MG. Magnetic resonance imaging features of pituicytomas: analysis of 10 cases. J Comput Assist Tomogr. 2010;34:757–61.
14. Nakasu Y, Nakasu S, Saito A, Horiguchi S, Kameya T. Pituicytoma. Two case reports. Neurol Med Chir (Tokyo). 2006;46:152–6.
15. Katsuta T, Inoue T, Nakagaki H, Takeshita M, Morimoto K, Iwaki T. Distinctions between pituicytoma and ordinary pilocytic astrocytoma. Case report. J Neurosurg. 2003;98:404–6.
16. Phillips JJ, Misra A, Feuerstein BG, Kunwar S, Tihan T. Pituicytoma: characterization of a unique neoplasm by histology, immunohistochemistry, ultrastructure, and array-based comparative genomic hybridization. Arch Pathol Lab Med. 2010;134:1063–9.
17. Wolfe SQ, Bruce J, Morcos JJ. Pituicytoma: case report. Neurosurgery. 2008;63:E173–4; discussion E174.
18. Kowalski RJ, Prayson RA, Mayberg MR. Pituicytoma. Ann Diagn Pathol. 2004;8:290–4.

Granular Cell Tumors

36

Gabriel Zada, M. Beatriz S. Lopes,
Srinivasan Mukundan Jr., and Edward Laws Jr.

36.1 Epidemiology and Clinical Presentation

- These tumors were previously referred to as choristomas, granular cell myoblastoma, granular cell pituicytoma, and granular cell schwannoma.
- Unlike granular cell tumors arising in the gastrointestinal tract and skin, which are thought to be of Schwann cell origin, pituitary granular cell tumors are considered to be unique neoplasms of the neurohypophysis and pituitary stalk; they have been suggested to derive from pituicytes [1].
- They are benign, indolent, and slow-growing tumors with little potential for invasion or malignant transformation [2].
- They are the most common lesions to arise primarily in the neurohypophysis and have been discovered in 9 % of routine neurohypophysis autopsy specimens [3, 4].
- Symptomatic tumors are quite rare, corresponding to less than 0.5 % of tumors involving this region [1].
- The tumors typically present in adult patients (mean age 48 years) with symptoms of mass effect, including headache and visual loss [5].
- They occur more frequently in women than in men (2:1) [2, 5].
- Granular cell tumors comprise 0.17 % of resected sellar lesions in major transsphenoidal series [6].

36.2 Imaging Features

- CT imaging demonstrates a hypodense or isodense mass that enhances with contrast, with occasional calcification. The dorsum sellae can infrequently demonstrate bony erosion. The tumors often appear hyperdense to the brain on CT imaging [3, 5, 7].
- MRI typically shows a well-defined, T1- and T2-isointense mass with homogenous enhancement and an epicenter near the dorsum sella, often extending into the suprasellar region (Fig. 36.1) [5, 7].
- Granular cell tumors frequently mimic the imaging features of pituitary adenomas and meningiomas.

G. Zada, MD, MS (✉)
Department of Neurological Surgery, Keck School of Medicine, University of Southern California, 1200 N State Street, #3300, Los Angeles, CA 90033, USA
e-mail: gzada@usc.edu

M.B.S. Lopes, MD, PhD
Department of Pathology (Neuropathology), University of Virginia School of Medicine, 1215 Lee Street, Room 3060–HEP, Charlottesville, VA 22908, USA
e-mail: msl2e@virginia.edu

S. Mukundan Jr., PhD, MD
Department of Radiology, Brigham and Women's Hospital, 75 Francis Street, Boston, MA 02115, USA
e-mail: smukundan@partners.org

E. Laws Jr., MD
Department of Neurosurgery, Brigham and Women's Hospital, 15 Francis Street, Boston, MA 02115, USA
e-mail: elaws@partners.org

G. Zada et al. (eds.), *Atlas of Sellar and Parasellar Lesions: Clinical, Radiologic, and Pathologic Correlations*, DOI 10.1007/978-3-319-22855-6_36

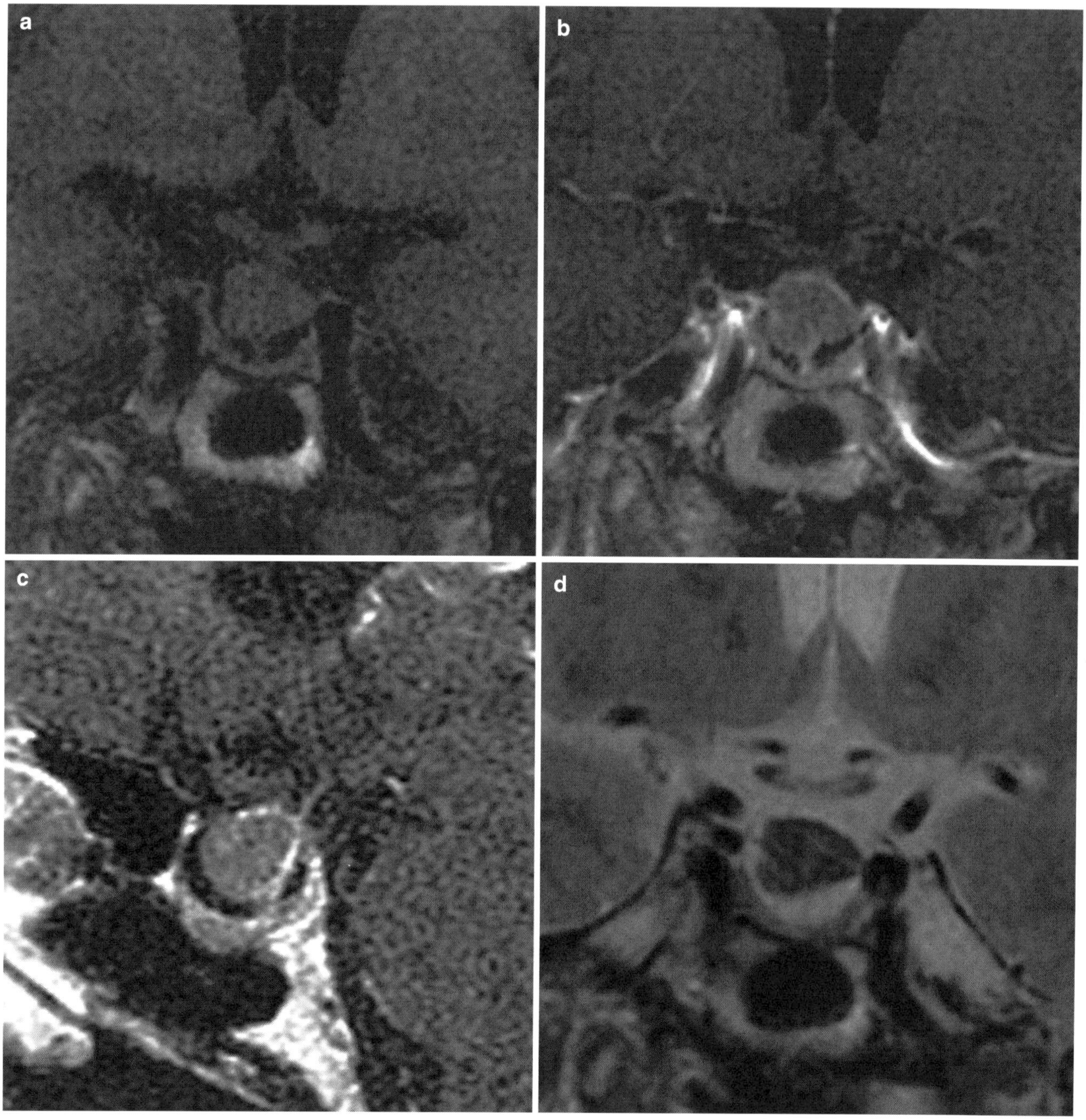

Fig. 36.1 Granular cell tumor. (**a**) Coronal T1-weighted pre-gadolinium image. (**b**) Coronal T1-weighted post-gadolinium image. (**c**) Sagittal T1-weighted post-gadolinium image. (**d**) Coronal T2-weighted image. There is a hypoenhancing mass in the suprasellar region anterior to and abutting the pituitary stalk. The mass appears separate from the pituitary gland

36.3 Histopathology

- Intraoperatively and grossly, granular cell tumors firm, vascular tumors that may bleed extensively during surgical resection [3].
- Histologically, granular cell tumors are characterized by uniform polygonal cells with distinct, eosinophilic granular cytoplasm. The nuclei are round with delicate chromatin and uniform nucleoli, and they tend to be located in the periphery of the cells.
- The cytoplasmic granules are positive for periodic acid–Schiff (PAS) stain and are diastase resistant (Fig. 36.2) [8].
- The tumor shows absent to low mitotic activity, and necrosis is rarely seen.
- A fine, delicate network of capillaries is present, with occasional perivascular lymphocytic infiltrates.
- Granular cell tumors are negative for neuroendocrine markers.
- The tumors show immunoreactivity for vimentin and S100 protein, but only occasionally show GFAP immunoreactivity [8].
- The macrophage/lysosome marker CD68 is consistently and strongly immunoreactive in all tumors.
- Most significantly, granular cell tumors are strongly immunoreactive for TTF-1, as are the other pituicyte-derived tumors [9, 10].
- Electron microscopy shows a typical rich, lysosomal population (Fig. 36.2c). Intermediate filaments are scarce, and neurosecretory granules are absent.
- Although very rare, there are some reported cases of atypical granular cell tumor [8, 11].

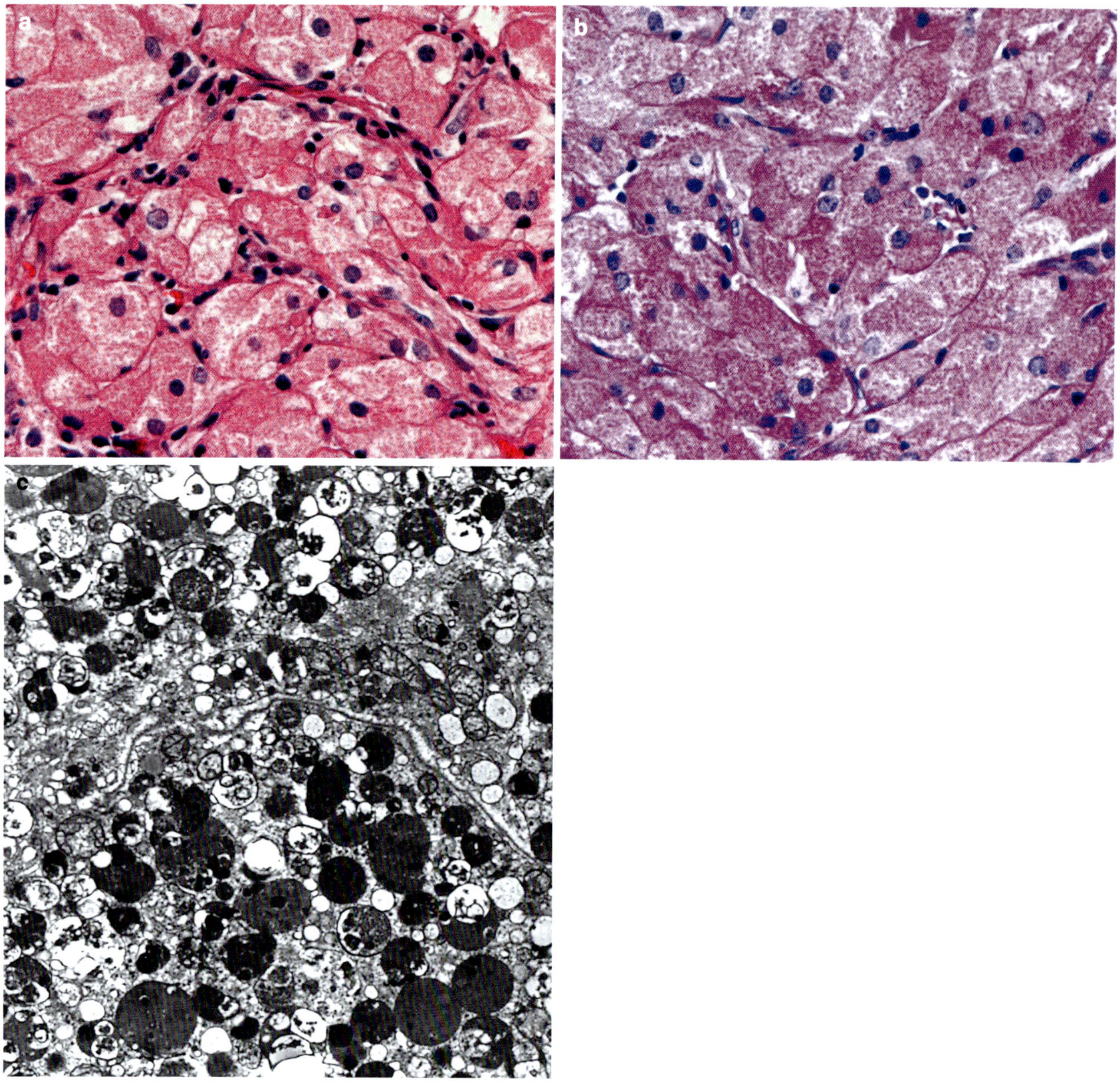

Fig. 36.2 Granular cell tumor. Granular cell tumors show characteristic plump, large cells with granular cytoplasm by H&E stain (**a**), which is strongly positive by periodic acid–Schiff (PAS) staining after diastase treatment (**b**). The granular cytoplasmic component is represented by lysosomal accumulation by electron microscopy (**c**). Similar to other tumors thought to be derived from pituicytes of the neurohypophysis, nuclear immunoreactivity for TTF-1 is present (*not shown*)

36.4 Clinical and Surgical Management

- Surgical resection, typically via a transsphenoidal approach, is the mainstay of treatment [3, 5].
- Granular cell tumors may be especially firm and not amenable to suction [3].
- The use of radiotherapy has been reported for residual or recurrent tumors, with excellent rates of long-term tumor control [3, 5].
- Recurrence has been reported in 14 % of tumors.

References

1. Lopes M, Scheithauer B, Saeger W. Granular cell tumor. In: DeLellis R, Lloyd R, Heitz P, Eng C, editors. WHO classification of tumours, pathology and genetic of tumours of endocrine organs. Lyon: IARC Press; 2004. p. 44–5.
2. Cone L, Srinivasan M, Romanul FC. Granular cell tumor (choristoma) of the neurohypophysis: two cases and a review of the literature. AJNR Am J Neuroradiol. 1990;11:403–6.
3. Schaller B, Kirsch E, Tolnay M, Mindermann T. Symptomatic granular cell tumor of the pituitary gland: case report and review of the literature. Neurosurgery. 1998;42:166–70; discussion 170–1.
4. Tomita T, Gates E. Pituitary adenomas and granular cell tumors. Incidence, cell type, and location of tumor in 100 pituitary glands at autopsy. Am J Clin Pathol. 1999;111:817–25.
5. Cohen-Gadol AA, Pichelmann MA, Link MJ, Scheithauer BW, Krecke KN, Young Jr WF, et al. Granular cell tumor of the sellar and suprasellar region: clinicopathologic study of 11 cases and literature review. Mayo Clin Proc. 2003;78:567–73.
6. Saeger W, Ludecke DK, Buchfelder M, Fahlbusch R, Quabbe HJ, Petersenn S. Pathohistological classification of pituitary tumors: 10 years of experience with the German Pituitary Tumor Registry. Eur J Endocrinol. 2007;156:203–16.
7. Covington MF, Chin SS, Osborn AG. Pituicytoma, spindle cell oncocytoma, and granular cell tumor: clarification and meta-analysis of the world literature since 1893. AJNR Am J Neuroradiol. 2011;32:2067–72.
8. Kasashima S, Oda Y, Nozaki J, Shirasaki M, Nakanishi I. A case of atypical granular cell tumor of the neurohypophysis. Pathol Int. 2000;50:568–73.
9. Lee EB, Tihan T, Scheithauer BW, Zhang PJ, Gonatas NK. Thyroid transcription factor 1 expression in sellar tumors: a histogenetic marker? J Neuropathol Exp Neurol. 2009;68:482–8.
10. Mete O, Lopes MB, Asa SL. Spindle cell oncocytomas and granular cell tumors of the pituitary are variants of pituicytoma. Am J Surg Pathol. 2013;37:1694–9.
11. Shuangshoti S, Chantra K, Navalitloha Y, Charoonwatanalaoha S. Atypical granular cell tumor of the neurohypophysis: a case report with review of the literature. J Med Assoc Thai. 1998;81: 641–6.

Germ Cell Tumors of the Sellar Region

37

Gabriel Zada, M. Beatriz S. Lopes, Srinivasan Mukundan Jr., and Edward Laws Jr.

37.1 Epidemiology and Clinical Presentation

- Germ cell tumors comprise 0.15 % of lesions in major transsphenoidal series [1].
- They frequently present in children and adolescents, with a mean age of 18 years [2, 3].
- Germ cell tumors of the sellar region often (6–13 % of cases) occur as synchronous lesions in association with pineal germinomas ("bifocal disease"). They typically arise in the suprasellar or hypothalamic region and may extend along the floor of the third ventricle [4–7].
- They often present with "idiopathic" diabetes insipidus, without evidence of a focal mass lesion on MRI (referred to as "occult neurohypophyseal germinoma"). Suprasellar germinoma may be a delayed diagnosis in patients with idiopathic diabetes insipidus who present with infundibular thickening [8–10].
- Levels of β-hCG are often elevated in the serum and CSF [8].
- Alpha-fetoprotein (AFP) may be elevated in some patients.
- Hyperprolactinemia and GH deficiency are the most frequently associated types of anterior pituitary dysfunction [9].
- Mature teratomas in the suprasellar region often present with symptoms related to mass effect, such as visual loss [2].
- Primary intrasellar germ cell tumors have been reported infrequently; they typically arise in the neurohypophysis [11, 12].
- They are frequently invasive tumors that may extend into the cavernous sinus or suprasellar space [13].

37.2 Imaging Features

- Germ cell tumors often present initially with thickening or enhancement of the infundibulum, which precedes development of a focal suprasellar mass [14].
- Germ cell tumors in the sellar region are often isointense to the brain on T1- and T2-weighted imaging and demonstrate avid contrast enhancement (Fig. 37.1) [15, 16].
- Intrasellar germ cell tumors frequently arise in the neurohypophysis and can be seen as distinct lesions posterior to the adenohypophysis [17].
- Invasion of the cavernous sinus and suprasellar region may occur (Fig. 37.2).

G. Zada, MD, MS (✉)
Department of Neurological Surgery, Keck School of Medicine, University of Southern California, 1200 N State Street, #3300, Los Angeles, CA 90033, USA
e-mail: gzada@usc.edu

M.B.S. Lopes, MD, PhD
Department of Pathology (Neuropathology), University of Virginia School of Medicine, 1215 Lee Street, Room 3060–HEP, Charlottesville, VA 22908, USA
e-mail: msl2e@virginia.edu

S. Mukundan Jr., PhD, MD
Department of Radiology, Brigham and Women's Hospital, 75 Francis Street, Boston, MA 02115, USA
e-mail: smukundan@partners.org

E. Laws Jr., MD
Department of Neurosurgery, Brigham and Women's Hospital, 15 Francis Street, Boston, MA 02115, USA
e-mail: elaws@partners.org

G. Zada et al. (eds.), *Atlas of Sellar and Parasellar Lesions: Clinical, Radiologic, and Pathologic Correlations*, DOI 10.1007/978-3-319-22855-6_37

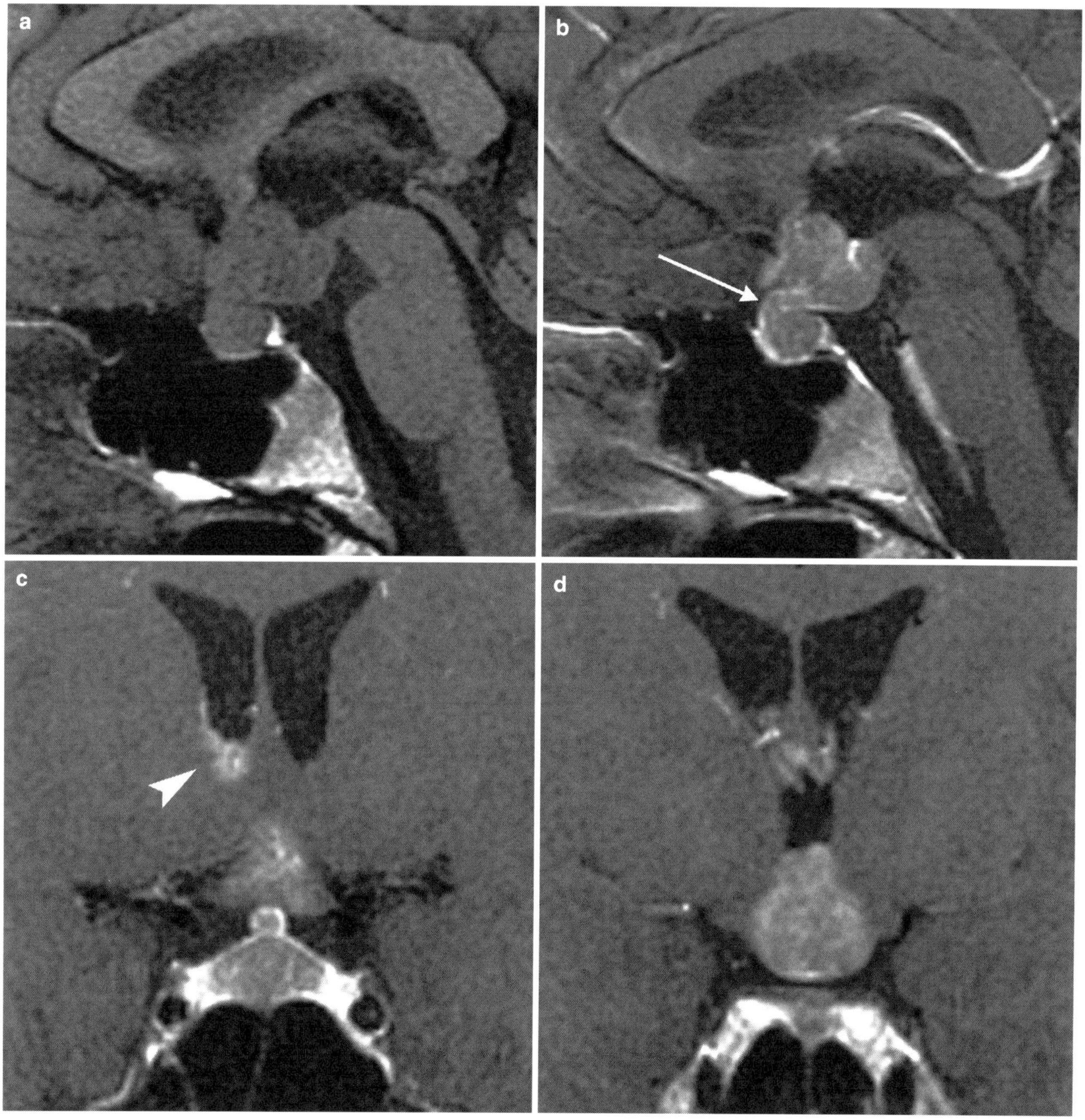

Fig. 37.1 Germ cell tumor. (**a**) Sagittal T1-weighted pre-gadolinium image. (**b**) Sagittal T1-weighted post-gadolinium image. (**c**, **d**) Coronal T1-weighted post-gadolinium image. There is a lobular, heterogeneously enhancing mass in the sella and suprasellar regions, with involvement of the pituitary stalk (**b**, *arrow*) and the floor of the third ventricle. Additional nodular enhancing lesion is seen in the right lateral ventricle (**c**, *arrowhead*), consistent with distant spread of tumor

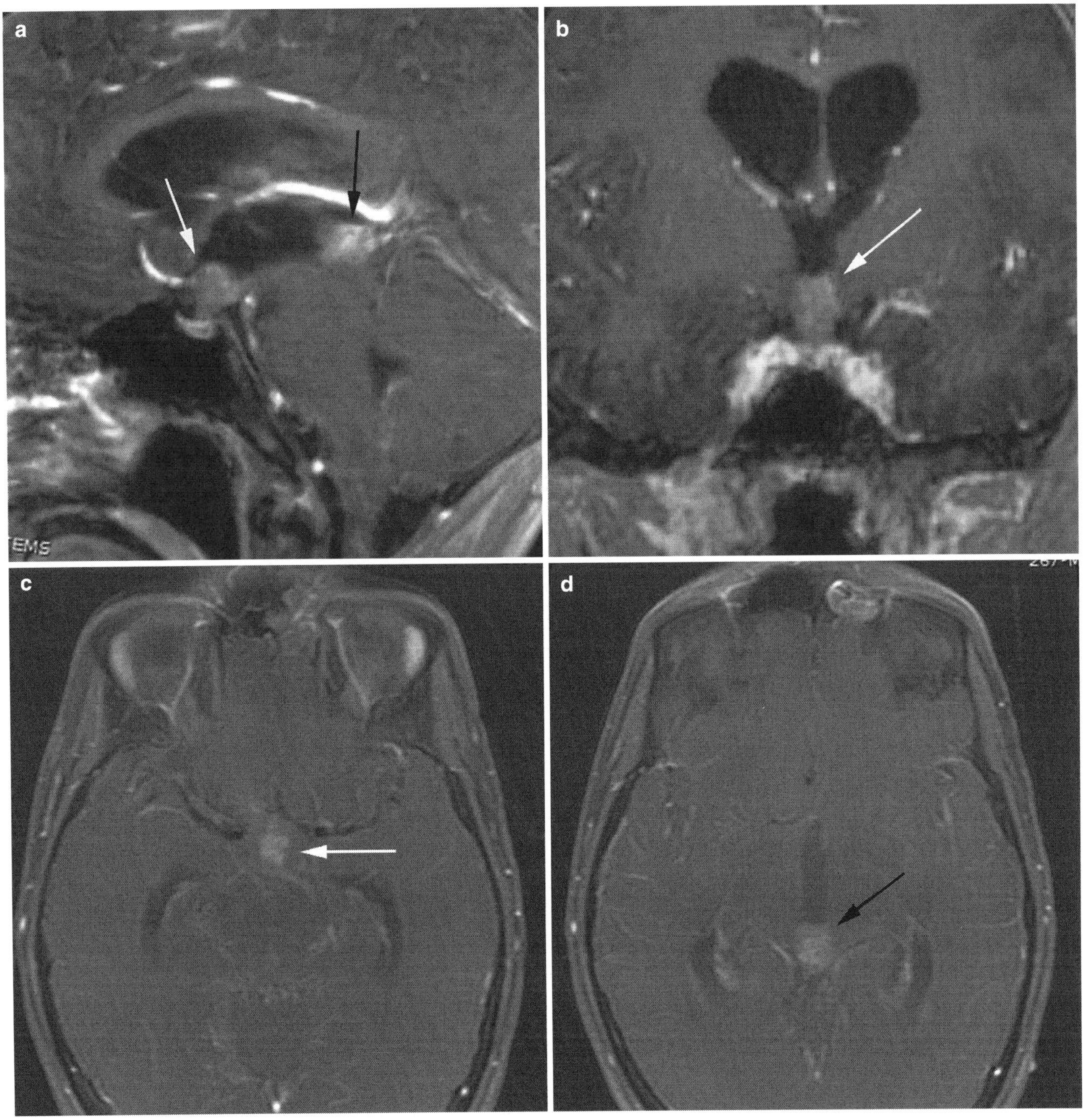

Fig. 37.2 Germinoma. (**a**) Sagittal T1-weighted post-gadolinium image. (**b**) Coronal T1-weighted post-gadolinium image. (**c, d**) Axial T1-weighted, fat-saturated, post-gadolinium image. There are nodular enhancing masses in both the suprasellar region (**a**, **d**, *white arrows*) and the pineal region (**a–c**, *black arrows*). The suprasellar lesion involves the pituitary stalk, but the pituitary gland appears separate from the mass. There is hydrocephalus with enlargement of the lateral and third ventricles

37.3 Histopathology

- Germ cell tumors of the sellar or suprasellar region are histologically identical to their gonadal and extragonadal counterparts.
- The tumors may be divided into two major groups: germinomas and nongerminomatous germ cell tumors. The nongerminomatous group includes embryonal carcinoma, endodermal sinus tumor (yolk-sac tumor), choriocarcinoma, and teratomas (mature, immature, or with malignant transformation) [18].
- In the sellar/suprasellar region, germinoma (Fig. 37.3) is the most frequent germ cell tumor, accounting for 61.5 % of cases, followed by teratomas and mixed germ cell tumors [19, 20].
- In addition to specific histopathologic patterns, several immunomarkers are helpful to differentiate these tumor subtypes (e.g. OCT4, c-kit).
- In children presenting with diabetes insipidus and hypopituitarism who undergo surgical biopsy, germ cell tumors may be masked by lymphocytic infiltration and demonstrate a pathology that is initially more consistent with hypophysitis. Delayed development of germ cell tumors frequently follows, however, even up to several years later [21, 22].

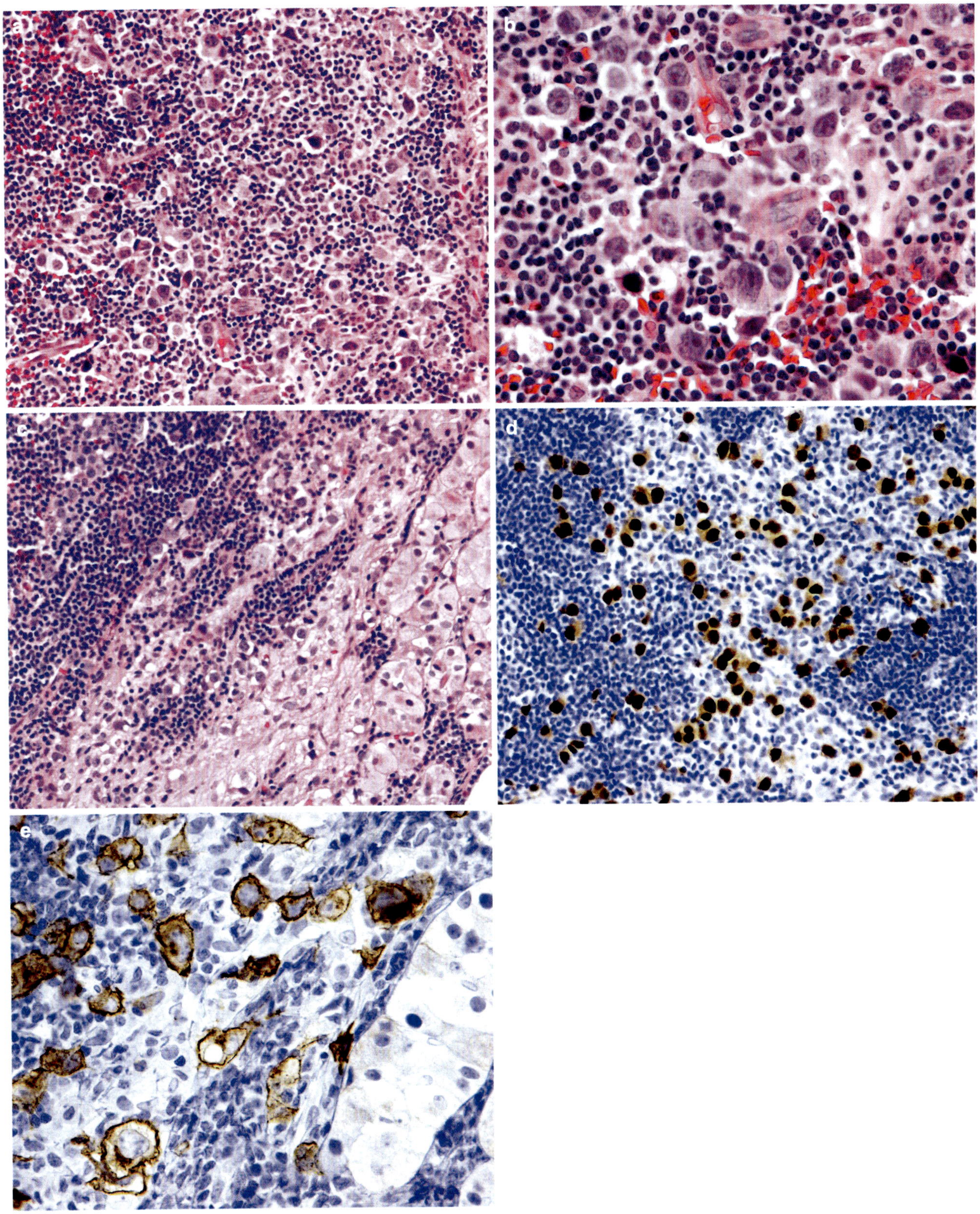

Fig. 37.3 Germinoma. An intrasellar germinoma showing large cells with prominent vesicular nuclei intermixed with a rich infiltrate of lymphocytes (**a**, **b**). The germinomatous and lymphocytic cells have obliterated the anterior pituitary parenchyma, with only a few remaining normal neuroendocrine acini (**c**). Immunohistochemical stains for OCT4 (**d**) and c-kit (**e**) highlight the neoplastic large cells in contrast to the stromal lymphocytes

37.4 Clinical and Surgical Management

- Patients should undergo serum and CSF evaluation for AFP, carcinoembryonic antigen (CEA), and β-hCG.
- Multimodal intervention is frequently required and depends on the histological tumor components [23, 24]:
  - Localized germinomas can be treated with radiation, frequently with good response rates [25].
  - Disseminated germinomas are typically treated with chemotherapy.
  - Mature teratoma components are treated with surgical resection.
- The endoscopic endonasal transsphenoidal approach has been used for biopsy or resection [26, 27].
- β-hCG and AFP levels in the serum and CSF may be used to monitor treatment progress.
- Prognosis is worse for embryonal carcinomas and choriocarcinomas than for germinomas or mature teratomas [23].
- The 5-year survival rate for patients undergoing radiation for germinomas is 85 %, compared with 46 % for patients with nongerminomatous germ cell tumors [6].

References

1. Saeger W, Ludecke DK, Buchfelder M, Fahlbusch R, Quabbe HJ, Petersenn S. Pathohistological classification of pituitary tumors: 10 years of experience with the German Pituitary Tumor Registry. Eur J Endocrinol. 2007;156:203–16.
2. Nishio S, Inamura T, Takeshita I, Fukui M, Kamikaseda K. Germ cell tumor in the hypothalamo-neurohypophysial region: clinical features and treatment. Neurosurg Rev. 1993;16:221–7.
3. Donat JF, Okazaki H, Gomez MR, Reagan TJ, Baker Jr HL, Laws Jr ER. Pineal tumors. A 53-year experience. Arch Neurol. 1978;35:736–40.
4. Lee L, Saran F, Hargrave D, Bodi I, Bassi S, Hortobagyi T. Germinoma with synchronous lesions in the pineal and suprasellar regions. Childs Nerv Syst. 2006;22:1513–8.
5. Sugiyama K, Uozumi T, Kiya K, Mukada K, Arita K, Kurisu K, et al. Intracranial germ-cell tumor with synchronous lesions in the pineal and suprasellar regions: report of six cases and review of the literature. Surg Neurol. 1992;38:114–20.
6. Hoffman HJ, Otsubo H, Hendrick EB, Humphreys RP, Drake JM, Becker LE, et al. Intracranial germ-cell tumors in children. J Neurosurg. 1991;74:545–51.
7. Cuccia V, Alderete D. Suprasellar/pineal bifocal germ cell tumors. Childs Nerv Syst. 2010;26:1043–9.
8. Kato T, Sawamura Y, Tada M, Murata J, Abe H, Shirato H, Fujieda K. Occult neurohypophyseal germinomas in patients presenting with central diabetes insipidus. Neurosurg Focus. 1998;5(1), e6.
9. Mootha SL, Barkovich AJ, Grumbach MM, Edwards MS, Gitelman SE, Kaplan SL, Conte FA. Idiopathic hypothalamic diabetes insipidus, pituitary stalk thickening, and the occult intracranial germinoma in children and adolescents. J Clin Endocrinol Metab. 1997;82:1362–7.
10. Robison NJ, Prabhu SP, Sun P, Chi SN, Kieran MW, Manley PE, et al. Predictors of neoplastic disease in children with isolated pituitary stalk thickening. Pediatr Blood Cancer. 2013;60:1630–5.
11. Cho DY, Wang YC, Ho WL. Primary intrasellar mixed germ-cell tumor with precocious puberty and diabetes insipidus. Childs Nerv Syst. 1997;13:42–6.
12. Oishi M, Iida T, Koide M, Akazawa Y, Azuma Y, Fujisawa I, Takeuchi J. Primary intrasellar microgerminoma detected by magnetic resonance imaging: case report. Neurosurgery. 1989;25: 458–62.
13. Andrew J, Kendall BE, Brook CD. Germinoma of the pituitary gland; a report of two cases. J Neurol Neurosurg Psychiatry. 1985;48:589–92.
14. Oishi M, Morii K, Okazaki H, Tamura T, Tanaka R. Neurohypophyseal germinoma traced from its earliest stage via magnetic resonance imaging: case report. Surg Neurol. 2001;56:236–41.
15. Fukushima T, Takemura Y, Tsugu H, Iwaasa M, Nabeshima K, Takano K, Utsunomiya H. Neurohypophyseal granulomatous germinoma invading the right cavernous sinus: case report and review of the literature. Pediatr Neurosurg. 2007;43:297–302.
16. Liang L, Korogi Y, Sugahara T, Ikushima I, Shigematsu Y, Okuda T, et al. MRI of intracranial germ-cell tumours. Neuroradiology. 2002;44:382–8.
17. Kidooka M, Okada T, Nakajima M, Handa J. Intra- and suprasellar germinoma mimicking a pituitary adenoma--case report. Neurol Med Chir (Tokyo). 1995;35:96–9.
18. Rosenblum M, Nakazato Y, Matsutani M. CNS germ cell tumors. In: Louis DN, Ohgaki H, Wiestler OD, Cavanee W, editors. WHO classification of tumours of the central nervous system. Lyon: IARC Press; 2007. p. 198–204.
19. Huang X, Zhang R, Mao Y, Zhou LF. Modified grading system for clinical outcome of intracranial non-germinomatous malignant germ cell tumors. Oncol Lett. 2010;1:627–31.

20. Villano JL, Virk IY, Ramirez V, Propp JM, Engelhard HH, McCarthy BJ. Descriptive epidemiology of central nervous system germ cell tumors: nonpineal analysis. Neuro Oncol. 2010;12:2 57–64.
21. Edouard T, Stafford DE, Oliver I, Jesuran M, Bertozzi AI, Cances C, et al. Isolated lymphocytic infiltration of pituitary stalk preceding the diagnosis of germinoma in 2 prepubertal children treated with growth hormone. Horm Res. 2009;72:57–62.
22. Fehn M, Bettendorf M, Ludecke DK, Sommer C, Saeger W. Lymphocytic hypophysitis masking a suprasellar germinoma in a 12-year-old girl--a case report. Pituitary. 1999;1:303–7.
23. Kyritsis AP. Management of primary intracranial germ cell tumors. J Neurooncol. 2010;96:143–9.
24. Bruce JN, Connelly ES, Sonabend AM. Pineal cell and germ cell tumors. In: Kaye AH, Laws Jr ER, editors. Brain tumors: an encyclopedic approach. 3rd ed. Amsterdam: Elsevier; 2011. p. 646–71.
25. Osuka S, Tsuboi K, Takano S, Ishikawa E, Matsushita A, Tokuuye K, et al. Long-term outcome of patients with intracranial germinoma. J Neurooncol. 2007;83:71–9.
26. de Divitiis E, Cappabianca P, Gangemi M, Cavallo LM. The role of the endoscopic transsphenoidal approach in pediatric neurosurgery. Childs Nerv Syst. 2000;16:692–6.
27. Dehdashti AR, Ganna A, Witterick I, Gentili F. Expanded endoscopic endonasal approach for anterior cranial base and suprasellar lesions: indications and limitations. Neurosurgery. 2009;64:677–87; discussion 687–9.

38 Olfactory Neuroblastoma and Sellar Neuroblastoma

Gabriel Zada, M. Beatriz S. Lopes, Srinivasan Mukundan Jr., and Edward Laws Jr.

38.1 Epidemiology and Clinical Presentation

- Olfactory neuroblastoma (ONB), also referred to as esthesioneuroblastoma, is an uncommonly occurring malignant tumor that arises from the olfactory neuroepithelium of the upper nasal cavity and anterior skull base. Tumors that are large enough may extend posteriorly to the sellar region.
- ONB represents 2–6 % of all sinonasal malignancies [1, 2].
- The incidence is 0.4 (per million persons per year).
- The age distribution of patients is bimodal, in the second and sixth decades of life [2].
- Common clinical symptoms include unilateral nasal obstruction and epistaxis, but may also include anosmia, visual symptoms, facial pain, lacrimation, headache, and rhinorrhea [2].
- Primary sellar neuroblastoma is extremely rare [3–6].

38.2 Imaging Features

- ONB classically appears as a "dumbbell-shaped" mass, with the waist centered at the cribriform plate.
- CT imaging will often show speckled calcifications and bony erosion of the lamina papyracea, cribriform plate, and/or the fovea ethmoidalis [2].
- T1-weighted MR images typically show hypointense to intermediate tumor signal intensity compared with brain. T2-weighted images may show hyperintense regions that often correlate to the cystic regions. There is often avid tumor contrast enhancement, which may be heterogeneous. Cerebral invasion and surrounding edema may occasionally be seen (Fig. 38.1) [2, 7–9].
- The diagnosis of olfactory neuroblastoma is supported by the MRI finding of peritumoral cysts capping the intracranial portion of the tumor (Fig. 38.2) [9].
- Cervical lymph node metastases are seen in approximately 36 % of patients at the time of diagnosis [7].
- 18F-FDG PET/CT is a useful adjunct in patients with ONB and may affect treatment decisions in up to 39 % of patients, when compared with conventional neuroimaging [10].
- ONB is often staged according to the Kadish criteria. According to this staging system, group A represents tumors limited to the nasal cavity, group B represents tumors localized to the nasal cavity and paranasal sinuses, and group C tumors extend beyond the nasal cavity and paranasal sinuses [11].

G. Zada, MD, MS (✉)
Department of Neurological Surgery, Keck School of Medicine, University of Southern California, 1200 N State Street, #3300, Los Angeles, CA 90033, USA
e-mail: gzada@usc.edu

M.B.S. Lopes, MD, PhD
Department of Pathology (Neuropathology), University of Virginia School of Medicine, 1215 Lee Street, Room 3060–HEP, Charlottesville, VA 22908, USA
e-mail: msl2e@virginia.edu

S. Mukundan Jr., PhD, MD
Department of Radiology, Brigham and Women's Hospital, 75 Francis Street, Boston, MA 02115, USA
e-mail: smukundan@partners.org

E. Laws Jr., MD
Department of Neurosurgery, Brigham and Women's Hospital, 15 Francis Street, Boston, MA 02115, USA
e-mail: elaws@partners.org

G. Zada et al. (eds.), *Atlas of Sellar and Parasellar Lesions: Clinical, Radiologic, and Pathologic Correlations*, DOI 10.1007/978-3-319-22855-6_38

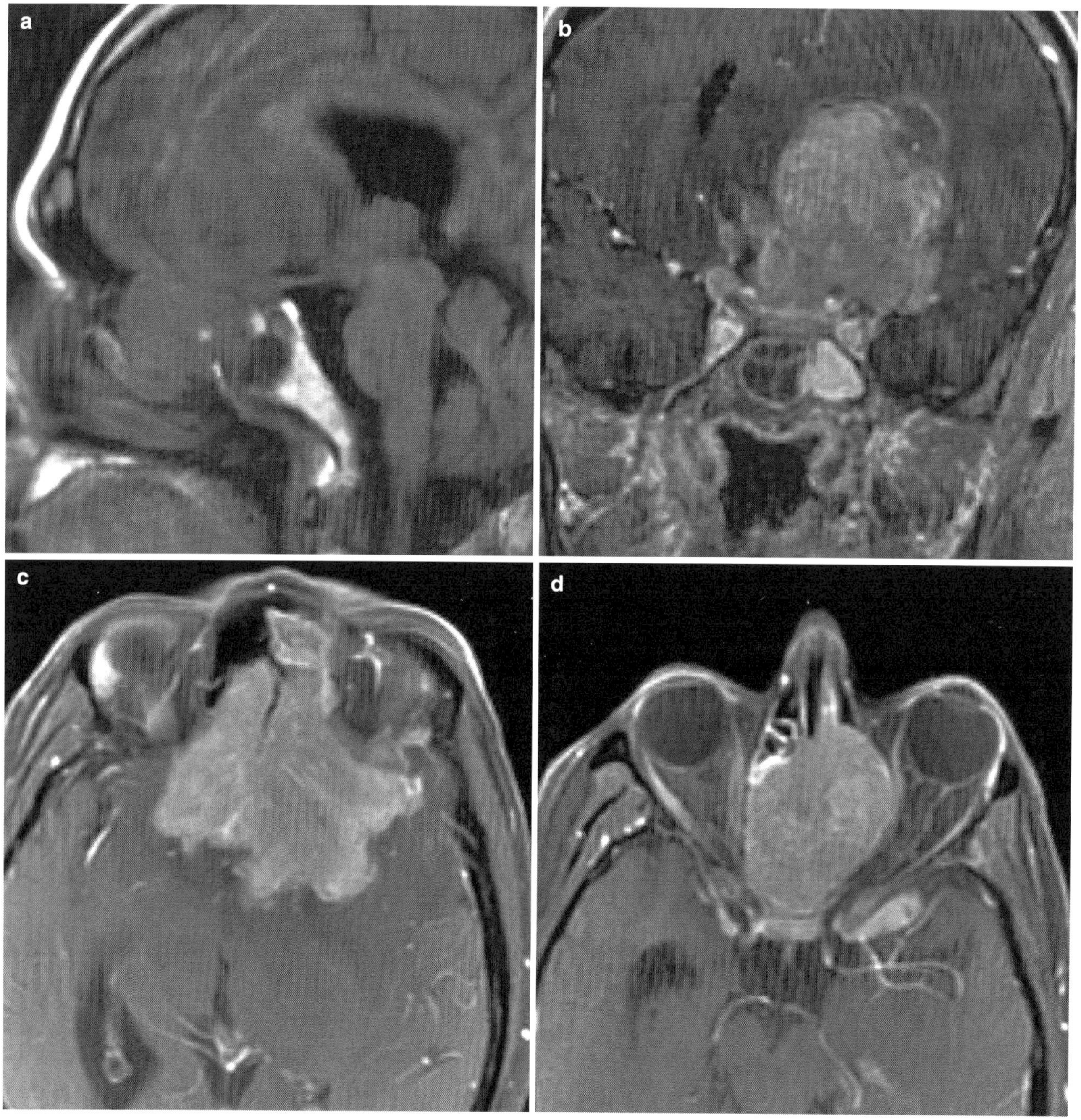

Fig. 38.1 Olfactory neuroblastoma. (**a**) Sagittal T1-weighted precontrast image. (**b**) Coronal T1-weighted gadolinium-enhanced image. (**c**, **d**) Axial fat-saturated T1-weighted gadolinium-enhanced image. There is a large, heterogeneously enhancing mass centered in the floor of the anterior cranial fossa. Nodular components are compressing the frontal lobes and are seen inferiorly within the nasal cavities. The mass extends to the left orbit, with medial displacement of the medial rectus. There is marked edema in the left frontal lobe, and the visualized parts of the lateral ventricles are dilated

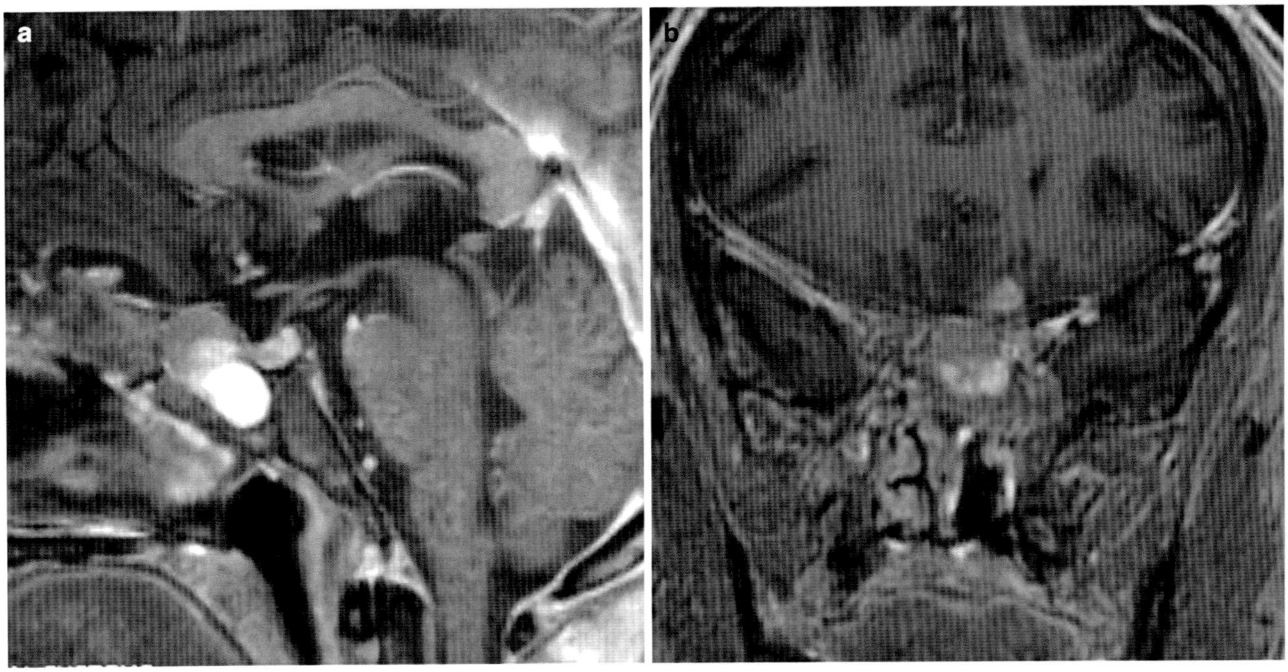

Fig. 38.2 Olfactory neuroblastoma. (**a**) Sagittal T1-weighted gadolinium-enhanced image. (**b**) Coronal T1-weighted gadolinium-enhanced image. A heterogeneously enhancing mass is centered in the floor of the anterior cranial fossa, with components eroding the nasal cavities, sphenoid sinuses, and anterior clivus. The pituitary gland is distinctly seen from the mass on the sagittal plane. There is a small cystic component superiorly abutting the left frontal lobe

38.3 Histopathology

- Classically, ONBs are characterized by small, round, blue cells slightly larger than mature lymphocytes, with a very high ratio of nucleus to cytoplasm, arranged in a lobular pattern (Fig. 38.3a, b).
- ONB is often graded according to Hyams criteria, which range from Grade I to Grade IV [12]. These criteria are based on several features, including architecture, pleomorphism, neurofibrillary matrix, rosettes, mitoses, necrosis, glands, and calcification. Grade I ONB is characterized by lobular cytoarchitecture, little pleomorphism, prominent neurofibrillary matrix, Homer-Wright pseudorosettes, no mitoses or necrosis, and variable calcification. On the other extreme, Grade IV ONB is characterized by loss of lobular cytoarchitecture, marked pleomorphism, necrosis, mitoses, Flexner-Wintersteiner rosettes, and absent calcification [12].
- ONBs are typically positive for synaptophysin (Fig. 38.3c), chromogranin, CD56, neuron-specific enolase, neurofilament protein (NFP), and S100 protein [2].
- The Ki-67 proliferative index is usually high, ranging between 10 and 50 % [2].

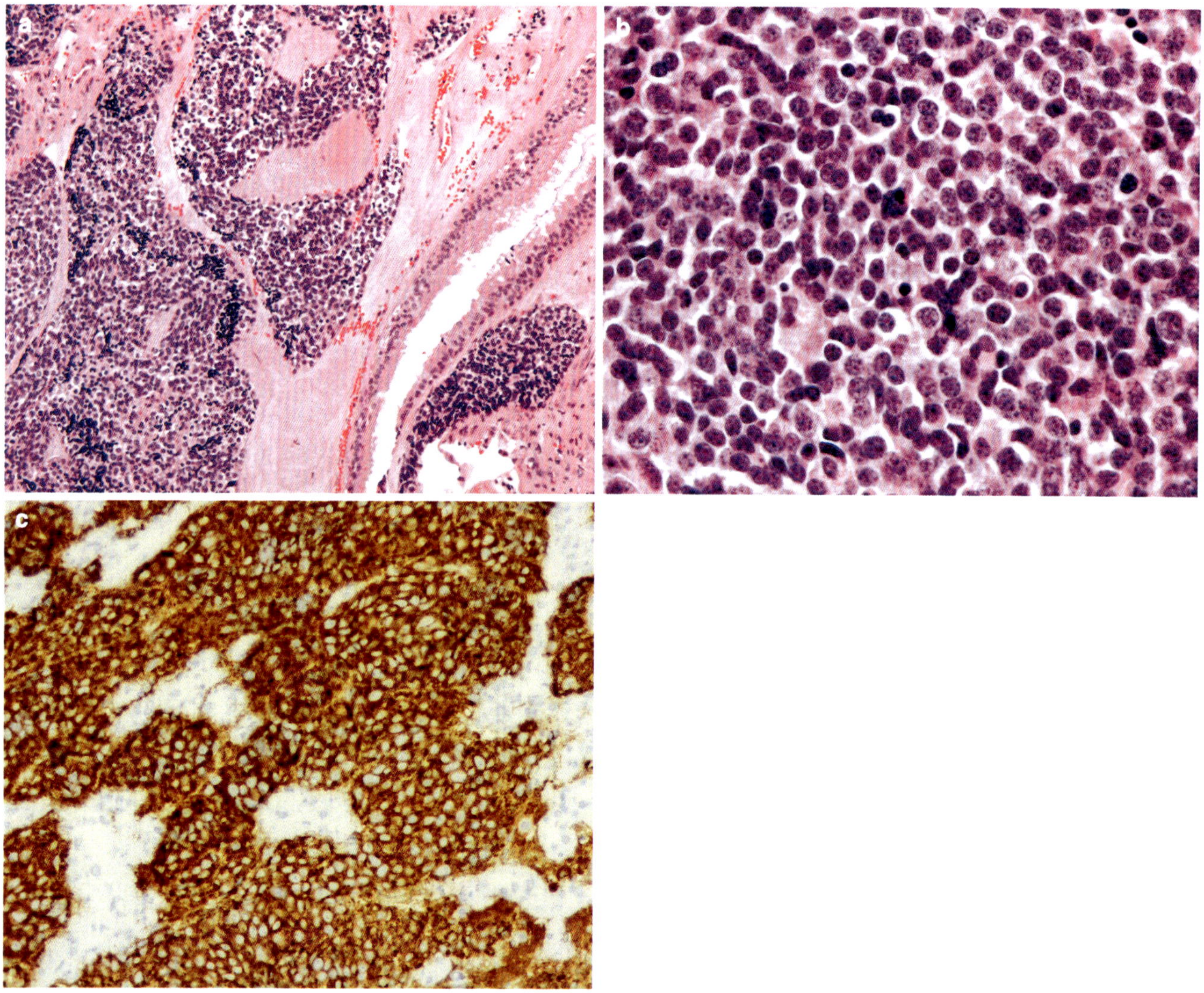

Fig. 38.3 Olfactory neuroblastoma. (**a**) Olfactory neuroblastomas are located in the sinonasal submucosa. (**b**) The tumors are composed of a uniform population of small cells with typical "salt and pepper" or dispersed chromatin. Mitotic activity may be high. (**c**) The tumors are characteristically strongly immunoreactive for synaptophysin

38.4 Clinical and Surgical Management

- Depending on the stage of disease at the time of diagnosis and the degree of tumor resection, multimodality treatment consisting of surgery, radiation, and chemotherapy is often implemented.
- One large meta-analysis showed no difference in survival between patients who underwent surgery alone and those who underwent surgery plus radiotherapy at 5 years (78 % vs. 75 %) or 10 years (67 % vs. 61 %) [13].
- Survival has been associated with Kadish stage and Hyams stage [11, 13]. According to the original Kadish staging, patients with Kadish A tumors had a 5-year survival of 75–91 %, compared with 41–47 % for patients harboring Kadish C tumors [11].
- Surgical resection may be performed via standard open craniotomy, craniofacial approaches, or more recently, extended endoscopic endonasal approaches [14].
- In a series of 11 patients by Gallia et al. [14], complete endoscopic endonasal surgical resection was possible in all patients, with no patients demonstrating recurrence at 28 months follow-up.
- Recent meta-analyses have lent support to equal or more favorable outcomes following endoscopic resection compared with open surgery, although some selection bias exists in the surgical approaches assigned to varying Kadish ONB subtypes [15, 16].
- The benefits of adjuvant radiation have been debated; some studies have shown a beneficial effect [17] and others have shown no major benefits [13].
- Recurrence develops in approximately 30–48 % of cases, with a median time to recurrence of 7 years [2, 17].
- Metastatic lesions to cervical lymph nodes, lungs, and bones may require additional surgery and multimodality treatment [18]. Platinum-based chemotherapy is often utilized [19]. Autologous bone marrow transplantation has helped achieve long-term survival in limited cases.

References

1. Bak M, Wein RO. Esthesioneuroblastoma: a contemporary review of diagnosis and management. Hematol Oncol Clin North Am. 2012;26:1185–207.
2. Thompson LD. Olfactory neuroblastoma. Head Neck Pathol. 2009;3:252–9.
3. Mariani L, Schaller B, Weis J, Ozdoba C, Seller RW. Esthesioneuroblastoma of the pituitary gland: a clinicopathological entity? Case report and review of the literature. J Neurosurg. 2004;101:1049–52.
4. Sajko T, Rumboldt Z, Talan-Hranilovic J, Radic I, Gnjidic Z. Primary sellar esthesioneuroblastoma. Acta Neurochir (Wien). 2005;147:447–8; discussion 448.
5. Sarwar M. Primary sellar-parasellar esthesioneuroblastoma. AJR Am J Roentgenol. 1979;133:140–1.
6. Dupuy M, Bonneville F, Grunenwald S, Breibach F, Delisle MB, Chaynes P, et al. Primary sellar neuroblastoma. A new case and review of literature. Ann Endocrinol (Paris). 2012;73:216–21.
7. Yu T, Xu YK, Li L, Jia FG, Duan G, Wu YK, et al. Esthesioneuroblastoma methods of intracranial extension: CT and MR imaging findings. Neuroradiology. 2009;51:841–50.
8. Raghavan P, Phillips CD. Magnetic resonance imaging of sinonasal malignancies. Top Magn Reson Imaging. 2007;18:259–67.
9. Schuster JJ, Phillips CD, Levine PA. MR of esthesioneuroblastoma (olfactory neuroblastoma) and appearance after craniofacial resection. AJNR Am J Neuroradiol. 1994;15:1169–77.
10. Broski SM, Hunt CH, Johnson GB, Subramaniam RM, Peller PJ. The added value of 18F-FDG PET/CT for evaluation of patients with esthesioneuroblastoma. J Nucl Med. 2012;53:1200–6.
11. Kadish S, Goodman M, Wang CC. Olfactory neuroblastoma. A clinical analysis of 17 cases. Cancer. 1976;37:1571–6.
12. Hyams V, Batsakis J, Michaels L. Tumors of the upper respiratory tract and ear. In: Armed Forces Institute of Pathology Fascicles, 2nd series. Washington: American Registry of Pathology Press; 1988. p. 240–8.
13. Kane AJ, Sughrue ME, Rutkowski MJ, Aranda D, Mills SA, Buencamino R, et al. Posttreatment prognosis of patients with esthesioneuroblastoma. J Neurosurg. 2010;113:340–51.
14. Gallia GL, Reh DD, Salmasi V, Blitz AM, Koch W, Ishii M. Endonasal endoscopic resection of esthesioneuroblastoma: the Johns Hopkins Hospital experience and review of the literature. Neurosurg Rev. 2011;34:465–75.
15. Devaiah AK, Andreoli MT. Treatment of esthesioneuroblastoma: a 16-year meta-analysis of 361 patients. Laryngoscope. 2009;119: 1412–6.
16. Komotar RJ, Starke RM, Raper DM, Anand VK, Schwartz TH. Endoscopic endonasal compared with anterior craniofacial and combined cranionasal resection of esthesioneuroblastomas. World Neurosurg. 2013;80:148–59.
17. Ow TJ, Hanna EY, Roberts DB, Levine NB, El-Naggar AK, Rosenthal DI, et al. Optimization of long-term outcomes for patients with esthesioneuroblastoma. Head Neck. 2014;36:524–30.
18. McElroy Jr EA, Buckner JC, Lewis JE. Chemotherapy for advanced esthesioneuroblastoma: the Mayo Clinic experience. Neurosurgery. 1998;42:1023–7; discussion 1027–8.
19. Turano S, Mastroianni C, Manfredi C, Biamonte R, Ceniti S, Liguori V, et al. Advanced adult esthesioneuroblastoma successfully treated with cisplatin and etoposide alternated with doxorubicin, ifosfamide and vincristine. J Neurooncol. 2010;98:131–5.

Hypothalamic Hamartoma

39

Gabriel Zada, M. Beatriz S. Lopes, Srinivasan Mukundan Jr., and Edward Laws Jr.

39.1 Epidemiology and Clinical Presentation

- Hypothalamic hamartomas are congenital lesions that present in the region of the floor of the third ventricle, hypothalamus, tuber cinereum, mammillary bodies, and infundibulum.
- The mean age at presentation is 10 years [1].
- Patients typically present with a classic triad [2]:
  - Precocious puberty
  - Gelastic seizures (uncontrollable laughter)
  - Developmental delay
- Central precocious puberty occurs in 30–45 % of patients and is often associated with obesity [1, 3].
- Serum levels of FSH, LH, estradiol, and testosterone can be elevated [4].
- Gelastic seizures often progress to more complex seizure disorders and finally to intractable epilepsy [5].
- The lesions may be associated with the Pallister–Hall syndrome (hypothalamic hamartoma, central polydactyly, pituitary hypoplasia, bifid epiglottis, imperforate anus) [6].
- Hypothalamic hamartomas comprise only 0.07 % of major transsphenoidal series [7].

39.2 Imaging Features

- Hypothalamic hamartomas can present as intraventricular lesions at the floor of the third ventricle or as sessile lesions arising from the tuber cinereum and infundibulum [3, 8].
- The hamartomas are typically hypointense on T1-weighted imaging and isointense or hyperintense on T2-weighted imaging (Fig. 39.1).
- They typically do not enhance following contrast administration on CT or MR imaging [9].
- The pituitary bright spot is typically preserved [9].

G. Zada, MD, MS (✉)
Department of Neurological Surgery, Keck School of Medicine, University of Southern California, 1200 N State Street, #3300, Los Angeles, CA 90033, USA
e-mail: gzada@usc.edu

M.B.S. Lopes, MD, PhD
Department of Pathology (Neuropathology), University of Virginia School of Medicine, 1215 Lee Street, Room 3060–HEP, Charlottesville, VA 22908, USA
e-mail: msl2e@virginia.edu

S. Mukundan Jr., PhD, MD
Department of Radiology, Brigham and Women's Hospital, 75 Francis Street, Boston, MA 02115, USA
e-mail: smukundan@partners.org

E. Laws Jr., MD
Department of Neurosurgery, Brigham and Women's Hospital, 15 Francis Street, Boston, MA 02115, USA
e-mail: elaws@partners.org

G. Zada et al. (eds.), *Atlas of Sellar and Parasellar Lesions: Clinical, Radiologic, and Pathologic Correlations*,
DOI 10.1007/978-3-319-22855-6_39

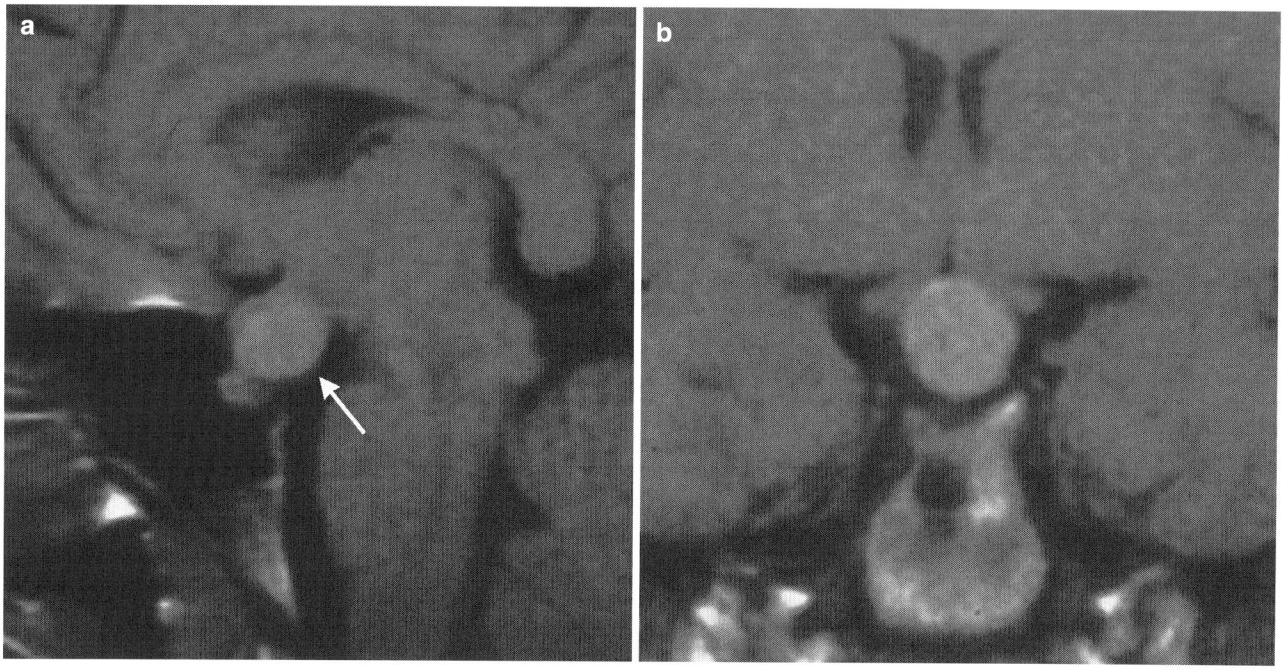

Fig. 39.1 Hypothalamic hamartoma. (**a**) Sagittal T1-weighted pre-gadolinium MR image. (**b**) Coronal T1-weighted pre-gadolinium image. A well-circumscribed mass with slight T1 hyperintensity (*arrow*) is seen in the suprasellar region posterior to and abutting the pituitary stalk. The mass appears separate from the pituitary gland

39.3 Histopathology

- These growths consist of abnormal distributions of histologically normal neuronal and glial cells [10].
- They have an overall resemblance to hypothalamic gray matter [9].
- The bulk of the lesions consist of mature, small neurons (Fig. 39.2) [10].
- Neuronal markers, such as synaptophysin, are typically positive.
- Positive immunostaining for luteinizing hormone–releasing hormone (LHRH) has been demonstrated in tumors from children with precocious puberty [11].

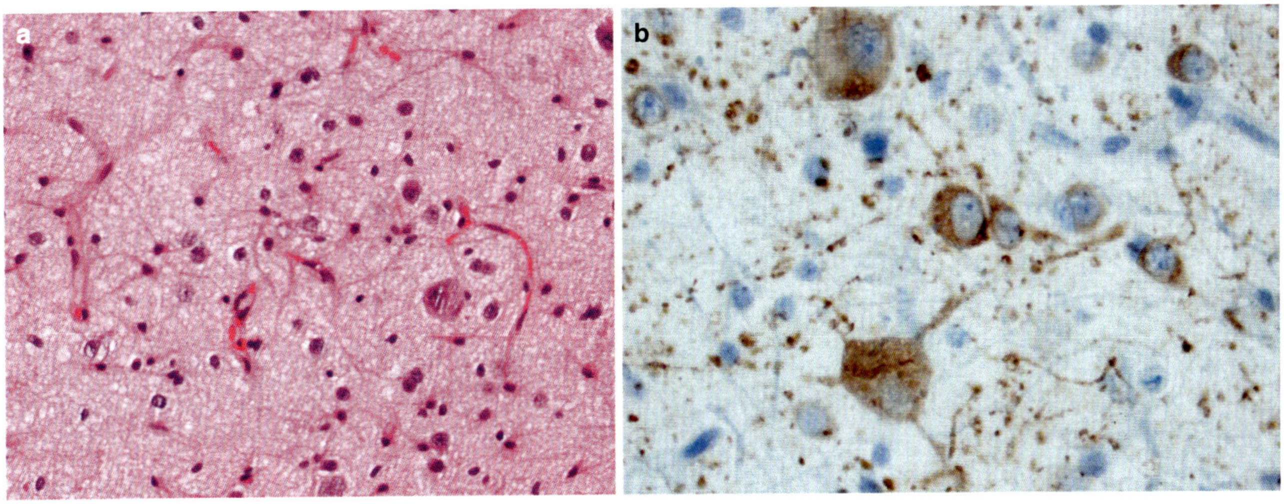

Fig. 39.2 Hypothalamic hamartoma. (**a**) Hypothalamic neuronal hamartoma is composed primarily of mature neurons arranged in a haphazard pattern or in small clusters. (**b**) The abnormally shaped neuronal cells are labeled with neuronal-associated markers, including microtubule-associated protein 2 (MAP2) (Courtesy of Dr. Carrie A. Mohila, Department of Pathology (Neuropathology), Texas Children's Hospital, Baylor College of Medicine, Houston, TX)

39.4 Clinical and Surgical Management

- Gonadotropin-releasing hormone (GnRH, LRH) analogues may be administered to successfully suppress central precocious puberty, making surgery for this particular indication somewhat obsolete [1, 12].
- The primary indication for surgical treatment of hypothalamic hamartoma is seizures.
- Video-EEG monitoring may demonstrate an associated epileptogenic cortical region that improves or normalizes following surgical resection [13, 14].
- Interhemispheric–transcallosal–interforniceal and pterional approaches have been the most widely utilized open approaches for hypothalamic hamartomas [2, 14–16].
- Complete seizure resolution has been reported in 49–54 % of patients following an interhemispheric approach, with another 24–35 % demonstrating some improvement in seizures [14–16].
- Endoscopic approaches for resection or disconnection of hamartomas have been reported with excellent outcomes in recent years [8, 17, 18].
- Complete resection via endoscopic intraventricular approaches has been reported in up to 32 % of patients, 93 % of whom were seizure-free at follow-up [17].
- Hypopituitarism and diabetes insipidus occur frequently following surgical resection [1].
- Short-term memory dysfunction may occur in up to 48 % of patients following surgical resection of hamartomas [14, 15].
- In recent years, stereotactic radiosurgery has been utilized with a low risk profile and seizure improvement in 60 % of patients (complete seizure resolution in 40 % and reduced frequency in 20 %) [16].
- Radiosurgery is more effective in treating smaller, noninvasive hamartomas, especially when the entire lesion can be covered [19–21].
- Stereotactic radiofrequency thermocoagulation also has been reported to improve seizure frequency with some success for hamartomas that are small (<10 mm in diameter) [22].

References

1. Freeman JL, Zacharin M, Rosenfeld JV, Harvey AS. The endocrinology of hypothalamic hamartoma surgery for intractable epilepsy. Epileptic Disord. 2003;5:239–47.
2. Maixner W. Hypothalamic hamartomas--clinical, neuropathological and surgical aspects. Childs Nerv Syst. 2006;22:867–73.
3. Debeneix C, Bourgeois M, Trivin C, Sainte-Rose C, Brauner R. Hypothalamic hamartoma: comparison of clinical presentation and magnetic resonance images. Horm Res. 2001;56:12–8.
4. Li CD, Luo SQ, Gong J, Ma ZY, Jia G, Zhang YQ, Li JF. Surgical treatment of hypothalamic hamartoma causing central precocious puberty: long-term follow-up. J Neurosurg Pediatr. 2013;12:151–4.
5. Tellez-Zenteno JF, Serrano-Almeida C, Moien-Afshari F. Gelastic seizures associated with hypothalamic hamartomas. An update in the clinical presentation, diagnosis and treatment. Neuropsychiatr Dis Treat. 2008;4:1021–31.
6. Biesecker LG, Abbott M, Allen J, Clericuzio C, Feuillan P, Graham Jr JM, et al. Report from the workshop on Pallister-Hall syndrome and related phenotypes. Am J Med Genet. 1996;65:76–81.
7. Saeger W, Ludecke DK, Buchfelder M, Fahlbusch R, Quabbe HJ, Petersenn S. Pathohistological classification of pituitary tumors: 10 years of experience with the German Pituitary Tumor Registry. Eur J Endocrinol. 2007;156:203–16.
8. Drees C, Chapman K, Prenger E, Baxter L, Maganti R, Rekate H, et al. Seizure outcome and complications following hypothalamic hamartoma treatment in adults: endoscopic, open, and Gamma Knife procedures. J Neurosurg. 2012;117:255–61.
9. Boyko OB, Curnes JT, Oakes WJ, Burger PC. Hamartomas of the tuber cinereum: CT, MR, and pathologic findings. AJNR Am J Neuroradiol. 1991;12:309–14.
10. Coons SW, Rekate HL, Prenger EC, Wang N, Drees C, Ng YT, et al. The histopathology of hypothalamic hamartomas: study of 57 cases. J Neuropathol Exp Neurol. 2007;66:131–41.
11. Judge DM, Kulin HE, Page R, Santen R, Trapukdi S. Hypothalamic hamartoma: a source of luteinizing-hormone-releasing factor in precocious puberty. N Engl J Med. 1977;296:7–10.
12. Comite F, Pescovitz OH, Rieth KG, Dwyer AJ, Hench K, McNemar A, et al. Luteinizing hormone-releasing hormone analog treatment of boys with hypothalamic hamartoma and true precocious puberty. J Clin Endocrinol Metab. 1984;59:888–92.
13. Kramer U, Spector S, Nasser W, Siomin V, Fried I, Constantini S. Surgical treatment of hypothalamic hamartoma and refractory seizures: a case report and review of the literature. Pediatr Neurosurg. 2001;34:40–2.
14. Harvey AS, Freeman JL, Berkovic SF, Rosenfeld JV. Transcallosal resection of hypothalamic hamartomas in patients with intractable epilepsy. Epileptic Disord. 2003;5:257–65.

15. Rosenfeld JV, Feiz-Erfan I. Hypothalamic hamartoma treatment: surgical resection with the transcallosal approach. Semin Pediatr Neurol. 2007;14:88–98.
16. Pati S, Sollman M, Fife TD, Ng YT. Diagnosis and management of epilepsy associated with hypothalamic hamartoma: an evidence-based systematic review. J Child Neurol. 2013;28:909–16.
17. Rekate HL, Feiz-Erfan I, Ng YT, Gonzalez LF, Kerrigan JF. Endoscopic surgery for hypothalamic hamartomas causing medically refractory gelastic epilepsy. Childs Nerv Syst. 2006;22:874–80.
18. Cappabianca P, Cinalli G, Gangemi M, Brunori A, Cavallo LM, de Devitiis E, et al. Application of neuroendoscopy to intraventricular lesions. Neurosurgery. 2008;62:575–97; discussion 597–8.
19. Quigg M, Barbaro NM. Stereotactic radiosurgery for treatment of epilepsy. Arch Neurol. 2008;65:177–83.
20. Regis J, Scavarda D, Tamura M, Villeneuve N, Bartolomei F, Brue T, et al. Gamma knife surgery for epilepsy related to hypothalamic hamartomas. Semin Pediatr Neurol. 2007;14:73–9.
21. Mathieu D, Deacon C, Pinard CA, Kenny B, Duval J. Gamma Knife surgery for hypothalamic hamartomas causing refractory epilepsy: preliminary results from a prospective observational study. J Neurosurg. 2010;113:215–21.
22. Homma J, Kameyama S, Masuda H, Ueno T, Fujimoto A, Oishi M, Fukuda M. Stereotactic radiofrequency thermocoagulation for hypothalamic hamartoma with intractable gelastic seizures. Epilepsy Res. 2007;76:15–21.

40 Plasmacytoma

Gabriel Zada, M. Beatriz S. Lopes, Srinivasan Mukundan Jr., and Edward Laws Jr.

40.1 Epidemiology and Clinical Presentation

- Plasmacytomas, or plasma cell tumors, are typically singular tumors that arise in the bone. They rarely occur in the sellar/parasellar region, where the clivus and sphenoid wing are most commonly affected [1].
- They may be solitary or the presenting tumor of multiple myeloma (MM), which often consists of multifocal osteolytic tumors, pathological fractures, hypercalcemia, and anemia.
- MM occurs much more frequently in the spine; an intracranial presentation accounts for only 3 % of MM [2].
- Conversely, occult MM is common in cases with a monofocal cranial presentation.
- Patients diagnosed with plasmacytoma are often older adults.
- Sellar region plasmacytoma is extremely uncommon, accounting for 0.02 % of major transsphenoidal series [3].
- Headache and visual complaints develop frequently and are often accompanied by cranial nerve paresis, which occurs in the majority of sellar region plasmacytomas [4].
- Cranial nerve VI is the most commonly affected.
- Anterior pituitary dysfunction is very uncommon for these lesions [5].

40.2 Imaging Features

- On CT or plain x-ray, significant bony destruction of the sella and clivus is common.
- On MRI, plasmacytomas are typically large, invasive lesions with bony destruction. They are usually hypointense on T2-weighted images, with homogeneous enhancement, and demonstrate a low apparent diffusion coefficient (ADC) (Figs. 40.1, 40.2, 40.3, 40.4, and 40.5).
- Infrasellar or parasellar extension is seen in 57 % of cases [4].
- Suprasellar extension occurs in 33 % of cases.
- Plasmacytomas frequently mimic nonfunctional macroadenomas or chordomas. FDG-PET/CT imaging may be used to differentiate plasmacytoma from less malignant entities [6].

G. Zada, MD, MS (✉)
Department of Neurological Surgery, Keck School of Medicine, University of Southern California, 1200 N State Street, #3300, Los Angeles, CA 90033, USA
e-mail: gzada@usc.edu

M.B.S. Lopes, MD, PhD
Department of Pathology (Neuropathology), University of Virginia School of Medicine, 1215 Lee Street, Room 3060–HEP, Charlottesville, VA 22908, USA
e-mail: msl2e@virginia.edu

S. Mukundan Jr., PhD, MD
Department of Radiology, Brigham and Women's Hospital, 75 Francis Street, Boston, MA 02115, USA
e-mail: smukundan@partners.org

E. Laws Jr., MD
Department of Neurosurgery, Brigham and Women's Hospital, 15 Francis Street, Boston, MA 02115, USA
e-mail: elaws@partners.org

G. Zada et al. (eds.), *Atlas of Sellar and Parasellar Lesions: Clinical, Radiologic, and Pathologic Correlations*, DOI 10.1007/978-3-319-22855-6_40

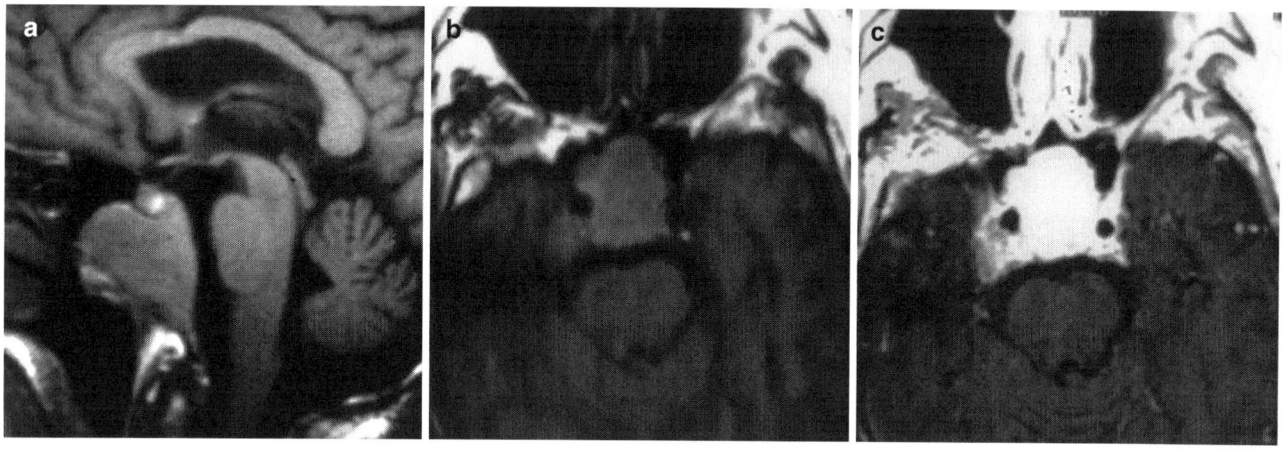

Fig. 40.1 Plasmacytoma. (**a**) Sagittal T1-weighted precontrast image. (**b**) Axial T1-weighted precontrast image. (**c**) Axial T1-weighted gadolinium-enhanced image. There is an expansile, homogeneously enhancing mass replacing the entire clivus. The pituitary gland appears normal within the sella

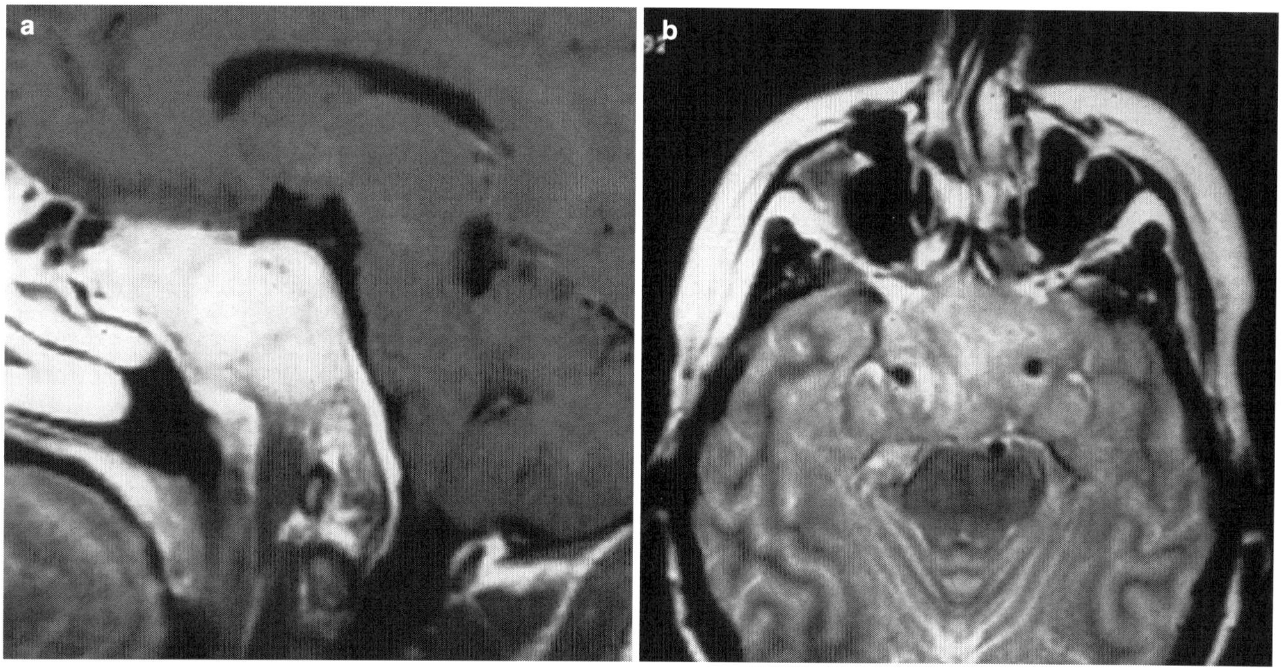

Fig. 40.2 Plasmacytoma. (**a**) Sagittal T1-weighted gadolinium-enhanced image. (**b**) Coronal T1-weighted gadolinium-enhanced image. There is a large, homogeneously enhancing mass replacing the clivus and obliterating the sella. The pituitary gland is not distinctly visualized. The mass extends to bilateral cavernous sinuses

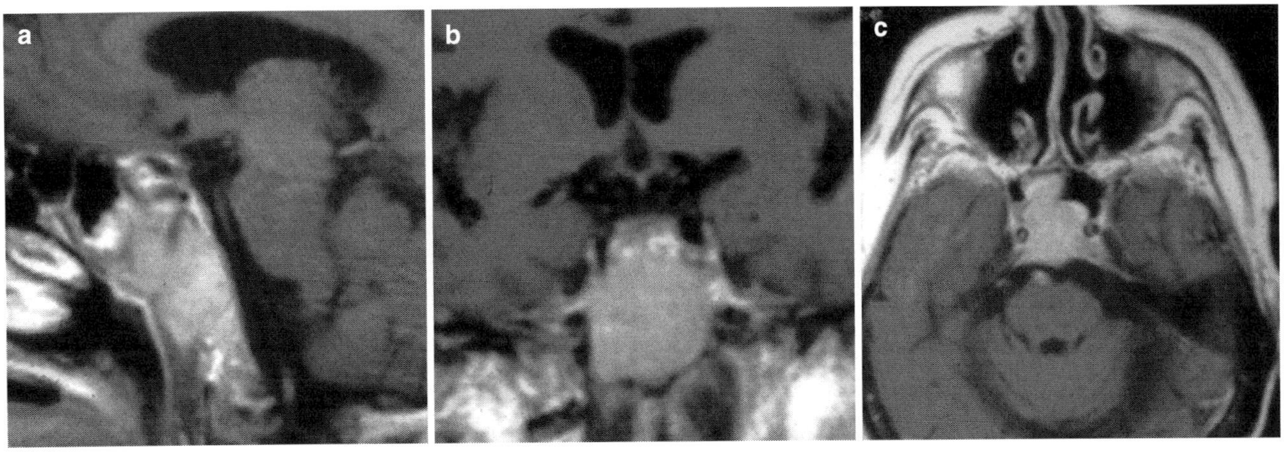

Fig. 40.3 Plasmacytoma. (**a**) Sagittal T1-weighted gadolinium-enhanced image. (**b**) Coronal T1-weighted gadolinium-enhanced image. (**c**) Axial T1-weighted gadolinium-enhanced image. There is a large, homogeneously enhancing mass replacing the clivus. The pituitary gland is not distinctly visualized

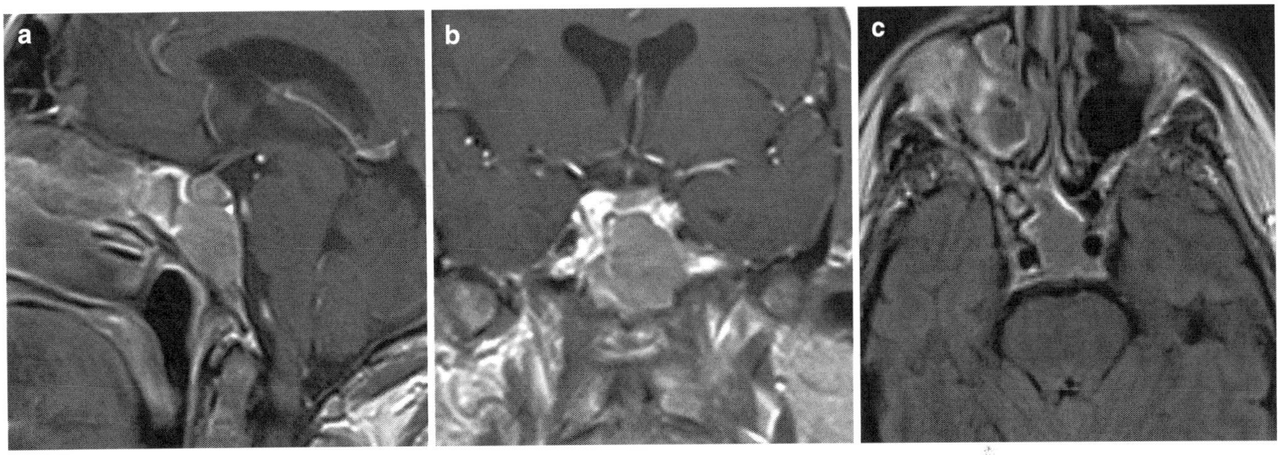

Fig. 40.4 Plasmacytoma. (**a**) Sagittal T1-weighted gadolinium-enhanced image. (**b**) Coronal T1-weighted gadolinium-enhanced image. (**c**) Axial T1-weighted gadolinium-enhanced image. There is a homogeneously enhancing mass centered in the clivus. The pituitary gland is not distinctly visualized

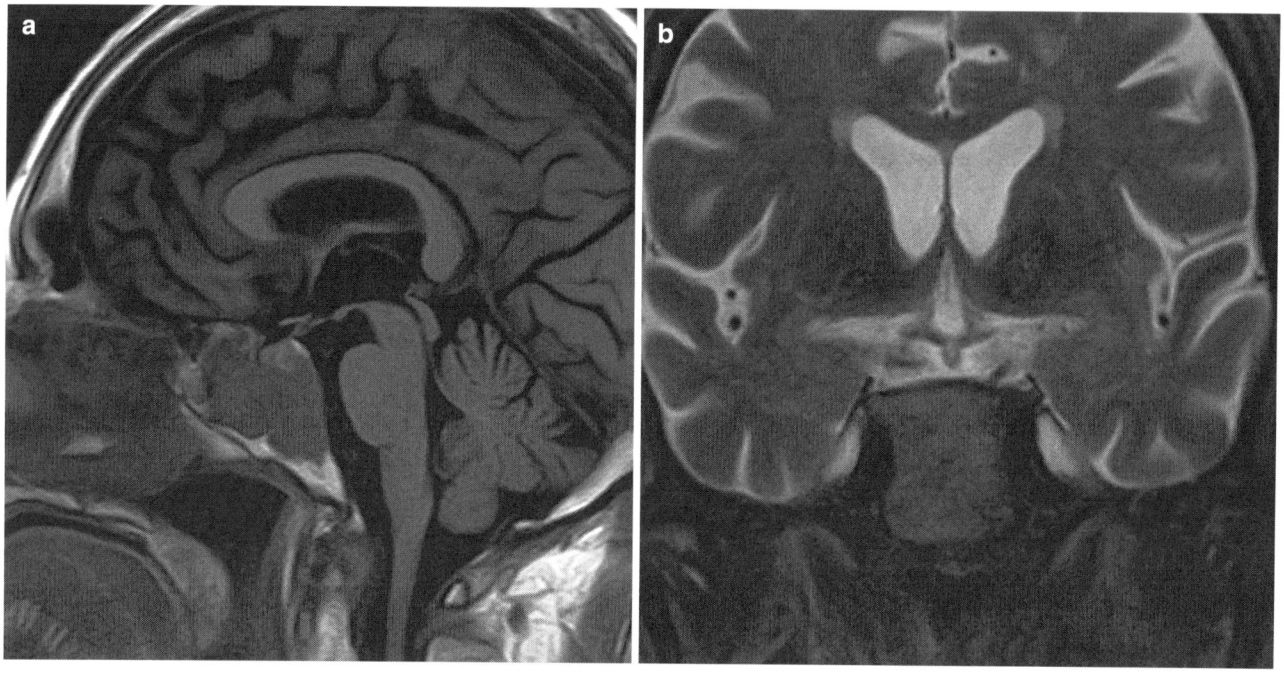

Fig. 40.5 Plasmacytoma. (**a**) Sagittal T1-weighted image. (**b**) Coronal T2-weighted image. There is a large mass centered in the clivus eroding into the sphenoid sinus. The mass is distinct from the pituitary gland

40.3 Histopathology

- Plasmacytomas are highly cellular tumors typically consisting of a monoclonal origin of plasma B cells (Fig. 40.6).
- They demonstrate positive immunoreactivity for CD138, CD43, and kappa light chain immunoglobulin. Negative immunoreactivity for chromogranin, synaptophysin, placental alkaline phosphatase (PLAP), EMA, CEA, and CAM52 is typically seen in plasmacytoma.
- This diagnosis requires differentiation from lymphocytic hypophysitis (polyclonal B-cell lineage).

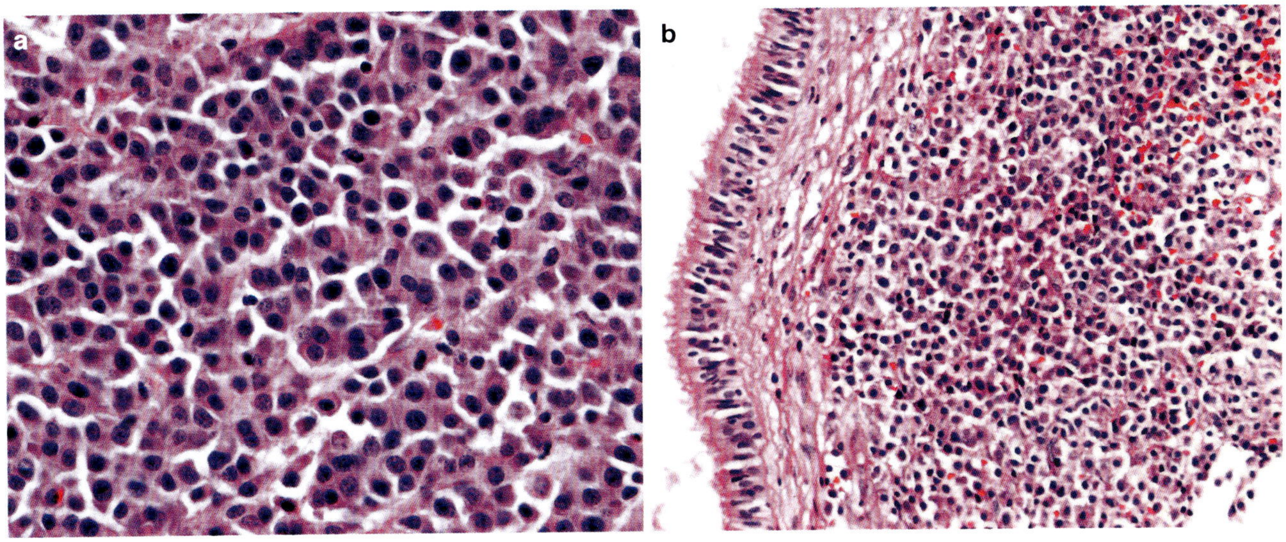

Fig. 40.6 Plasmacytomas and other hematologic neoplasms of the skull base and sellar bones may infiltrate the sella, mimicking pituitary adenomas on neuroimaging and causing signs of hypopituitarism. Plasmacytomas are histologically characterized by a proliferation of plasma with a moderate degree of cellular pleomorphism and numerous mitotic figures (**a**). In the present case, infiltration of the sphenoid mucosa is evident (**b**)

40.4 Clinical and Surgical Management

- Sellar plasmacytoma is often mistaken preoperatively for a nonfunctional pituitary adenoma or chordoma [7, 8].
- A systemic search for additional bony lesions should be undertaken.
- Blood IgG K levels and urine analysis for Bence-Jones proteins and IgG K should be performed.
- Transsphenoidal surgery has been reported for biopsy or surgical debulking. Aggressive gross total resection is not recommended, as plasmacytoma is often a highly invasive and radiosensitive tumor.
- Postoperative adjuvant radiation and/or chemotherapy is typically required following surgery.
- Some patients will undergo autologous bone marrow stem cell transplantation.
- Long-term clinical outcomes vary. Most patients will progress to systemic multiple myeloma. Patients treated with surgical debulking followed by adjunctive chemotherapy and irradiation may have favorable long-term outcomes [9].

References

1. Losa M, Terreni MR, Tresoldi M, Marcatti M, Campi A, Triutzi F, et al. Solitary plasmacytoma of the sphenoid sinus involving the pituitary fossa: a case report and review of the literature. Surg Neurol. 1992;37:388–93.
2. Silverstein A, Doniger DE. Neurologic complications of myelomatosis. Arch Neurol. 1963;9:534–43.
3. Saeger W, Ludecke DK, Buchfelder M, Fahlbusch R, Quabbe HJ, Petersenn S. Pathohistological classification of pituitary tumors: 10 years of experience with the German Pituitary Tumor Registry. Eur J Endocrinol. 2007;156:203–16.
4. Sinnott BP, Hatipoglu B, Same DH. Intrasellar plasmacytoma presenting as a non-functional invasive pituitary macro-adenoma: case report and literature review. Pituitary. 2006;9:65–72.
5. Evans PJ, Jones MK, Hall R, Scanlon MF. Pituitary function with a solitary intrasellar plasmacytoma. Postgrad Med J. 1985;61:513–4.
6. Cistaro A, Durando S, Pazè F, Limberti A, Cogoni M, Juenemann C, et al. Expansive masses arising from the clivus: the role of FDG-PET/CT in the metabolic assessment of skeletal lesions. J Radiol Case Rep. 2009;3:33–40.
7. Joukhadar R, Chiu K. Sellar plasmacytomas: a concise review. Pituitary. 2012;15:146–9.
8. Pitini V, Arrigo C, Alafaci C, Altavilla G. Extramedullary plasmacytoma presented as a non-functional invasive pituitary macroadenoma. J Neurooncol. 2008;88:227–9.
9. McLaughlin DM, Gray WJ, Jones FG, Mirakhur M, McCance DR, Sheridan B, Atkinson AB. Plasmacytoma: an unusual cause of a pituitary mass lesion. A case report and a review of the literature. Pituitary. 2004;7:179–81.

Lymphoma

41

Gabriel Zada, M. Beatriz S. Lopes, Srinivasan Mukundan Jr., and Edward Laws Jr.

41.1 Epidemiology and Clinical Presentation

- Sellar region lymphoma may arise as primary CNS lymphoma (PCNSL) or systemic lymphoma (often non-Hodgkin's lymphoma) metastasizing to the pituitary gland [1, 2]. (*See* Metastases to the Pituitary Gland, Chap. 50).
- Overall, PCNSL accounts for approximately 1 % of all intracranial neoplasms [2, 3].
- This entity is more common in men [4] and can occur in immunocompromised or immunocompetent individuals. The mean age in immunocompetent patients is 60–70 years, compared with 30–40 years in immunocompromised individuals [3].
- PCNSL develops more commonly in immunocompromised individuals, especially those with HIV/AIDS, although the incidence of this disease has declined in the past decade [3].
- Primary intrasellar lymphoma, a rare presentation of PCNSL, frequently presents with fever, endocrine dysfunction (in over half of patients), cranial nerve paresis, and diabetes insipidus [3, 5, 6].
- This condition occasionally may mimic pituitary apoplexy [7].
- Sellar region PCNSL comprises less than 0.1 % of all lesions undergoing transsphenoidal surgery, according to major series [8, 9].
- In some cases, PCNSL may arise in the infundibulum and may present with diabetes insipidus [10, 11].

G. Zada, MD, MS (✉)
Department of Neurological Surgery, Keck School of Medicine, University of Southern California, 1200 N State Street, #3300, Los Angeles, CA 90033, USA
e-mail: gzada@usc.edu

M.B.S. Lopes, MD, PhD
Department of Pathology (Neuropathology), University of Virginia School of Medicine, 1215 Lee Street, Room 3060–HEP, Charlottesville, VA 22908, USA
e-mail: msl2e@virginia.edu

S. Mukundan Jr., PhD, MD
Department of Radiology, Brigham and Women's Hospital, 75 Francis Street, Boston, MA 02115, USA
e-mail: smukundan@partners.org

E. Laws Jr., MD
Department of Neurosurgery, Brigham and Women's Hospital, 15 Francis Street, Boston, MA 02115, USA
e-mail: elaws@partners.org

G. Zada et al. (eds.), *Atlas of Sellar and Parasellar Lesions: Clinical, Radiologic, and Pathologic Correlations*,
DOI 10.1007/978-3-319-22855-6_41

41.2 Imaging Features

- On MRI, PCNSL typically appears as an isointense or hypointense mass on T1-weighted imaging and is hypointense on T2 imaging (Fig. 41.1).
- Homogeneous contrast enhancement is generally observed [3].
- Because of hypercellularity, lymphomas often exhibit low diffusivity (low intensity on ADC maps).
- These tumors are often erosive, with infrasellar, suprasellar, and cavernous sinus invasion.
- FDG PET/CT can be used to support the diagnosis [12].

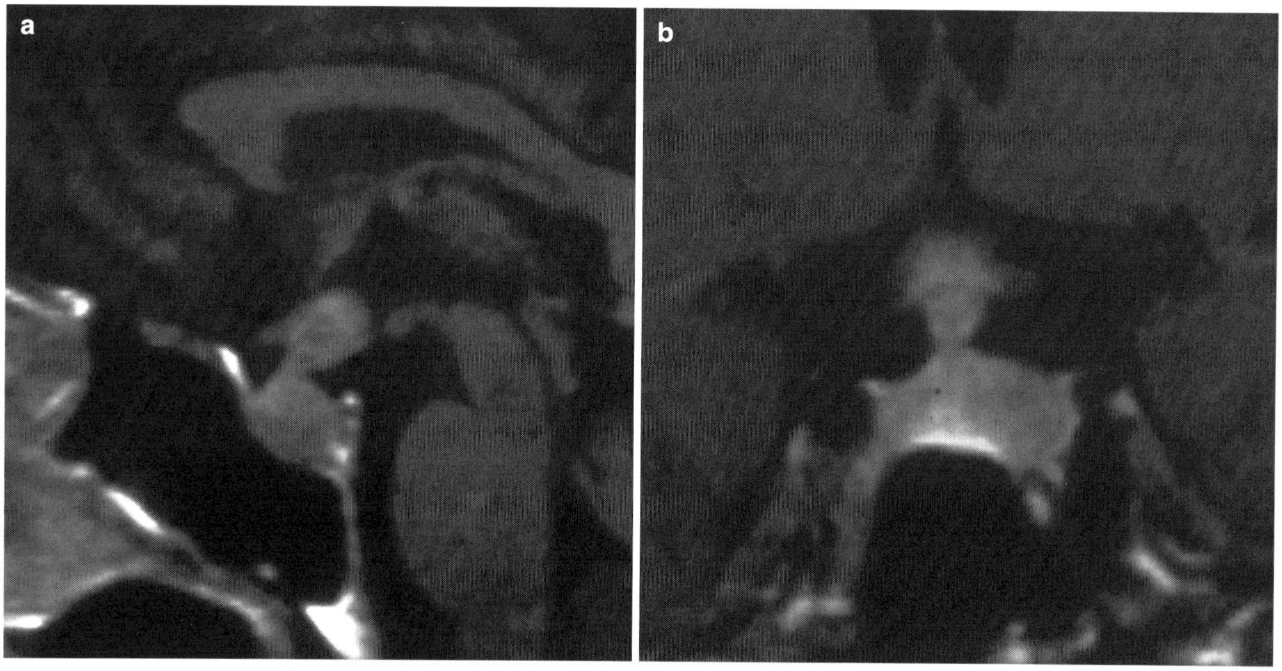

Fig. 41.1 Sellar region lymphoma. (**a**) Sagittal T1-weighted image. (**b**) Coronal T1-weighted image. There is nodular thickening of the pituitary stalk with diffuse enlargement of the gland

41.3 Histopathology

- Sellar lymphoma represents large, B-cell non-Hodgkin's lymphoma in 54 % of cases [3, 5, 13] (Fig. 41.2).
- Less frequently, sellar lymphoma can have a T-cell origin (24 % of cases), may be T-cell lymphoma with reactive B-cell lymphocytes or rarely may be the Burkitt's variety [1, 4, 5, 14].
- It is typically characterized by dense cellularity with a high nuclear/cytoplasmic ratio.
- B-cell varieties demonstrate positive immunostaining for CD20, CD79a and CD45 [3].
- T-cell varieties are frequently positive for CD3, CD5, and CD8 immunostains.
- The lymphoma may occur with concomitant hypophysitis [15].
- There is generally a lack of immunoreactivity for hormonal cell markers.

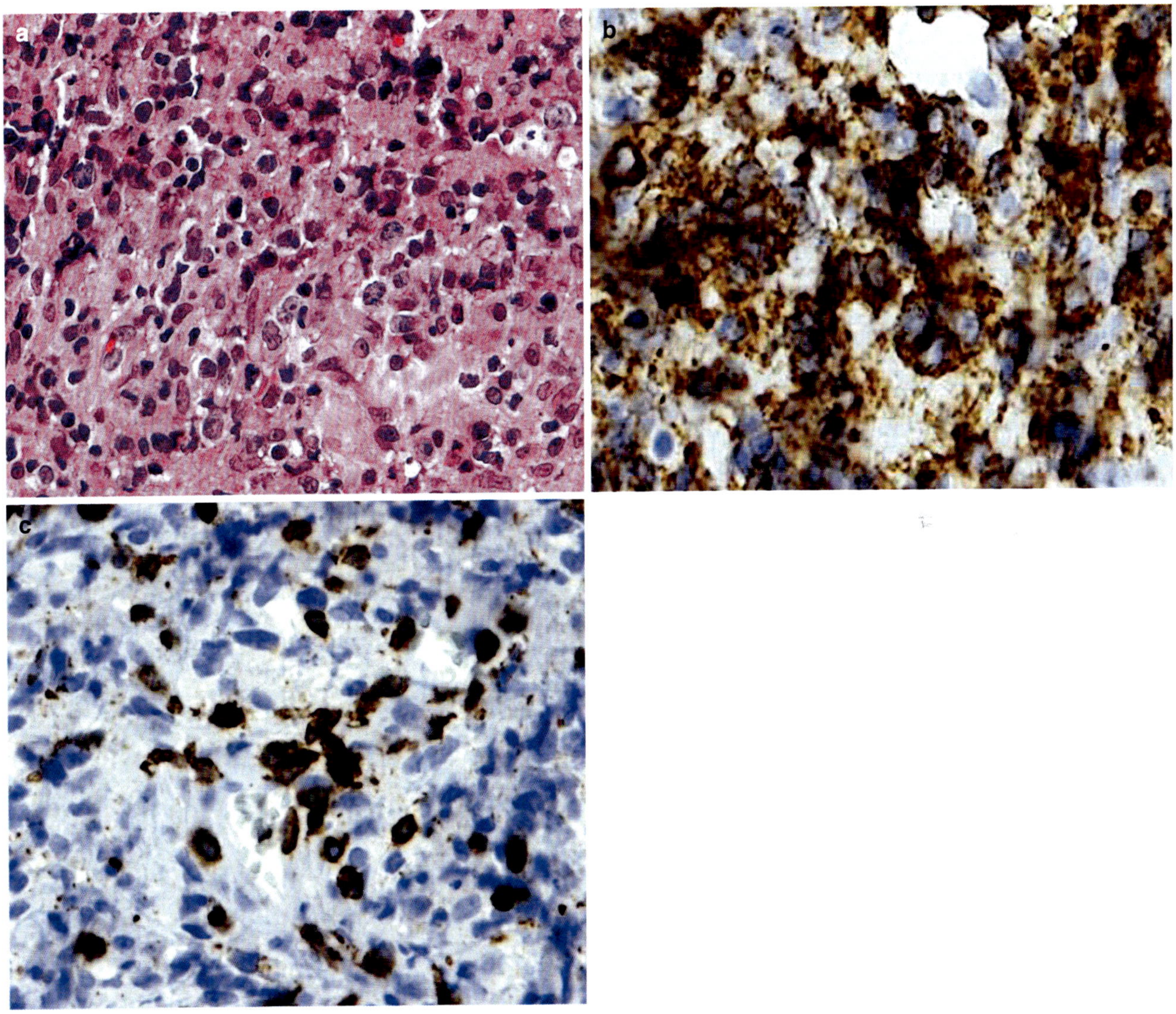

Fig. 41.2 Large B-cell lymphomas may involve the pituitary as primarily tumors or by secondary involvement of bone marrow disease. (**a–c**) In this case of a disseminated, diffuse, large B-cell lymphoma, the pituitary and the sellar soft tissues were invaded by a population of large cells with pleomorphic nuclei (**a**) immunoreactive for CD20 (**b**); small, reactive T cells may be present, as demonstrated by CD3 (**c**)

41.4 Clinical and Surgical Management

- The role of surgery is primarily biopsy and perhaps partial tumor debulking, especially in patients with visual loss [5].
- Transsphenoidal resection has been reported for patients with primary intrasellar lymphoma [3, 16].
- Radiation and chemotherapy are the mainstays of treatment.
- On average, survival is increased from 4 months with surgery alone to 12–18 months with whole-brain radiotherapy [17].
- The most common chemotherapy regimens include high-dose methotrexate and cyclophosphamide, doxorubicin, vincristine, and prednisone (CHOP), followed by whole-brain radiotherapy [18, 19].
- Approximately 70 % of examined patients with primary pituitary lymphoma survive more than 6 months after diagnosis, whereas survival is often less than 6 months for patients with cerebral lymphomas [5].

References

1. Megan Ogilvie C, Payne S, Evanson J, Lister TA, Grossman AB. Lymphoma metastasizing to the pituitary: an unusual presentation of a treatable disease. Pituitary. 2005;8:139–46.
2. Da Silva AN, Lopes MB, Schiff D. Rare pathological variants and presentations of primary central nervous system lymphomas. Neurosurg Focus. 2006;21(5), E7.
3. Kaufmann TJ, Lopes MB, Laws Jr ER, Lipper MH. Primary sellar lymphoma: radiologic and pathologic findings in two patients. AJNR Am J Neuroradiol. 2002;23:364–7.
4. Liu JK, Sayama C, Chin SS, Couldwell WT. Extranodal NK/T-cell lymphoma presenting as a pituitary mass. Case report and review of the literature. J Neurosurg. 2007;107:660–5.
5. Giustina A, Gola M, Doga M, Rosei EA. Clinical review 136: primary lymphoma of the pituitary: an emerging clinical entity. J Clin Endocrinol Metab. 2001;86:4567–75.
6. Yasuda M, Akiyama N, Miyamoto S, Warabi M, Takahama Y, Kitamura M, et al. Primary sellar lymphoma: intravascular large B-cell lymphoma diagnosed as a double cancer and improved with chemotherapy, and literature review of primary parasellar lymphoma. Pituitary. 2010;13:39–47.
7. Rizek P, Seitelbach M, Alturkustani M, Leung A, Fraser JA. Sellar and parasellar intravascular lymphoma mimicking pituitary apoplexy. J Neuroophthalmol. 2012;32:33–7.
8. Saeger W, Ludecke DK, Buchfelder M, Fahlbusch R, Quabbe HJ, Petersenn S. Pathohistological classification of pituitary tumors: 10 years of experience with the German Pituitary Tumor Registry. Eur J Endocrinol. 2007;156:203–16.
9. Freda PU, Post KD. Differential diagnosis of sellar masses. Endocrinol Metab Clin North Am. 1999;28:81–117.
10. Robison NJ, Prabhu SP, Sun P, Chi SN, Kieran MW, Manley PE, et al. Predictors of neoplastic disease in children with isolated pituitary stalk thickening. Pediatr Blood Cancer. 2013;60:1630–5.
11. Zheng WL, Zhang GS, Tan CL, Shen JK, Yang JJ, Zhong HY. Diabetes insipidus as main presentation of non-Hodgkin's lymphoma with hypophyseal involvement: two case reports. Leuk Res. 2010;34:e32–4.
12. Soussan M, Wartski M, Ezra J, Glaisner S, Pecking AP, Alberini JL. Non-Hodgkin lymphoma localization in the pituitary gland: diagnosis by FDG-PET/CT. Clin Nucl Med. 2008;33:111–2.
13. Mathiasen RA, Jarrahy R, Cha ST, Kovacs K, Herman VS, Ginsberg E, Shahinian HK. Pituitary lymphoma: a case report and literature review. Pituitary. 2000;2:283–7.
14. Wiens AL, Hagen MC, Bonnin JM, Rizzo KA. T-cell lymphoblastic lymphoma/leukemia presenting as a pituitary mass lesion: a case report and review of the literature. Neuropathology. 2012;32:668–74.
15. Huang YY, Lin SF, Dunn P, Wai YY, Hsueh C, Tsai JS. Primary pituitary lymphoma presenting as hypophysitis. Endocr J. 2005;52:543–9.
16. Moshkin O, Muller P, Scheithauer BW, Juco J, Horvath E, Patterson BJ, et al. Primary pituitary lymphoma: a histological, immunohistochemical, and ultrastructural study with literature review. Endocr Pathol. 2009;20:46–9.
17. Deangelis LM. Current management of primary central nervous system lymphoma. Oncology (Williston Park). 1995;9:63–71; discussion 71, 75–6, 78.
18. Schultz C, Scott C, Sherman W, Donahue B, Fields J, Murray K, et al. Preirradiation chemotherapy with cyclophosphamide, doxorubicin, vincristine, and dexamethasone for primary CNS lymphomas: initial report of Radiation Therapy Oncology Group protocol 88–06. J Clin Oncol. 1996;14:556–64.
19. Omuro AM, Abrey LE. Chemotherapy for primary central nervous system lymphoma. Neurosurg Focus. 2006;21(5):E12.

Gangliocytoma and Ganglioglioma

42

Gabriel Zada, M. Beatriz S. Lopes, Srinivasan Mukundan Jr., and Edward Laws Jr.

42.1 Epidemiology and Clinical Presentation

42.1.1 Gangliocytoma

- Gangliocytomas originating in the posterior pituitary are rare [1].
- The majority of gangliocytomas of the neurohypophysis are actually a composite tumor with gangliocytic and pituitary adenomatous elements, forming so-called mixed gangliocytoma-pituitary adenomas [1].
- The term "pituitary adenoma with adenohypophyseal neuronal choristoma" (PANCH) has also been used by some investigators [2], but it is discouraged by the current WHO classification [1].
- Clinically, gangliocytomas present with hormonal oversecretion syndromes in 74 % of reported cases [5]. These tumors are associated with neuroendocrine disorders, mainly acromegaly, although fewer cases with Cushing's disease and hyperprolactinemia have been described [1].
- Hypothalamic factors such as growth hormone (GH)–releasing hormone (GHRH) and corticotropin-releasing hormone (CRH) are often secreted, resulting in clinical syndromes such as acromegaly or Cushing's syndrome [6–8].
- They are associated with pituitary adenomas in 65 % of cases [5, 7, 9].
- Intrasellar gangliocytoma is more closely associated with coexisting pituitary adenomas, whereas suprasellar gangliocytomas are more closely associated with pituitary hyperplasia [5].
- Secretion of hypothalamic hormones is thought to play a major role in the growth of the coexisting adenoma [5].
- According to major series, gangliocytomas comprise approximately 0.3–0.5 % of all sellar lesions treated via a transsphenoidal approach [3, 10].
- Mixed gangliocytoma-pituitary adenomas are estimated to correspond to 0.5–1.25 % of all sellar region tumors [3, 4].

42.1.2 Ganglioglioma

- Ganglioglioma is a mixed glioneuronal tumor that is comprised of cells resembling hypothalamic neurons and astrocytes.
- Ganglioglioma is an exceedingly rare glioneuronal tumor arising from the neurohypophysis; only a few cases have been reported in the literature [11, 12].
- Clinically, these tumors may result in oversecretion of vasopressin and the syndrome of inappropriate antidiuretic hormone (SIADH) [11, 13].
- Knowledge of these neoplasms is limited primarily to case reports.
- Gangliogliomas comprise approximately 0.02 % of all sellar lesions treated surgically, according to major transsphenoidal series [10].

G. Zada, MD, MS (✉)
Department of Neurological Surgery, Keck School of Medicine, University of Southern California, 1200 N State Street, #3300, Los Angeles, CA 90033, USA
e-mail: gzada@usc.edu

M.B.S. Lopes, MD, PhD
Department of Pathology (Neuropathology), University of Virginia School of Medicine, 1215 Lee Street, Room 3060–HEP, Charlottesville, VA 22908, USA
e-mail: msl2e@virginia.edu

S. Mukundan Jr., PhD, MD
Department of Radiology, Brigham and Women's Hospital, 75 Francis Street, Boston, MA 02115, USA
e-mail: smukundan@partners.org

E. Laws Jr., MD
Department of Neurosurgery, Brigham and Women's Hospital, 15 Francis Street, Boston, MA 02115, USA
e-mail: elaws@partners.org

G. Zada et al. (eds.), *Atlas of Sellar and Parasellar Lesions: Clinical, Radiologic, and Pathologic Correlations*, DOI 10.1007/978-3-319-22855-6_42

42.2 Imaging Features

- Sellar gangliocytomas and gangliogliomas are often indistinguishable from pituitary adenomas, as the majority of cases are associated with pituitary adenomas and may be masked by them (Fig. 42.1).
- Suprasellar ganglioglioma may invade the optic apparatus and mimic an astrocytoma or germ cell tumor (Fig. 42.2) [15].

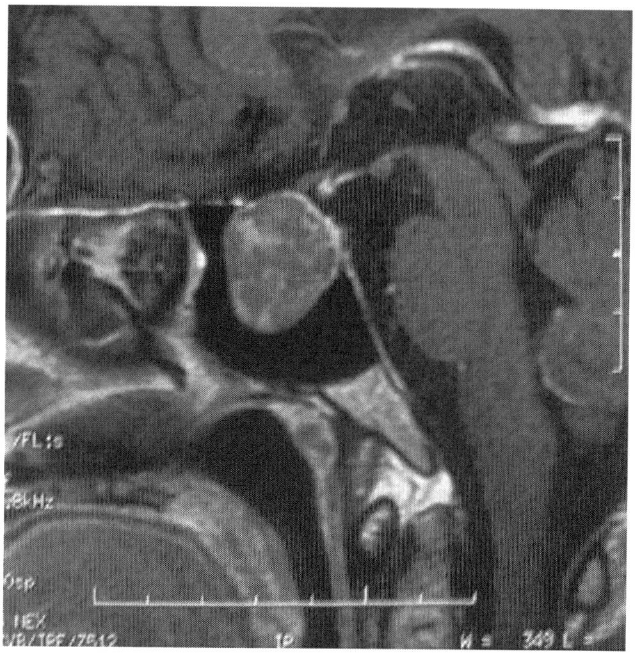

Fig. 42.1 Gangliocytoma in the presence of a prolactinoma. This sagittal T1-weighted gadolinium-enhanced MR image shows a heterogeneously enhancing mass of the sellar region with sellar expansion (Adapted with permission from Mikami et al. [14])

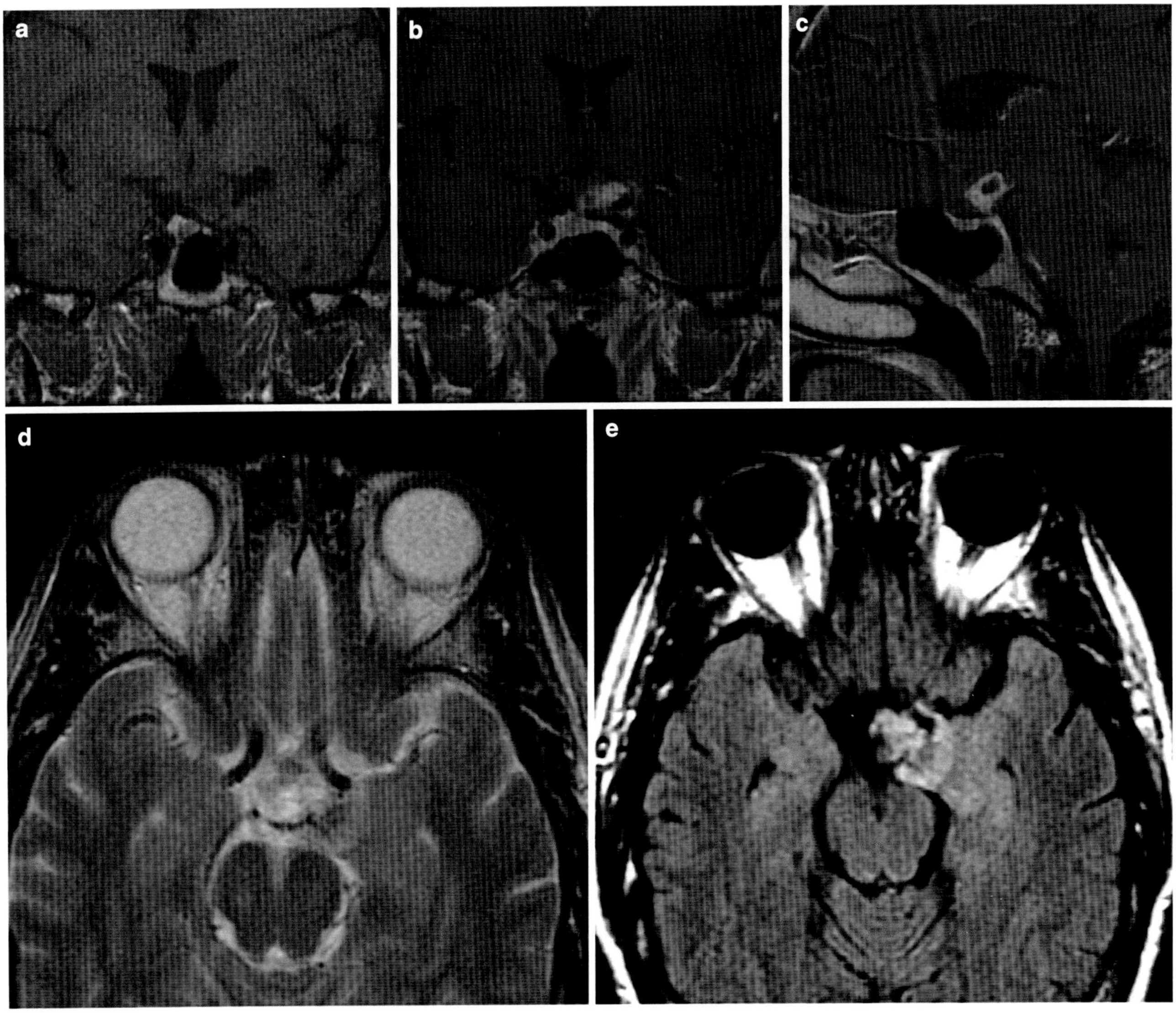

Fig. 42.2 Ganglioglioma. (**a**) Coronal T1-weighted precontrast MR image. (**b**) Coronal T1-weighted gadolinium-enhanced image. (**c**) Sagittal T1-weighted gadolinium-enhanced image. (**d**) Axial T2-weighted image. (**e**) Axial T2-FLAIR image. An enhancing mass is located in the left suprasellar region, contiguous with the left temporal lobe uncus. The mass mildly elevates the optic chiasm on the left and abuts the pituitary stalk and supraclinoid left internal carotid artery

42.3 Histopathology

42.3.1 Gangliocytoma

- In most cases, an intimate microscopic association between gangliocytomatous elements and pituitary adenoma cells is observed. The proportion of pituitary adenoma and neuronal elements may vary widely [16, 17].
- The ganglion cells are mostly large, pyramidal neurons immersed within variably prominent neuropil-like stroma.
- Ganglion cells are readily identified by immunoreactivity for neuronal-associated proteins such as neurofilament proteins (NFPs) and synaptophysin and silver impregnation preparations (Fig. 42.3) [3].
- Glial elements are not present, confirming the pure ganglionic derivation of these tumors.
- The ganglion cells may also express hypothalamic hormones including GHRH, somatostatin, CRH, or GnRH [16].
- The most frequently associated pituitary adenoma is a GH-secreting adenoma, particularly the sparsely granulated and GH/PRL cell subtypes [3, 4, 16].
- These tumors have also been reported to coexist with adrenocorticotropic hormone (ACTH) cell adenomas and prolactinomas [14, 18–20].
- The origin of sellar gangliocytomas is not completely understood [1, 2, 21, 22].
- Three major hypotheses have been considered for the histogenesis of such tumors:
  1. Displaced hypothalamic neurons in the sellar region might produce hypothalamic-releasing factors that would stimulate the proliferation of an adenoma [1].
  2. The ganglionic components originate from neuronal differentiation within adenomatous cells of sparsely granulated adenomas, in a process suggestive of transdifferentiation [2, 22].
  3. Both neuronal and adenomatous components may have a common origin from progenitor/stem cells present in the adult adenohypophysis that are capable of multidirectional differentiation [21].

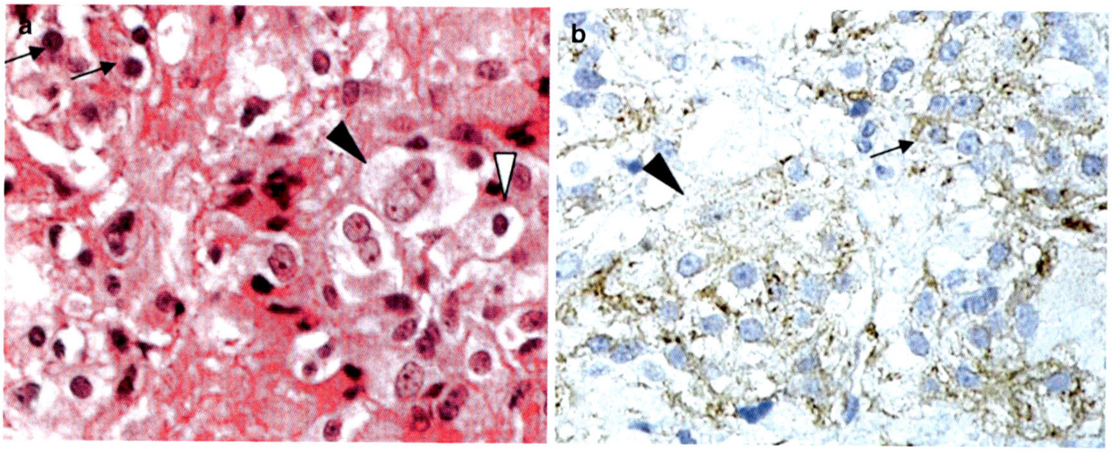

Fig. 42.3 Gangliocytoma in the presence of a prolactinoma. (**a**) With H&E staining, the tumor can be seen to be composed of small, round cells corresponding to the pituitary adenoma (*arrows*) and large ganglions (*black arrowhead*). Tumor cells showing intermediate features (*white arrowhead*) are also observed. (**b**) With PRL staining, adenoma cells (*arrow*) are immunoreactive for PRL. Ganglions are also weakly positive for PRL (*black arrowhead*). (**c**) GH staining is negative. (**d**) NF staining is positive in the fibrillary substrates of ganglions. (**e**) Synaptophysin (SYN) staining is observed in the ganglions. (**f**, **g**) Double immunostaining shows that the regional distribution of PRL (*brown*) and NF (*blue*) overlaps in some areas. (**h**) Cytokeratin stain CAM5.2 is strongly positive in fibrillary structures and rather weak in adenoma cells (Adapted with permission from Mikami et al. [14])

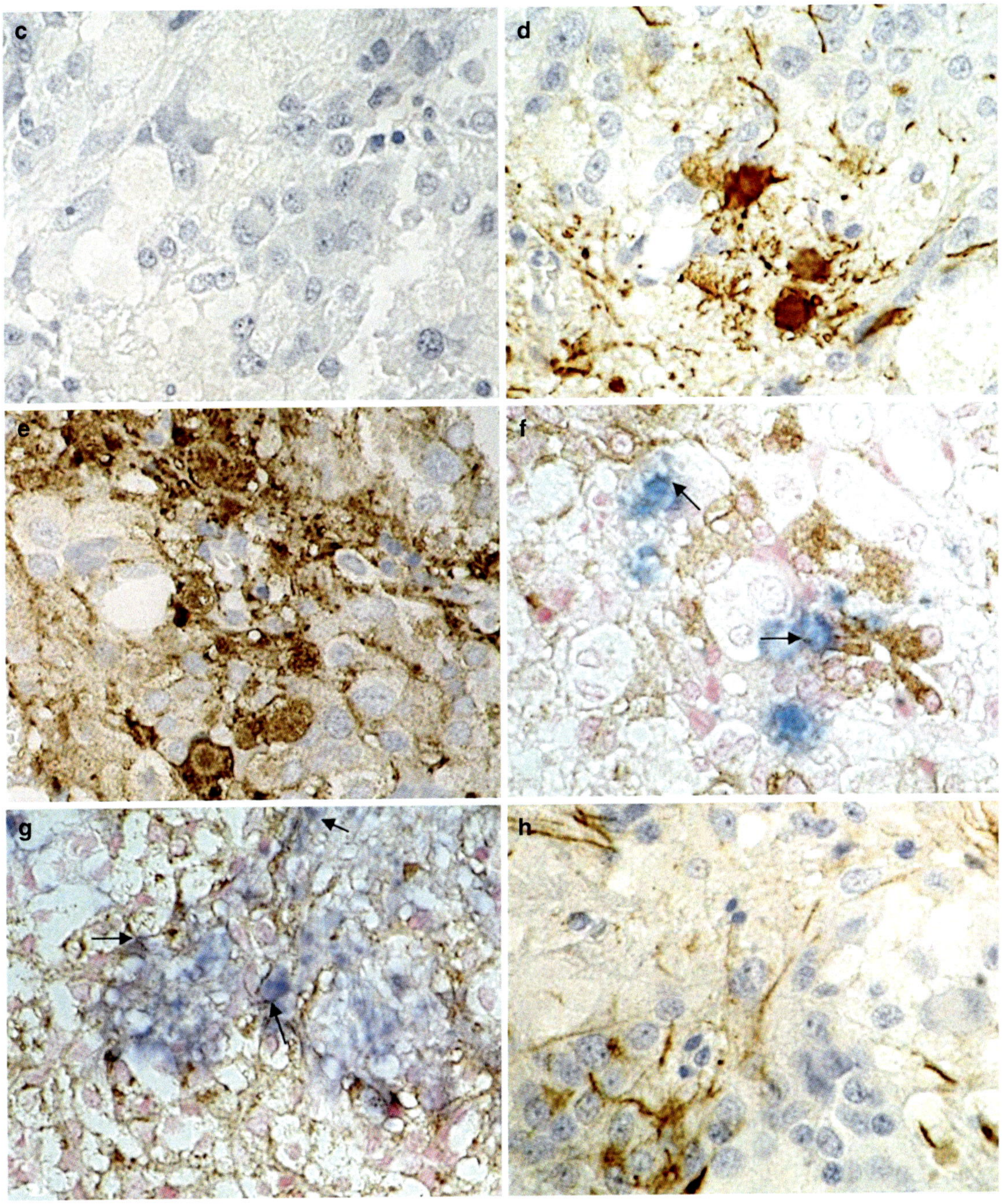

Fig. 42.3 (continued)

42.3.2 Ganglioglioma

- Gangliogliomas of the sellar region appear to have similar histopathological features as those tumors arriving in other locations of the CNS—i.e., a variable combination of ganglionic and glial cells (Fig. 42.4).
- A case of ganglioglioma was reported to demonstrate immunoreactivity for vasopressin in a patient presenting with signs of SIADH [13]. In both gangliocytomas and gangliogliomas, ultrastructural findings on electron microscopy may be useful to confirm the presence of synaptic vesicles corresponding to neuronal elements [11].

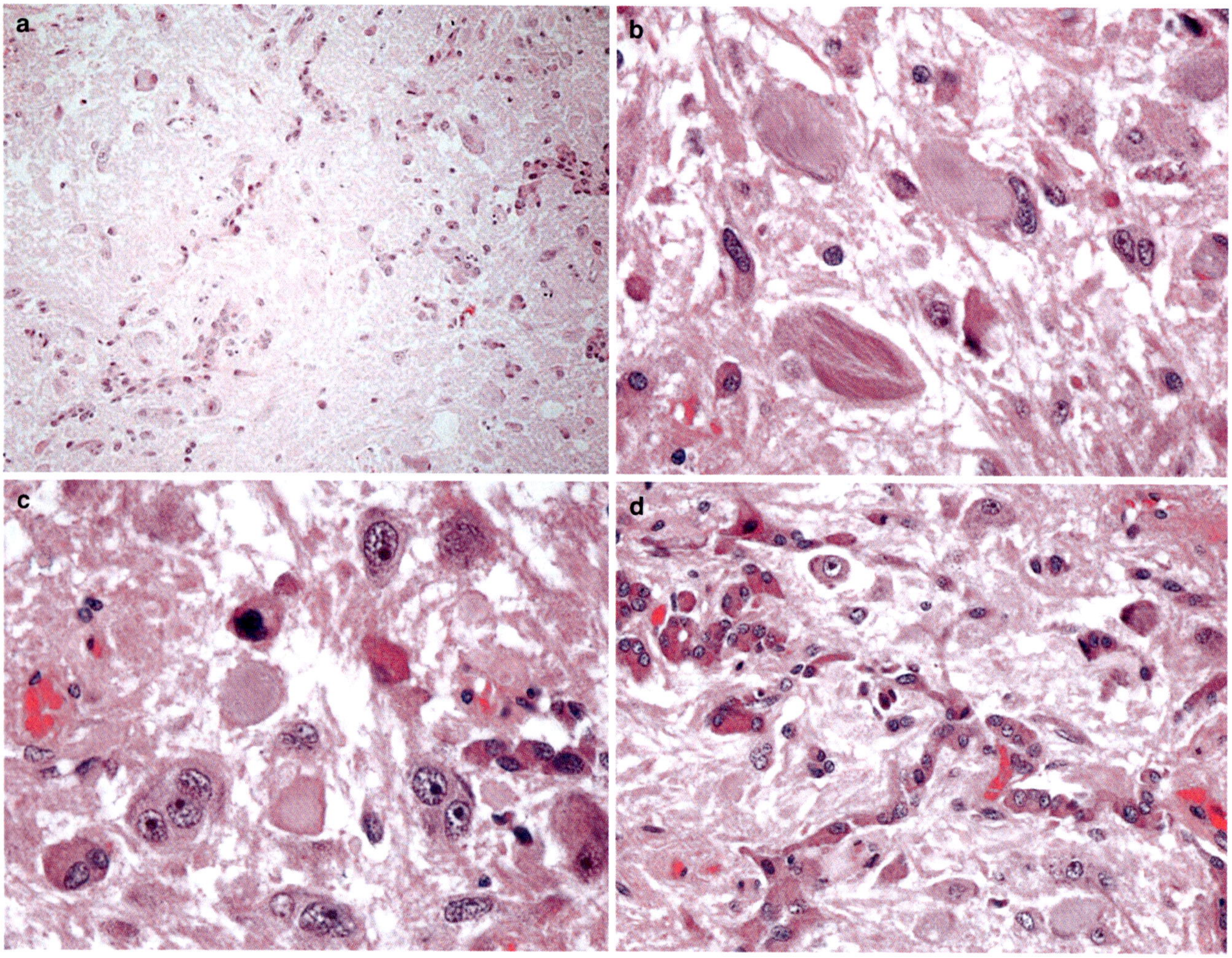

Fig. 42.4 Ganglioglioma. Microsections of the expanded asymmetric posterior lobe show accumulation of ganglion cells and scant astrocytes (**a**). Ganglion cells are dysmorphic (**b**) and feature neurofibrillary tangles (**c**). Note the association of ganglion cells with basophil invasion (**d**) (Adapted with permission from Scheithauer et al. [12])

42.4 Clinical and Surgical Management

- Resection of gangliocytoma and ganglioglioma via trans-sphenoidal approaches and open craniotomy has been reported [23, 24].
- The transitional or "collision" nature of gangliocytomas may make them more resistant to medical therapy when they are associated with functional pituitary adenomas [18].
- Management strategies are similar to those utilized for pituitary adenomas: adjunctive medications and/or radiation therapy may be used, especially for gangliocytomas coexisting with functional pituitary adenomas.
- The appropriate medical management of any underlying hormonal excess syndrome, as well as SIADH or diabetes insipidus, should be carried out in all patients.
- There have been no major series for pituitary gangliogliomas, but long-term outcomes for intracranial ganglioglioma are reported to be excellent. Per one large series, the 15-year overall survival rate was 94 %. Progression-free survival was affected by the degree of resection, and the administration of adjunctive radiation therapy delayed progression [25].

References

1. Asa SL, Kovacs K, Tindall GT, Barrow DL, Horvath E, Vecsei P. Cushing's disease associated with an intrasellar gangliocytoma producing corticotrophin-releasing factor. Ann Intern Med. 1984;101:789–93.
2. Horvath E, Kovacs K, Scheithauer BW, Lloyd RV, Smyth HS. Pituitary adenoma with neuronal choristoma (PANCH): composite lesion or lineage infidelity? Ultrastruct Pathol. 1994;18:565–74.
3. Kontogeorgos G, Mourouti G, Kyrodimou E, Liapi-Avgeri G, Parasi E. Ganglion cell containing pituitary adenomas: signs of neuronal differentiation in adenoma cells. Acta Neuropathol. 2006;112:21–8.
4. Kurosaki M, Saeger W, Ludecke DK. Intrasellar gangliocytomas associated with acromegaly. Brain Tumor Pathol. 2002;19:63–7.
5. Puchner MJ, Ludecke DK, Saeger W, Riedel M, Asa SL. Gangliocytomas of the sellar region--a review. Exp Clin Endocrinol Diabetes. 1995;103:129–49.
6. Baysefer A, Gezen F, Kayali H, Erdogan E, Timurkaynak E, Celasun B. Intrasellar gangliocytoma resembling pituitary adenoma. Minim Invasive Neurosurg. 1997;40:107–9.
7. Geddes JF, Jansen GH, Robinson SF, Gomori E, Holton JL, Monson JP, et al. 'Gangliocytomas' of the pituitary: a heterogeneous group of lesions with differing histogenesis. Am J Surg Pathol. 2000;24:607–13.
8. Saeger W, Puchner MJ, Ludecke DK. Combined sellar gangliocytoma and pituitary adenoma in acromegaly or Cushing's disease. A report of 3 cases. Virchows Arch. 1994;425:93–9.
9. Towfighi J, Salam MM, McLendon RE, Powers S, Page RB. Ganglion cell-containing tumors of the pituitary gland. Arch Pathol Lab Med. 1996;120:369–77.
10. Saeger W, Ludecke DK, Buchfelder M, Fahlbusch R, Quabbe HJ, Petersenn S. Pathohistological classification of pituitary tumors: 10 years of experience with the German Pituitary Tumor Registry. Eur J Endocrinol. 2007;156:203–16.
11. Saeger W, Ludecke DK, Losa M. Combined neuronal and endocrine tumors of the sellar region. Pathologe. 1997;18:419–24.
12. Scheithauer BW, Silva AI, Parisi JE, Kovacs K, Horvath E. Ganglioglioma of the neurohypophysis. Endocr Pathol. 2008;19:112–6.
13. Fehn M, Lohmann F, Ludecke DK, Rudorff KH, Saeger W. Ganglioglioma of the neurohypophysis with secretion of vasopressin. Exp Clin Endocrinol Diabetes. 1998;106:425–30.
14. Mikami S, Kameyama K, Takahashi S, Yoshida K, Kawase T, Sano T, Mukai M. Combined gangliocytoma and prolactinoma of the pituitary gland. Endocr Pathol. 2008;19:117–21.
15. Jalali R, Deopujari CE, Bhutani R, Suhas U, Rajasekharan P, Kane SV, Gupta T. Suprasellar ganglioglioma with unusual diffuse involvement of the entire optico-chiasmal hypothalamic pathway. J Cancer Res Ther. 2008;4:140–3.
16. Asa SL, Scheithauer BW, Bilbao JM, Horvath E, Ryan N, Kovacs K, et al. A case for hypothalamic acromegaly: a clinicopathological study of six patients with hypothalamic gangliocytomas producing growth hormone-releasing factor. J Clin Endocrinol Metab. 1984;58:796–803.
17. Sy J, Ang LC. Cytomorphologic spectrum of mixed pituitary adenoma-gangliocytomas: a report of two cases. Acta Cytol. 2010;54:981–4.
18. McCowen KC, Glickman JN, Black PM, Zervas NT, Lidov HG, Garber JR. Gangliocytoma masquerading as a prolactinoma. Case report. J Neurosurg. 1999;91:490–5.
19. Serri O, Berthelet F, Belair M, Vallette S, Asa SL. An unusual association of a sellar gangliocytoma with a prolactinoma. Pituitary. 2008;11:85–7.
20. Puchner MJ, Ludecke DK, Valdueza JM, Saeger W, Willig RP, Stalla GK, Odink RJ. Cushing's disease in a child caused by a corticotropin-releasing hormone-secreting intrasellar gangliocytoma associated

with an adrenocorticotropic hormone-secreting pituitary adenoma. Neurosurgery. 1993;33:920–4; discussion 924–5.
21. Chen J, Hersmus N, Van Duppen V, Caesens P, Denef C, Vankelecom H. The adult pituitary contains a cell population displaying stem/progenitor cell and early embryonic characteristics. Endocrinology. 2005;146:3985–98.
22. Vidal S, Horvath E, Kovacs K, Lloyd RV, Smyth HS. Reversible transdifferentiation: interconversion of somatotrophs and lactotrophs in pituitary hyperplasia. Mod Pathol. 2001;14:20–8.
23. Fischer EG, Morris JH, Kettyle WM. Intrasellar gangliocytoma and syndromes of pituitary hypersecretion. Case report. J Neurosurg. 1983;59:1071–5.
24. Morikawa M, Tamaki N, Kokunai T, Imai Y. Intrasellar pituitary gangliocyto-adenoma presenting with acromegaly: case report. Neurosurgery. 1997;40:611–4; discussion 614–5.
25. Compton JJ, Long term outcomes for low-grade intracranial ganglioglioma: 30 year experience from the mayo. Clinic J Nevrojury. 2012(5) 825–30.

Spindle Cell Oncocytoma

43

Gabriel Zada, M. Beatriz S. Lopes, Srinivasan Mukundan Jr., and Edward Laws Jr.

43.1 Epidemiology and Clinical Presentation

- Spindle cell oncocytoma (SCO) is an exceedingly rare, nonfunctioning, nonadenomatous tumor that arises in the pituitary gland. In 2007, it was classified as a separate pathological entity by the WHO [1].
- SCOs are thought to arise from folliculostellate cells [2]. However, recent data on the shared immunoreactivity for TTF-1 of normal pituicytes and pituicytomas, granular cell tumors, and spindle cell oncocytomas may suggest an alternative and common histogenesis (See Chap. 4)
- In many cases, an SCO may mimic a nonfunctioning pituitary adenoma. As nonadenomatous sellar lesions, however, SCOs also require differentiation from pituicytomas or granular cell tumors [3, 4].
- SCOs typically present with visual loss, hypopituitarism, and headaches [5].
- The mean age at diagnosis is 61 years [2].

G. Zada, MD, MS (✉)
Department of Neurological Surgery, Keck School of Medicine, University of Southern California, 1200 N State Street, #3300, Los Angeles, CA 90033, USA
e-mail: gzada@usc.edu

M.B.S. Lopes, MD, PhD
Department of Pathology (Neuropathology), University of Virginia School of Medicine, 1215 Lee Street, Room 3060–HEP, Charlottesville, VA 22908, USA
e-mail: msl2e@virginia.edu

S. Mukundan Jr., PhD, MD
Department of Radiology, Brigham and Women's Hospital, 75 Francis Street, Boston, MA 02115, USA
e-mail: smukundan@partners.org

E. Laws Jr., MD
Department of Neurosurgery, Brigham and Women's Hospital, 15 Francis Street, Boston, MA 02115, USA
e-mail: elaws@partners.org

G. Zada et al. (eds.), *Atlas of Sellar and Parasellar Lesions: Clinical, Radiologic, and Pathologic Correlations*, DOI 10.1007/978-3-319-22855-6_43

43.2 Imaging Features

- SCOs often appear quite similar to nonfunctioning pituitary adenomas [2].
- Most SCOs are both intrasellar and suprasellar, infiltrating tumors (Fig. 43.1) [2, 3].
- Many SCOs demonstrate heterogeneous enhancement, and some show evidence of intratumoral hemorrhage [3, 6].

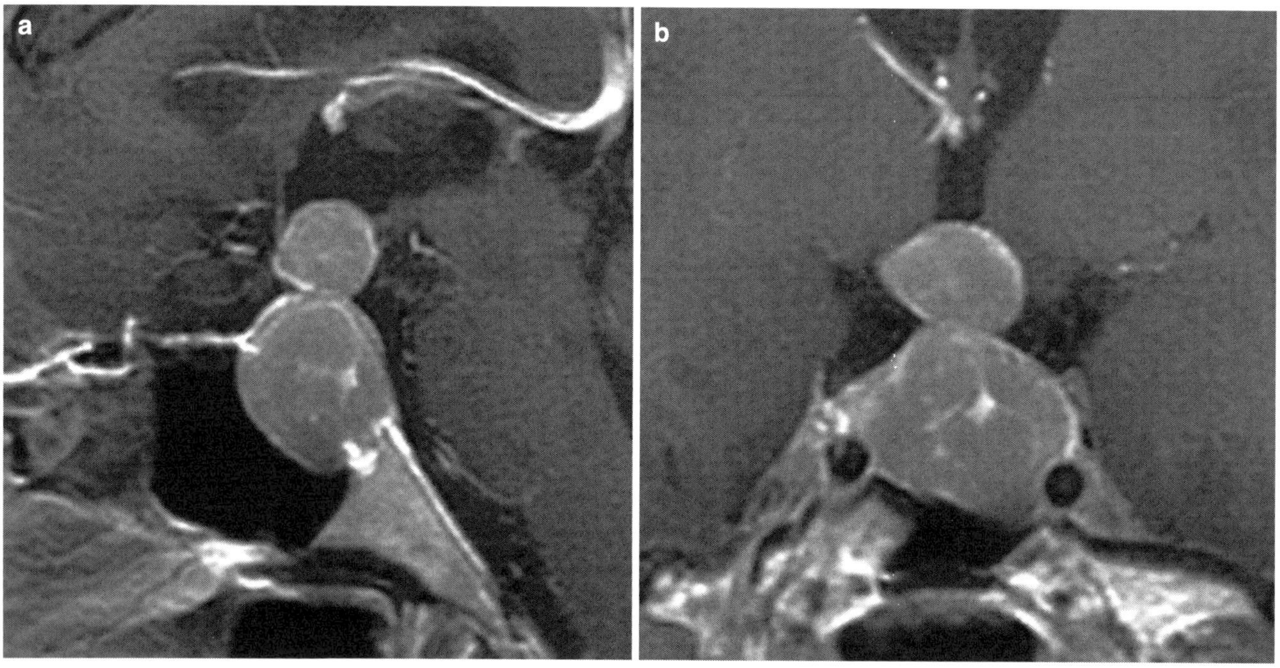

Fig. 43.1 Spindle cell oncocytoma. (**a**) Sagittal T1-weighted gadolinium-enhanced MR image. (**b**) Coronal T1-weighted gadolinium-enhanced image. An enhancing mass centered in the sella is eroding the upper clivus, with suprasellar extension to the anterior floor of the third ventricle. The pituitary gland is not seen distinct from the mass

43.3 Histopathology

- SCO is classified as a WHO Grade I neoplasm.
- SCOs are composed of fusiform, mitochondrion-rich spindle cells alternating with areas of epithelioid-like cells that exhibit eosinophilic, granular cytoplasm [7, 8].
- SCOs demonstrate immunoreactivity for the S100 protein, vimentin, EMA, Bcl-2, galectin-3, nestin, and TTF-1, as well as the antimitochondrial antibody 113-1 (Fig. 43.2). Conversely, they do not stain for GFAP, follicular-epithelial cytokeratin, neurofilament, synaptophysin, carcinoembryonic antigen, or anterior pituitary hormones [6, 7, 9].
- The Ki-67 labeling index may be as high as 20 % in SCOs [8].

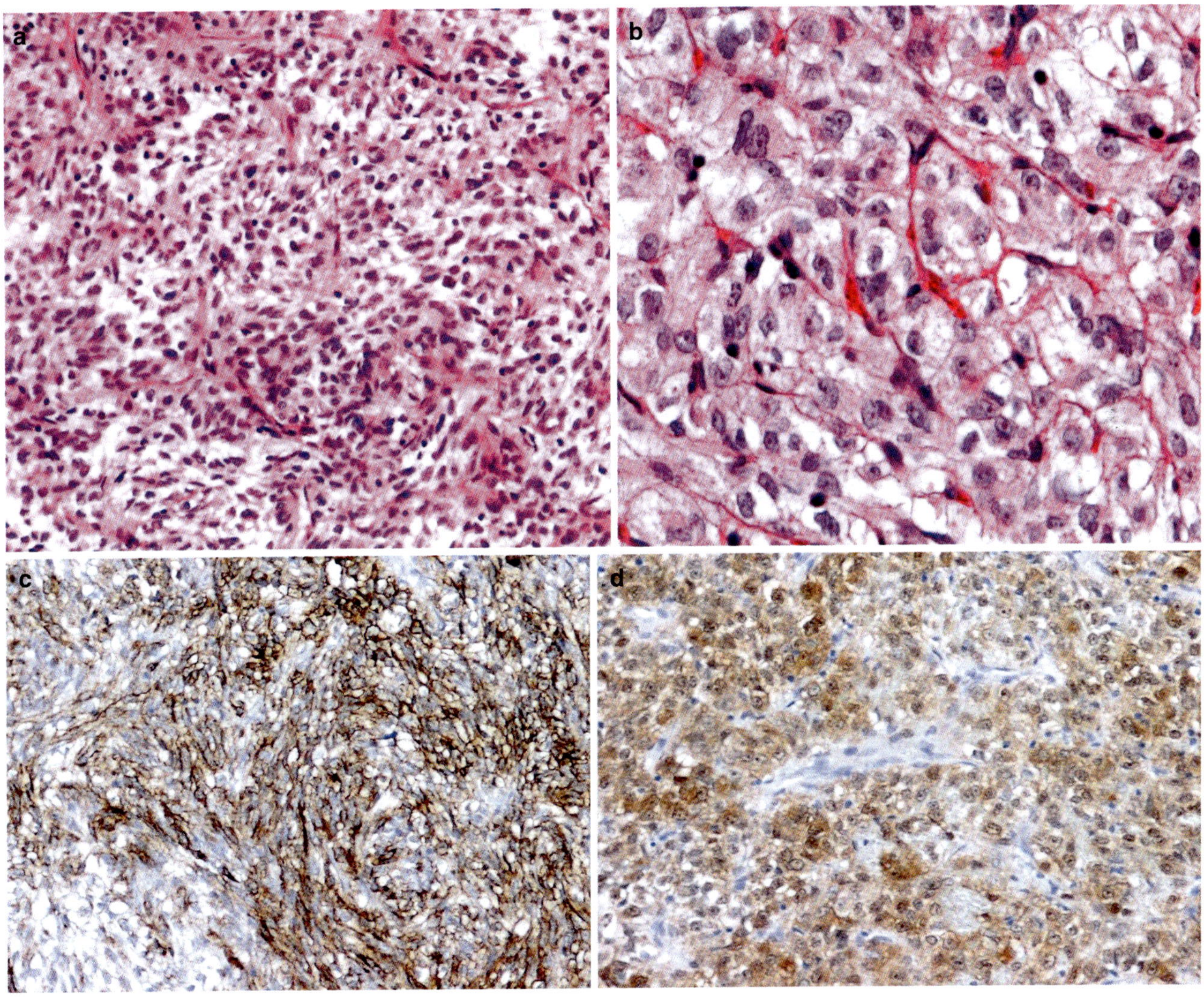

Fig. 43.2 Spindle cell oncocytoma. These tumors are characterized by spindle cells arranged in interwoven fascicles (**a**) intermixed with plump cells with eosinophilic, finely granular cytoplasm consistent with an oncocytic cellular component (**b**) (H&E stain). The tumor cells are immunoreactive for EMA (**c**), vimentin, S100 (**d**), and TTF-1 and are mostly negative for GFAP. The recent observation of TTF-1 expression in normal pituicytes and tumors of the pituitary region—including pituicytomas, granular cell tumors, and spindle cell oncocytoma—raises the possibility that these tumors may represent different variants of a common pathogenetic origin

43.4 Clinical and Surgical Management

- SCOs are often mistaken for nonfunctioning pituitary adenomas. They are typically treated via transsphenoidal resection [7, 8].
- SCOs are notably characterized by high vascularity and firm consistency, often limiting the degree of safe tumor resection [4, 10].
- Recurrence of SCOs following transsphenoidal resection appears to be common [6, 8, 11–13].
- Only limited anecdotal reports are available pertaining to adjunctive radiation or medical management of SCOs.

References

1. Roncaroli F, Scheithauer BW. Papillary tumor of the pineal region and spindle cell oncocytoma of the pituitary: new tumor entities in the 2007 WHO Classification. Brain Pathol. 2007;17:314–8.
2. Roncaroli F, Scheithauer BW, Cenacchi G, Horvath E, Kovacs K, Lloyd RV, et al. 'Spindle cell oncocytoma' of the adenohypophysis: a tumor of folliculostellate cells? Am J Surg Pathol. 2002;26:1048–55.
3. Covington MF, Chin SS, Osborn AG. Pituicytoma, spindle cell oncocytoma, and granular cell tumor: clarification and meta-analysis of the world literature since 1893. AJNR Am J Neuroradiol. 2011;32:2067–72.
4. Ogiwara H, Dubner S, Shafizadeh S, Raizer J, Chandler JP. Spindle cell oncocytoma of the pituitary and pituicytoma: two tumors mimicking pituitary adenoma. Surg Neurol Int. 2011;2:116.
5. Matyja E, Maksymowicz M, Grajkowska W, Olszewski W, Zielinski G, Bonicki W. Spindle cell oncocytoma of the adenohypophysis – a clinicopathological and ultrastructural study of two cases. Folia Neuropathol. 2010;48:175–84.
6. Borges MT, Lillehei KO, Kleinschmidt-DeMasters BK. Spindle cell oncocytoma with late recurrence and unique neuroimaging characteristics due to recurrent subclinical intratumoral bleeding. J Neurooncol. 2011;101:145–54.
7. Vajtai I, Beck J, Kappeler A, Hewer E. Spindle cell oncocytoma of the pituitary gland with follicle-like component: organotypic differentiation to support its origin from folliculo-stellate cells. Acta Neuropathol. 2011;122:253–8.
8. Kloub O, Perry A, Tu PH, Lipper M, Lopes MB. Spindle cell oncocytoma of the adenohypophysis: report of two recurrent cases. Am J Surg Pathol. 2005;29:247–53.
9. Alexandrescu S, Brown RE, Tandon N, Bhattacharjee MB. Neuron precursor features of spindle cell oncocytoma of adenohypophysis. Ann Clin Lab Sci. 2012;42:123–9.
10. Fujisawa H, Tohma Y, Muramatsu N, Kida S, Kaisaki Y, Tamamura H. Spindle cell oncocytoma of the adenohypophysis with marked hypervascularity. Case report. Neurol Med Chir (Tokyo). 2012;52:594–8.
11. Borota OC, Scheithauer BW, Fougner SL, Hald JK, Ramm-Pettersen J, Bollerslev J. Spindle cell oncocytoma of the adenohypophysis: report of a case with marked cellular atypia and recurrence despite adjuvant treatment. Clin Neuropathol. 2009;28:91–5.
12. Coiré CI, Horvath E, Smyth HS, Kovacs K. Rapidly recurring folliculostellate cell tumor of the adenohypophysis with the morphology of a spindle cell oncocytoma: case report with electron microscopic studies. Clin Neuropathol. 2009;28:303–8.
13. Demssie YN, Joseph J, Dawson T, Roberts G, de Carpentier J, Howell S. Recurrent spindle cell oncocytoma of the pituitary, a case report and review of literature. Pituitary. 2011;14:367–70.

Nasopharyngeal Carcinoma and Squamous Cell Carcinoma of the Paranasal Sinuses

44

Gabriel Zada, M. Beatriz S. Lopes, Srinivasan Mukundan Jr., and Edward Laws Jr.

44.1 Epidemiology and Clinical Presentation

- *Nasopharyngeal carcinoma (NPC)* is the most common primary malignancy of the nasopharynx. The WHO divides NPC into three subtypes: Type 1 (I) is squamous cell carcinoma; Type 2a (II) is keratinizing undifferentiated carcinoma; Type 2b (III) is nonkeratinizing undifferentiated carcinoma.
- NPC is associated with the Epstein-Barr virus (EBV), and therefore, it is more commonly seen in parts of Eastern and Southeast Asia.
- In most countries, the incidence is less than 1 per 100,000 persons per year. In some parts of Southeast Asia, however, the incidence may be as high as 30 per 100,000 persons per year [1].
- On occasion, NPC may arise in the sphenoid sinus and invade the sellar or parasellar spaces. In rare cases, NPC metastases to the pituitary gland have been reported [2].
- The median age at diagnosis is 58 years [3].
- In general, patients with NPC most commonly present with a palpable neck lump (76 %), nasal obstruction (73 %), epistaxis, or nasal discharge. Some patients with skull base erosion will have headache and cranial nerve dysfunction, especially of cranial nerves III, V, VI, and XII. Some patients have signs of Eustachian tube dysfunction [4].
- *Squamous cell carcinoma of the paranasal sinuses (PNSSCC)* is the most common sinonasal malignancy, accounting for approximately 60 % of such cancers [5].
- The mean age at diagnosis is 59–63 years [6, 7].
- Known risk factors for PNSSCC include an immunocompromised state, papilloma, and occupational exposures to nickel, chromium, isopropyl alcohol, Thorotrast, radium, and toxins such as mustard gas [8].
- PNSSCC most commonly arises in the maxillary sinus (67 %), ethmoid sinus (20 %), nasal cavity (9 %), and sphenoid sinus (4 %) [6].
- Squamous cell carcinoma may occasionally present as a sellar mass [9].
- Common clinical presentation includes nasal obstruction, epistaxis, nasal discharge, headache, facial pain, and cranial nerve paresis.

G. Zada, MD, MS (✉)
Department of Neurological Surgery, Keck School of Medicine, University of Southern California, 1200 N State Street, #3300, Los Angeles, CA 90033, USA
e-mail: gzada@usc.edu

M.B.S. Lopes, MD, PhD
Department of Pathology (Neuropathology), University of Virginia School of Medicine, 1215 Lee Street, Room 3060–HEP, Charlottesville, VA 22908, USA
e-mail: msl2e@virginia.edu

S. Mukundan Jr., PhD, MD
Department of Radiology, Brigham and Women's Hospital, 75 Francis Street, Boston, MA 02115, USA
e-mail: smukundan@partners.org

E. Laws Jr., MD
Department of Neurosurgery, Brigham and Women's Hospital, 15 Francis Street, Boston, MA 02115, USA
e-mail: elaws@partners.org

G. Zada et al. (eds.), *Atlas of Sellar and Parasellar Lesions: Clinical, Radiologic, and Pathologic Correlations*,
DOI 10.1007/978-3-319-22855-6_44

44.2 Imaging Features

- MRI is the modality of choice for evaluating local tumor burden and soft tissue disease.
- On MRI, NPC is typically characterized by hypointense to intermediate T2 signal intensity that is higher than muscle signal, low signal intensity on T1-weighted images, and less contrast enhancement than in normal mucosa.
- Most NPCs (82 %) arise in the posterolateral recess of the pharyngeal wall (Rosenmüller fossa); 12 % arise in the midline (Fig. 44.1) [10]. Obstruction of Eustachian tube drainage can also manifest as unilateral middle ear and mastoid effusion, which occasionally can be detected incidentally during head imaging with prompt clinical evaluation of the nasopharynx.
- Nonenhanced T1-weighted imaging is helpful in detecting tumor between the tensor and levator, in the parapharyngeal space and retropharyngeal space, owing to a loss of normally observed high-intensity fat.
- Perineural spread can be detected by enlargement of nerves, including cranial nerve V in the pterygopalatine fossa, masticator space, foramen ovale, and cavernous sinus and cranial nerve VII near the stylomastoid foramen. Tumor can spread intracranially through the skull base foramina.
- The presence of more than 2 mm of dural thickening and nodular dural enhancement associated with sinonasal squamous cell carcinoma is predictive of dural invasion [11].
- CT imaging is helpful in identifying skull base erosion and bony destruction, which is found in 30–80 % of patients at presentation (Fig. 44.2) [12].
- NPCs and PNSSCC are staged according to standard TNM criteria. MRI and FDG PET/CT are commonly used for these purposes [13]. They may invade the skull base, sella, orbits, dura, and brain (Figs. 44.3 and 44.4). Staging for local invasion and distant metastases is crucial [14].

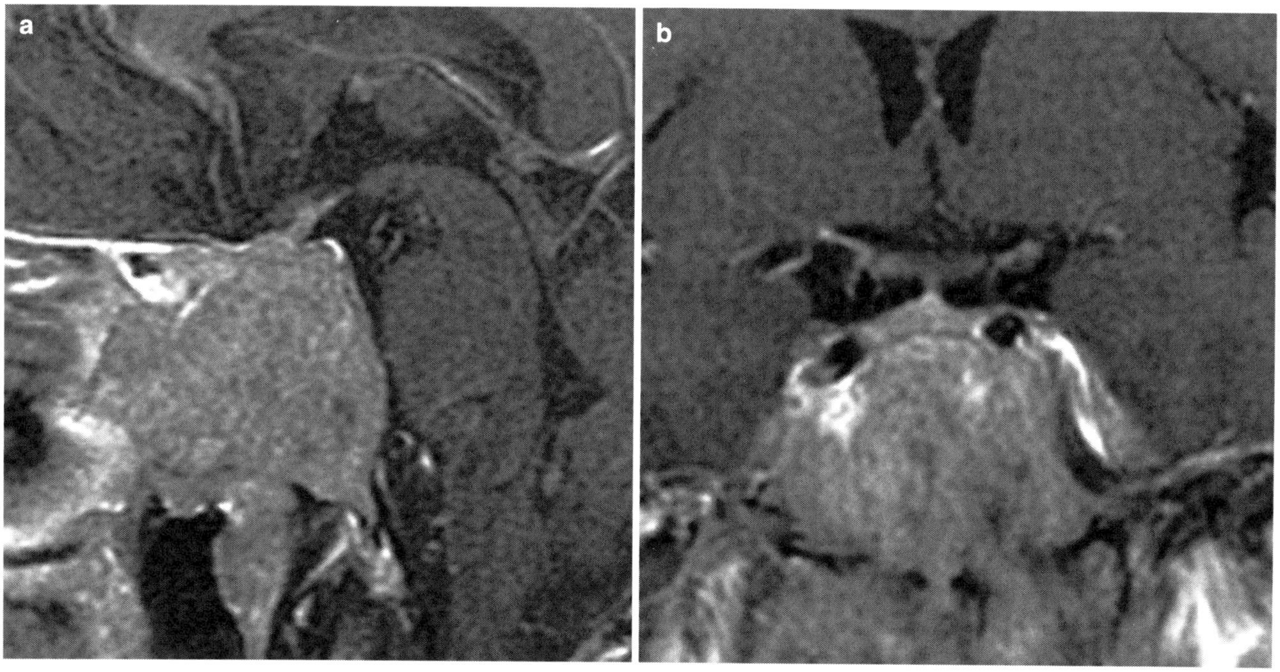

Fig. 44.1 Nasopharyngeal carcinoma (NPC). (**a**) Sagittal T1-weighted gadolinium-enhanced MR image. (**b**) Coronal T1-weighted gadolinium-enhanced image. A large enhancing mass is centered in the sphenoid sinus, replacing most of the clivus body. The pituitary gland is immediately above the mass

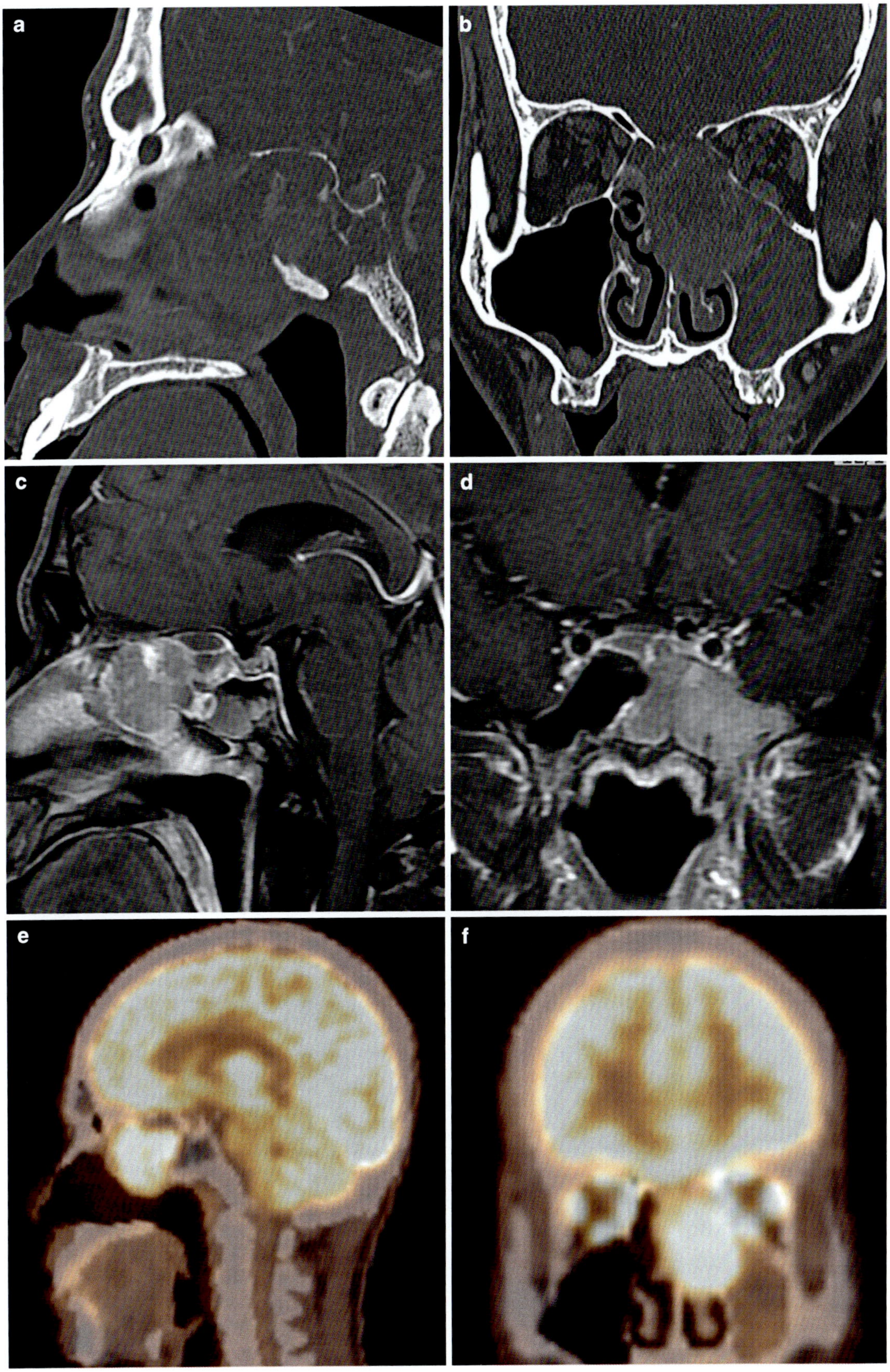

Fig. 44.2 NPC. (**a**) Sagittal CT image with contrast enhancement. (**b**) Coronal CT image with contrast enhancement. (**c**) Sagittal T1-weighted gadolinium-enhanced MR image. (**d**) Coronal T1-weighted gadolinium-enhanced image. A large enhancing mass is centered in the nasopharynx, eroding the septa and roofs of the ethmoid, the wall of the left maxillary antrum, and the upper body of the clivus. The mass extends laterally below the cavernous sinus to the floor of the middle cranial fossa and pterygopalatine fossa. The pituitary gland is distinctly seen above the mass. (**e**, **f**) FDG PET/CT shows the hypermetabolic sinus mass

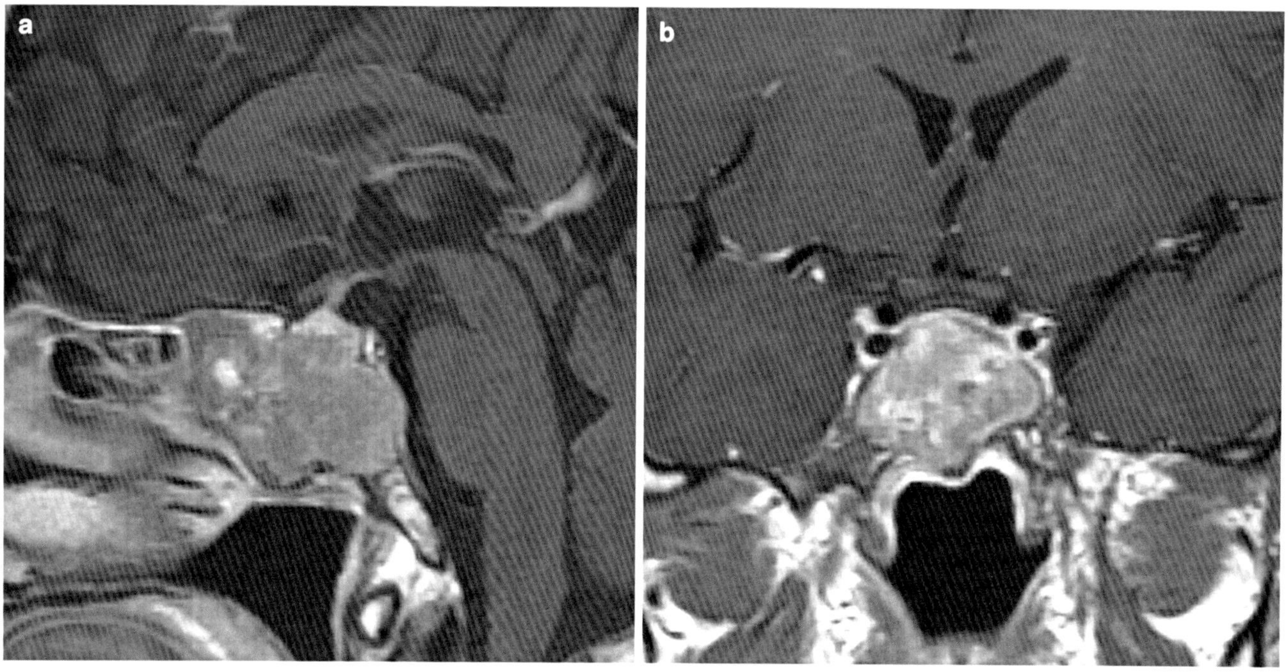

Fig. 44.3 Squamous cell carcinoma of the paranasal sinuses (PNSSCC). (**a**) Sagittal T1-weighted gadolinium-enhanced MR image. (**b**) Coronal T1-weighted gadolinium-enhanced image. An enhancing mass is centered in the sphenoid sinus, eroding the upper clivus, including the sellar floor. The pituitary gland is surrounded by the mass

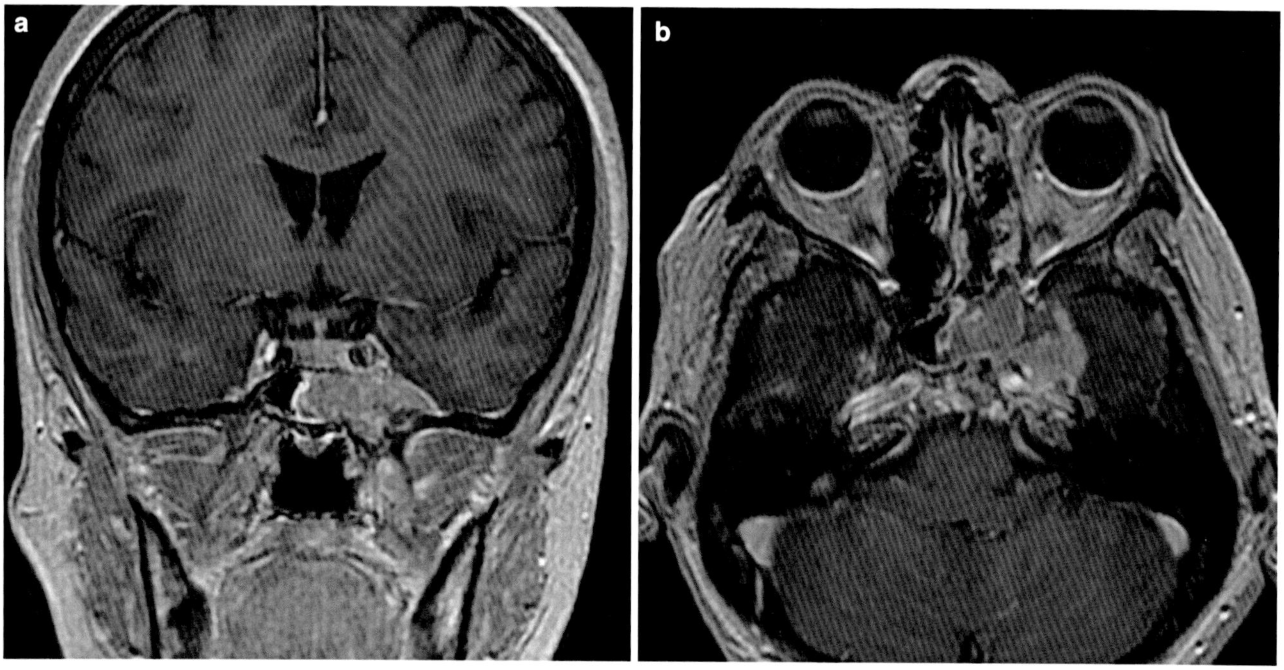

Fig. 44.4 PNSSCC. (**a**) Coronal T1-weighted gadolinium-enhanced MR image. (**b**) Axial T1-weighted gadolinium-enhanced image. An enhancing mass is seen centered in the left sphenoid sinus and middle fossa floor. The mass is highly invasive, with extension into the left medial/anterior temporal lobe

44.3 Histopathology

- The current WHO classification of NPC includes keratinizing squamous cell carcinomas (WHO I) or nonkeratinizing carcinomas. Nonkeratinizing carcinomas are further subdivided into differentiated (WHO II) and undifferentiated (WHO III) carcinomas.
- Latent EBV infection often leads to the development of NPC [1].
- NPCs are characterized by polygonal epithelial cells intermixed with lymphoid cells.
- Latent membrane protein 1 (LMP-1) has been noted to be highly expressed in EBV-associated NPC [1, 15].
- PNSSCCs are often associated with (and may arise from) inverted epithelial papillomas of the paranasal sinuses [16].
- They may be characterized by sheets of epithelial cells with varying degrees of keratin production, often with prominent palisading and intraepithelial nesting (Fig. 44.5) [8, 16].
- Some PNSSCCs are associated with the human papillomavirus (HPV) [17].
- The pituitary tumor-transforming gene (*PTTG*) is overexpressed in almost all cases of PNSSCC [18, 19].

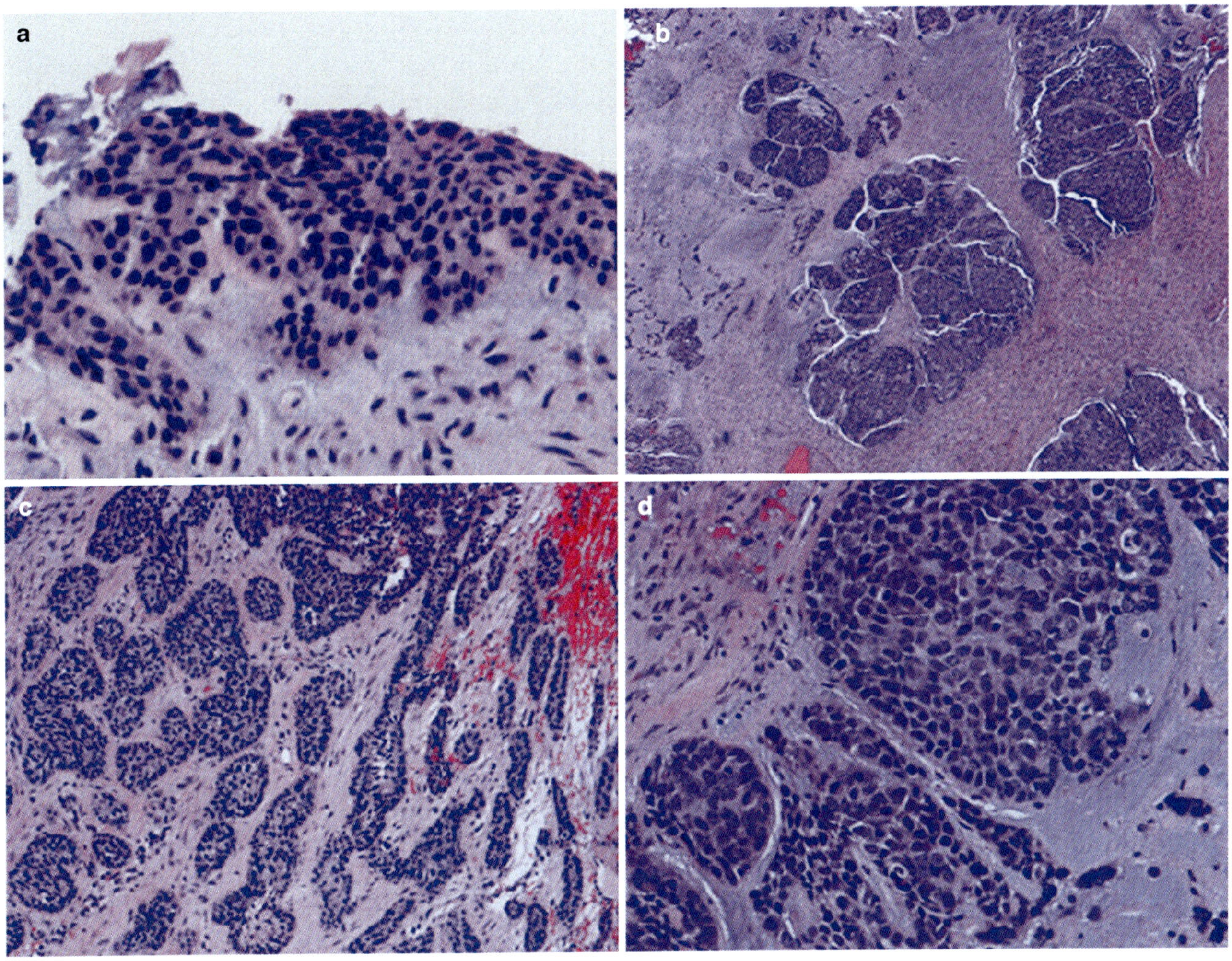

Fig. 44.5 Squamous cell carcinoma of the sphenoid sinus and sella. (**a**) Light microscopy revealed squamous dysplasia and carcinoma in situ of the mucosal surface (H&E, original magnification ×100). (**b**) Light microscopy revealed an invasive basaloid squamous cell carcinoma (BSCC). The BCSS grew as nested lobules in a fibrotic background. Large lobules showed compacted nests with a jigsaw-like pattern (H&E, original magnification ×40). (**c**) In this region, the BSCC grew as cords and trabeculae with peripheral palisading (H&E, original magnification ×100). (**d**) In a high-power view, the tumor was composed of closely packed, moderately pleomorphic basaloid cells with hyperchromatic nuclei and scant cytoplasm (H&E, original magnification ×200) (Adapted from Gu et al. [9], with permission)

44.4 Clinical and Surgical Management

- In patients diagnosed with NPC, EBV DNA can often be detected by blood serology tests. The quantity of EBV DNA detected in blood indicates the stage and prognosis of the disease [1].
- Standard TNM staging systems are typically applied at the time of diagnosis.
- Endoscopic endonasal biopsy can often be performed to confirm the diagnosis.
- Patients will commonly undergo biopsy or surgical debulking followed by radiation therapy and chemotherapy. Common chemotherapeutic regimens generally include cisplatin, 5-fluorouracil, and folinic acid [1, 20].
- Intensity-modulated radiation therapy (IMRT) doses of greater than 66 Gy have been associated with improved progression-free survival [21].
- The rate of hypopituitarism following radiation treatment for NPC is as high as 62 % in the 5 years following radiation. The growth hormone, cortisol, and thyroid hormonal axes were the ones most often affected. Vigilant monitoring and replacement of anterior pituitary hormones are recommended [1, 22].
- The median overall survival for patients undergoing chemoradiotherapy was 80.3 months, versus 28.5 months with radiotherapy alone [3].
- In a major series of patients with mostly stage III/IV NPC, the overall survival at 30 months was 97 % [20].
- The primary mode of treatment failure is the development of distant metastases.
- For PNSSCC, the 2-year overall survival for patients with a partial response after induction chemotherapy is 77 % [6].
- The overall 5-year survival ranges between 37 and 64 % [7, 23, 24].

References

1. Wei WI, Sham JS. Nasopharyngeal carcinoma. Lancet. 2005;365:2041–54.
2. Gunn GB, Villa RD, Sedler RR, Hardwicke F, Gomari GA, Mark RJ. Nasopharyngeal carcinoma metastasis to the pituitary gland: a case report and literature review. J Neurooncol. 2004;68:87–90.
3. Colaco RJ, Betts G, Donne A, Swindell R, Yap BK, Sykes AJ, et al. Nasopharyngeal carcinoma: a retrospective review of demographics, treatment and patient outcome in a single centre. Clin Oncol (R Coll Radiol). 2013;25:171–7.
4. Ansa B, Goodman M, Ward K, Kono SA, Owonikoko TK, Higgins K, et al. Paranasal sinus squamous cell carcinoma incidence and survival based on Surveillance, Epidemiology, and End Results Data, 1973 to 2009. Cancer. 2013;119:2602–10.
5. Hermans R, De Vuysere S, Marchal G. Squamous cell carcinoma of the sinonasal cavities. Semin Ultrasound CT MR. 1999;20:150–61.
6. Hanna EY, Cardenas AD, DeMonte F, Roberts D, Kupferman M, Weber R, et al. Induction chemotherapy for advanced squamous cell carcinoma of the paranasal sinuses. Arch Otolaryngol Head Neck Surg. 2011;137:78–81.
7. Kermer C, Poeschl PW, Wutzl A, Schopper C, Klug C, Poeschl E. Surgical treatment of squamous cell carcinoma of the maxilla and nasal sinuses. J Oral Maxillofac Surg. 2008;66:2449–53.
8. Raghavan P, Phillips CD. Magnetic resonance imaging of sinonasal malignancies. Top Magn Reson Imaging. 2007;18:259–67.
9. Gu X, Eskandari F, Fowler M. Sphenoid sinus basaloid squamous cell carcinoma presenting as a sellar mass: report a case with review of the literature. Head Neck Pathol. 2011;5:81–5.
10. Abdel Khalek Abdel Razek A, King A. MRI and CT of nasopharyngeal carcinoma. AJR Am J Roentgenol. 2012;198:11–8.
11. McIntyre JB, Perez C, Penta M, Tong L, Truelson J, Batra PS. Patterns of dural involvement in sinonasal tumors: prospective correlation of magnetic resonance imaging and histopathologic findings. Int Forum Allergy Rhinol. 2012;2:336–41.
12. Cheung YK, Sham J, Cheung YL, Chan FL. Evaluation of skull base erosion in nasopharyngeal carcinoma: comparison of plain radiography and computed tomography. Oncology. 1994;51:42–6.
13. Chang MC, Chen JH, Liang JA, Yang KT, Cheng KY, Kao CH. Accuracy of whole-body FDG-PET and FDG-PET/CT in M staging of nasopharyngeal carcinoma: a systematic review and meta-analysis. Eur J Radiol. 2013;82:366–73.
14. Eggesbo HB. Imaging of sinonasal tumours. Cancer Imaging. 2012;12:136–52.
15. Burgos JS. Involvement of the Epstein-Barr virus in the nasopharyngeal carcinoma pathogenesis. Med Oncol. 2005;22:113–21.
16. Lasser A, Rothfeld PR, Shapiro RS. Epithelial papilloma and squamous cell carcinoma of the nasal cavity and paranasal sinuses: a clinicopathological study. Cancer. 1976;38:2503–10.
17. Bishop JA, Guo TW, Smith DF, Wang H, Ogawa T, Pai SI, Westra WH. Human papillomavirus-related carcinomas of the sinonasal tract. Am J Surg Pathol. 2013;37:185–92.
18. Solbach C, Roller M, Eckerdt F, Peters S, Knecht R. Pituitary tumor-transforming gene expression is a prognostic marker for tumor recurrence in squamous cell carcinoma of the head and neck. BMC Cancer. 2006;6:242.
19. Zhou C, Liu S, Zhou X, Xue L, Quan L, Lu N, et al. Overexpression of human pituitary tumor transforming gene (hPTTG), is regulated by beta-catenin/TCF pathway in human esophageal squamous cell carcinoma. Int J Cancer. 2005;113:891–8.
20. Buehrlen M, Zwaan CM, Granzen B, Lassay L, Deutz P, Vorwerk P, et al. Multimodal treatment, including interferon beta, of nasopharyngeal carcinoma in children and young adults: preliminary results from the prospective, multicenter study NPC-2003-GPOH/DCOG. Cancer. 2012;118:4892–900.

21. Kam MK, Teo PM, Chau RM, Cheung KY, Choi PH, Kwan WH, et al. Treatment of nasopharyngeal carcinoma with intensity-modulated radiotherapy: the Hong Kong experience. Int J Radiat Oncol Biol Phys. 2004;60:1440–50.
22. Lam KS, Tse VK, Wang C, Yeung RT, Ho JH. Effects of cranial irradiation on hypothalamic-pituitary function--a 5-year longitudinal study in patients with nasopharyngeal carcinoma. Q J Med. 1991;78:165–76.
23. Haylock BJ, John DG, Paterson IC. The treatment of squamous cell carcinoma of the paranasal sinuses. Clin Oncol (R Coll Radiol). 1991;3:17–21.
24. Lavertu P, Roberts JK, Kraus DH, Levine HL, Wood BG, Medendorp SV, Tucker HM. Squamous cell carcinoma of the paranasal sinuses: the Cleveland Clinic experience 1977–1986. Laryngoscope. 1989;99:1130–6.

Sinonasal Melanoma

45

Gabriel Zada, M. Beatriz S. Lopes, Srinivasan Mukundan Jr., and Edward Laws Jr.

45.1 Epidemiology and Clinical Presentation

- Sinonasal melanoma is a relatively common skull base malignancy that can arise in the nasal cavity (often along the nasal septum) or paranasal sinuses and occasionally primarily in the sphenoid sinus [1, 2].
- The mean age at presentation is 63–67 years [3, 4].
- The most common clinical presentation is epistaxis and airway obstruction.
- In rare circumstances, melanoma can arise primarily in the sellar region [5–7].
- In other rare cases, melanoma can metastasize to the pituitary gland [8–10].
- Melanoma in this region may cause visual loss, hypopituitarism, headache, and cranial nerve paresis [2, 11].

45.2 Imaging Features

- On MRI, melanoma is typically characterized by an avidly enhancing mass, often with evidence of intratumoral hemorrhage [12, 13].
- The most common locations of sinonasal melanoma are the nasal septum and the maxillary sinus, near the maxillary antrum [14].
- Increased T1 signal may be seen in sinonasal melanoma, typically attributed to the presence of paramagnetic melanin and/or coexistent hemorrhage (Fig. 45.1) [13, 14].

G. Zada, MD, MS (✉)
Department of Neurological Surgery, Keck School of Medicine, University of Southern California, 1200 N State Street, #3300, Los Angeles, CA 90033, USA
e-mail: gzada@usc.edu

M.B.S. Lopes, MD, PhD
Department of Pathology (Neuropathology), University of Virginia School of Medicine, 1215 Lee Street, Room 3060–HEP, Charlottesville, VA 22908, USA
e-mail: msl2e@virginia.edu

S. Mukundan Jr., PhD, MD
Department of Radiology, Brigham and Women's Hospital, 75 Francis Street, Boston, MA 02115, USA
e-mail: smukundan@partners.org

E. Laws Jr., MD
Department of Neurosurgery, Brigham and Women's Hospital, 15 Francis Street, Boston, MA 02115, USA
e-mail: elaws@partners.org

G. Zada et al. (eds.), *Atlas of Sellar and Parasellar Lesions: Clinical, Radiologic, and Pathologic Correlations*,
DOI 10.1007/978-3-319-22855-6_45

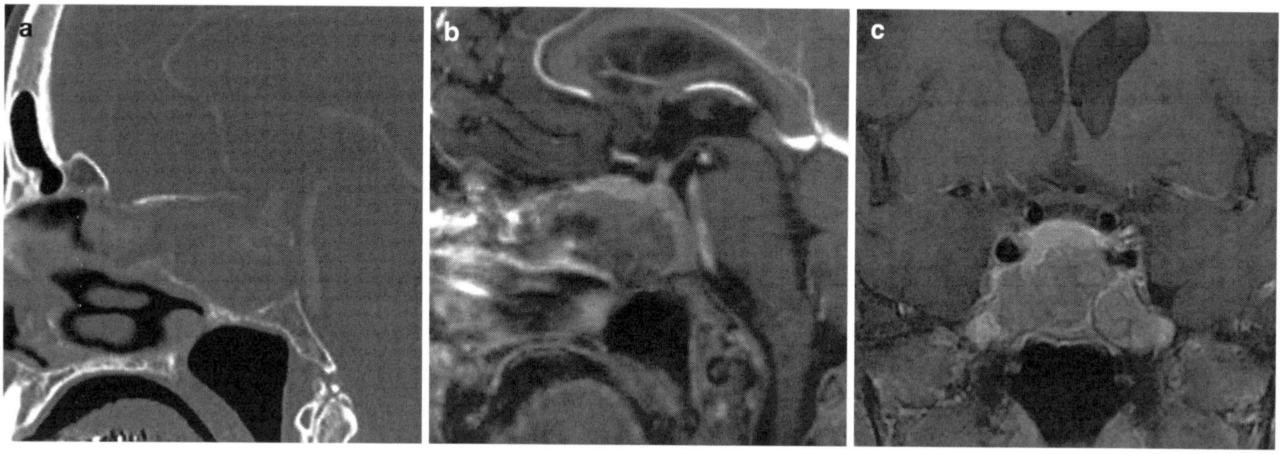

Fig. 45.1 Sinus malignancy: melanoma. (**a**) Sagittal CT image with contrast enhancement. (**b**) Sagittal T1-weighted gadolinium-enhanced MR image. (**c**) Coronal T1-weighted gadolinium-enhanced image. A heterogeneously enhancing mass is centered in the sphenoid sinus, eroding the upper clivus. The pituitary gland is immediately along the superior/posterior margin of the mass

45.3 Histopathology

- Melanoma is characterized as a malignant melanocytic tumor with immunopositivity for S100 protein and HMB-45 (Fig. 45.2).
- Common histopathological features include necrosis, pigmentation, vascular invasion (68 %), and a lymphocytic response (63 %) [15].
- Tumor pigmentation and papillary pseudoarchitecture are associated with a worse outcome [16].

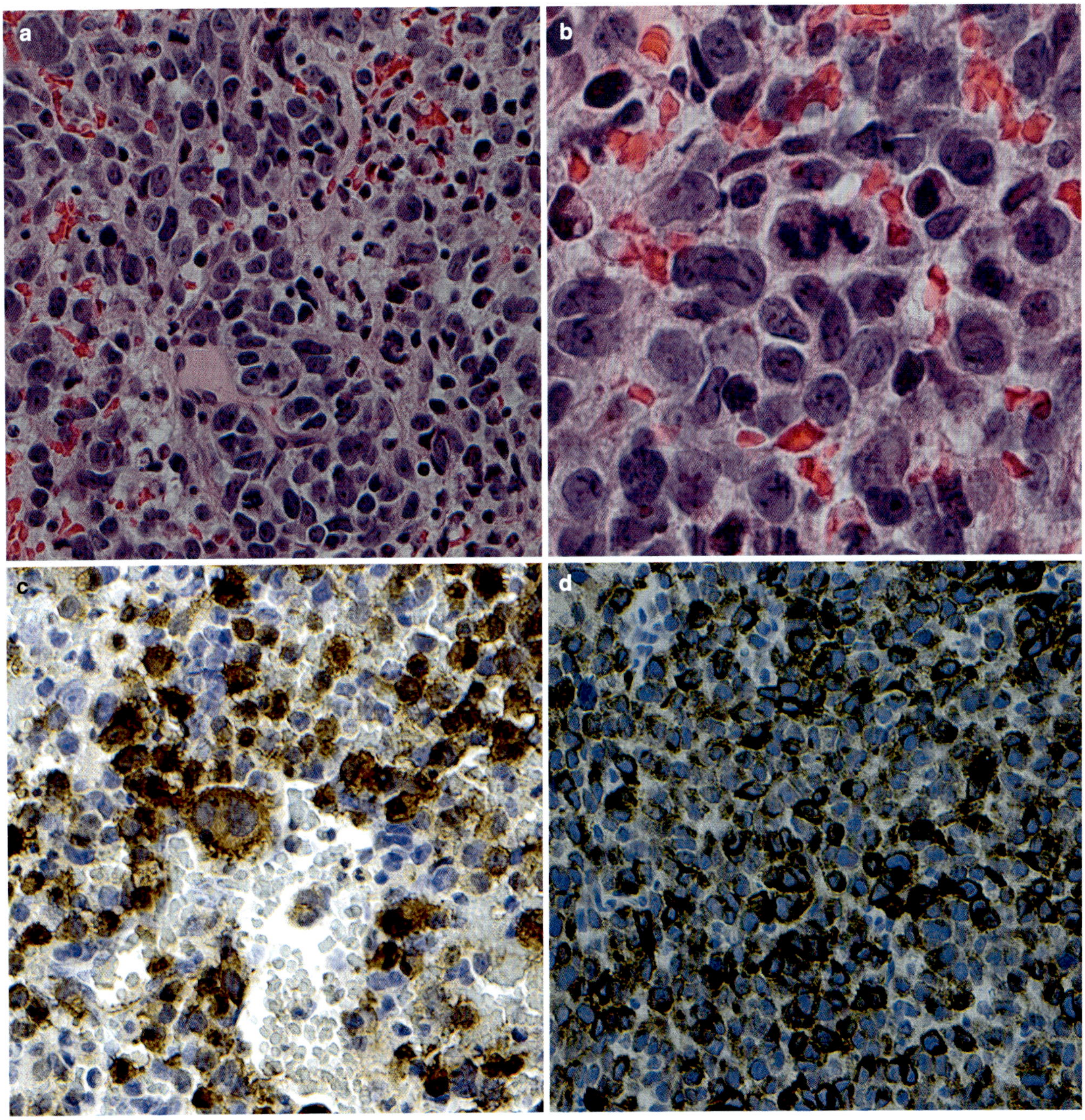

Fig. 45.2 Sinus malignancy: melanoma. H&E staining demonstrates epithelioid-shaped cells with numerous mitoses, prominent "cherry-red" nucleoli, and weakly eosinophilic and slightly blue-gray cytoplasm (**a**). This lesion had associated hemorrhage and microhemorrhage (×40 objective). A high-power view (**b**) demonstrates the same features (×100). Malignant cells were stained positively by anti-S100 antibodies (**c**) and by anti-MelanA/MART1 antibodies (×20) (**d**). Binucleate forms may also be seen in melanoma (**c**)

45.4 Clinical and Surgical Management

- A standard TNM classification system is used to stage patients and has been shown to correlate with outcomes [17].
- Maximal safe tumor debulking is recommended, followed by adjunctive chemotherapy, radiation, or both. When possible, obtaining tumor-free margins is recommended.
- Chemotherapy has been shown to offer a greater survival benefit than radiation [18].
- Current options for chemotherapy include dacarbazine, temozolomide, paclitaxel, and others. Chemotherapy may be administered with or without interferon-alpha.
- Craniofacial approaches have traditionally been used to achieve maximal safe tumor resection [4].
- Endoscopic approaches have become the mainstay of surgical treatment for many patients with skull base melanoma [19, 20].
- Recurrence and the development of distant metastases are common.
- Overall 5-year survival is approximately 24–30 %, with a mean survival time of 23–44 months [3, 20–22].

References

1. Busaba NY. Primary melanoma of the sphenoid sinus. Otolaryngol Head Neck Surg. 2000;123:748–9.
2. Lynch SC, Lee AG, Graham SM, Kirby PA. Primary melanoma of the sphenoid sinus presenting with a third cranial nerve palsy. J Neuroophthalmol. 2005;25:289–92.
3. Clifton N, Harrison L, Bradley PJ, Jones NS. Malignant melanoma of nasal cavity and paranasal sinuses: report of 24 patients and literature review. J Laryngol Otol. 2011;125:479–85.
4. Ganly I, Patel SG, Singh B, Kraus DH, Bridger PG, Cantu G, et al. Craniofacial resection for malignant melanoma of the skull base: report of an international collaborative study. Arch Otolaryngol Head Neck Surg. 2006;132:73–8.
5. Sidiropoulos M, Syro LV, Rotondo F, Scheithauer BW, Penagos LC, Uribe H, et al. Melanoma of the sellar region mimicking pituitary adenoma. Neuropathology. 2013;33:175–8.
6. Scholtz CL, Siu K. Melanoma of the pituitary. Case report. J Neurosurg. 1976;45:101–3.
7. Tüttenberg J, Fink W, Back W, Wenz F, Schadendorf D, Thomé C. A rare primary sellar melanoma. Case report. J Neurosurg. 2004;100:931–4.
8. Leung GK, Chow WS, Tan KC, Fan YW, Lam KS. Metastatic melanoma of the pituitary gland. Case report. J Neurosurg. 2003;99:913–5.
9. McCutcheon IE, Waguespack SG, Fuller GN, Couldwell WT. Metastatic melanoma to the pituitary gland. Can J Neurol Sci. 2007;34:322–7.
10. Wang YY, Norris A, de Plessis D, Gnanalingham KK. Melanoma of the sellar region. J Clin Neurosci. 2011;18:154–6.
11. Neilson JM, Moffat AD. Hypopituitarism caused by a melanoma of the pituitary gland. J Clin Pathol. 1963;16:144–9.
12. Chappell PM, Kelly WM, Ercius M. Primary sellar melanoma simulating hemorrhagic pituitary adenoma: MR and pathologic findings. AJNR Am J Neuroradiol. 1990;11:1054–6.
13. Yousem DM, Li C, Montone KT, Montgomery L, Loevner LA, Rao V, et al. Primary malignant melanoma of the sinonasal cavity: MR imaging evaluation. Radiographics. 1996;16:1101–10.
14. Raghavan P, Phillips CD. Magnetic resonance imaging of sinonasal malignancies. Top Magn Reson Imaging. 2007;18:259–67.
15. Kerr EH, Hameed O, Lewis Jr JS, Bartolucci AA, Wang D, Said-Al-Naief N. Head and neck mucosal malignant melanoma: clinicopathologic correlation with contemporary review of prognostic indicators. Int J Surg Pathol. 2012;20:37–46.
16. Moreno MA, Roberts DB, Kupferman ME, DeMonte F, El-Naggar AK, Williams M, et al. Mucosal melanoma of the nose and paranasal sinuses, a contemporary experience from the M. D. Anderson Cancer Center. Cancer. 2010;116:2215–23.
17. Koivunen P, Bäck L, Pukkila M, Laranne J, Kinnunen I, Grénman R, Mäkitie AA. Accuracy of the current TNM classification in predicting survival in patients with sinonasal mucosal melanoma. Laryngoscope. 2012;122:1734–8.
18. Gore MR, Zanation AM. Survival in sinonasal melanoma: a meta-analysis. J Neurol Surg B Skull Base. 2012;73:157–62.
19. Suh JD, Ramakrishnan VR, Chi JJ, Palmer JN, Chiu AG. Outcomes and complications of endoscopic approaches for malignancies of the paranasal sinuses and anterior skull base. Ann Otol Rhinol Laryngol. 2013;122:54–9.
20. Lund VJ, Chisholm EJ, Howard DJ, Wei WI. Sinonasal malignant melanoma: an analysis of 115 cases assessing outcomes of surgery, postoperative radiotherapy and endoscopic resection. Rhinology. 2012;50:203–10.
21. Roth TN, Gengler C, Huber GF, Holzmann D. Outcome of sinonasal melanoma: clinical experience and review of the literature. Head Neck. 2010;32:1385–92.
22. Gal TJ, Silver N, Huang B. Demographics and treatment trends in sinonasal mucosal melanoma. Laryngoscope. 2011;121:2026–33.

Sinonasal Adenocarcinoma

46

Gabriel Zada, M. Beatriz S. Lopes, Srinivasan Mukundan Jr., and Edward Laws Jr.

46.1 Epidemiology and Clinical Presentation

- Sinus adenocarcinoma (including salivary tumors, acinic tumors, and adenoid cystic carcinoma) is a relatively uncommon primary malignancy of the paranasal sinuses, accounting for 10–20 % of primary sinonasal cancers [1].
- These tumors have been associated with environmental and occupation exposures including tobacco, wood dust, and metal dust [2, 3].
- The mean age at diagnosis in patients with sinonasal adenocarcinoma is 64 years. On average, patients with the adenoid cystic carcinoma subtype have a slightly lower age (mean 54 years.) [4].
- Clinical symptoms frequently include airway obstruction, nasal discharge, epistaxis, facial pain, and visual complaints.
- Sinonasal adenocarcinoma is typically classified as salivary type, intestinal type (ITAC), or nonintestinal type (non-ITAC).
- The salivary type is by far the most common. It includes adenoid cystic carcinoma and acinic cell tumors. Adenoid cystic carcinoma is the second most common sinonasal cancer [5].

G. Zada, MD, MS (✉)
Department of Neurological Surgery, Keck School of Medicine, University of Southern California, 1200 N State Street, #3300, Los Angeles, CA 90033, USA
e-mail: gzada@usc.edu

M.B.S. Lopes, MD, PhD
Department of Pathology (Neuropathology), University of Virginia School of Medicine, 1215 Lee Street, Room 3060–HEP, Charlottesville, VA 22908, USA
e-mail: msl2e@virginia.edu

S. Mukundan Jr., PhD, MD
Department of Radiology, Brigham and Women's Hospital, 75 Francis Street, Boston, MA 02115, USA
e-mail: smukundan@partners.org

E. Laws Jr., MD
Department of Neurosurgery, Brigham and Women's Hospital, 15 Francis Street, Boston, MA 02115, USA
e-mail: elaws@partners.org

G. Zada et al. (eds.), *Atlas of Sellar and Parasellar Lesions: Clinical, Radiologic, and Pathologic Correlations*, DOI 10.1007/978-3-319-22855-6_46

46.2 Imaging Features

- Adenocarcinoma typically arises in the region of the ethmoid sinus, but it often invades the orbits, bony skull base, dura, and occasionally brain (Figs. 46.1 and 46.2) [3, 6, 7].
- Adenoid cystic carcinoma typically arises in the maxillary sinus [8].
- These tumors often demonstrate T2 hyperintensity and heterogeneous enhancement, often delineating solid tumor from cystic regions [9].

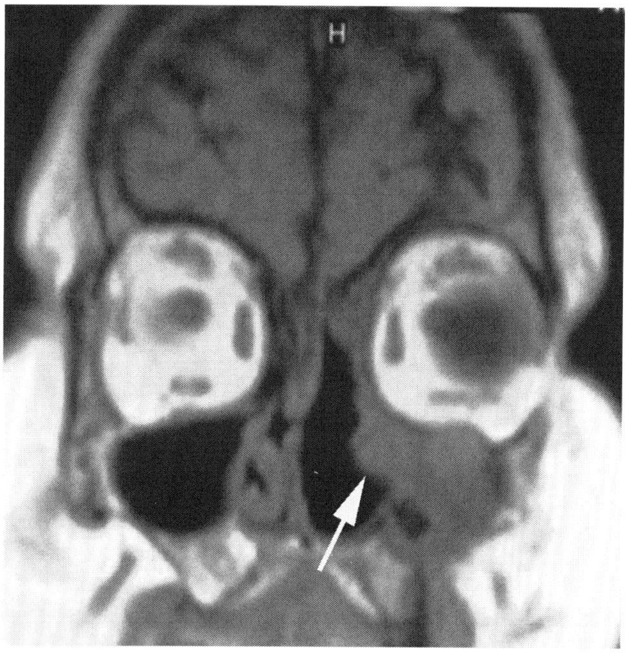

Fig. 46.1 Sinonasal adenocarcinoma. Coronal MRI shows an invasive mass (*arrow*) arising from the left middle turbinate, with extension to the ethmoid sinus, maxillary sinus, and floor of the orbit (Adapted with permission from Villar et al. [6])

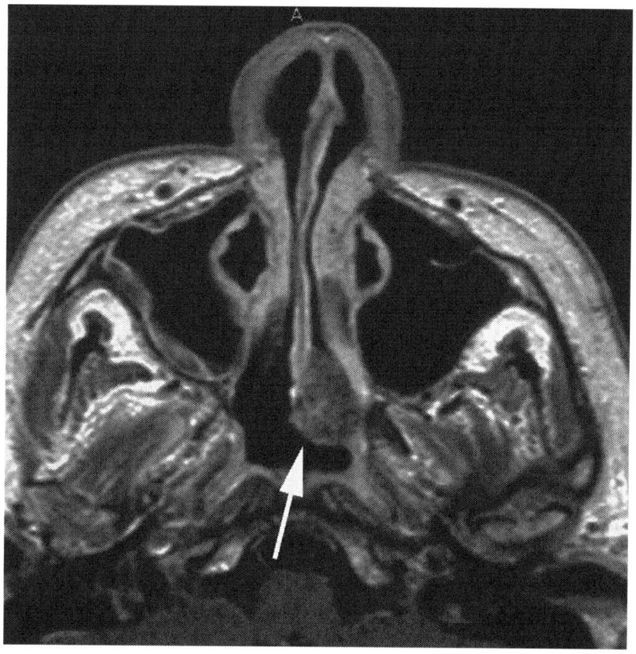

Fig. 46.2 Sinonasal adenocarcinoma. Axial MR image shows a left, intranasal low-grade adenocarcinoma (*arrow*) (Adapted with permission from Orvidas et al. [7])

46.3 Histopathology

- ITAC, which bears a close resemblance to colon adenocarcinoma, is commonly located in the ethmoid sinus (Fig. 46.3). ITAC tumors demonstrate immunoreactivity for CK7, CK20, CDX2, and MUC [2].
- Low-grade non-ITAC tumors may vary from tubular and simple glandular tumors to papillary or cystic types. Higher-grade non-ITAC neoplasms are characterized by necrosis, cellular pleomorphism, and a high mitotic rate [2].
- Adenoid cystic carcinoma is often characterized by basaloid cells with small, hyperchromatic nuclei, and scant cytoplasm arranged into three subtypes: cribriform, tubular, and solid. Perineural invasion is seen in up to 70 % of these tumors. They classically have a "Swiss cheese" or sieve-like pattern. Immunoreactivity for c-kit is often positive [10, 11].

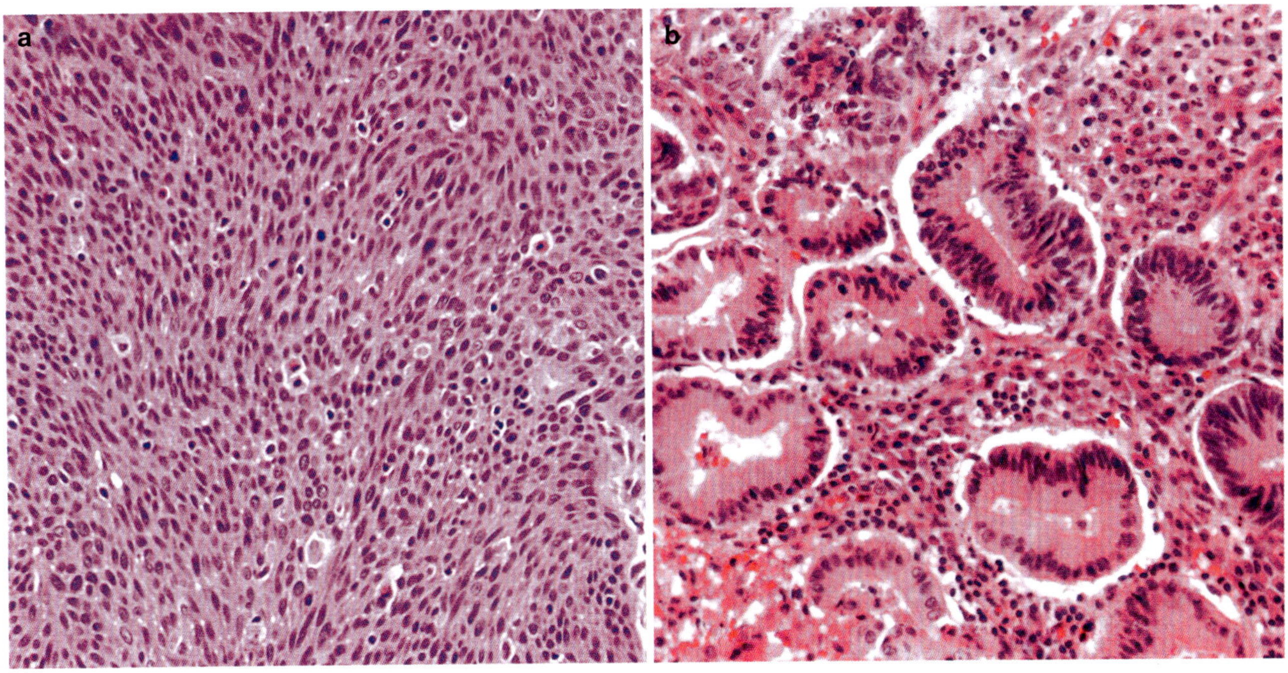

Fig. 46.3 Adenocarcinomas of the nasal and paranasal cavities are divided into two main categories: intestinal-type adenocarcinoma (ITAC) and non-ITAC. (**a**) In this example of a low-grade, non-ITAC sinonasal carcinoma, the tumor cells are arranged in lobules and show a moderate degree of pleomorphism and mitotic activity. (**b**) A tumor from the sphenoethmoidal recess shows moderately differentiated ITAC

46.4 Clinical and Surgical Management

- Maximal safe tumor resection followed by adjuvant radiation and possibly chemotherapy is the mainstay of treatment.
- Endoscopic endonasal resection is now widely and effectively used to treat this and other sinonasal malignancies [1].
- Sinonasal adenoid cystic carcinomas have a notoriously high recurrence rate, over 90 % [4].
- Overall survival rates for sinonasal adenocarcinoma are approximately 48–63 % [1, 2, 4].

References

1. Lund VJ, Chisholm EJ, Takes RP, Suarez C, Mendenhall WM, Rinaldo A, et al. Evidence for treatment strategies in sinonasal adenocarcinoma. Head Neck. 2012;34:1168–78.
2. Slootweg PJ, Ferlito A, Cardesa A, Thompson LD, Hunt JL, Strojan P, et al. Sinonasal tumors: a clinicopathologic update of selected tumors. Eur Arch Otorhinolaryngol. 2013;270:5–20.
3. Breheret R, Laccourreye L, Jeufroy C, Bizon A. Adenocarcinoma of the ethmoid sinus: retrospective study of 42 cases. Eur Ann Otorhinolaryngol Head Neck Dis. 2011;128:211–7.
4. Husain Q, Kanumuri VV, Svider PF, Radvansky BM, Boghani Z, Liu JK, Eloy JA. Sinonasal adenoid cystic carcinoma: systematic review of survival and treatment strategies. Otolaryngol Head Neck Surg. 2013;148:29–39.
5. Lupinetti AD, Roberts DB, Williams MD, Kupferman ME, Rosenthal DI, Demonte F, et al. Sinonasal adenoid cystic carcinoma: the M. D Anderson Cancer Center experience. Cancer. 2007;110:2726–31.
6. Villar R, Ramos B, Acosta M, Haro JJ, Gomez A. Recurrent adenocarcinoma of the sinonasal tract. Oral Maxillofac Surg. 2013;17:155–8.
7. Orvidas LJ, Lewis JE, Weaver AL, Bagniewski SM, Olsen KD. Adenocarcinoma of the nose and paranasal sinuses: a retrospective study of diagnosis, histologic characteristics, and outcomes in 24 patients. Head Neck. 2005;27:370–5.
8. Sanghvi S, Patel NR, Patel CR, Kalyoussef E, Baredes S, Eloy JA. Sinonasal adenoid cystic carcinoma: comprehensive analysis of incidence and survival from 1973 to 2009. Laryngoscope. 2013;123:1592–7.
9. Raghavan P, Phillips CD. Magnetic resonance imaging of sinonasal malignancies. Top Magn Reson Imaging. 2007;18:259–67.
10. Lin YC, Chen KC, Lin CH, Kuo KT, Ko JY, Hong RL. Clinicopathological features of salivary and non-salivary adenoid cystic carcinomas. Int J Oral Maxillofac Surg. 2012;41:354–60.
11. Jaso J, Malhotra R. Adenoid cystic carcinoma. Arch Pathol Lab Med. 2011;135:511–5.

Sinonasal Undifferentiated Carcinoma (SNUC)

47

Gabriel Zada, M. Beatriz S. Lopes, Srinivasan Mukundan Jr., and Edward Laws Jr.

47.1 Epidemiology and Clinical Presentation

- Sinonasal undifferentiated carcinoma (SNUC) is a rare and aggressive primary malignancy that often presents with intracranial invasion and advanced disease [1, 2].
- In rare circumstances, patients can develop distant metastases or leptomeningeal involvement [3, 4].
- The median age at presentation is 52 years [5].
- Clinical symptoms are similar to those of other sinonasal malignancies, including airway obstruction, epistaxis, nasal discharge, facial pain, headache, visual symptoms, and diplopia [2].

47.2 Imaging Features

- SNUCs are characterized by highly aggressive and infiltrative disease, often with intracranial invasion (Fig. 47.1) [5].
- Tumors are generally large and advanced ant the time of diagnosis, with most patients having tumors over 4 cm in diameter. The tumors tend to arise in the ethmoid sinuses and superior nasal cavity. They generally have poorly defined margins [6].
- CT scans often show bony erosion of the paranasal sinuses and skull base.
- On MRI, SNUC is characterized by T1 signal that is isointense to muscle and T2 images that are isointense or hyperintense. Heterogeneous contrast enhancement is common [6].
- SNUCs have a high propensity for neural invasion and dural involvement.

G. Zada, MD, MS (✉)
Department of Neurological Surgery, Keck School of Medicine, University of Southern California, 1200 N State Street, #3300, Los Angeles, CA 90033, USA
e-mail: gzada@usc.edu

M.B.S. Lopes, MD, PhD
Department of Pathology (Neuropathology), University of Virginia School of Medicine, 1215 Lee Street, Room 3060–HEP, Charlottesville, VA 22908, USA
e-mail: msl2e@virginia.edu

S. Mukundan Jr., PhD, MD
Department of Radiology, Brigham and Women's Hospital, 75 Francis Street, Boston, MA 02115, USA
e-mail: smukundan@partners.org

E. Laws Jr., MD
Department of Neurosurgery, Brigham and Women's Hospital, 15 Francis Street, Boston, MA 02115, USA
e-mail: elaws@partners.org

G. Zada et al. (eds.), *Atlas of Sellar and Parasellar Lesions: Clinical, Radiologic, and Pathologic Correlations*,
DOI 10.1007/978-3-319-22855-6_47

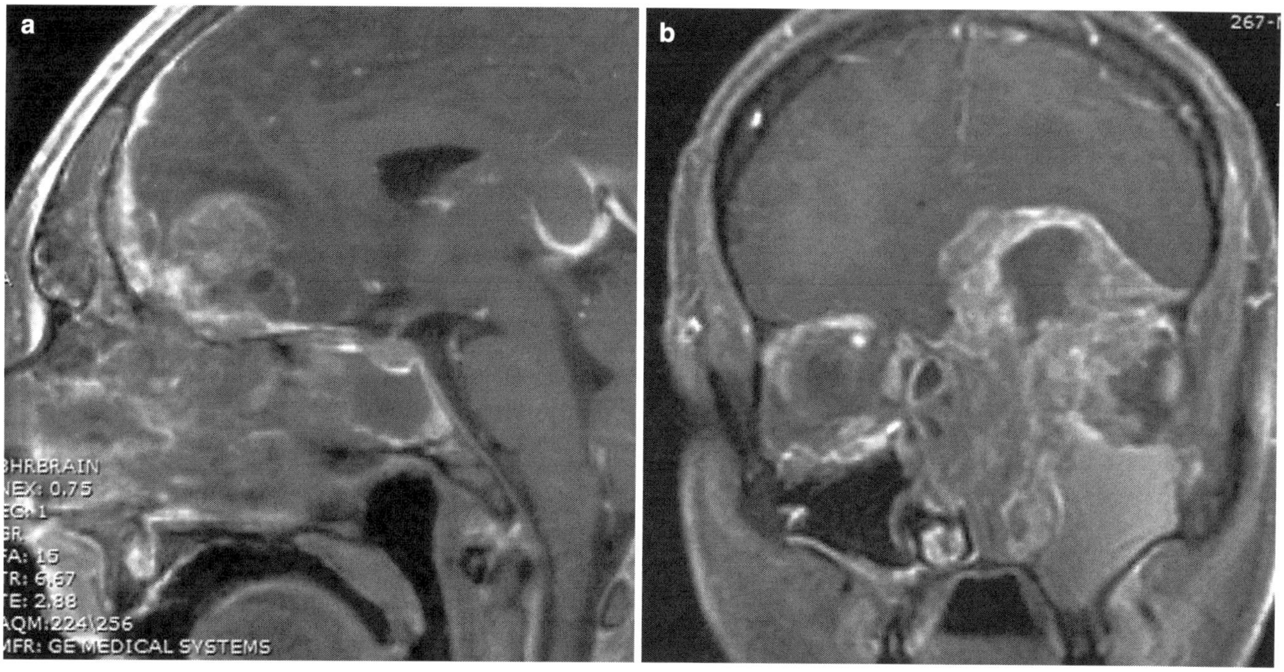

Fig. 47.1 Sinonasal undifferentiated carcinoma (SNUC). (**a**) Sagittal T1-weighted gadolinium-enhanced MR image. (**b**) Coronal T1-weighted gadolinium-enhanced image. A large, heterogeneously enhancing mass involves the nasal cavity and ethmoid and sphenoid sinuses, invades the left orbit, and extends through the cribriform plate and left orbital roof to the left anterior cranial fossa, with displacement of the left frontal lobe

47.3 Histopathology

- SNUC is a highly aggressive carcinoma characterized by medium-sized cells with small to moderate amounts of eosinophilic cytoplasm, frequent mitoses, necrosis, and prominent vasculature (Fig. 47.2) [2].
- Positive immunoreactivity for pancytokeratins, simple keratin, EMA, and neuron-specific enolase is common [2].

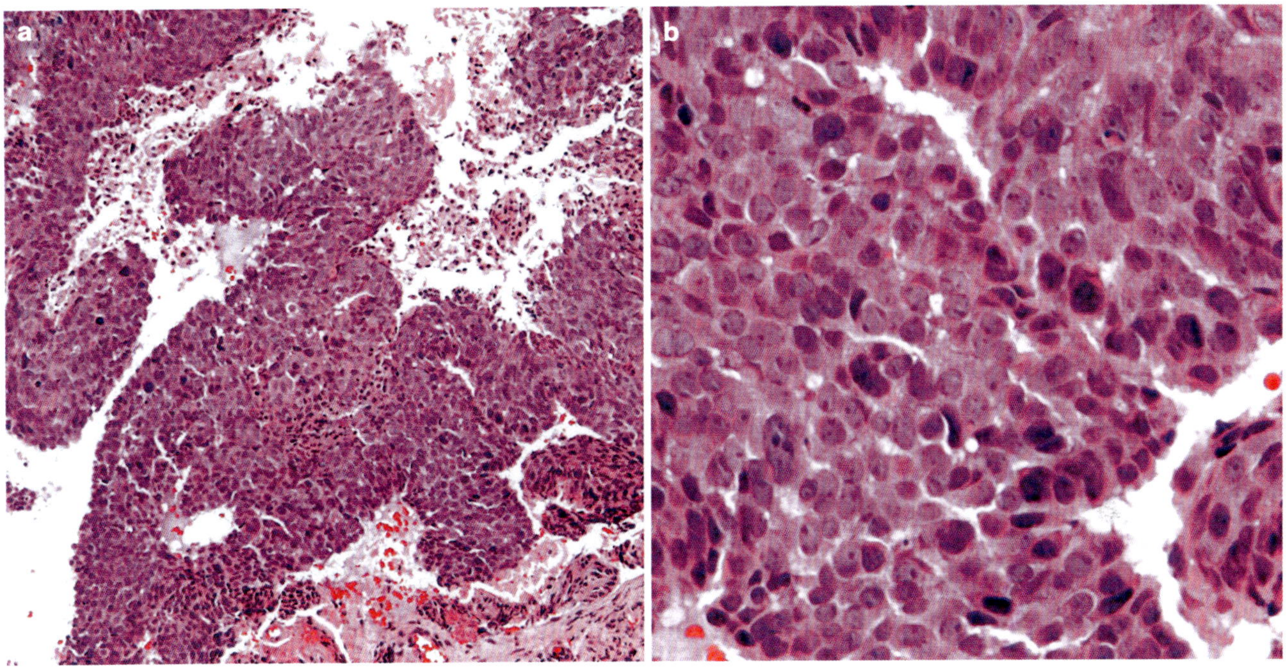

Fig. 47.2 SNUC. (**a**) SNUCs are composed of nests and lobules of undifferentiated cells with no squamous or glandular differentiation. Necrosis may be prominent. (**b**) The cells are medium to large in size, with a large nucleus and prominent nucleoli

47.4 Clinical and Surgical Management

- Both the Kadish staging system and Hyams grading system can be adapted to predict outcome in SNUC [7, 8].
- Multimodal treatment consisting of maximal safe tumor resection, chemotherapy, and radiation is recommended and has been shown to extend patient survival [9].
- Intensity-modulated radiation therapy (IMRT) is the recommended treatment modality for radiation [10].
- Clinical outcomes in patients with SNUC remain poor, with survival times typically extending just beyond 1 year [1, 9].

References

1. Gorelick J, Ross D, Marentette L, Blaivas M. Sinonasal undifferentiated carcinoma: case series and review of the literature. Neurosurgery. 2000;47:750–4; discussion 754–5.
2. Frierson Jr HF, Mills SE, Fechner RE, Taxy JB, Levine PA. Sinonasal undifferentiated carcinoma. An aggressive neoplasm derived from schneiderian epithelium and distinct from olfactory neuroblastoma. Am J Surg Pathol. 1986;10:771–9.
3. Liu SV. Leptomeningeal carcinomatosis in sinonasal undifferentiated carcinoma. Head Neck. 2013;35:E343–5.
4. Kim BS, Vongtama R, Juillard G. Sinonasal undifferentiated carcinoma: case series and literature review. Am J Otolaryngol. 2004;25:162–6.
5. Mourad WF, Hauerstock D, Shourbaji RA, Hu KS, Culliney B, Li Z, et al. Trimodality management of sinonasal undifferentiated carcinoma and review of the literature. Am J Clin Oncol. 2013;36:584–8.
6. Phillips CD, Futterer SF, Lipper MH, Levine PA. Sinonasal undifferentiated carcinoma: CT and MR imaging of an uncommon neoplasm of the nasal cavity. Radiology. 1997;202:477–80.
7. Miyamoto RC, Gleich LL, Biddinger PW, Gluckman JL. Esthesioneuroblastoma and sinonasal undifferentiated carcinoma: impact of histological grading and clinical staging on survival and prognosis. Laryngoscope. 2000;110:1262–5.
8. Hyams V, Batsakis J, Michaels L. Tumors of the upper respiratory tract and ear. In: Armed forces institute of pathology fascicles, vol. 2. Washington: American Registry of Pathology Press; 1988. p. 240–8.
9. Xu CC, Dziegielewski PT, McGaw WT, Seikaly H. Sinonasal undifferentiated carcinoma (SNUC): the Alberta experience and literature review. J Otolaryngol Head Neck Surg. 2013;42:2.
10. Al-Mamgani A, van Rooij P, Mehital R, Tans L, Levendag PC. Combined-modality treatment improved outcome in sinonasal undifferentiated carcinoma: single-institutional experience of 21 patients and review of the literature. Eur Arch Otorhinolaryngol. 2013;270:293–9.

Fibrosarcoma of the Sellar Region

48

Gabriel Zada, M. Beatriz S. Lopes, Srinivasan Mukundan Jr., and Edward Laws Jr.

48.1 Epidemiology and Clinical Presentation

- Malignant mesenchymal tumors rarely arise in the sellar region. Most of them are either spread of a primary skull base lesion or are secondary to radiation therapy for a sellar tumor [1].
- The most common primary sarcoma of the sellar region is the chondrosarcoma, followed by fibrosarcoma and rhabdomyosarcoma, each with a few case reports [2]. Postradiation fibrosarcomas are the most common of these malignant neoplasms [2].
- Pituitary fibrosarcoma is a rare cancer that is often associated with prior radiation exposure or therapy [3–6].
- Secondary pituitary fibrosarcomas commonly develop 10–15 years after treatment for a separate tumor, often a pituitary adenoma [3, 5].
- Undifferentiated sarcoma of the cavernous sinus has been reported 15 years following Gamma Knife radiosurgery for a pituitary adenoma [7].
- Primary pituitary fibrosarcoma (without a prior history of radiation) is exceedingly rare, but it has been reported [8, 9].
- It typically presents clinically with headache, visual loss, cranial nerve paresis, and hypopituitarism [4, 7, 9].
- Fibrosarcomas typically comprise 0.05 % of lesions treated in major transsphenoidal series [10].

G. Zada, MD, MS (✉)
Department of Neurological Surgery, Keck School of Medicine, University of Southern California, 1200 N State Street, #3300, Los Angeles, CA 90033, USA
e-mail: gzada@usc.edu

M.B.S. Lopes, MD, PhD
Department of Pathology (Neuropathology), University of Virginia School of Medicine, 1215 Lee Street, Room 3060–HEP, Charlottesville, VA 22908, USA
e-mail: msl2e@virginia.edu

S. Mukundan Jr., PhD, MD
Department of Radiology, Brigham and Women's Hospital, 75 Francis Street, Boston, MA 02115, USA
e-mail: smukundan@partners.org

E. Laws Jr., MD
Department of Neurosurgery, Brigham and Women's Hospital, 15 Francis Street, Boston, MA 02115, USA
e-mail: elaws@partners.org

G. Zada et al. (eds.), *Atlas of Sellar and Parasellar Lesions: Clinical, Radiologic, and Pathologic Correlations*,
DOI 10.1007/978-3-319-22855-6_48

48.2 Imaging Features

- Pituitary fibrosarcomas are highly infiltrating tumors, which often invade the cavernous sinuses, suprasellar region, and clivus (Fig. 48.1) [8, 11, 12].
- They often demonstrate avid contrast enhancement in a heterogeneous pattern (Fig. 48.2) [5].

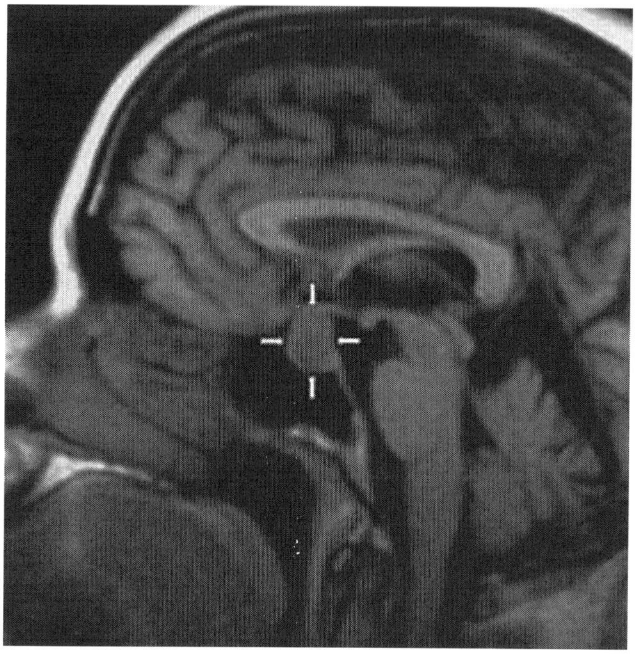

Fig. 48.1 Fibrosarcoma. Sagittal noncontrast MRI of the pituitary (*arrows*) shows a spontaneously sclerosing epithelioid fibrosarcoma extending superiorly to the optic chiasm (Adapted with permission from Massier et al. [11].)

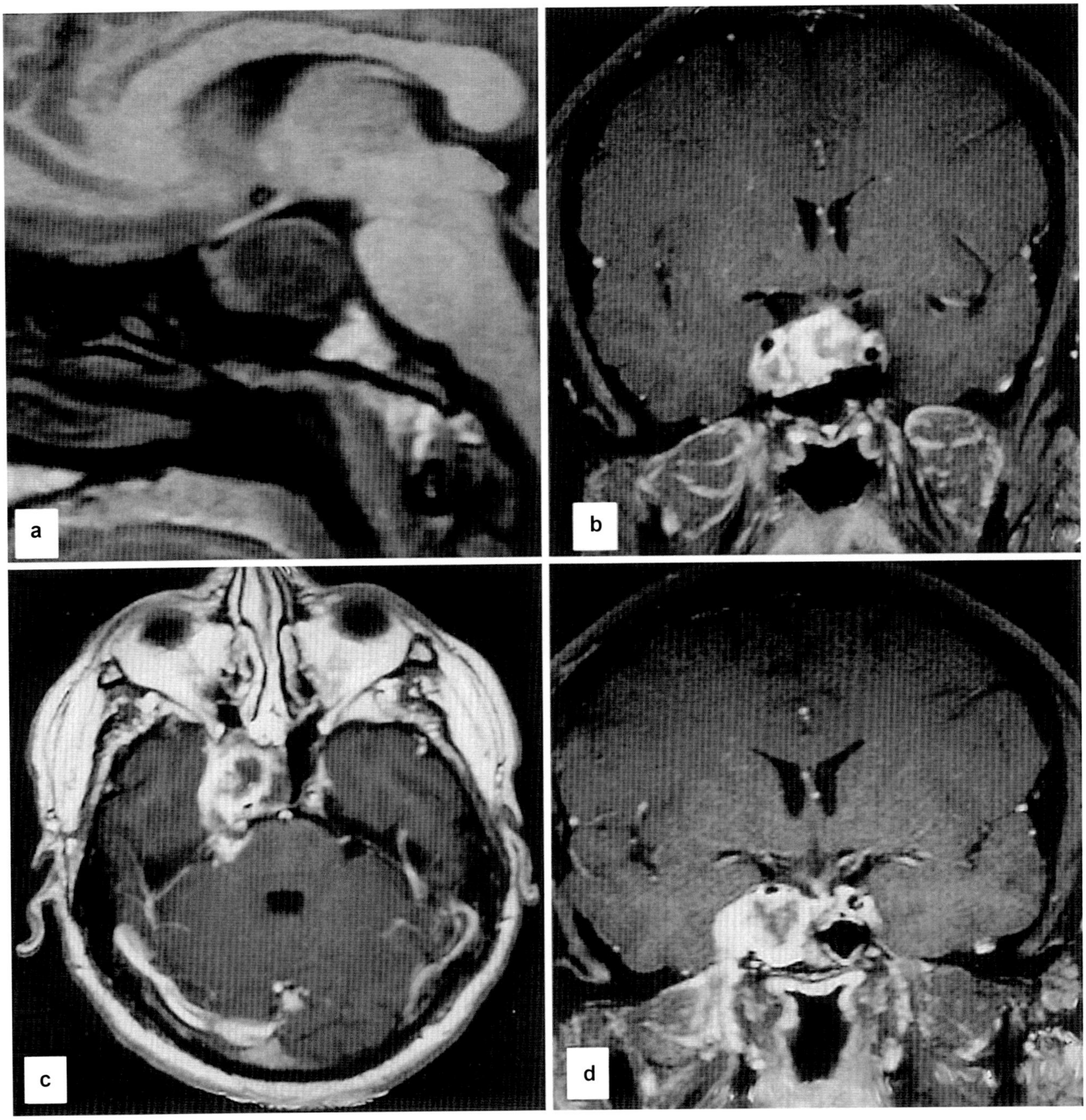

Fig. 48.2 MRI of a patient with a radiation-induced sellar fibrosarcoma. (**a**) Sagittal MRI (T1-weighted) showing the partially cystic tumor with extension toward the optic chiasm and the brainstem. (**b**) Coronal MRI (T1-weighted, gadolinium-enhanced) showing inhomogeneous enhancement of the tumor with extensive intrasellar growth, suprasellar extension into the right cavernous sinus, and mild dislocation of the right internal carotid artery; there is also growth into the sphenoid sinus. (**c**) Axial MRI scan 5 months after radiosurgery (T1-weighted, gadolinium-enhanced), showing further tumor growth with infiltration of the pterygopalatine fossa and the lateral and medial pterygoid muscle on the right side. (**d**) Coronal MRI scan 5 months after radiosurgery (T1-weighted, gadolinium-enhanced), showing further infiltration of the right cavernous sinus and the right sphenoid sinus, with perineural growth along the mandibular branch of cranial nerve V (Adapted with permission from Berkmann et al. [2].)

48.3 Histopathology

- The histopathological features of fibrosarcoma of the pituitary region are similar to those arising in soft tissues.
- The tumors are composed of spindle-shaped cells with nuclear pleomorphism, and frequent mitoses are commonly observed (Fig. 48.3) [13].
- Immunoreactivity for vimentin is seen in fibrosarcomas. These tumors lack immunostaining for S100, cytokeratin, desmin, and CD34 [5].
- If the fibrosarcoma is a secondary tumor following treatment of a primary pituitary adenoma, some retained areas of pituitary adenoma pathology may be interspersed with the fibrosarcoma [5].

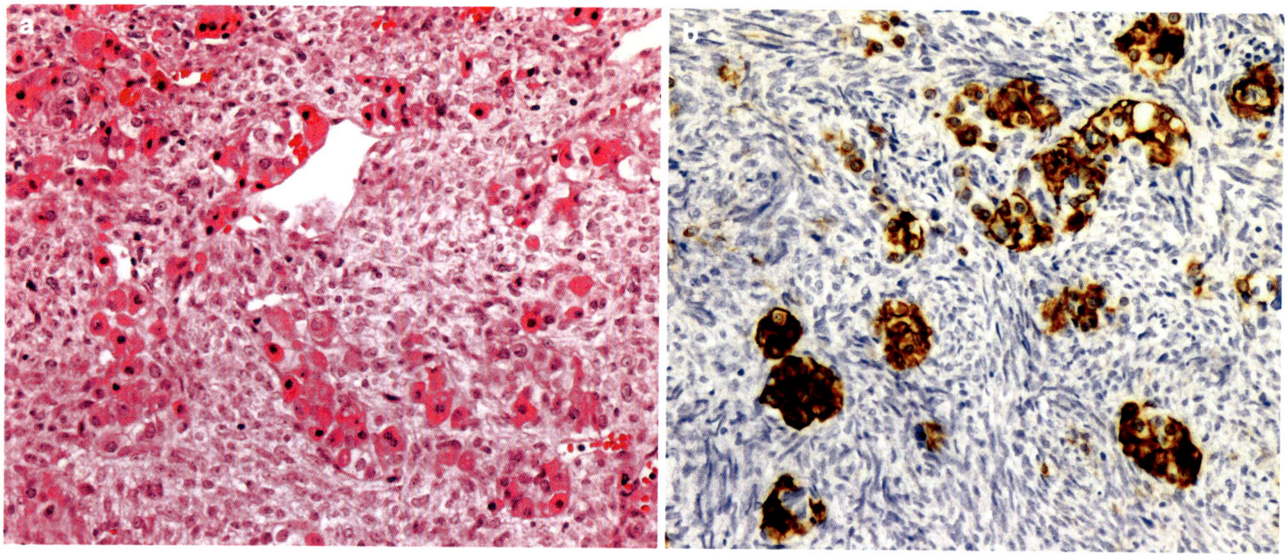

Fig. 48.3 Primary fibrosarcoma of the sella turcica diffusely involving the anterior pituitary. The tumor is composed of spindle cells with elongated nuclei arranged in fascicles. Note the pituitary neuroendocrine cells entrapped by the tumor, as seen by H&E (**a**) and highlighted by chromogranin (**b**)

48.4 Clinical and Surgical Management

- Transsphenoidal approaches and craniotomy have been used for partial debulking. The consistency of these tumors is typically quite firm [8].
- Despite multimodality therapy with surgical debulking, chemotherapy, and radiation, outcomes for patients with pituitary fibrosarcoma remain poor [8].
- Overall survival is generally less than 1 year [9, 12].

References

1. Lopes M, Scheithauer B, Saeger W. Granular cell tumor. In: DeLellis R, Lloyd R, Heitz P, Eng C, editors. WHO classification of tumours, pathology and genetic of tumours of endocrine organs. Lyon: IARC Press; 2004. p. 41–3.
2. Berkmann S, Tolnay M, Hanggi D, Ghaffari A, Gratzl O. Sarcoma of the sella after radiotherapy for pituitary adenoma. Acta Neurochir (Wien). 2010;152:1725–35.
3. Ahmad K, Fayos JV. Pituitary fibrosarcoma secondary to radiation therapy. Cancer. 1978;42:107–10.
4. Coppeto JR, Roberts M. Fibrosarcoma after proton-beam pituitary ablation. Arch Neurol. 1979;36:380–1.
5. Gnanalingham KK, Chakraborty A, Galloway M, Revesz T, Powell M. Osteosarcoma and fibrosarcoma caused by postoperative radiotherapy for a pituitary adenoma. Case report. J Neurosurg. 2002;96:960–3.
6. Martin WH, Cail WS, Morris JL, Constable WC. Fibrosarcoma after high energy radiation therapy for pituitary adenoma. AJR Am J Roentgenol. 1980;135:1087–90.
7. Sasagawa Y, Tachibana O, Iizuka H. Undifferentiated sarcoma of the cavernous sinus after gamma knife radiosurgery for pituitary adenoma. J Clin Neurosci. 2013;20:1152–4.
8. Lopes MB, Lanzino G, Cloft HJ, Winston DC, Vance ML, Laws Jr ER. Primary fibrosarcoma of the sella unrelated to previous radiation therapy. Mod Pathol. 1998;11:579–84.
9. Li ZJ, Sun P, Guo Y, Wang RZ. Primary pituitary fibrosarcoma presenting with multiple metastases: a case report and literature review. Neurol India. 2010;58:316–8.
10. Saeger W, Ludecke DK, Buchfelder M, Fahlbusch R, Quabbe HJ, Petersenn S. Pathohistological classification of pituitary tumors: 10 years of experience with the German pituitary tumor registry. Eur J Endocrinol. 2007;156:203–16.
11. Massier A, Scheithauer BW, Taylor HC, Clark C, Llerena L. Sclerosing epithelioid fibrosarcoma of the pituitary. Endocr Pathol. 2007;18:233–8.
12. Shi T, Farrell MA, Kaufmann JC. Fibrosarcoma complicating irradiated pituitary adenoma. Surg Neurol. 1984;22:277–84.
13. Ahmed M, Kanaan I, Rifai A, Tulbah A, Ghannam N. An unusual treatment-related complication in a patient with growth hormone-secreting pituitary tumor. J Clin Endocrinol Metab. 1997;82: 2816–20.

Juvenile Nasopharyngeal Angiofibroma (JNA)

49

Gabriel Zada, M. Beatriz S. Lopes, Srinivasan Mukundan Jr., and Edward Laws Jr.

49.1 Epidemiology and Clinical Presentation

- Juvenile nasopharyngeal angiofibroma (JNA) is a rare, histologically benign skull base tumor that develops in adolescents and young adults, almost exclusively in males [1, 2].
- JNAs represent less than 1 % of head and neck tumors.
- The median age at diagnosis is 15 years [3].
- The incidence rate of JNA is 0.4 per million persons per year and as high as 3.7 per million males per year [3].
- Patients typically present with epistaxis and nasal obstruction [2].
- JNA may be related to familial adenomatous polyposis (FAP) [4].

G. Zada, MD, MS (✉)
Department of Neurological Surgery, Keck School of Medicine, University of Southern California, 1200 N State Street, #3300, Los Angeles, CA 90033, USA
e-mail: gzada@usc.edu

M.B.S. Lopes, MD, PhD
Department of Pathology (Neuropathology), University of Virginia School of Medicine, 1215 Lee Street, Room 3060–HEP, Charlottesville, VA 22908, USA
e-mail: msl2e@virginia.edu

S. Mukundan Jr., PhD, MD
Department of Radiology, Brigham and Women's Hospital, 75 Francis Street, Boston, MA 02115, USA
e-mail: smukundan@partners.org

E. Laws Jr., MD
Department of Neurosurgery, Brigham and Women's Hospital, 15 Francis Street, Boston, MA 02115, USA
e-mail: elaws@partners.org

G. Zada et al. (eds.), *Atlas of Sellar and Parasellar Lesions: Clinical, Radiologic, and Pathologic Correlations*, DOI 10.1007/978-3-319-22855-6_49

49.2 Imaging Features

- JNAs typically arise in the region of the pterygopalatine fossa, and erosion of the bone posterior to the sphenopalatine foramen is a common sign on CT scans (Fig. 49.1) [5].
- The cancellous bone of the sphenoid is commonly involved (68 % of patients), and the degree of involvement of the sphenoid bone correlates with outcome [5, 6].
- On MRI, intratumoral flow voids and strong contrast enhancement are hallmarks of the vascularity typically seen with JNAs [5].
- On angiographic studies, unilateral blood supply is seen in up to 85 % of JNAs and is typically from the internal maxillary artery (Fig. 49.1f) [7].
- The most common staging system for JNA is the system proposed by Chandler et al. [8]:
  - Stage I tumor remains confined to the nasopharynx.
  - Stage II tumor extends into the nasal cavity and/or sphenoid sinus.
  - Stage III tumor extends into one or more of the following: antrum, ethmoid sinus, pterygomaxillary and infratemporal fossae, orbit, and/or cheek.
  - Stage IV tumor extends into the cranial cavity.

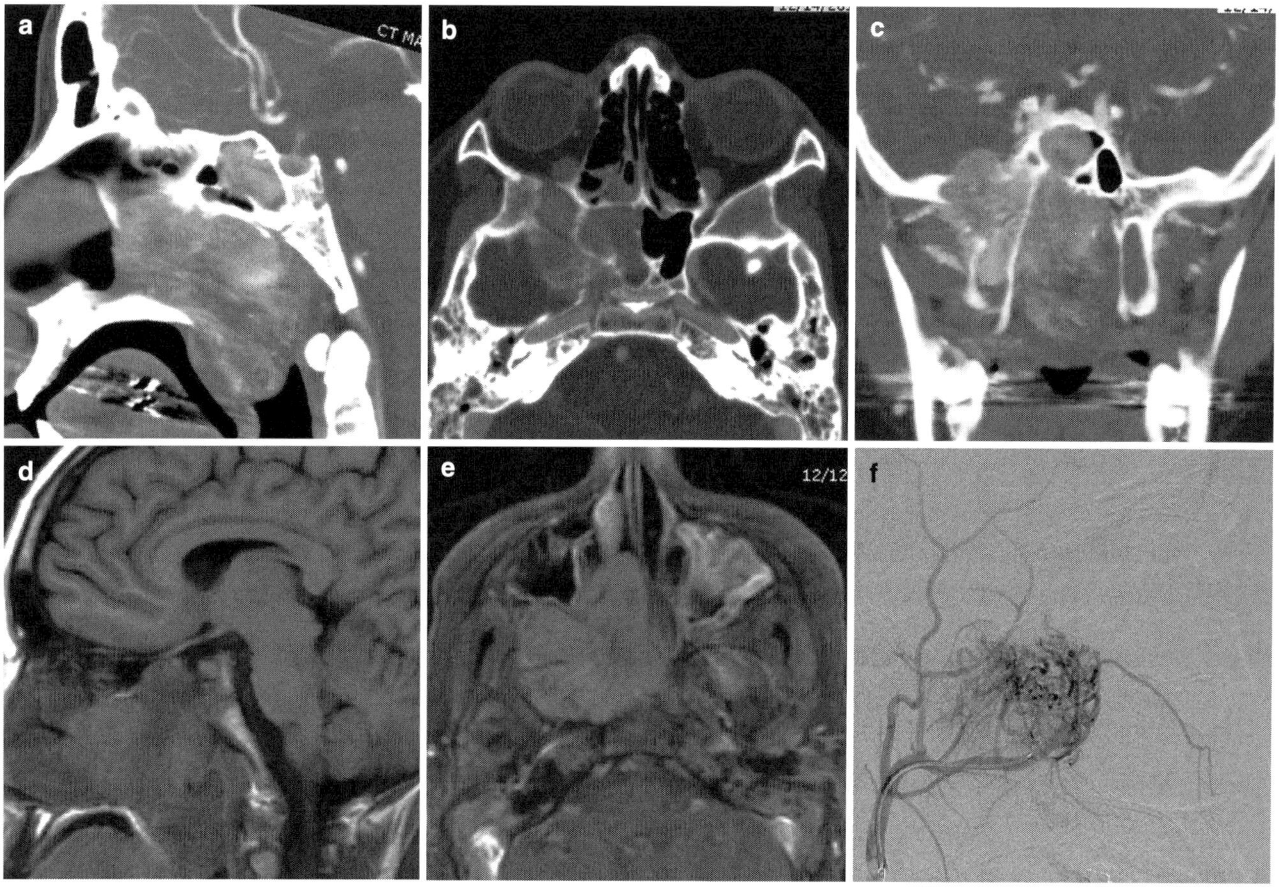

Fig. 49.1 Juvenile nasopharyngeal angiofibroma (JNA). (**a**) Sagittal contrast-enhanced CT image. (**b**) Axial contrast-enhanced CT image. (**c**) Coronal contrast-enhanced CT image. (**d**) Sagittal precontrast T1-weighted MR image. (**e**) Axial T1-weighted post-gadolinium, fat-saturated MR image. There is an avidly enhancing mass in the posterior right nasal cavity and pterygopalatine fossa, eroding the floor of the right middle cranial fossa (**c**) and the clivus (**d**) and extending into the sphenoid sinus. (**f**) Digital subtraction cerebral angiography with the catheter in the right internal maxillary artery, showing markedly increased vascularity within the tumor

49.3 Histopathology

- JNA is characterized by highly vascular capillary-like channels within a fibrous stroma (Fig. 49.2). Blood vessels typically lack smooth muscle and elastic fibers. Staghorn-shaped vessels may be seen.
- Immunostaining for vimentin and vascular endothelial growth factor (VEGF) is typically positive [9].
- Immunostaining for c-kit is almost always negative [9].
- Immunoreactivity for the testosterone and estrogen receptors may play a key role in development.

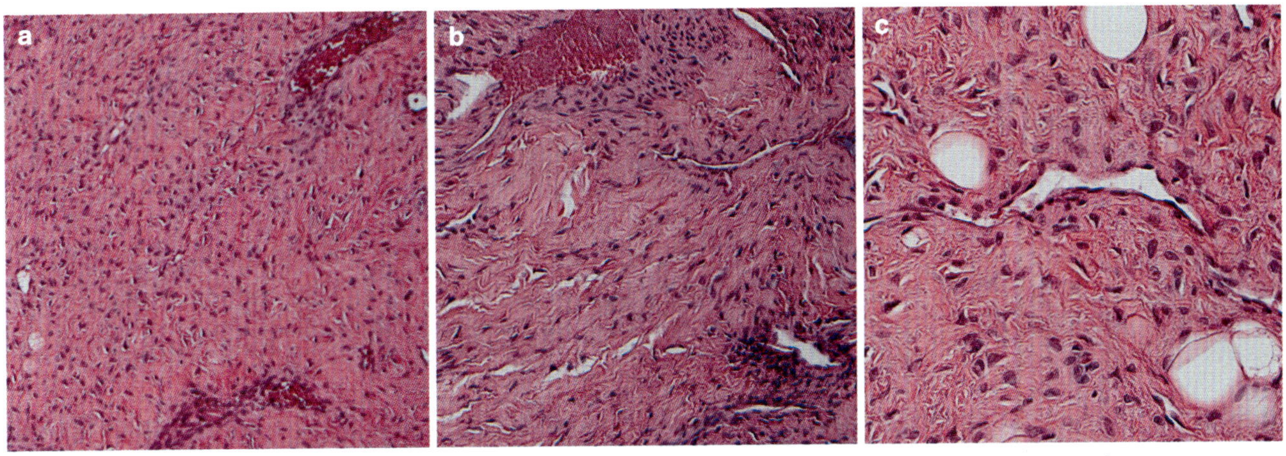

Fig. 49.2 JNA. (**a**) Low-power view (×10 objective) of an angiofibroma, showing haphazardly arranged fibrous tissue and thin, wavy collagen. (**b**) Medium-power (×20) view of the same lesion showing multiple thin-walled blood vessels compressed by fibrous tissue. (**c**) High-power (×40) image of thin-walled blood vessel with a flattened endothelial cell lining surrounded by fibrous tissue containing cells with thin strands of wavy collagen. This lesion also had associated adipose tissue, evidenced by the presence of several mature adipocytes, and could be seen infiltrating adjacent adipose tissue (*not shown*)

49.4 Clinical and Surgical Management

- The primary treatment for JNA is surgical resection. Possible approaches include open craniofacial, orbitozygomatic, endoscopic-assisted, and pure endonasal endoscopic approaches. In recent years, endoscopic approaches have been more widely explored for this indication [1, 7, 10, 11].
- JNAs are often tumors highly vascular, firm, and rubbery.
- Preoperative embolization of JNAs is an effective strategy for reducing intraoperative blood loss associated with resection [3, 12].
- Neoadjuvant use of the testosterone receptor blocker flutamide has demonstrated some success in the preoperative treatment of JNA [13].
- Although some degree of selection bias likely exists regarding assignment of the approach to varying tumors, endoscopic approaches have been associated with decreased intraoperative blood loss and lower recurrence rates [10].
- Complete resections may be possible in over 90 % of patients; they are generally limited by the degree of internal carotid artery involvement. For higher-stage JNAs, neoadjuvant treatment or primary radiation may be a safe alternative [7].
- Radiation therapy may be effectively employed for residual or recurrent disease and typically offers reductions in tumor volume of 30–50 %. Local tumor control is achieved in up to 85 % of patients [14–17].
- Most patients have excellent outcomes, with 86 % experiencing disease freedom at a mean follow-up time of 47 months [12].

References

1. Cherekaev VA, Golbin DA, Kapitanov DN, Roginsky VV, Yakovlev SB, Arustamian SR. Advanced craniofacial juvenile nasopharyngeal angiofibroma. Description of surgical series, case report, and review of literature. Acta Neurochir (Wien). 2011;153:499–508.
2. Witt TR, Shah JP, Sternberg SS. Juvenile nasopharyngeal angiofibroma. A 30 year clinical review. Am J Surg. 1983;146:521–5.
3. Glad H, Vainer B, Buchwald C, Petersen BL, Theilgaard SA, Bonvin P, et al. Juvenile nasopharyngeal angiofibromas in Denmark 1981–2003: diagnosis, incidence, and treatment. Acta Otolaryngol. 2007;127:292–9.
4. Valanzano R, Curia MC, Aceto G, Veschi S, De Lellis L, Catalano T, et al. Genetic evidence that juvenile nasopharyngeal angiofibroma is an integral FAP tumour. Gut. 2005;54:1046–7.
5. Lloyd G, Howard D, Lund VJ, Savy L. Imaging for juvenile angiofibroma. J Laryngol Otol. 2000;114:727–30.
6. Lloyd G, Howard D, Phelps P, Cheesman A. Juvenile angiofibroma: the lessons of 20 years of modern imaging. J Laryngol Otol. 1999;113:127–34.
7. Nicolai P, Villaret AB, Farina D, Nadeau S, Yakirevitch A, Berlucchi M, Galtelli C. Endoscopic surgery for juvenile angiofibroma: a critical review of indications after 46 cases. Am J Rhinol Allergy. 2010;24:e67–72.
8. Chandler JR, Goulding R, Moskowitz L, Quencer RM. Nasopharyngeal angiofibromas: staging and management. Ann Otol Rhinol Laryngol. 1984;93:322–9.
9. Pauli J, Gundelach R, Vanelli-Rees A, Rees G, Campbell C, Dubey S, Perry C. Juvenile nasopharyngeal angiofibroma: an immunohistochemical characterisation of the stromal cell. Pathology. 2008;40:396–400.
10. Boghani Z, Husain Q, Kanumuri VV, Khan MN, Sangvhi S, Liu JK, Eloy JA. Juvenile nasopharyngeal angiofibroma: a systematic review and comparison of endoscopic, endoscopic-assisted, and open resection in 1047 cases. Laryngoscope. 2013;123:859–69.
11. Zanation AM, Mitchell CA, Rose AS. Endoscopic skull base techniques for juvenile nasopharyngeal angiofibroma. Otolaryngol Clin North Am. 2012;45:711–30.
12. Leong SC. A systematic review of surgical outcomes for advanced juvenile nasopharyngeal angiofibroma with intracranial involvement. Laryngoscope. 2013;123:1125–31.
13. Gates GA, Rice DH, Koopmann Jr CF, Schuller DE. Flutamide-induced regression of angiofibroma. Laryngoscope. 1992;102:641–4.
14. Gullane PJ, Davidson J, O'Dwyer T, Forte V. Juvenile angiofibroma: a review of the literature and a case series report. Laryngoscope. 1992;102:928–33.
15. Kasper ME, Parsons JT, Mancuso AA, Mendenhall WM, Stringer SP, Cassisi NJ, Million RR. Radiation therapy for juvenile angiofibroma: evaluation by CT and MRI, analysis of tumor regression, and selection of patients. Int J Radiat Oncol Biol Phys. 1993;25:689–94.
16. Lee JT, Chen P, Safa A, Juillard G, Calcaterra TC. The role of radiation in the treatment of advanced juvenile angiofibroma. Laryngoscope. 2002;112:1213–20.
17. Reddy KA, Mendenhall WM, Amdur RJ, Stringer SP, Cassisi NJ. Long-term results of radiation therapy for juvenile nasopharyngeal angiofibroma. Am J Otolaryngol. 2001;22:172–5.

Metastatic Tumors to the Pituitary Gland

50

Gabriel Zada, M. Beatriz S. Lopes, Srinivasan Mukundan Jr., and Edward Laws Jr.

50.1 Epidemiology and Clinical Presentation

- Metastatic tumors to the pituitary gland frequently present in the sixth and seventh decades of life [1, 2].
- Microscopic pituitary metastases have been reported in 1–3 % of all cancer patients on routine autopsy studies. They are thought to be common on account of the rich blood supply to the pituitary gland [3].
- Metastases to the pituitary gland may be identified in up to 6–29 % of breast cancer patients [3–5].
- Diagnosis of a metastatic tumor to the pituitary may represent the initial presentation of a primary cancer and can present without systemic clinical symptoms [3, 6].
- This entity is relatively rare and comprises 0.6–1 % of patients in major transsphenoidal series [1, 3, 7].
- The most common clinical symptoms are headache, fatigue, polyuria, and visual loss [2].
- Diabetes insipidus is the most common presenting endocrine symptom, occurring in about 50–70 % of patients. It is thought to occur more frequently secondary to the rich vascular supply to the posterior pituitary gland [1, 2, 6, 8–10].
- Visual loss, anterior hypopituitarism, and cranial nerve paresis are other frequent findings [1, 10, 11].
- Cranial nerve paresis and diabetes insipidus occur much more frequently in association with metastatic tumors than with pituitary adenomas; thus, they may provide clinical support for assigning the diagnosis prior to surgery [1, 8, 10].

G. Zada, MD, MS (✉)
Department of Neurological Surgery, Keck School of Medicine, University of Southern California, 1200 N State Street, #3300, Los Angeles, CA 90033, USA
e-mail: gzada@usc.edu

M.B.S. Lopes, MD, PhD
Department of Pathology (Neuropathology), University of Virginia School of Medicine, 1215 Lee Street, Room 3060–HEP, Charlottesville, VA 22908, USA
e-mail: msl2e@virginia.edu

S. Mukundan Jr., PhD, MD
Department of Radiology, Brigham and Women's Hospital, 75 Francis Street, Boston, MA 02115, USA
e-mail: smukundan@partners.org

E. Laws Jr., MD
Department of Neurosurgery, Brigham and Women's Hospital, 15 Francis Street, Boston, MA 02115, USA
e-mail: elaws@partners.org

G. Zada et al. (eds.), *Atlas of Sellar and Parasellar Lesions: Clinical, Radiologic, and Pathologic Correlations*,
DOI 10.1007/978-3-319-22855-6_50

50.2 Imaging Features

- On MRI, metastases frequently mimic pituitary macroadenomas.
- They are typically isointense on T1- and T2-weighted imaging, with avid contrast enhancement (Figs. 50.1, 50.2, 50.3, 50.4, 50.5, and 50.6).
- MRI may show some differentiating features [3]:
  - Thickening of the infundibulum
  - Loss of high T1 signal intensity in the posterior pituitary (posterior pituitary bright spot)
  - Sclerosis of the sella turcica
- Metastases are frequently noted to have cavernous sinus invasion (Fig. 50.7) [11].
- They are often characterized by a classic "blush" on cerebral angiography, demonstrating recruitment of vasculature from the hypophyseal arteries [11].
- FDG PET/CT imaging may be used to support the diagnosis [12].

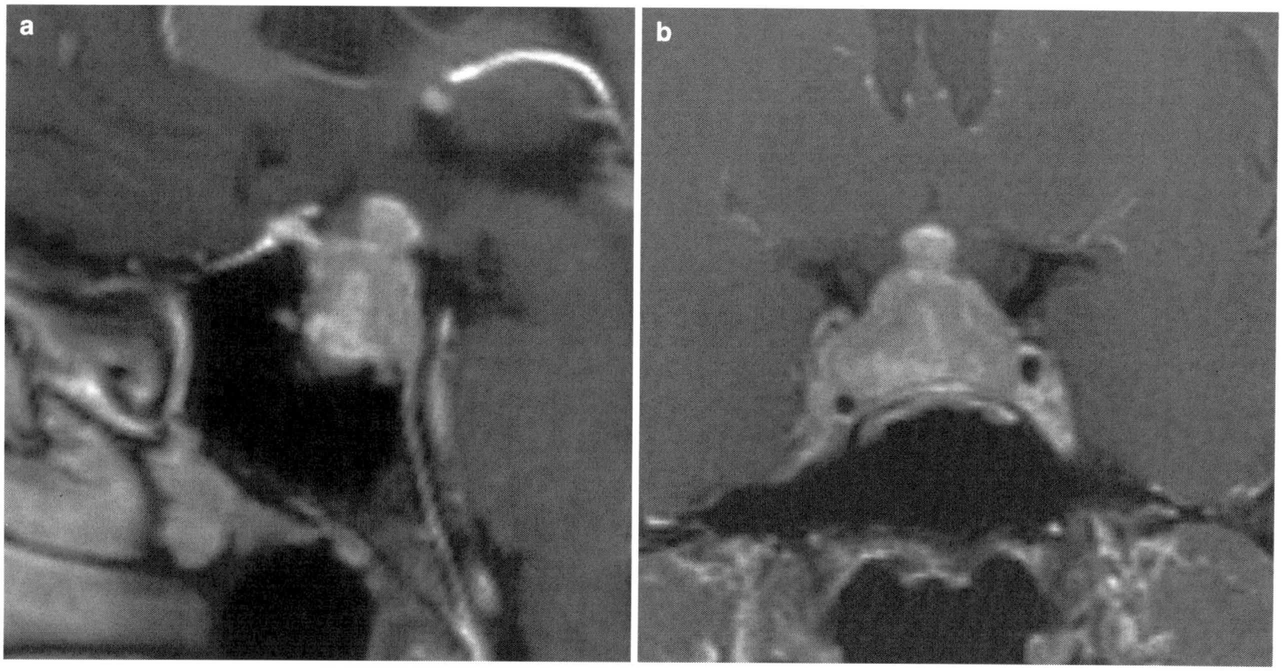

Fig. 50.1 Metastasis from breast cancer. (**a**) Sagittal T1-weighted gadolinium-enhanced MR image. (**b**) Coronal T1-weighted gadolinium-enhanced image. A large, heterogeneously enhancing mass is centered in the sella with suprasellar extension. The mass abuts the cavernous internal carotid arteries (ICAs) bilaterally. The normal pituitary gland cannot be distinguished from the mass

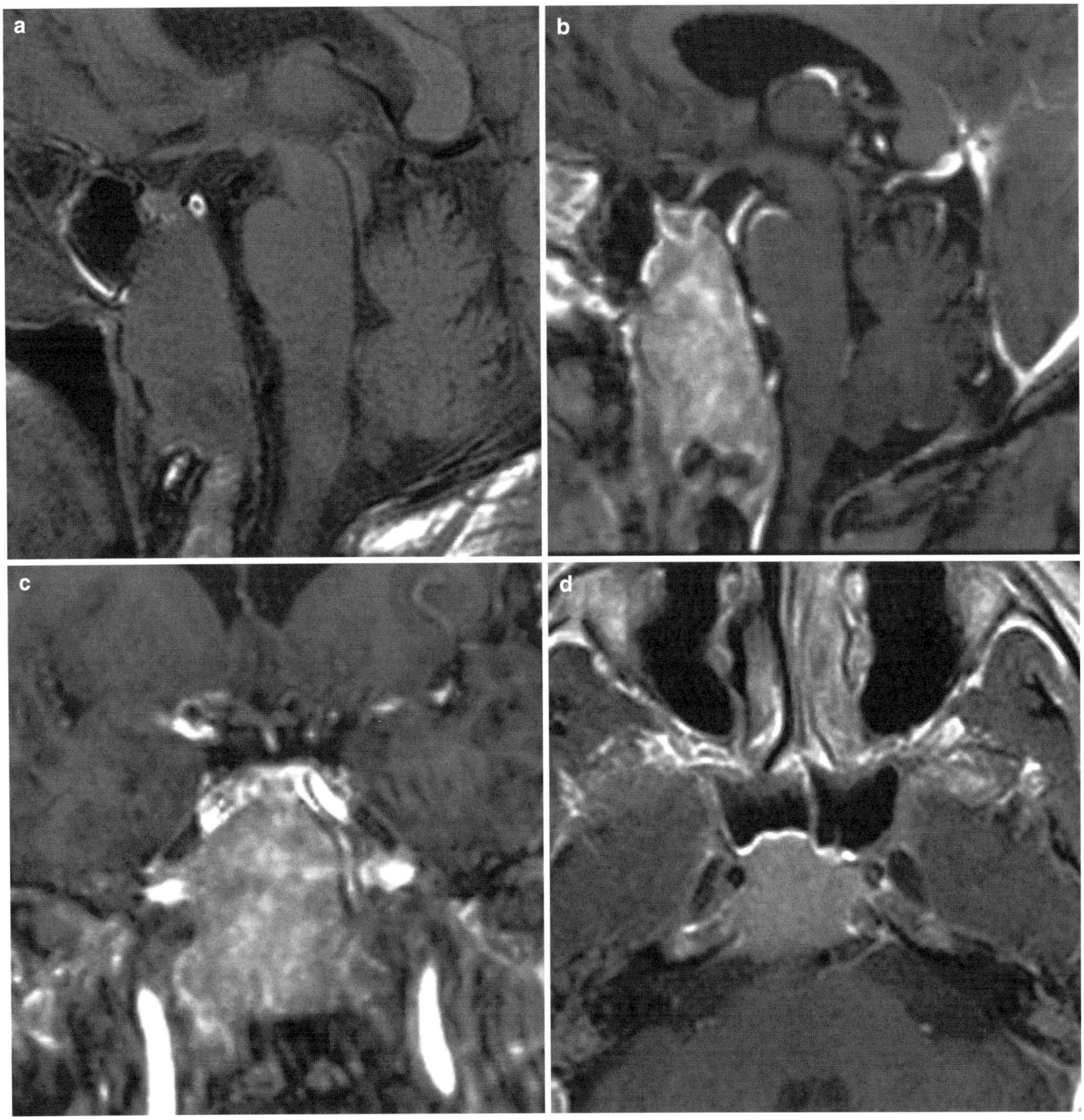

Fig. 50.2 Metastasis. (**a**) Sagittal T1-weighted precontrast MR image. (**b**) Sagittal T1-weighted gadolinium-enhanced image. (**c**) Coronal T1-weighted gadolinium-enhanced image. (**d**) Axial T1-weighted gadolinium-enhanced image. There is a large, heterogeneously enhancing mass replacing most of the clivus. The mass abuts the cavernous ICAs bilaterally. The normal pituitary gland is seen within the sella, above the mass

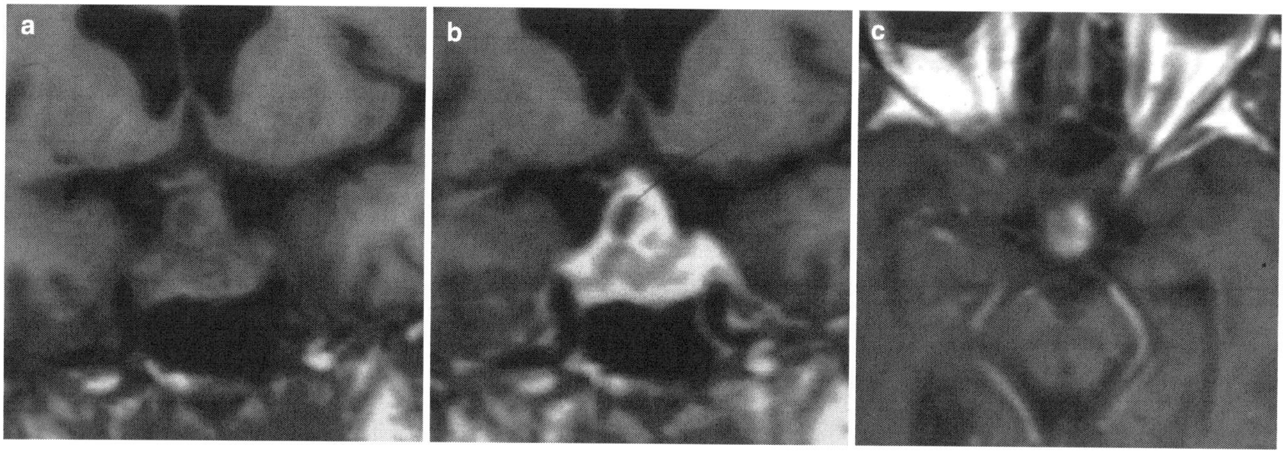

Fig. 50.3 Metastasis. (**a**) Coronal T1-weighted precontrast MR image. (**b**) Coronal T1-weighted gadolinium-enhanced image. (**c**) Axial T1-weighted gadolinium-enhanced image. There is an enhancing mass in the sella, with suprasellar extension abutting the optic chiasm. The mass abuts the cavernous ICAs bilaterally. The normal pituitary gland cannot be distinguished from the mass

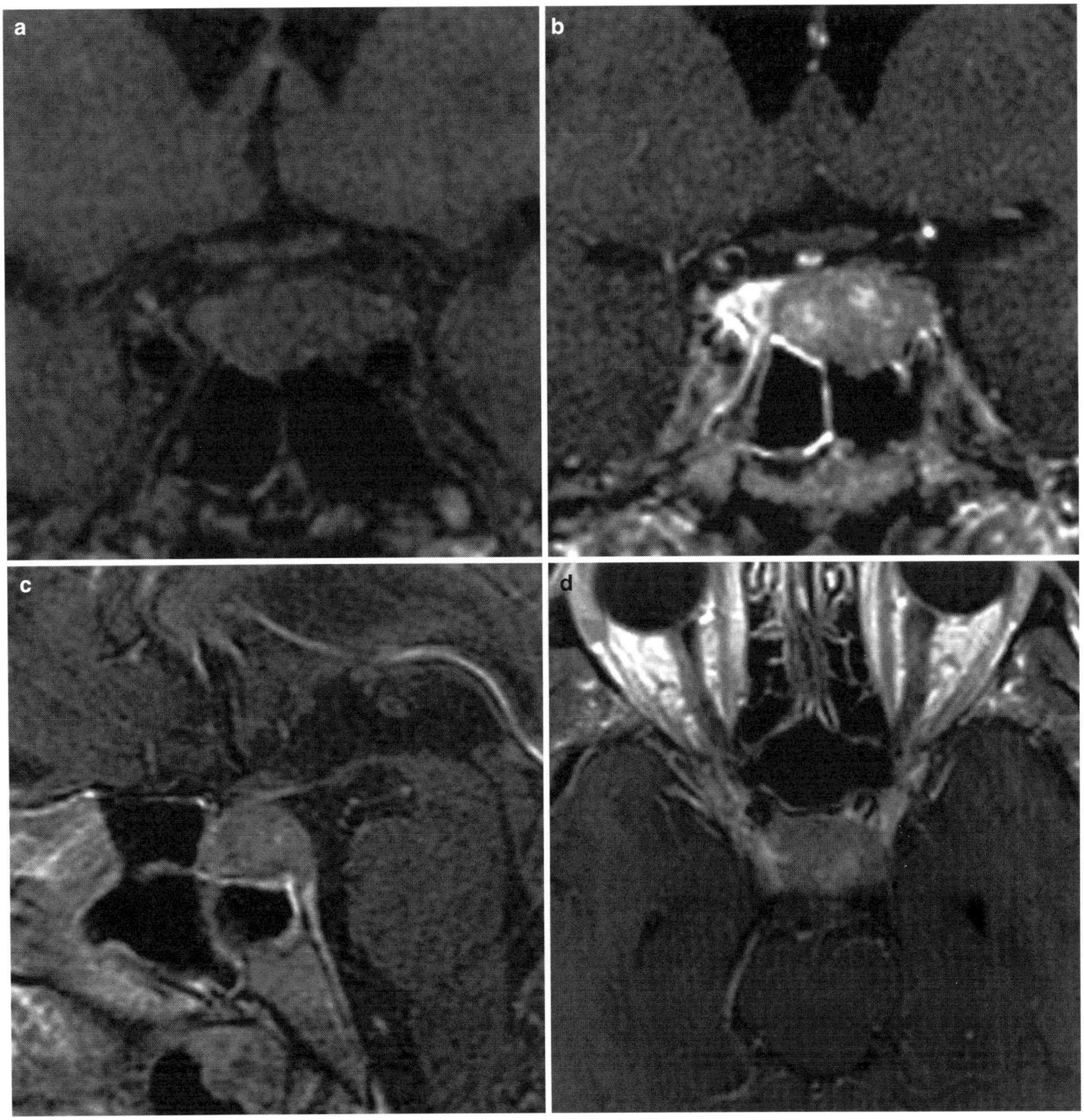

Fig. 50.4 Metastasis. (**a**) Coronal T1-weighted precontrast MR image. (**b**) Coronal T1-weighted gadolinium-enhanced image. (**c**) Sagittal T1-weighted gadolinium-enhanced image. (**d**) Axial T1-weighted gadolinium-enhanced image. An enhancing mass in the left aspect of the sella abuts the left cavernous ICA. The normal pituitary gland is to the right of the mass

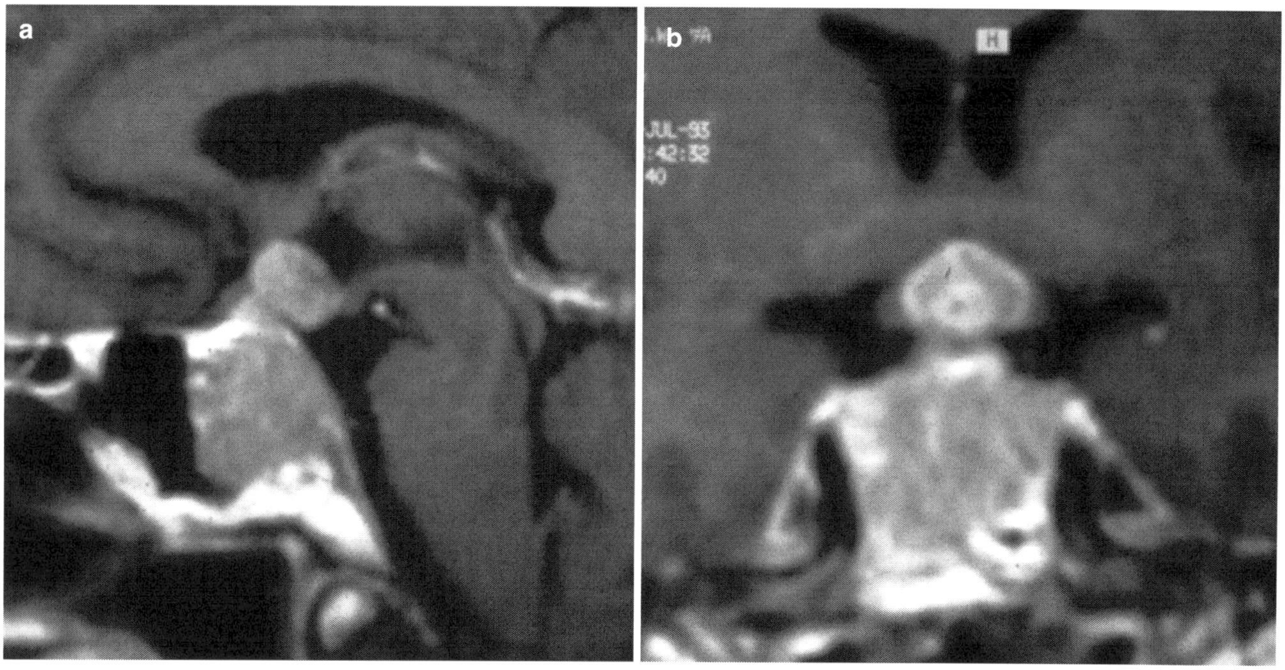

Fig. 50.5 Metastasis. (**a**) Sagittal T1-weighted gadolinium-enhanced MR image. (**b**) Coronal T1-weighted gadolinium-enhanced image. There is an enhancing mass replacing the superior clivus, extending to the sella and the anterior floor of the third ventricle. The normal pituitary gland cannot be distinguished from the mass

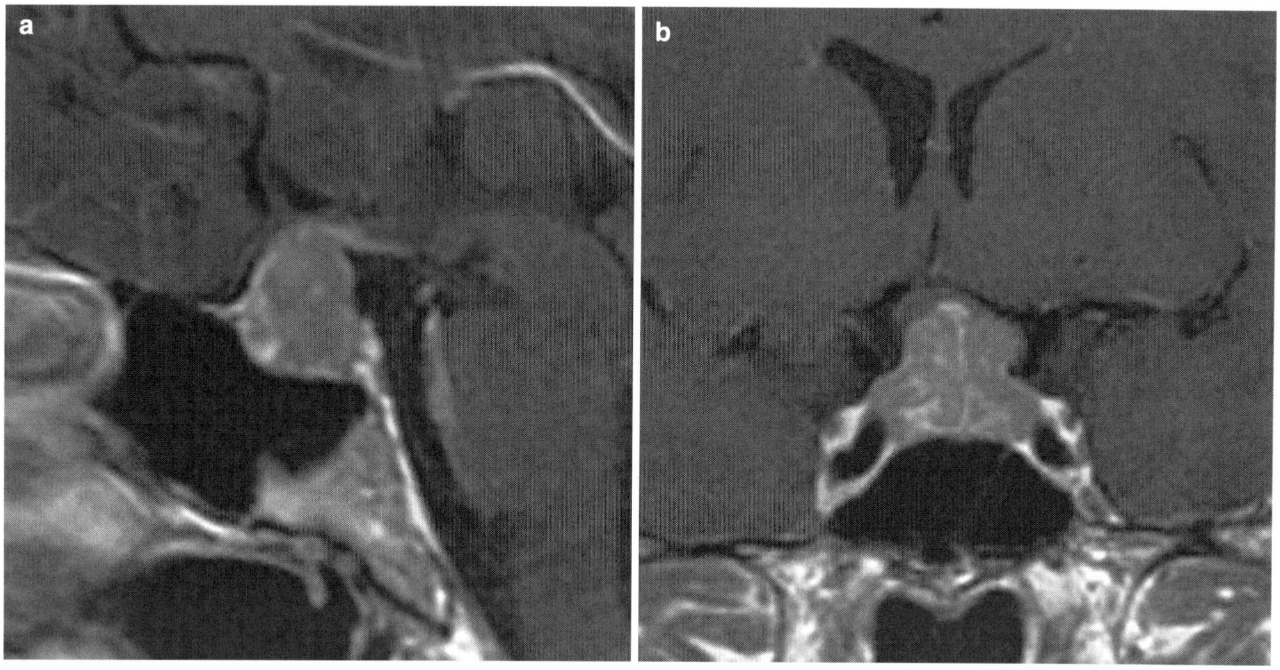

Fig. 50.6 Metastasis from breast cancer. (**a**) Sagittal T1-weighted gadolinium-enhanced MR image. (**b**) Coronal T1-weighted gadolinium-enhanced image. A sellar/suprasellar enhancing mass displaces the optic chiasm superiorly and abuts the cavernous ICAs bilaterally. The normal pituitary gland cannot be distinguished from the mass

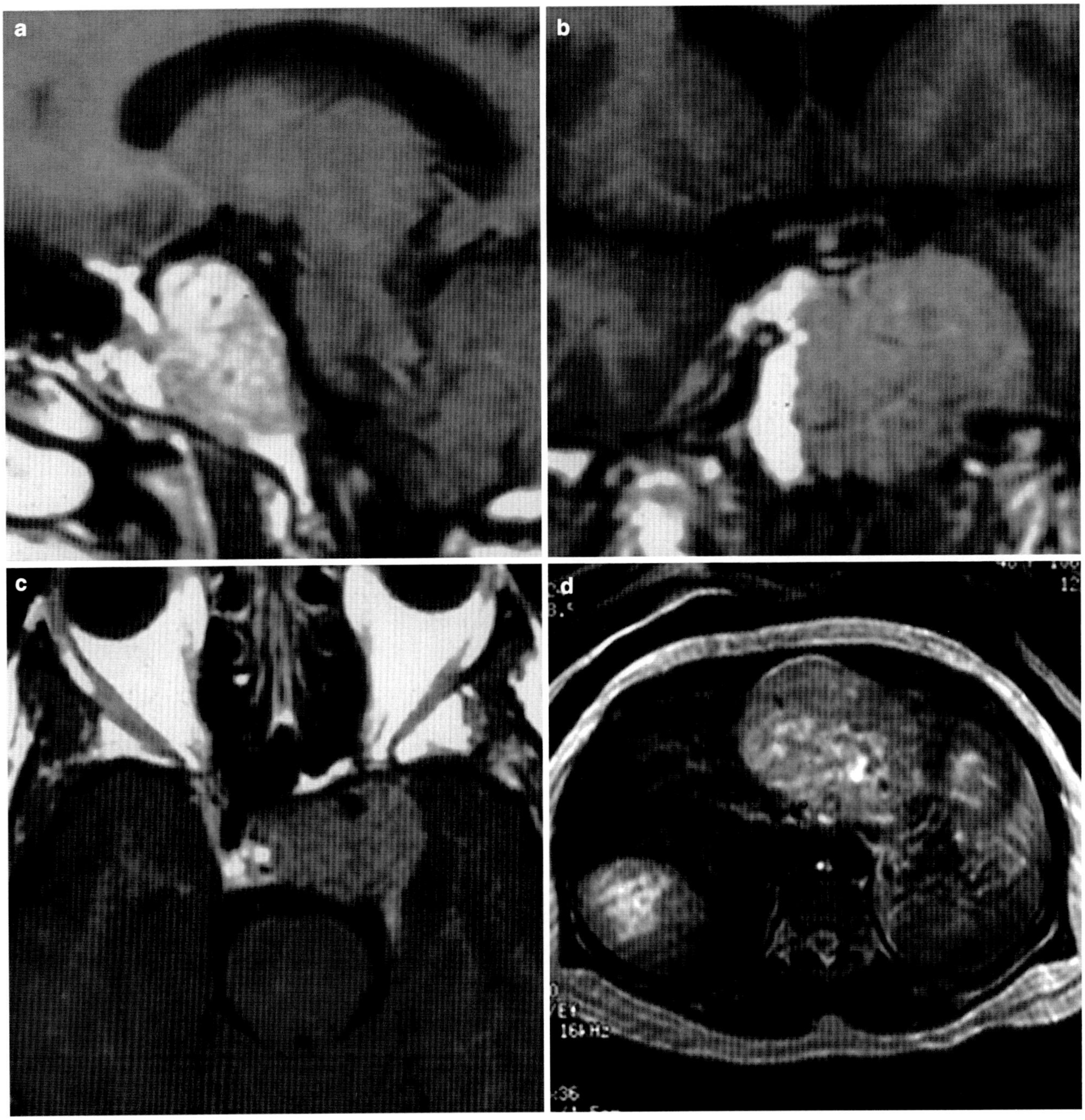

Fig. 50.7 Metastasis from pheochromocytoma. (**a**) Sagittal T1-weighted gadolinium-enhanced MR image. (**b**) Coronal T1-weighted gadolinium-enhanced image. (**c**) Axial T1-weighted gadolinium-enhanced image. (**d**) Axial T1-weighted, gadolinium-enhanced image showing a heterogeneously enhancing left adrenal mass. An enhancing mass is centered in the upper clivus, involving the sella and extending to the left cavernous sinus and encasing the left ICA (**c**). The normal pituitary gland cannot be distinguished from the mass

50.3 Histopathology

- Metastatic tumors to the pituitary gland have been reported to spread from many primary cancers, including breast, lung, gastrointestinal, prostate, renal, melanoma, and thyroid cancers [6].
- Metastases from breast and lung primaries are the most common (Fig. 50.8) [3, 6, 9, 13].
- In some cases, it may be difficult to differentiate metastatic tumors from pituitary adenomas. Special immunomarkers, such as thyroid transcription factor 1, cdx-2, or peptides of gut or lung origin, can be used to screen for a primary source [14].
- Primary carcinomas metastasize to various regions [3, 13]:
  - Posterior pituitary gland alone (57 %)
  - Anterior pituitary gland alone (13 %)
  - Both anterior and posterior gland lobes (12 %)
- The remainder of tumors metastasize to parasellar regions, including the pituitary stalk.

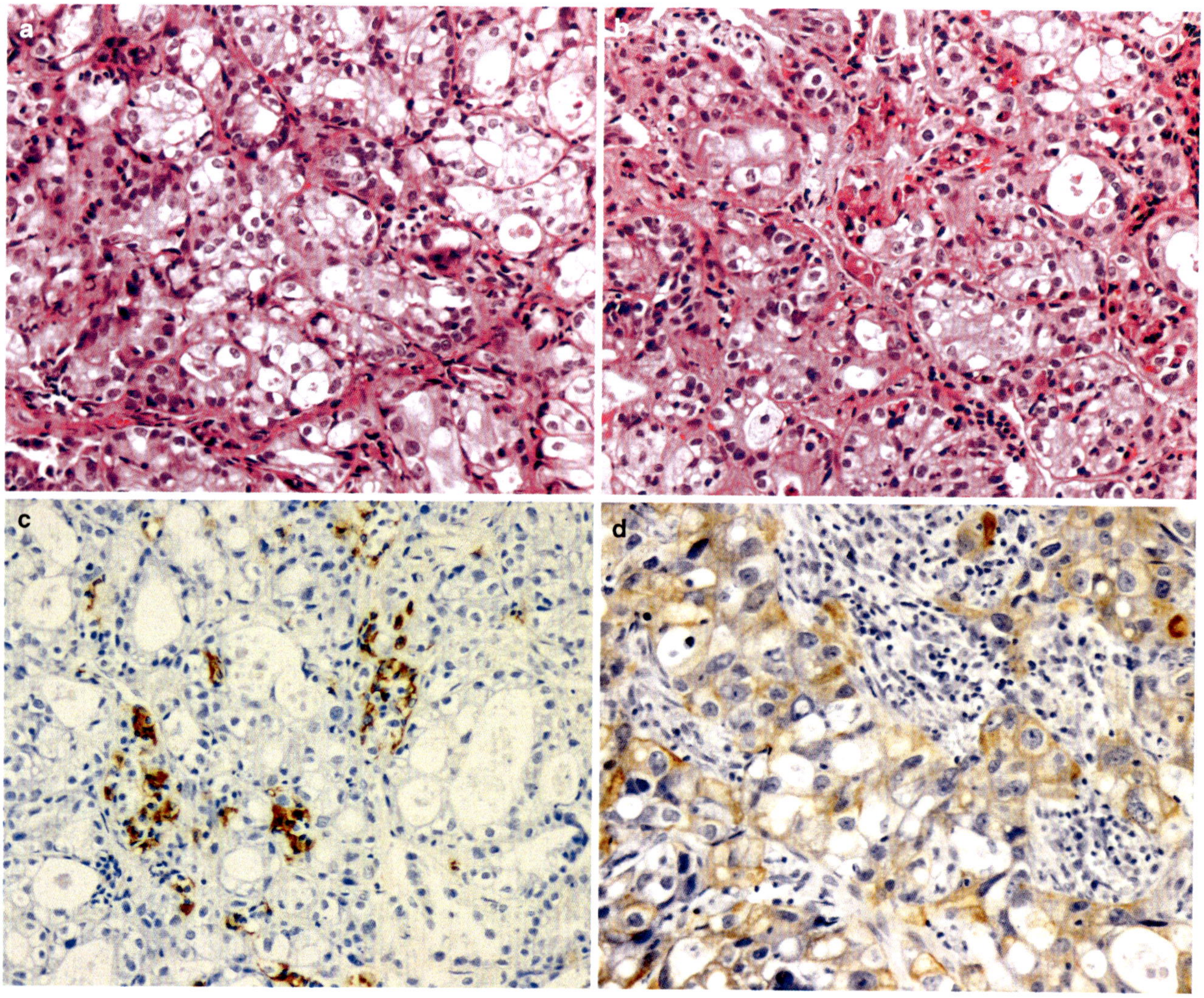

Fig. 50.8 Metastatic adenocarcinoma to the pituitary gland. A metastatic, moderately differentiated adenocarcinoma of the lung in the sellar region shows formation of glands and intracytoplasmic secretory vacuoles (**a**). Intermixed with the neoplastic glands, entrapped anterior pituitary cells can be seen; in this field, several acidophilic cells (**b**) immunoreactive for GH (**c**) are present. The neoplastic glands are immunoreactive for cytokeratin (**d**)

50.4 Clinical and Surgical Management

- Transsphenoidal surgery can be used for a biopsy and maximal safe tumor resection [1, 9].
- Gross total resection is often difficult to achieve, especially with highly invasive and vascular metastatic tumors.
- Metastatic tumors to the sella are often highly vascular and firm tumors, with recruitment of blood supply from the hypophyseal arterial system, as demonstrated by the angiographic "blush" characteristic of these lesions [11].
- Surgical resection does not improve overall survival, but may improve quality of life, especially as it pertains to preservation of vision and palliation of headaches [3, 15].
- Local control of metastatic tumors in the sellar region via multimodality intervention may significantly improve survival times [9].
- Monitoring and appropriate treatment of diabetes insipidus should be carried out in all patients with this diagnosis [8].
- Stereotactic radiosurgery has been reported in patients with pituitary metastases, many of whom had improvements in diabetes insipidus and neurological symptoms [16].
- Appropriate systemic chemotherapy and radiation should be administered as indicated.
- Clinical outcomes remain poor following the diagnosis, as the majority of patients already have (or will soon develop) systemic lesions following the diagnosis of a pituitary metastatic tumor.
- The mean survival time following diagnosis is approximately 1 year; it ranges from 6 to 22 months [3, 9, 15, 16].

References

1. Branch Jr CL, Laws Jr ER. Metastatic tumors of the sella turcica masquerading as primary pituitary tumors. J Clin Endocrinol Metab. 1987;65:469–74.
2. Ariel D, Sung H, Coghlan N, Dodd R, Gibbs IC, Katznelson L. Clinical characteristics and pituitary dysfunction in patients with metastatic cancer to the sella. Endocr Pract. 2013;19:914–9.
3. Fassett DR, Couldwell WT. Metastases to the pituitary gland. Neurosurg Focus. 2004;16(4):E8.
4. Marin F, Kovacs KT, Scheithauer BW, Young Jr WF. The pituitary gland in patients with breast carcinoma: a histologic and immunocytochemical study of 125 cases. Mayo Clin Proc. 1992;67:949–56.
5. Gurling KJ, Scott GB, Baron DN. Metastases in pituitary tissue removed at hypophysectomy in women with mammary carcinoma. Br J Cancer. 1957;11:519–22.
6. Komninos J, Vlassopoulou V, Protopapa D, Korfias S, Kontogeorgos G, Sakas DE, et al. Tumors metastatic to the pituitary gland: case report and literature review. J Clin Endocrinol Metab. 2004;89:574–80.
7. Saeger W, Ludecke DK, Buchfelder M, Fahlbusch R, Quabbe HJ, Petersenn S. Pathohistological classification of pituitary tumors: 10 years of experience with the German Pituitary Tumor Registry. Eur J Endocrinol. 2007;156:203–16.
8. Sioutos P, Yen V, Arbit E. Pituitary gland metastases. Ann Surg Oncol. 1996;3:94–9.
9. Morita A, Meyer FB, Laws Jr ER. Symptomatic pituitary metastases. J Neurosurg. 1998;89:69–73.
10. Aaberg Jr TM, Kay M, Sternau L. Metastatic tumors to the pituitary. Am J Ophthalmol. 1995;119:779–85.
11. Nelson PB, Robinson AG, Martinez AJ. Metastatic tumor of the pituitary gland. Neurosurgery. 1987;21:941–4.
12. Agarwal KK, Sharma P, Singla S, Suman Kc S, Bal C, Kumar R. A rare case of non-small cell lung cancer metastasizing to the pituitary gland: detection with (18)F-FDG PET-CT. Clin Nucl Med. 2014;39:e318–9.
13. Teears RJ, Silverman EM. Clinicopathologic review of 88 cases of carcinoma metastatic to the pituitary gland. Cancer. 1975;36:216–20.
14. Al-Brahim NY, Asa SL. My approach to pathology of the pituitary gland. J Clin Pathol. 2006;59:1245–53.
15. Zoli M, Mazzatenta D, Faustini-Fustini M, Pasquini E, Frank G. Pituitary metastases: role of surgery. World Neurosurg. 2013;79:327–30.
16. Kano H, Niranjan A, Kondziolka D, Flickinger JC, Lunsford LD. Stereotactic radiosurgery for pituitary metastases. Surg Neurol. 2009;72:248–55; discussion 255–6.

Part VII

Inflammatory and Infectious Lesions of the Anterior Skull Base, Sellar and Parasellar Region

Spontaneous Abscess of the Sellar Region

51

Gabriel Zada, M. Beatriz S. Lopes, Srinivasan Mukundan Jr., and Edward Laws Jr.

51.1 Epidemiology and Clinical Presentation

- Spontaneous pituitary abscesses are rare, representing less than 0.6 % of patients with sellar lesions undergoing surgical treatment [1–3].
- Pituitary abscesses may also be acquired or iatrogenic conditions, rarely following cerebral trauma or transsphenoidal surgery. (See Chap. 75 for information regarding acquired pituitary abscesses.)
- Spontaneous pituitary abscesses may be bacterial, fungal, or mycobacterial, with the former being much less common. Later sections of this chapter give more details on abscesses related to invasive fungal sinusitis or sellar tuberculosis.
- Spontaneous abscesses typically develop secondary to extension from paranasal sinus disease and sphenoid sinusitis or from a spontaneous or traumatic cerebrospinal fluid (CSF) leak. Sepsis is also known to be an inciting factor [2, 4–7].
- Spontaneous pituitary abscesses also have been reported to occur in association with other sellar lesions, including pituitary adenoma, craniopharyngioma, or Rathke cleft cyst [2, 8, 9].
- Sellar abscesses and other infections develop more frequently following surgery, especially in the presence of a CSF leak. These iatrogenic cases are usually bacterial [10–12].
- Pituitary abscesses may present clinically with headache, fever, hypopituitarism (85 %), meningitis, diabetes insipidus, visual loss, cranial nerve paresis, altered mental status, and/or toxemia [2, 7].
- Diabetes insipidus tends to be quite common in patients with sellar abscess; it is present in up to 70 % of patients at the time of diagnosis [7].
- The most common offending bacterial organisms are staphylococcus, streptococcus, and pneumococcus species [3, 7, 12].
- An increased peripheral white blood cell (WBC) count is observed in only one third of patients [12].

G. Zada, MD, MS (✉)
Department of Neurological Surgery, Keck School of Medicine, University of Southern California, 1200 N State Street, #3300, Los Angeles, CA 90033, USA
e-mail: gzada@usc.edu

M.B.S. Lopes, MD, PhD
Department of Pathology (Neuropathology), University of Virginia School of Medicine, 1215 Lee Street, Room 3060–HEP, Charlottesville, VA 22908, USA
e-mail: msl2e@virginia.edu

S. Mukundan Jr., PhD, MD
Department of Radiology, Brigham and Women's Hospital, 75 Francis Street, Boston, MA 02115, USA
e-mail: smukundan@partners.org

E. Laws Jr., MD
Department of Neurosurgery, Brigham and Women's Hospital, 15 Francis Street, Boston, MA 02115, USA
e-mail: elaws@partners.org

G. Zada et al. (eds.), *Atlas of Sellar and Parasellar Lesions: Clinical, Radiologic, and Pathologic Correlations*, DOI 10.1007/978-3-319-22855-6_51

51.2 Imaging Features

- CT scan generally shows a homogenous, low-density mass with rim enhancement following contrast administration.
- MRI typically demonstrates a cystic mass with homogenous, low-intensity or isointense signals on T1-weighted imaging and high-intensity signals on T2-weighted images, with rim enhancement following gadolinium administration (Figs. 51.1, 51.2, and 51.3) [13–15].
- Sellar abscess may infrequently resemble a cystic or hemorrhagic pituitary adenoma, a Rathke cleft cyst, or a cystic craniopharyngioma [13].
- Restricted diffusion-weighted imaging (DWI) often supports the presence of a sellar abscess, but its usefulness is somewhat limited along the skull base and paranasal sinuses [16, 17].
- A thickened, enhancing infundibulum may be associated with sellar abscess on MRI with contrast [18, 19].

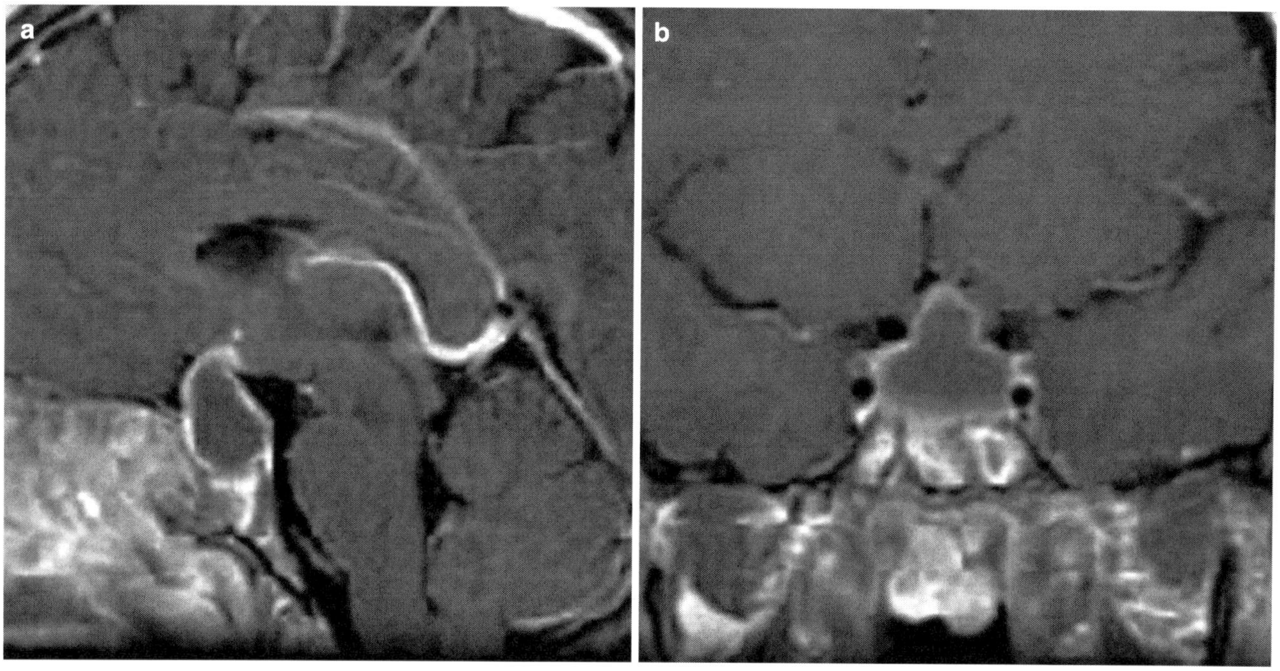

Fig. 51.1 Bacterial sellar abscess. Preoperative MR images of a patient with a history of remote prior transsphenoidal surgery for a pituitary tumor and a bacterial sellar abscess: Sagittal (**a**) and coronal (**b**) T1-weighted images demonstrate an isointense lesion in the pituitary fossa, with ring enhancement after contrast injection (Adapted from Ciapetta et al. [20] with permission)

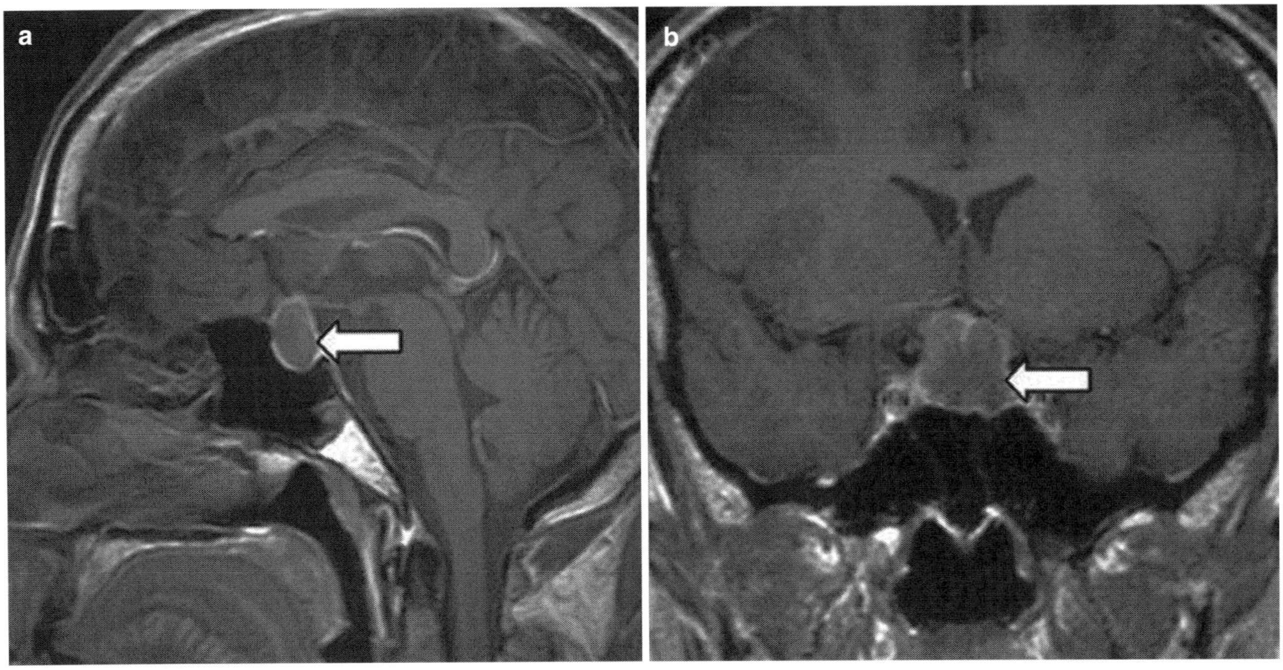

Fig. 51.2 Spontaneous pituitary abscess. Preoperative (postcontrast) MR images in a patient with a spontaneous pituitary abscess. (**a**) Sagittal section shows a sellar cystic mass with suprasellar extension (*arrow*). The lesion is seen pushing the optic chiasm upward. The pituitary stalk is intact. (**b**) Coronal section shows the pituitary sellar mass with suprasellar extension (*arrow*). The lesion is seen pushing the optic chiasm upward (Adapted from Dalan and Leow [14], with permission)

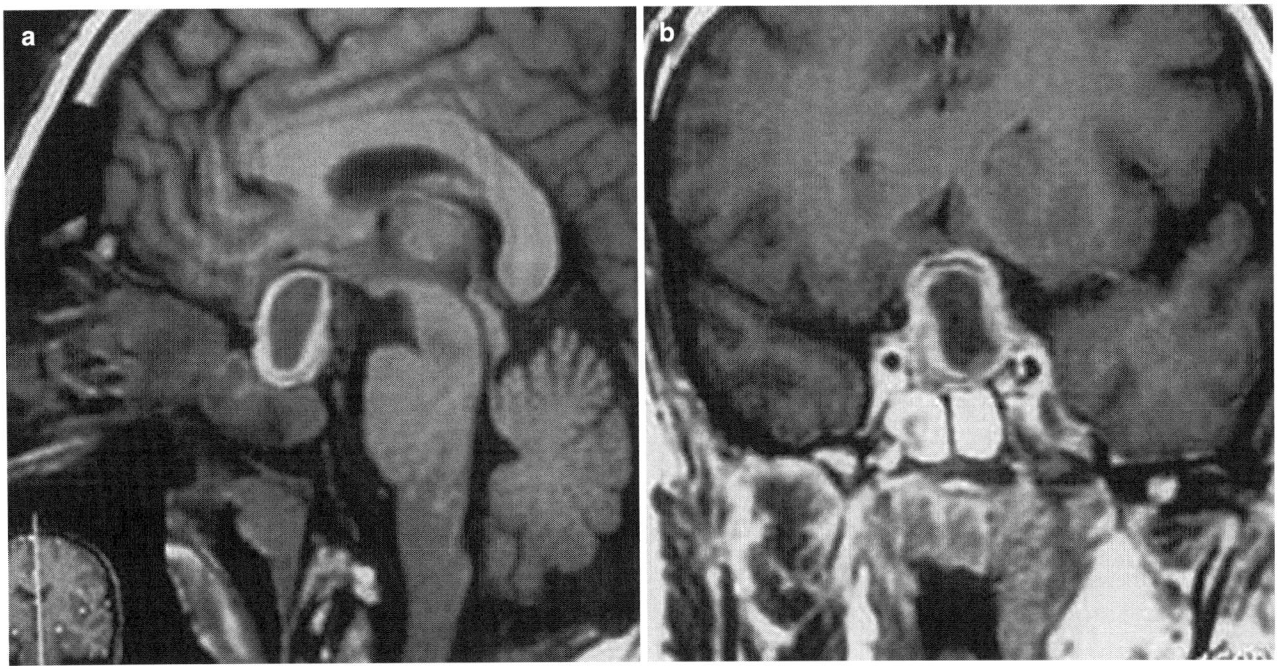

Fig. 51.3 Spontaneous abscess. Preoperative post-gadolinium T1-weighted MRI scans in a patient with a spontaneous aspergillosis abscess. A sellar and suprasellar mass with peripheral contrast enhancement is seen on sagittal (**a**) and coronal (**b**) sections. Marked compression of the optic chiasm and thickened sphenoid sinus mucosa (suggesting sinusitis) can also be seen (Adapted with permission from Iplikcioglu AC et al., Acta Neurochir (Wien) (2004) 146:521–524)

51.3 Histopathology

- A wide variety of bacterial and fungal organisms have been implicated in the formation of sellar abscesses.
- Histopathology may demonstrate necrosis and abscess wall, with infiltration by polymorphonuclear leukocytes or macrophages [2].
- In most cases (over 80 %), organisms are not isolated on cultures [7].
- Polymerase chain reaction (PCR) techniques may be useful in establishing a definitive diagnosis.

51.4 Clinical and Surgical Management

- The diagnosis of sellar abscess is often missed prior to surgery [7].
- Transsphenoidal surgical drainage and marsupialization of the abscess wall is the standard management [7, 20].
- In some cases, conservative management with antibiotics may be attempted, although there is little evidence to support this strategy [21].
- Intraoperative cultures for aerobic, anaerobic, fungal, and acid-fast bacilli should be sent.
- Sellar floor reconstruction is not recommended unless a CSF leak is present.
- For bacterial abscesses, intravenous antibiotics are typically required for at least 6 weeks after drainage.
- Tubercular or fungal abscess should be treated with the appropriate antibiotic regimens.
- Symptoms from mass effect generally improve following drainage, whereas hypopituitarism typically fails to do so [12, 22].
- Recurrence rates varying from 0 to 18 % have been reported after surgical and antibiotic management of sellar abscess [7, 12].

References

1. Saeger W, Ludecke DK, Buchfelder M, Fahlbusch R, Quabbe HJ, Petersenn S. Pathohistological classification of pituitary tumors: 10 years of experience with the German pituitary tumor registry. Eur J Endocrinol. 2007;156:203–16.
2. Dutta P, Bhansali A, Singh P, Kotwal N, Pathak A, Kumar Y. Pituitary abscess: report of four cases and review of literature. Pituitary. 2006;9:267–73.
3. Jain KC, Varma A, Mahapatra AK. Pituitary abscess: a series of six cases. Br J Neurosurg. 1997;11:139–43.
4. Verdalle P, Roquet E, Hor F, Raynal M, Courtois A, Bauduceau B, et al. Pituitary abscess. A rare complication of sinusitis. Rev Laryngol Otol Rhinol (Bord). 1997;118:327–9.
5. Somali MH, Anastasiou AL, Goulis DG, Polyzoides C, Avramides A. Pituitary abscess presenting with cranial nerve paresis. Case report and review of literature. J Endocrinol Invest. 2001;24:45–50.
6. Shono T, Nishio S, Muratani H, Yasuda T, Fukui M, Moutai K. Pituitary abscess secondary to isolated sphenoid sinusitis. Minim Invasive Neurosurg. 1999;42:204–6.
7. Zhang X, Sun J, Shen M, Shou X, Qiu H, Qiao N, et al. Diagnosis and minimally invasive surgery for the pituitary abscess: a review of twenty nine cases. Clin Neurol Neurosurg. 2012;114:957–61.
8. Nelson PB, Haverkos H, Martinez AJ, Robinson AG. Abscess formation within pituitary tumors. Neurosurgery. 1983;12:331–3.
9. Arseni C, Dănăilă L, Carp N, Ghitescu M, Istrati C. Intrasellar abscess. Neurochirurgia (Stuttg). 1975;18:207–13.
10. Henegar MM, Koby MB, Silbergeld DL, Rich KM, Moran CJ. Intrasellar abscess following transsphenoidal surgery. Surg Neurol. 1996;45:183–8.
11. Sudhakar N, Ray A, Vafidis JA. Complications after transsphenoidal surgery: our experience and a review of the literature. Br J Neurosurg. 2004;18:507–12.
12. Vates GE, Berger MS, Wilson CB. Diagnosis and management of pituitary abscess: a review of twenty-four cases. J Neurosurg. 2001;95:233–41.
13. Wolansky LJ, Gallagher JD, Heary RF, Malantic GP, Dasmahapatra A, Shaderowfsky PD, Budhwani N. MRI of pituitary abscess: two cases and review of the literature. Neuroradiology. 1997;39:499–503.
14. Dalan R, Leow MK. Pituitary abscess: our experience with a case and a review of the literature. Pituitary. 2008;11:299–306.
15. Sabbah P, Bonardel G, Herve R, Marjou F, Hor F, Pharaboz C, Bauduceau B. CT and MRI findings in primitive pituitary abscess: a case report and review of literature. J Neuroradiol. 1999;26:196–9.
16. Takayasu T, Yamasaki F, Tominaga A, Hidaka T, Arita K, Kurisu K. A pituitary abscess showing high signal intensity on diffusion-weighted imaging. Neurosurg Rev. 2006;29:246–8.
17. Taguchi Y, Yoshida K, Takashima S, Tanaka K. Diffusion-weighted MRI findings in a patient with pituitary abscess. Intern Med. 2012;51:683.
18. Sinha S, Singh AK, Tatke M, Singh D. Hypophyseal tuberculoma: direct radiosurgery is contraindicated for a lesion with a thickened pituitary stalk: case report. Neurosurgery. 2000;46:735–8; discussion 738–9.
19. Patankar T, Patkar D, Bunting T, Castillo M, Mukherji SK. Imaging in pituitary tuberculosis. Clin Imaging. 2000;24:89–92.
20. Ciappetta P, Calace A, D'Urso PI, De Candia N. Endoscopic treatment of pituitary abscess: two case reports and literature review. Neurosurg Rev. 2008;31:237–46; discussion 246.
21. Uchida Y, Tsuchimochi N, Oku M, Fujihara N, Shimono N, Okada K, Harada M. Successful treatment of pituitary abscess with oral administration of Sparfloxacin. Intern Med. 2008;47:1147–51.
22. Hernández I, Garcia L, Guinto G, Cabrera L, Mercado M. Bacterial pituitary abscess: an unusual cause of panhypopituitarism. Endocr Pract. 2002;8:424–8.

Invasive Fungal Sinusitis and Fungal Abscess of the Sella

52

Gabriel Zada, M. Beatriz S. Lopes,
Srinivasan Mukundan Jr., and Edward Laws Jr.

52.1 Epidemiology and Clinical Presentation

- Fungal disease of the pituitary and parasellar region can present as a fungal abscess or as an invasive fungal sinusitis. Rhino-orbito-cerebral involvement is typically an extreme form of invasive fungal sinusitis seen in patients with mucormycosis. Allergic fungal sinusitis (AFS) is another manifestation of sinonasal fungal disease that is typically not invasive.
- Fungal sellar abscesses can be caused by a wide variety of species, including *Aspergillus* (most common), *Candida*, and *Brucella* species [1–5].
- Invasive fungal sinusitis accounts for 6–12 % of chronic sinusitis. It commonly presents with facial swelling, fever, and nasal congestion [6, 7].
- Invasive fungal sinusitis is typically caused by *Aspergillus* species or mucormycosis and may invade through the skull base. Isolated sphenoid sinus aspergilloma is a distinct entity that typically presents with postnasal drip and headache [8–12].
- Rhinocerebral mucormycosis and rhino-orbital-cerebral mucormycosis are lethal diseases that typically develop in immunocompromised patients. Uncontrolled diabetes mellitus is a major risk factor. Isolated sphenoid sinus mucormycosis with visual loss has been reported [13, 14].
- Common clinical manifestations in patients with rhino-orbital-cerebral mucormycosis are exophthalmia, rhinorrhea, altered mental status, and ophthalmoplegia [15].
- Pituitary apoplexy, internal carotid artery thrombosis, cavernous sinus thrombosis, and stroke have all been described in association with invasive mucormycosis [16, 17].

G. Zada, MD, MS (✉)
Department of Neurological Surgery,
Keck School of Medicine, University of Southern California,
1200 N State Street, #3300, Los Angeles,
CA 90033, USA
e-mail: gzada@usc.edu

M.B.S. Lopes, MD, PhD
Department of Pathology (Neuropathology),
University of Virginia School of Medicine,
1215 Lee Street, Room 3060–HEP, Charlottesville,
VA 22908, USA
e-mail: msl2e@virginia.edu

S. Mukundan Jr., PhD, MD
Department of Radiology, Brigham and Women's Hospital,
75 Francis Street, Boston, MA 02115, USA
e-mail: smukundan@partners.org

E. Laws Jr., MD
Department of Neurosurgery, Brigham and Women's Hospital,
15 Francis Street, Boston, MA 02115, USA
e-mail: elaws@partners.org

G. Zada et al. (eds.), *Atlas of Sellar and Parasellar Lesions: Clinical, Radiologic, and Pathologic Correlations*,
DOI 10.1007/978-3-319-22855-6_52

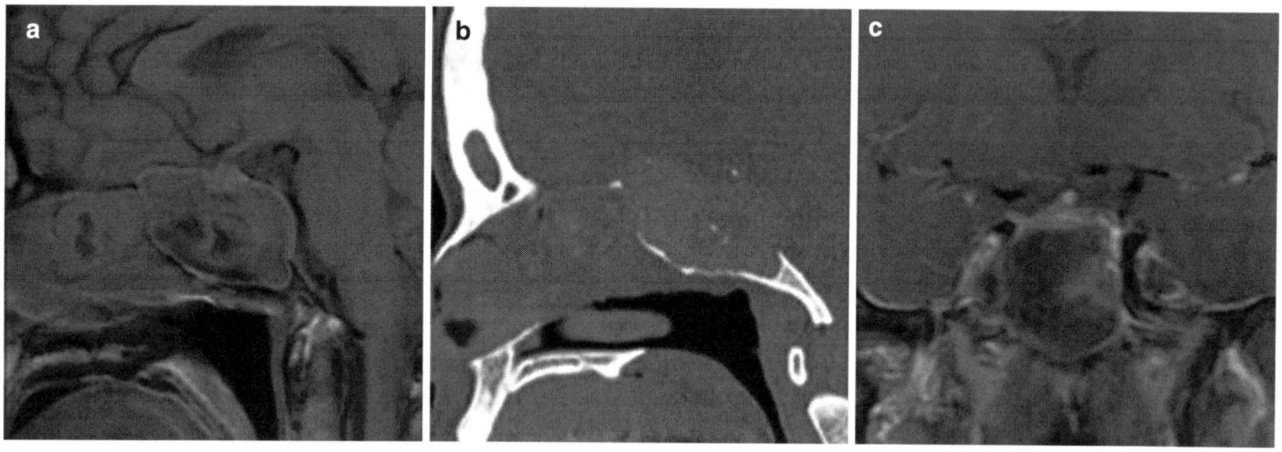

Fig. 52.1 Allergic fungal sinusitis. (**a**) Sagittal T1-weighted precontrast image. (**b**) Sagittal CT image with contrast enhancement. (**c**) Coronal T1-weighted gadolinium-enhanced image. There is expansion of the sphenoid sinus containing heterogeneous-appearing, hyperdense, and partly calcified material

52.2 Imaging Features

- Fungal pituitary abscesses are typically rim-enhancing lesions on CT scans or MRI, often with associated sinus disease (Figs. 52.1 and 52.2). Bony erosion may be seen on CT. Fungal abscesses are typically hypointense or isointense on T1-weighted MR images and are T2 hypointense, which has been attributed to an increase in paramagnetic substances in the fungal elements. Diffusion-weighted imaging may be used to support the diagnosis of pituitary abscess [5].
- Rhinocerebral mucormycosis is characterized by a poorly circumscribed and invasive mass, typically arising in the nasal cavity and ethmoid sinuses and extending into the orbit(s), frontal lobes, and/or temporal lobes. Bony erosion on CT images is quite common. On MRI, T1 isointensity and variable T2 signal are common [18].
- Other less common findings include pneumocephalus and thrombosis of the internal carotid artery or cavernous sinus. The "black turbinate sign" may be pathognomonic for mucormycosis when it is seen on MRI [19].

52.3 Histopathology

- The most common causes of fungal abscesses are *Aspergillus* and *Candida* species.
- Mucormycosis is caused by fungi of the order Mucorales, most commonly the *Rhizopus* species.
- Typical staining for diagnosis of fungal disease includes hematoxylin and eosin (H&E), Gomori's methenamine silver, and periodic acid–Schiff stains.
- Histologically, *Aspergillus* species are characterized by hyaline, uniform, septate, and dichotomously branched hyphae. Purulent, necrotizing inflammation is commonly observed.
- Grossly, mucormycosis is characterized by black, necrotic lesions and occasional tumefaction [15].
- Histologically, mucormycosis is characterized by broad-based and nonseptate hyphae with irregular branching that may occur at right angles. Vascular invasion and necrosis are common. Pyogenic inflammation and suppurative necrosis are commonly observed.

52.4 Clinical and Surgical Management

- Transsphenoidal surgery is the mainstay of treatment for achieving biopsy, cultures, and drainage or resection of sellar region fungal abscesses [20].
- In patients with invasive fungal sinusitis and rhinocerebral mucormycosis, early diagnosis and intervention are critical. Management typically consists of aggressive surgical debridement, glucose control, and antifungal therapy.
- Following surgical management and diagnosis, long-term antifungal agents are administered. The most common agents include amphotericin B, caspofungin, itraconazole, and voriconazole.
- Most patients with fungal pituitary abscesses treated in a timely manner will have a good long-term outcome [5, 20].
- On the other hand, outcomes for patients with invasive fungal sinusitis are poor, with an overall survival rate of less than 50 % [6].
- Outcomes in patients with invasive rhinocerebral mucormycosis are extremely poor, with a majority of patients dying from the disease.

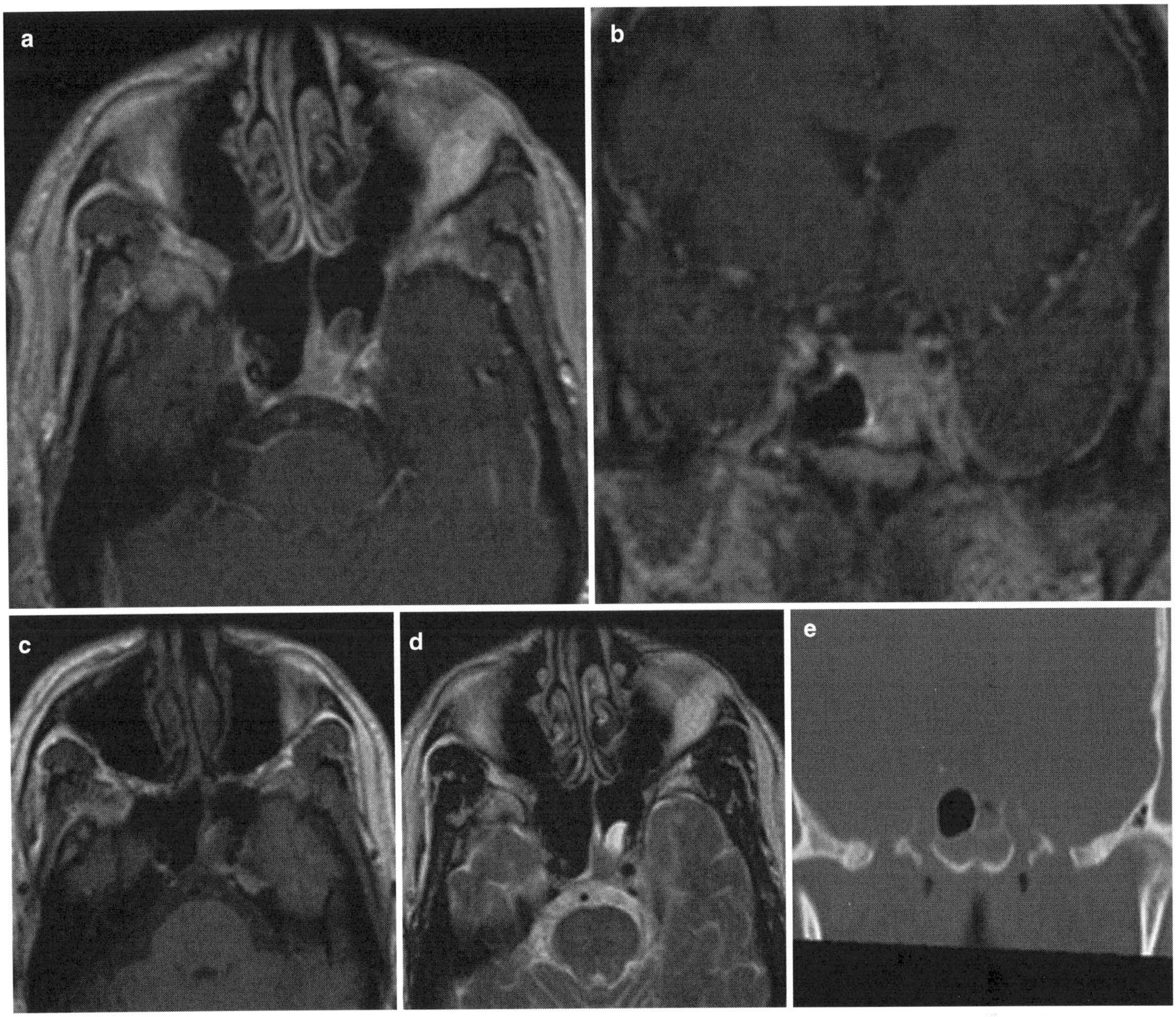

Fig. 52.2 Invasive fungal sinusitis. (**a**) Axial T1-weighted gadolinium-enhanced image. (**b**) Coronal T1-weighted gadolinium-enhanced image. (**c**) Axial T1-weighted precontrast image. (**d**) Axial T2-weighted image. (**e**) Coronal CT image in bone window. On (**a**–**c**), enhancing tissue is present along the superior medial margin of the left sphenoid sinus. Image (**d**) reveals erosion through the roof of the left sphenoid

References

1. Hao L, Jing C, Bowen C, Min H, Chao Y. Aspergillus sellar abscess: case report and review of the literature. Neurol India. 2008;56:186–8.
2. Heary RF, Maniker AH, Wolansky LJ. Candidal pituitary abscess: case report. Neurosurgery. 1995;36:1009–12; discussion 1012–3.
3. Iplikcioglu AC, Bek S, Bikmaz K, Ceylan D, Gökduman CA. Aspergillus pituitary abscess. Acta Neurochir (Wien). 2004; 146:521–4.
4. Güven MB, Cirak B, Kutluhan A, Ugras S. Pituitary abscess secondary to neurobrucellosis. Case illustration. J Neurosurg. 1999;90:1142.
5. Liu J, You C, Tang J, Chen L. Fungal pituitary abscess: case report and review of the literature. Neurol India. 2013;61:210–2.
6. Turner JH, Soudry E, Nayak JV, Hwang PH. Survival outcomes in acute invasive fungal sinusitis: a systematic review and quantitative synthesis of published evidence. Laryngoscope. 2013;123:1112–8.
7. Challa S, Uppin SG, Hanumanthu S, Panigrahi MK, Purohit AK, Sattaluri S, et al. Fungal rhinosinusitis: a clinicopathological study from South India. Eur Arch Otorhinolaryngol. 2010;267:1239–45.
8. Pinzer T, Reiss M, Bourquain H, Krishnan KG, Schackert G. Primary aspergillosis of the sphenoid sinus with pituitary invasion - a rare differential diagnosis of sellar lesions. Acta Neurochir (Wien). 2006;148:1085–90; discussion 1090.
9. Boutarbouch M, Arkha Y, El Ouahabi A, Derraz S, El Khamlichi A. Sphenoid sinus aspergillosis simulating pituitary tumor in immunocompetent patient. J Clin Neurosci. 2009;16:840–1.
10. Parker KM, Nicholson JK, Cezayirli RC, Biggs PJ. Aspergillosis of the sphenoid sinus: presentation as a pituitary mass and postoperative gallium-67 imaging. Surg Neurol. 1996;45:354–8.
11. Fuchs HA, Evans RM, Gregg CR. Invasive aspergillosis of the sphenoid sinus manifested as a pituitary tumor. South Med J. 1985;78:1365–7.
12. Lee TJ, Huang SF, Chang PH. Characteristics of isolated sphenoid sinus aspergilloma: report of twelve cases and literature review. Ann Otol Rhinol Laryngol. 2009;118:211–7.
13. Bansal S, Grover G, Grover M, Gupta AK. Isolated sphenoid mucormycosis presenting as visual impairment: changing trends? Am J Otolaryngol. 2010;31:64–6.
14. Del Valle ZA, Rubio Suárez A, Mellado Encinas P, Morales Angulo C, Cabrera PE. Mucormycosis of the sphenoid sinus in an otherwise healthy patient. Case report and literature review. J Laryngol Otol. 1996;110:471–3.
15. Mbarek C, Zribi S, Khamassi K, Hariga I, Ouni H, Ben Amor M, et al. Rhinocerebral mucormycosis: five cases and a literature review. B-ENT. 2011;7:189–93.
16. Simmons JH, Zeitler PS, Fenton LZ, Abzug MJ, Fiallo-Scharer RV, Klingensmith GJ. Rhinocerebral mucormycosis complicated by internal carotid artery thrombosis in a pediatric patient with type 1 diabetes mellitus: a case report and review of the literature. Pediatr Diabetes. 2005;6:234–8.
17. Anaissie EJ, Shikhani AH. Rhinocerebral mucormycosis with internal carotid occlusion: report of two cases and review of the literature. Laryngoscope. 1985;95:1107–13.
18. Herrera DA, et al. Imaging findings of rhinocerebral mucormycosis. Skull Base. 2009;19(2):117–25.
19. Safder S, et al. The "Black Turbinate" sign: An early MR imaging finding of nasal mucormycosis. AJNR Am J Neuroradiol. 2010; 31(4):771–4.
20. Liu W, et al. Successful treatment of sellar aspergillus abscess. J Clin Neurosci. 2010;17(12):1587–9.

Mucocele and Mucopyocele

53

Gabriel Zada, M. Beatriz S. Lopes,
Srinivasan Mukundan Jr., and Edward Laws Jr.

53.1 Epidemiology and Clinical Presentation

- Mucoceles and mucopyoceles are rare cystic and cavitated collections originating in the paranasal sinuses. They most commonly occur in the frontal and ethmoid sinuses. A mucocele contains mucinous secretions, whereas a mucopyocele is an abscess-like formation that also contains purulent material.
- Risk factors for development of a paranasal sinus mucocele include prior surgery, trauma, radiation, and sinusitis.
- Sphenoid sinus mucoceles comprise only 1–2 % of all paranasal sinus mucoceles [1].
- Mucoceles comprise only 0.05 % of lesions treated in major transsphenoidal series [2].
- Most commonly, sphenoid sinus mucocele and mucopyocele are iatrogenic conditions seen after transsphenoidal surgery for pituitary adenomas [3–5].
- The mean age at diagnosis is 53 years [1].
- Headaches, facial pain, and nasal discharge are the most common clinical presentations. Visual loss and cranial nerve paresis have been reported (more frequently with mucopyoceles) [1, 6–9].
- Infrequently, they erode through the sellar floor or clivus, or they are located purely in the intrasellar and suprasellar region. Spontaneous mucoceles and mucopyoceles of the sellar region are rare and have been confined primarily to case reports [6, 10, 11].
- In rare cases, mucopyocele of the anterior clinoid process may cause visual loss and cavernous sinus syndrome [12].

G. Zada, MD, MS (✉)
Department of Neurological Surgery, Keck School of Medicine, University of Southern California, 1200 N State Street, #3300, Los Angeles, CA 90033, USA
e-mail: gzada@usc.edu

M.B.S. Lopes, MD, PhD
Department of Pathology (Neuropathology), University of Virginia School of Medicine, 1215 Lee Street, Room 3060–HEP, Charlottesville, VA 22908, USA
e-mail: msl2e@virginia.edu

S. Mukundan Jr., PhD, MD
Department of Radiology, Brigham and Women's Hospital, 75 Francis Street, Boston, MA 02115, USA
e-mail: smukundan@partners.org

E. Laws Jr., MD
Department of Neurosurgery, Brigham and Women's Hospital, 15 Francis Street, Boston, MA 02115, USA
e-mail: elaws@partners.org

G. Zada et al. (eds.), *Atlas of Sellar and Parasellar Lesions: Clinical, Radiologic, and Pathologic Correlations*, DOI 10.1007/978-3-319-22855-6_53

53.2 Imaging Features

- Intrasellar and suprasellar mucoceles are rare and may be misdiagnosed as a pituitary adenoma or craniopharyngioma [13].
- CT scans show a nonenhancing mass with bony expansion. The cortical margins can become imperceptible with significant expansion.
- On MRI, the content of mucoceles is often T2 hyperintense with variable T1 intensity [14]. Following contrast administration, a thin layer of mucosal enhancement is expected along the periphery. Nodular enhancement should raise the possibility of an obstructive lesion causing secondary mucocele formation (Figs. 53.1 and 53.2).
- Intraorbital extension is a common finding, which develops in over 60 % of primary paranasal sinus mucoceles [15].
- Intracranial involvement is infrequent, occurring in 12–20 % of paranasal sinus mucoceles [1, 15].

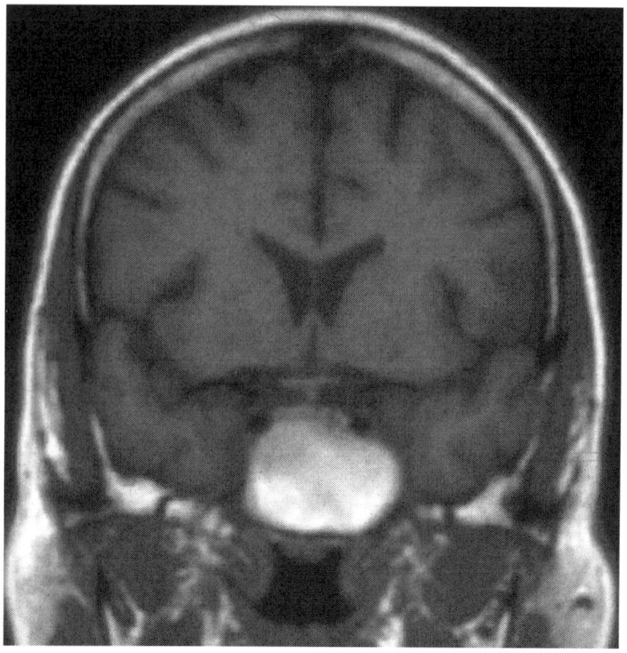

Fig. 53.1 Mucocele. Coronal T1-weighted precontrast MR image. The sphenoid is expanded and contains T1-hyperintense material. The normal pituitary gland is seen superior to the expanded sinus

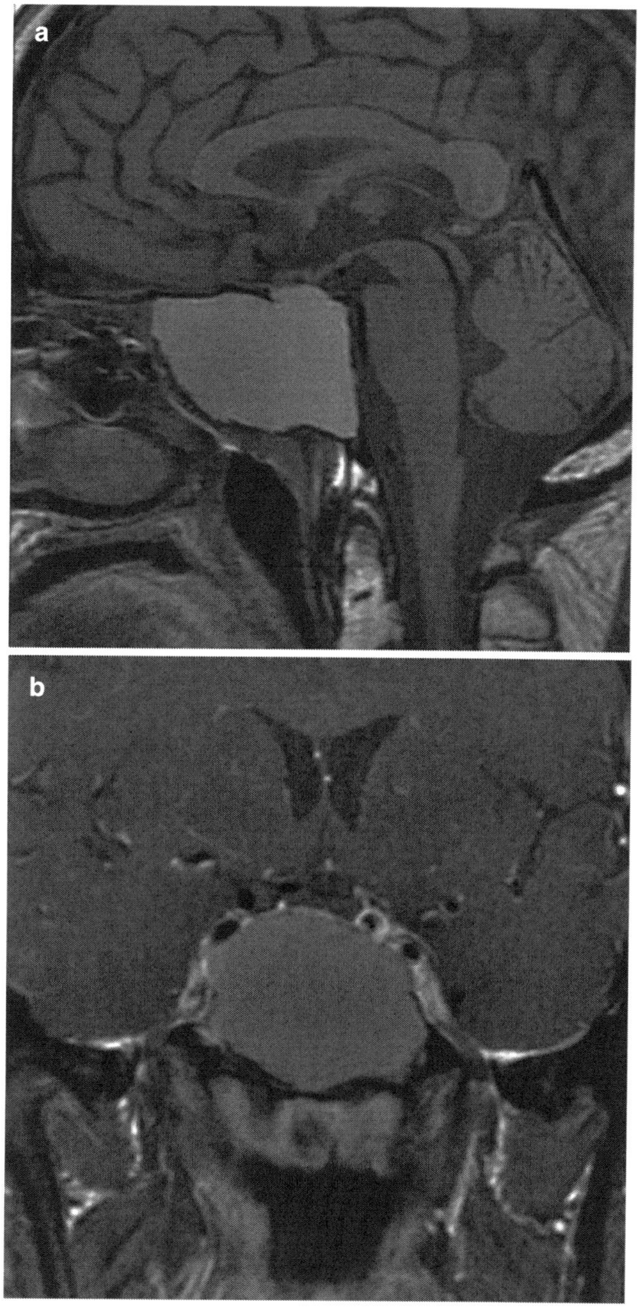

Fig. 53.2 Mucopyocele. (**a**) Sagittal T1-weighted pre-gadolinium MR image. (**b**) Coronal T1-weighted post-gadolinium image. The sphenoid is markedly expanded, containing T1 shortening material. The superior margin of the expanded sinus effaces the sella, and the pituitary gland is not clearly visible

53.3 Histopathology

- Mucoceles are epithelial-lined cystic masses demonstrating an inflammatory reaction and mucinous material. Pseudostratified, ciliated, columnar epithelium is commonly noted, often with metaplasia in recurrent or chronic lesions.
- Mucoceles share many features with respiratory mucosa and may contain areas of granulation changes, necrosis, and hemorrhage [3, 14].

53.4 Clinical and Surgical Management

- The mainstay of treatment is endonasal transsphenoidal marsupialization and drainage.
- Endoscopic endonasal management with the use of angled lenses is the gold standard surgical procedure, which facilitates maximal drainage of disease located in the lateral sphenoid recesses [16].
- Antibiotics are typically used to augment therapy.
- Outcomes are usually excellent, with low recurrence rates if the lesion is treated early [1, 17, 18].

References

1. Soon SR, Lim CM, Singh H, Sethi DS. Sphenoid sinus mucocele: 10 cases and literature review. J Laryngol Otol. 2010;124:44–7.
2. Saeger W, Ludecke DK, Buchfelder M, Fahlbusch R, Quabbe HJ, Petersenn S. Pathohistological classification of pituitary tumors: 10 years of experience with the German pituitary tumor registry. Eur J Endocrinol. 2007;156:203–16.
3. Herman P, Lot G, Guichard JP, Marianowski R, Assayag M, Tran BA, Huy P. Mucocele of the sphenoid sinus: a late complication of transsphenoidal pituitary surgery. Ann Otol Rhinol Laryngol. 1998;107:765–8.
4. Giordano M, Gerganov VM, Draf W, Fahlbusch R. Sphenoid sinus pyocele after transsphenoidal approach for pituitary adenoma. Pituitary. 2012;15:188–92.
5. Lu YJ, Chang CN, Pai PC, Wei KC, Chuang CC. Isolated sphenoid sinusitis or mucocele: a potential complication of endonasal transsphenoidal surgery. J Neurooncol. 2009;91:63–7.
6. Chua R, Shapiro S. A mucopyocele of the clivus: case report. Neurosurgery. 1996;39:589–90; discussion 590–1.
7. Lavezzi E, Fatti LM, Bucciarelli L, Bettinelli A, Scacchi M, Cavagnini F. Monolateral visual loss due to sphenoid sinus mucocele: a rare complication of transsphenoidal surgery. J Endocrinol Invest. 2006;29:1021–2.
8. Heylbroeck P, Watelet JB, Delbeke P, Van Cauwenberge P, Bachert C. Vision impairment as presenting symptom of a sphenoidal mucocele. Rhinology. 2003;41:187–91.
9. Pompili A, Mastrostefano R, Caroli F, Cattani F, Cianfriglia F, Nardis PF, et al. Mucocele of neurosurgical interest: clinical considerations on five cases. Acta Neurochir (Wien). 1990; 102:114–21.
10. El-Fiki ME, Abdel-Fattah HM, El-Deeb AK. Sphenoid sinus mucopyocele with marked intracranial extension: a more common phenomenon in the third world? Surg Neurol. 1993;39:115–9.
11. Simms NM, Brown WE, French LA. Mucocele of the sphenoid sinus presenting as an intrasellar mass. Case report. J Neurosurg. 1970;32:708–10.
12. Chagla AS, Bhaganagare A, Kansal R, Tyagi D. Complete recovery of visual loss following surgical treatment of mucopyocele of the anterior clinoid process. J Clin Neurosci. 2010;17:670–2.
13. Abla AA, Maroon JC, Wilberger Jr JE, Kennerdell JS, Deeb ZL. Intrasellar mucocele simulating pituitary adenoma: case report. Neurosurgery. 1986;18:197–9.
14. Capra GG, Carbone PN, Mullin DP. Paranasal sinus mucocele. Head Neck Pathol. 2012;6:369–72.
15. Fu CH, Chang KP, Lee TJ. The difference in anatomical and invasive characteristics between primary and secondary paranasal sinus mucoceles. Otolaryngol Head Neck Surg. 2007;136:621–5.
16. Giovannetti F, Filiaci F, Ramieri V, Ungari C. Isolated sphenoid sinus mucocele: etiology and management. J Craniofac Surg. 2008;19:1381–4.
17. Razmpa E, Naghibzadeh B, Bagheri A, Sadeghi M, Khak M. The clinical manifestation, evaluation and surgical management of sphenoid sinus mucoceles: a case series and literature review. B-ENT. 2011;7:87–90.
18. Hejazi N, Witzmann A, Hassler W. Ocular manifestations of sphenoid mucoceles: clinical features and neurosurgical management of three cases and review of the literature. Surg Neurol. 2001;56:338–43.

Sellar Tuberculosis

54

Gabriel Zada, M. Beatriz S. Lopes,
Srinivasan Mukundan Jr., and Edward Laws Jr.

54.1 Epidemiology and Clinical Presentation

- Tuberculosis (TB), an infectious disease caused by mycobacteria, rarely presents in the sellar or suprasellar region.
- TB in the sellar region typically presents as a granulomatous mass (tuberculoma) or tubercular abscess, with or without pachymeningitis.
- Overall, tuberculomas comprise 0.15–2 % of all intracranial lesions [1].
- Sellar tuberculomas make up at most 1–2 % of lesions in major transsphenoidal series, even in areas where TB is much more common [2].
- Patients are often young, with a mean age of 36 years [3].
- A female preponderance has been reported [2, 3].
- Isolated intrasellar tuberculomas are rare, with fewer than 50 cases reported.
- Only 25 % of patients show systemic evidence of tuberculosis at the time of diagnosis [1, 3].
- Clinical symptoms often include chronic headache, visual loss, and hypopituitarism [2, 4].
- The clinical presentation may mimic pituitary apoplexy [5].

G. Zada, MD, MS (✉)
Department of Neurological Surgery,
Keck School of Medicine, University of Southern California,
1200 N State Street, #3300, Los Angeles, CA 90033, USA
e-mail: gzada@usc.edu

M.B.S. Lopes, MD, PhD
Department of Pathology (Neuropathology),
University of Virginia School of Medicine,
1215 Lee Street, Room 3060–HEP, Charlottesville,
VA 22908, USA
e-mail: msl2e@virginia.edu

S. Mukundan Jr., PhD, MD
Department of Radiology, Brigham and Women's Hospital,
75 Francis Street, Boston, MA 02115, USA
e-mail: smukundan@partners.org

E. Laws Jr., MD
Department of Neurosurgery, Brigham and Women's Hospital,
15 Francis Street, Boston, MA 02115, USA
e-mail: elaws@partners.org

G. Zada et al. (eds.), *Atlas of Sellar and Parasellar Lesions: Clinical, Radiologic, and Pathologic Correlations*,
DOI 10.1007/978-3-319-22855-6_54

54.2 Imaging Features

- Sellar tuberculomas are frequently mistaken for pituitary adenomas [2].
- They may be intrasellar, suprasellar, or both [6].
- Tuberculomas typically appear as rim-enhancing masses on CT and MRI [7] (Figs. 54.1 and 54.2).
- CT scans may show intralesional calcifications [1].
- Concomitant imaging findings of pachymeningitis may be present with tubercular abscesses [8].
- Thickening of the infundibulum is a common MRI finding, evident in over 80 % of cases [9–11].

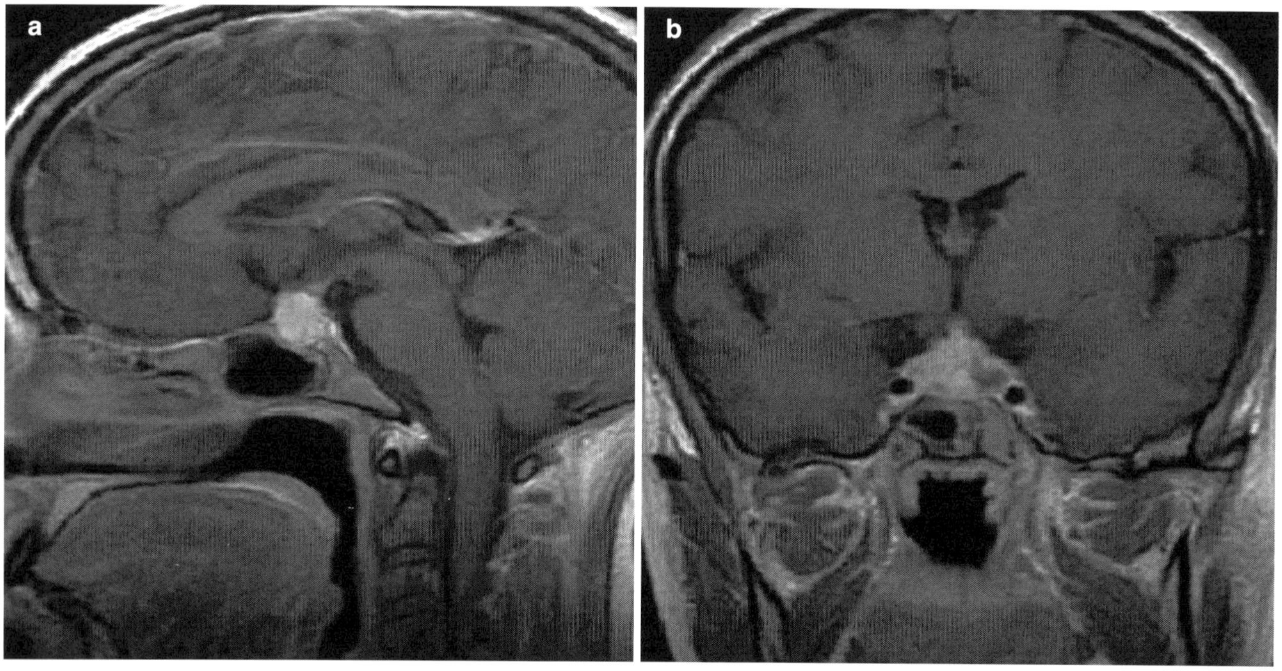

Fig. 54.1 Sellar tuberculoma. (**a**) Sagittal T1-weighted gadolinium-enhanced image. (**b**) Coronal T1-weighted gadolinium-enhanced image. A heterogeneously enhancing mass of the sella and suprasellar region is visualized. A patchy area of hypoenhancement is seen in the left aspect of the pituitary gland

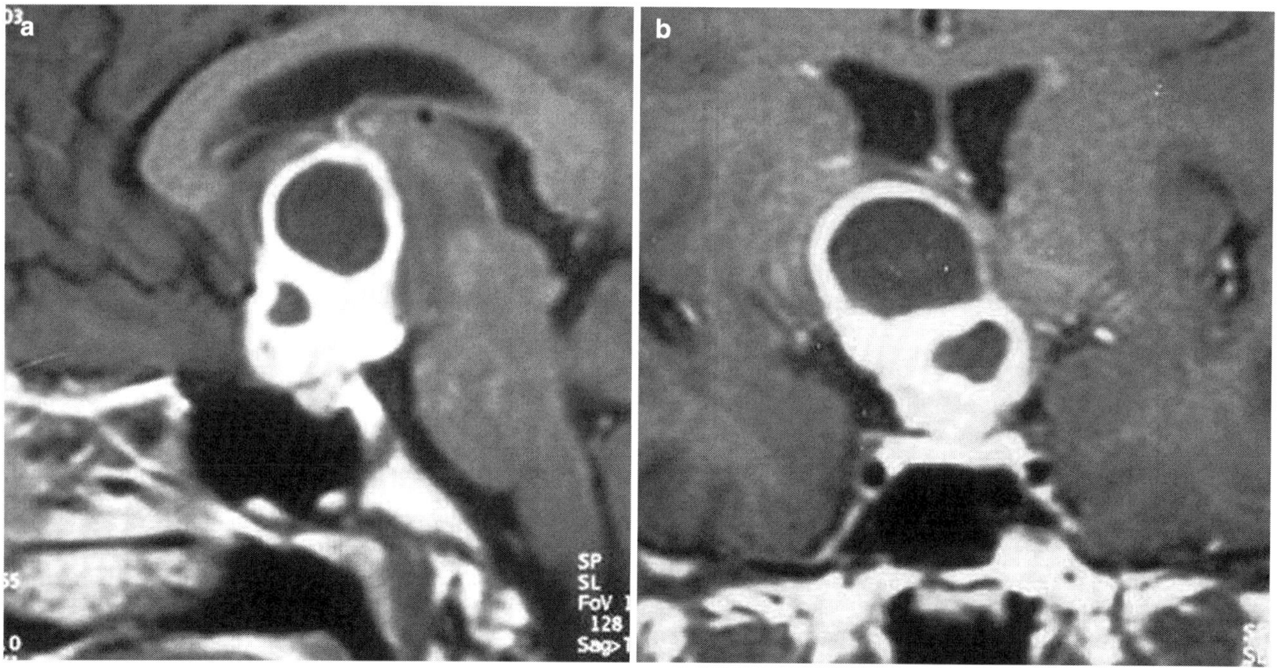

Fig. 54.2 Sellar tuberculoma. Sagittal (**a**) and coronal (**b**) post-contrast MRI shows a large sellar and suprasellar cystic and solid mass with marked enhancement of the peripheral solid part and a nonenhancing central liquefied area (Adapted from Dutta et al. [7], with permission)

54.3 Histopathology

- Tuberculous abscesses are characterized by chronic inflammation, granulomatous change, central caseating necrosis, Langhans giant cells, and epithelioid cells (Fig. 54.3).
- Polymerase chain reaction (PCR) techniques may aid in the diagnosis of tuberculosis.
- CSF analysis may show a lymphocytic reaction with elevated protein.

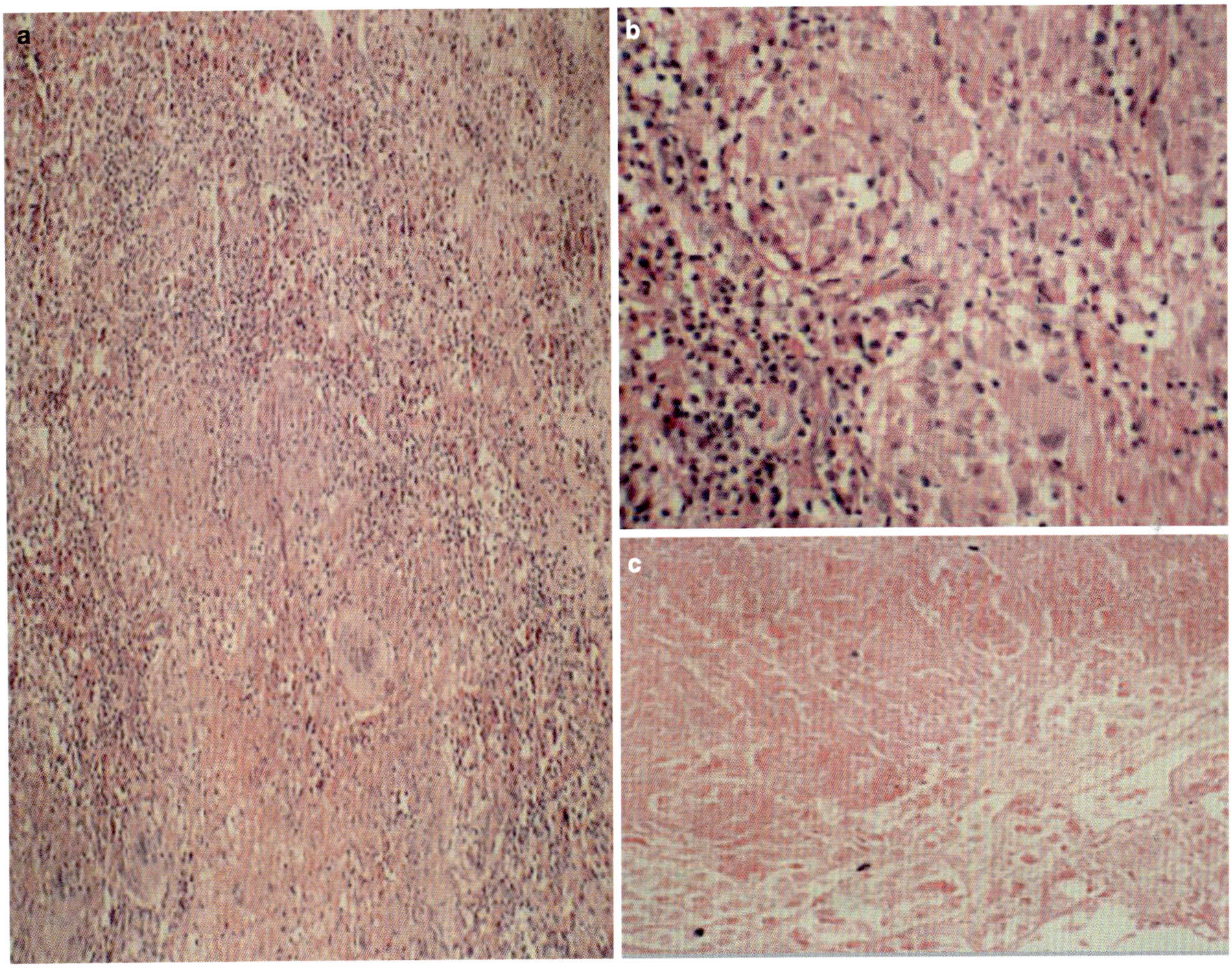

Fig. 54.3 Tuberculous abscess. Paraffin sections showing multiple epithelioid cell granulomas with Langhans type of giant cell (**a**) (H&E ×100), epithelioid cells with slipper-shaped nuclei (**b**) (H&E ×400), and focal areas of necrosis (**c**) (H&E ×400) (From Furtado et al. [3], with permission)

54.4 Clinical and Surgical Management

- Clinical management typically consists of transsphenoidal drainage or resection of the tubercular lesion.
- In many cases, dense adhesion to the optic apparatus is noted, and subtotal resection or simple fenestration should be employed.
- Following diagnosis and surgical management, patients are placed on long-term antitubercular treatment—typically consisting of rifampin, isoniazid, pyrazinamide, and ethambutol (RIPE therapy)—for 6–18 months.
- Outcomes following surgical and antibiotic management are typically good, with few reports of recurrence [2, 12].

References

1. Domingues FS, de Souza JM, Chagas H, Chimelli L, Vaisman M. Pituitary tuberculoma: an unusual lesion of sellar region. Pituitary. 2002;5:149–53.
2. Sharma MC, Arora R, Mahapatra AK, Sarat-Chandra P, Gaikwad SB, Sarkar C. Intrasellar tuberculoma--an enigmatic pituitary infection: a series of 18 cases. Clin Neurol Neurosurg. 2000;102:72–7.
3. Furtado SV, Venkatesh PK, Ghosal N, Hegde AS. Isolated sellar tuberculoma presenting with panhypopituitarism: clinical, diagnostic considerations and literature review. Neurol Sci. 2011;32:301–4.
4. Shukla S, Trivedi A, Singh K, Sharma V. Pituitary tuberculoma. J Neurosci Rural Pract. 2010;1:30–1.
5. Arunkumar MJ, Rajshekhar V. Intrasellar tuberculoma presenting as pituitary apoplexy. Neurol India. 2001;49:407–10.
6. Stalldecker G, Diez S, Carabelli A, Reynoso R, Rey R, Hofmann N, Beresñak A. Pituitary stalk tuberculoma. Pituitary. 2002;5:155–62.
7. Dutta P, Bhansali A, Singh P, Bhat MH. Suprasellar tubercular abscess presenting as panhypopituitarism: a common lesion in an uncommon site with a brief review of literature. Pituitary. 2006;9:73–7.
8. Behari S, Shinghal U, Jain M, Jaiswal AK, Wadwekar V, Das KB, Jha S. Clinicoradiological presentation, management options and a review of sellar and suprasellar tuberculomas. J Clin Neurosci. 2009;16:1560–6.
9. Chandy MJ. Thickening of the pituitary stalk: suggestive of intrasellar tuberculoma. Neurosurgery. 1995;37:1232–3.
10. Mittal P, Dua S, Saggar K, Gupta K. Magnetic resonance findings in sellar and suprasellar tuberculoma with hemorrhage. Surg Neurol Int. 2010;1:73.
11. Ashkan K, Papadopoulos MC, Casey AT, Thompson DN, Jarvis S, Powell M, Thomas DG. Sellar tuberculoma: report of two cases. Acta Neurochir (Wien). 1997;139:523–5.
12. Yilmazlar S, Bekar A, Taskapilioglu O, Tolunay S. Isolated intrasellar tuberculoma mimicking pituitary adenoma. J Clin Neurosci. 2007;14:477–81.

Neurocysticercosis of the Sellar Region

55

Gabriel Zada, M. Beatriz S. Lopes, Srinivasan Mukundan Jr., and Edward Laws Jr.

55.1 Epidemiology and Clinical Presentation

- Neurocysticercosis is the most common parasitic disease affecting the central nervous system (CNS).
- A higher degree of suspicion should be maintained for patients originating from regions where the disease is endemic (typically, developing countries).
- Cysticercosis is caused by the parasite *Taenia solium*, the tissue-invading larval form of the pork tapeworm.
- Cysticercosis can arise almost anywhere in the CNS (intraparenchymal, cisternal, intraventricular) and in rare cases has been described in the sellar or suprasellar region [1].
- Common clinical symptoms and signs of cysticercosis in the sellar region include headache, vision loss, hypopituitarism, seizures, and meningitis [2–4].
- Hydrocephalus is another common finding in patients with intracranial cysticercosis [2].
- Forms of the disease include colloidal, nodular–granular, and racemose (multiple cysts, typically in the basal cisterns) (Fig. 55.1).

G. Zada, MD, MS (✉)
Department of Neurological Surgery, Keck School of Medicine, University of Southern California, 1200 N State Street, #3300, Los Angeles, CA 90033, USA
e-mail: gzada@usc.edu

M.B.S. Lopes, MD, PhD
Department of Pathology (Neuropathology), University of Virginia School of Medicine, 1215 Lee Street, Room 3060–HEP, Charlottesville, VA 22908, USA
e-mail: msl2e@virginia.edu

S. Mukundan Jr., PhD, MD
Department of Radiology, Brigham and Women's Hospital, 75 Francis Street, Boston, MA 02115, USA
e-mail: smukundan@partners.org

E. Laws Jr., MD
Department of Neurosurgery, Brigham and Women's Hospital, 15 Francis Street, Boston, MA 02115, USA
e-mail: elaws@partners.org

G. Zada et al. (eds.), *Atlas of Sellar and Parasellar Lesions: Clinical, Radiologic, and Pathologic Correlations*, DOI 10.1007/978-3-319-22855-6_55

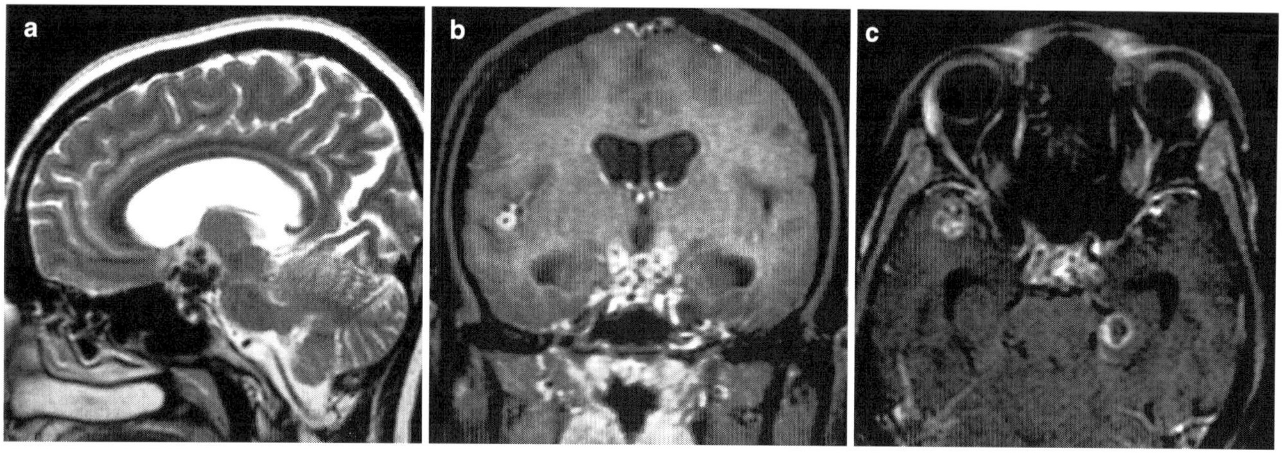

Fig. 55.1 Racemose neurocysticercosis in the pituitary gland. (**a**) Sagittal MR section showing many cystic membranes without a scolex in grapelike clusters in the sellar and suprasellar regions, suggesting racemose neurocysticercosis. Also shown are some single cysts in the cerebellum and brainstem. (**b**) Coronal section showing racemose neurocysticercosis of sellar and suprasellar regions. Some single cysts are also present in the grey–white matter junction of the cerebral cortex. (**c**) Axial section showing racemose neurocysticercosis of sellar and suprasellar regions. Single cysts can be seen in the grey–white matter junction of the cerebral cortex (Adapted from Dutta et al. [1], with permission)

55.2 Imaging Features

- Sellar region cysticercosis may be identified in the sella, in the suprasellar region near the infundibulum and hypothalamus, or in the basal cisterns adjacent to the suprasellar space.
- Isolated sellar cysticercosis cysts represent nearly half of cases, with the remaining patients having evidence of extrasellar or disseminated CNS involvement [3].
- Sellar region cysticercosis may mimic a cystic pituitary adenoma, arachnoid cyst, Rathke cleft cyst, or craniopharyngioma [5, 6].
- CT images often demonstrate bony expansion and erosion of the sella, a hypodense cystic lesion, and occasionally calcification in the mass or in other brain regions, lending support to the diagnosis of cysticercosis [5].
- On MRI, cysticercosis cysts typically have low or high T1 signal and heterogeneous contents [2, 5].
- Enhancement and thickening of the infundibulum may be seen on MRI [7].
- Leptomeningeal enhancement in the parasellar region also may be seen [2].

55.3 Histopathology

- The parasitic wall is characterized microscopically by wavy, dense cuticle and focal globular structures, often suggesting the scolex of the cysticercus [7].
- A surrounding inflammatory, mononuclear lymphocytic reaction with plasma cells is often observed.
- A variable degree of eosinophilia may be seen.

55.4 Clinical and Surgical Management

- Definitive diagnosis of neurocysticercosis may be a challenge.
- Several absolute criteria can establish the diagnosis [8]:
  - Histological evidence of cysticerci
  - Neuroimaging studies showing cystic lesions with a scolex
  - Subretinal parasites on funduscopic examination
- Other criteria can be considered major:
  - Lesions on neuroimaging studies that are highly suggestive of neurocysticercosis
  - Positive serum enzyme-linked immunoelectrotransfer blot (EITB) for the detection of anticysticercal antibodies
  - Resolution of intracranial cystic lesions after cysticidal drug therapy
  - Spontaneous resolution of single enhancing lesions
- The diagnosis can be supported by minor criteria:
  - Lesions on neuroimaging studies that are compatible with neurocysticercosis
  - Suggestive clinical manifestations
  - Positive CSF ELISA for detection of anticysticercal antibodies or cysticercal antigens
  - Cysticercosis outside the nervous system
- Also supporting the diagnosis is epidemiological evidence:
  - A household contact with *Taenia solium* infection
  - History of travel or residence in disease-endemic areas
- For sellar and suprasellar cysticercosis cysts, the transsphenoidal and extended transsphenoidal surgical approaches have been successfully used to achieve fenestration or resection. Open craniotomy has also been used to treat cysticercosis cysts of the suprasellar region.
- Intraventricular cysts may be fenestrated or resected via endoscopic intraventricular approaches.
- The antiparasitic agents albendazole and praziquantel are often administered following the diagnosis.
- In addition to hormonal replacement for hypopituitarism, corticosteroids should be used to decrease local inflammation and edema caused by surgical or medical treatment, as well as any element of meningitis caused by the infection.
- Effective seizure management is critical.
- Visual loss from a cysticercosis cyst may be partially induced by arachnoiditis in addition to compression, so it may fail to improve following surgical decompression [3].

References

1. Dutta D, Kumar M, Ghosh S, Mukhopadhyay S, Chowdhury S. Pituitary hormone deficiency due to racemose neurocysticercosis. Lancet Diabetes Endocrinol. 2013;1(2):e13.
2. Arriada-Mendicoa N, Celis-López MA, Higuera-Calleja J, Corona-Vázquez T. Imaging features of sellar cysticercosis. AJNR Am J Neuroradiol. 2003;24:1386–9.
3. Del Brutto OH, Del Brutto VJ. Intrasellar cysticercosis: a systematic review. Acta Neurol Belg. 2013;113:225–7.
4. Rafael H, Gomez-Llata S. Intrasellar cysticercosis. Case report. J Neurosurg. 1985;63:975–6.
5. Boecher-Schwarz HG, Hey O, Higer HP, Perneczky A. Intrasellar cysticercosis mimicking a pituitary adenoma. Br J Neurosurg. 1991;5:405–7.
6. Del Brutto OH, Guevara J, Sotelo J. Intrasellar cysticercosis. J Neurosurg. 1988;69:58–60.
7. Cheong JH, Kim JM, Kim CH. Neurocysticercosis involving the pituitary stalk: case report and literature review. J Korean Neurosurg Soc. 2010;48:91–3.
8. Del Brutto OH. Diagnostic criteria for neurocysticercosis, revisited. Pathog Glob Health. 2012;106:299–304.

Granulomatous Conditions of the Sellar Region

56

Gabriel Zada, M. Beatriz S. Lopes, Srinivasan Mukundan Jr., and Edward Laws Jr.

- Granulomatous conditions comprise a spectrum of diseases that include granulomatous pseudotumors and abscesses, granulomatous and xanthogranulomatous hypophysitis (see Inflammatory Hypophysitis, Chap. 57), and xanthogranulomas (see Chap. 23).
- Noncaseating, inflammatory granulomatous pseudotumors may be associated with many different conditions [1, 2]:
  - Neurosarcoidosis (see below)
  - Wegener's granulomatosis (see below) [3, 4]
  - Idiopathic giant cell granulomatous hypophysitis [5, 6]
  - Takayasu's disease [7]
  - Cogan's syndrome [8]
  - Crohn's disease [9]
  - Histiocytosis (see Langerhans Cell Histiocytosis, below)
  - Inflammatory pseudotumor (a diagnosis of exclusion) [2]

G. Zada, MD, MS (✉)
Department of Neurological Surgery, Keck School of Medicine, University of Southern California, 1200 N State Street, #3300, Los Angeles, CA 90033, USA
e-mail: gzada@usc.edu

M.B.S. Lopes, MD, PhD
Department of Pathology (Neuropathology), University of Virginia School of Medicine, 1215 Lee Street, Room 3060–HEP, Charlottesville, VA 22908, USA
e-mail: msl2e@virginia.edu

S. Mukundan Jr., PhD, MD
Department of Radiology, Brigham and Women's Hospital, 75 Francis Street, Boston, MA 02115, USA
e-mail: smukundan@partners.org

E. Laws Jr., MD
Department of Neurosurgery, Brigham and Women's Hospital, 15 Francis Street, Boston, MA 02115, USA
e-mail: elaws@partners.org

G. Zada et al. (eds.), *Atlas of Sellar and Parasellar Lesions: Clinical, Radiologic, and Pathologic Correlations*,
DOI 10.1007/978-3-319-22855-6_56

56.1 Neurosarcoidosis of the Sellar and Suprasellar Region

56.1.1 Epidemiology and Clinical Presentation

- Sarcoidosis is an inflammatory multisystem disorder of unknown cause, which is characterized by the formation of noncaseating granulomas. The symptoms of the disease vary according to the location of involvement and its severity.
- Sarcoidosis typically affects the pulmonary system; it manifests in the sellar and suprasellar region in 5–15 % of patients [10–12].
- Neurosarcoidosis involves mostly young and middle-aged adults, with a slightly higher prevalence in women [1, 13].
- It is more common in African-Americans.
- Neurosarcoidosis is often diagnosed in patients with known systemic sarcoidosis who subsequently develop neurological symptoms.
- It has been reported as the primary finding in patients with no evidence of intrathoracic or systemic disease, however [14]. Other sites within the CNS that are more commonly involved than the suprasellar region include the basal meninges, cranial nerves, and posterior fossa.
- Neurosarcoidosis has a subacute or chronic course with neurological and endocrinological signs and symptoms depending on the extension of the lesions. Patients with extensive involvement of the base of the brain and meninges may have hydrocephalus and cranial nerve palsies (including visual dysfunctions) owing to involvement of the optic tract and chiasm [11, 12].
- Isolated pituitary and suprasellar sarcoidosis has been infrequently reported [9, 15].
- The most common endocrinological symptoms of the disease are related to hypothalamic–pituitary system dysfunction, including hypogonadism, diabetes insipidus, and hyperprolactinemia [13, 16].

56.1.2 Imaging Features

- Neurosarcoidosis is often described as a solid or cystic mass of the sellar and suprasellar region, with a thickened capsule wall [17].
- Variable imaging findings may be found on MRI. Lesions are frequently reported to be isointense on T1 imaging and hyperintense on T2 imaging (Fig. 56.1) [18].
- A considerable contrast enhancement pattern of granulomatous component is typical, which may respond to treatment [19].
- Thickening of the infundibulum and attenuation of the posterior pituitary bright spot are frequently associated [20, 21].
- Lesions may be solid or cystic, depending on the contents and degree of necrosis [17].
- Adjacent meningeal enhancement may be identified [19, 22].

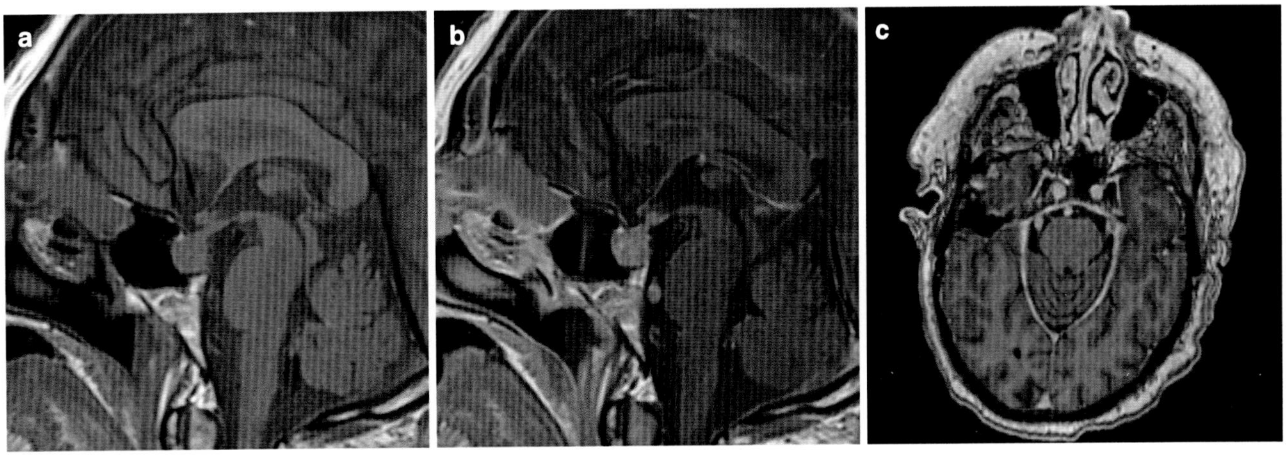

Fig. 56.1 Neurosarcoidosis. (**a**) Sagittal T1-weighted precontrast MR image. (**b**) Sagittal T1-weighted gadolinium-enhanced image. (**c**) Axial T1-weighted gadolinium-enhanced image. On (**a**) and (**b**), the pituitary stalk and gland are diffusely enlarged, with relatively homogeneous enhancement. On (**c**), the cisternal segments of the cranial nerve V demonstrate enhancement

56.1.3 Histopathology

- The histopathology of sarcoidosis involving the hypothalamic–pituitary region is similar to that in other systemic locations, characterized by collections of well-formed, noncaseating granulomas admixed with a moderate amount of lymphoplasmacytic inflammatory infiltrates [23]. Aggregates of activated epithelioid histiocytes with foreign body–type or Langhans multinucleated giant cells are characteristic of the granulomas. The inflammatory infiltrate shows a predominance of CD4+ lymphocytes. Tissue destruction may be extensive, and chronic lesions may present extensive stromal fibrosis and even calcification (Fig. 56.2).
- The diagnosis of sarcoidosis may be difficult and requires the exclusion of other diseases (mainly infectious), by clinical and laboratory means. Histochemical stains for fungi and mycobacteria, microbiological cultures of the tissues, and/or PCR-based tests are mandatory. Likewise, microbiological studies of CSF and serum should be performed to exclude more systemic infectious causes.
- Other causes of systemic granulomatous diseases (such as Churg–Strauss syndrome, lymphomatoid granulomatosis, and Wegener's granulomatosis) should also be ruled out. Detailed clinical and laboratory correlation is significant for the differential diagnosis.
- Involvement of the sella and suprasellar structures in Wegener's granulomatosis is uncommon. Radiologically, the gland is diffusely enlarged and exhibits a more homogeneous pattern of enhancement [21].
- Tuberculosis of the sellar and parasellar region is extremely rare. It has been reported to present in many ways, such as a thickened stalk, a hypophysitis with contiguous involvement of the stalk, a mass similar to a pituitary adenoma, and even a pituitary abscess.
- Neurosarcoidosis can be differentiated from tuberculous granulomas or abscesses via caseating necrosis and positive acid-fast bacillus (AFB) cultures.
- Xanthogranulomas are a separate entity that may be related to chronic inflammation in the setting of a craniopharyngioma or Rathke cleft cyst. (See Chaps. 21 and 22.)

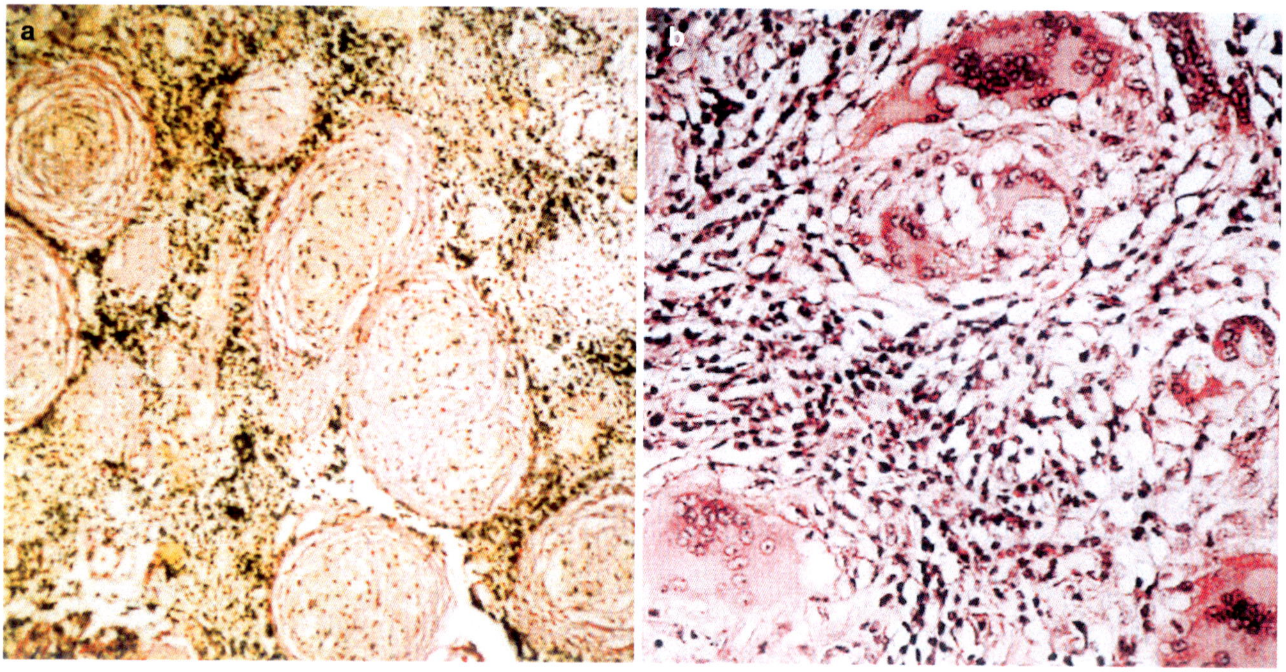

Fig. 56.2 Neurosarcoidosis. (**a**) Characteristic noncaseating sarcoid granulomas embedded within a fibrous stroma (Van Gieson, original magnification ×80). (**b**) Sarcoid granulomas consisting of follicles with central, multinucleated giant cells (some with polymorph, conchoid inclusion bodies) surrounded by epithelioid macrophages and fibroblasts (H&E, original magnification ×200) (Adapted from Nowak and Widenka [23], with permission)

56.1.4 Clinical and Surgical Management

- Surgical intervention, often via a transsphenoidal approach, can be utilized for biopsy or debulking, especially for drainage of cystic masses.
- For any granulomatous lesions, tuberculosis should be ruled out with PPD and chest x-ray.
- Upon diagnosis of a noncaseating granuloma without previously known systemic disease, a thorough workup for systemic conditions should be performed. For neurosarcoidosis, this workup includes a serum angiotensin-converting enzyme (ACE) level, erythrocyte sedimentation rate (ESR), calcium levels, gallium-67 lung scan, and bronchoalveolar lavage [24].
- CSF studies also should be performed, including cytology, cell counts, and ACE levels [16].
- Medical therapy typically includes corticosteroids and perhaps cyclosporine A or chloroquine [25, 26].
- Up to 87 % of neurosarcoidosis lesions will improve with steroid treatment, especially in regard to demonstration of contrast enhancement [27].
- Central diabetes insipidus and hypopituitarism typically fail to improve after treatment [16].

56.2 Wegener's Granulomatosis of the Sellar Region

56.2.1 Epidemiology and Clinical Presentation

- Wegener's granulomatosis (WG), a type of autoimmune vasculitis of small- and medium-sized blood vessels, rarely has intracranial manifestations. It typically manifests in the lungs, skin, and kidneys, but in rare cases, WG has been described to involve the pituitary gland and parasellar region.
- Pituitary WG is almost always diagnosed in the presence of other systemic findings [28].
- The mean age of patients with pituitary WG is 38 years [28].
- Diabetes insipidus and hypopituitarism are common features of WG involving the pituitary gland [4, 28–30].
- Involvement of the cavernous sinus presenting with cranial nerve paresis has also been described [31].
- Systemic manifestations of WG may also be evident, including fevers, rash, and pulmonary features [29].

56.2.2 Imaging Features

- On MRI, WG of the pituitary gland typically appears as an enhancing mass that is hypointense on T1-weighted imaging and hyperintense on T2 imaging (Fig. 56.3) [28, 29, 32].
- MRI also may show extension from the paranasal sinuses into the sella and cavernous sinus, often with meningeal thickening [31].
- Infundibular thickening and cystic changes also may be seen on MRI [28].
- Loss of the normal posterior pituitary bright spot may be seen, especially in patients with WG and diabetes insipidus (Fig. 56.4) [21, 32].
- The disease may be characterized by exacerbations and periods of quiescence during which MRI findings may appear essentially normal [21].

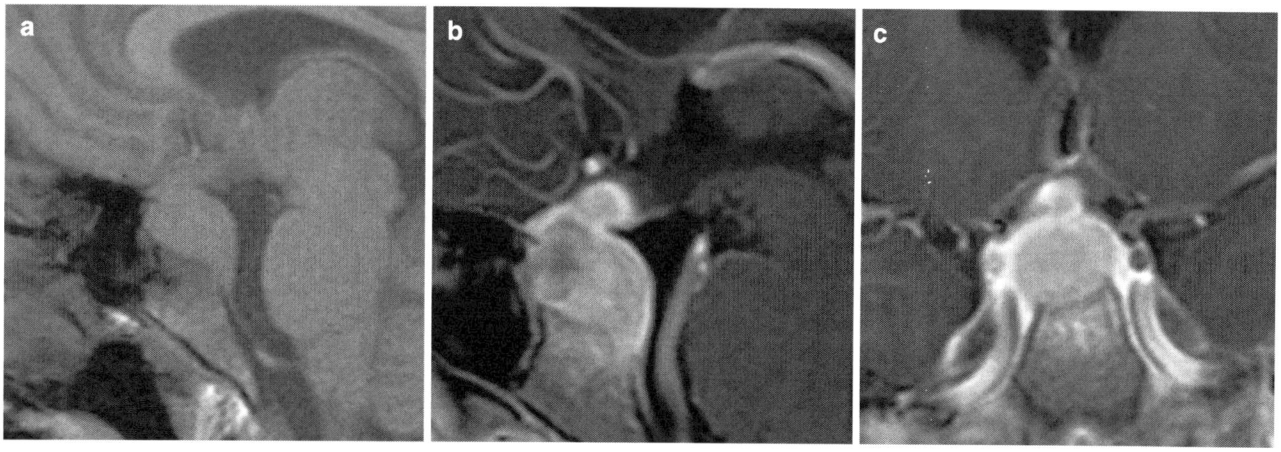

Fig. 56.3 Wegener's granulomatosis. (**a**) Sagittal T1-weighted precontrast MR image. (**b**) Sagittal T1-weighted gadolinium-enhanced image. (**c**) Coronal T1-weighted gadolinium-enhanced image. The pituitary stalk and gland are diffusely enlarged, with homogeneous enhancement. On (**b**), erosion of the sellar floor and enhancement of the upper clivus are visible

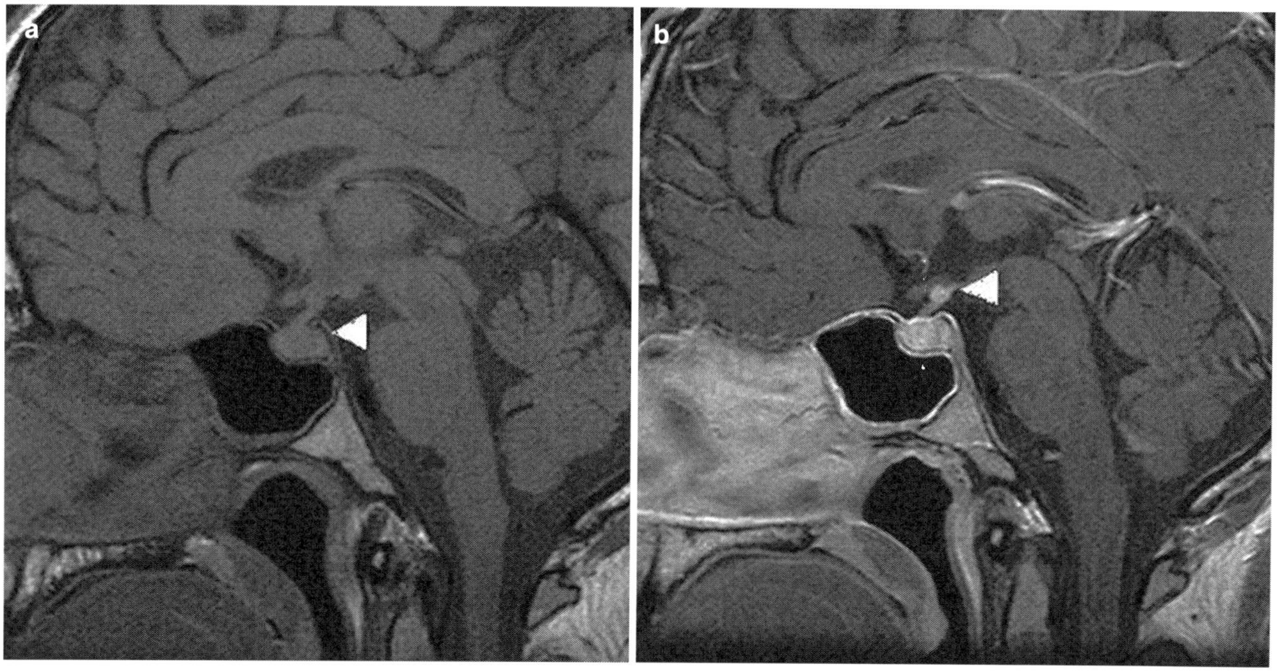

Fig. 56.4 Wegener's granulomatosis. (**a**) An unenhanced T1-weighted sagittal MR image through the pituitary gland shows the absence of the "bright spot" of the posterior pituitary (*white arrowhead*), typically seen with central diabetes insipidus. (**b**) A post-gadolinium T1-weighted sagittal image shows an enhancing nodule at the superior aspect of the infundibulum (*white arrowhead*) (Adapted from Yong et al. [28], with permission)

56.2.3 Histopathology

- WG is characterized by inflammation of the small blood vessels (polyangiitis).
- Granulomatous necrotizing inflammation of the pituitary gland can be seen [33].
- The disease is characterized histologically by an inflammatory infiltrate comprising neutrophils, lymphocytes, plasma cells, histiocytes, and eosinophils.

56.2.4 Clinical and Surgical Management

- The diagnosis of WG can be made by confirming c-antineutrophil cytoplasmic antibodies (c-ANCA) and positive skin lesions showing leukocytoclastic vasculitis [29].
- ANCA is positive in 80–95 % of cases [28].
- Proteinase 3 (PR3) positivity is seen in 70–80 % of ANCA-positive patients [28].
- The role of surgery is minimal in this disease; it may be limited to biopsy and/or sellar decompression.
- Systemic treatment often includes high-dose corticosteroids and immunosuppressive medications such as cyclophosphamide. Most patients respond favorably to cyclophosphamide, although one review reported relapse in 27 % of patients [28].
- The monoclonal antibody rituximab has recently been used successfully to treat refractory pituitary WG [34].
- Hypopituitarism and diabetes insipidus rarely improve after remission of pituitary WG, making vigilant endocrinological follow-up imperative [28].

56.3 Langerhans Cell Histiocytosis

56.3.1 Epidemiology and Clinical Presentation

- Langerhans cell histiocytosis (LCH), previously called histiocytosis X, is a clonal neoplastic proliferation of Langerhans-type histiocytes that typically develops in childhood.
- The estimated incidence of LCH in children is 1–5 per million per year [35].
- In children, the median age at diagnosis is 30 months.
- LCH may present in young adult patients (mean age 34 years), typically with diabetes insipidus and hypopituitarism [36].
- LCH is more common in males overall, but isolated hypothalamic–pituitary involvement may be more common in females [37].
- The wide spectrum of clinical presentation includes many syndromes [38]:
  - Eosinophilic granuloma: unifocal or multifocal lytic bony disease
  - Hand–Schuller–Christian disease: diabetes insipidus, exophthalmos, and bony lesions
  - Letterer–Siwe disease: fulminant disease occurring in infants
- Most children present with monostotic (61 %) or polyostotic lesions (27 %).
- Isolated skull lesions are the most common presentation.
- A unifocal hypothalamic–pituitary lesion (Gagel granuloma) is the presentation in 5 % [38].
- LCH granulomas comprise approximately 0.05 % of cases in major transsphenoidal series [39].
- The most common (and often the first) manifestation is central diabetes insipidus, occurring in 11–25 % of patients with LCH [37, 40–42].
- Anterior pituitary dysfunction occurs in up to 24 % of patients overall, almost always in association with diabetes insipidus [37, 43].
- Growth hormone (GH) deficiency develops in more than half of patients with diabetes insipidus [44].

56.3.2 Imaging Features

- LCH patients with sellar region findings on MRI often present with:
  - Thickening of the pituitary stalk (50–86 %) (Fig. 56.5) [45, 46]
  - Infundibular atrophy (8–29 %) [45, 46]
  - Suprasellar granuloma: typically isointense on T1-weighted images and hyperintense on T2-weighted images (10 %) [47]
  - Loss of hyperintensity of the neurohypophysis (posterior pituitary bright spot) on T1-weighted imaging [36, 45, 48]
- Intracranial involvement can be multifocal, frequently involving the cerebellum with enhancing or nonenhancing signal abnormalities.

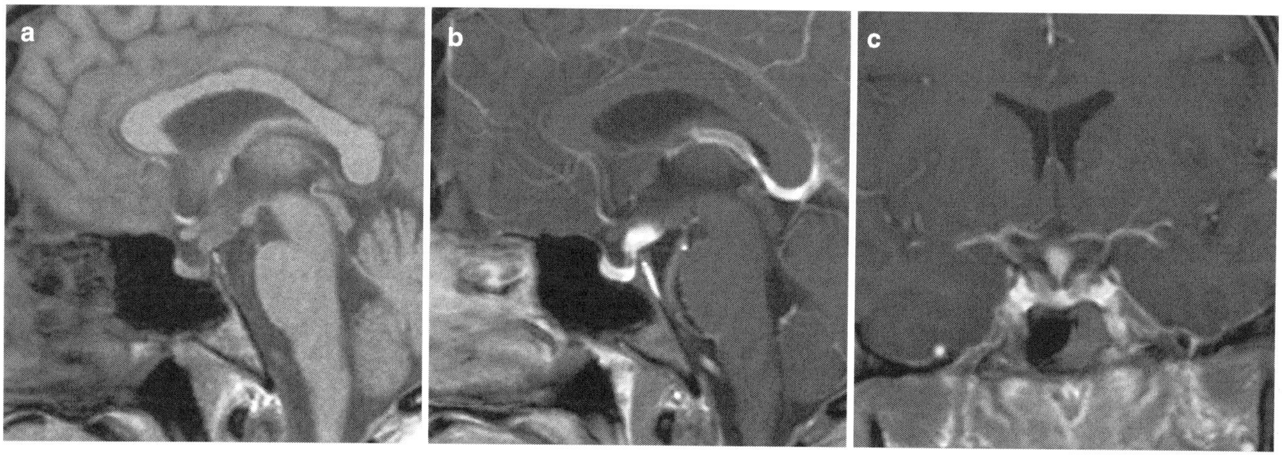

Fig. 56.5 Langerhans cell histiocytosis. (**a**) Sagittal T1-weighted precontrast MR image. (**b**) Sagittal T1-weighted gadolinium-enhanced image. (**c**) Coronal T1-weighted gadolinium-enhanced image. The pituitary stalk demonstrates nodular enhancement superiorly. The pituitary gland is normal in size

56.3.3 Histopathology

- Langerhans cell histiocytosis is characterized by a proliferation of Langerhans histiocytes admixed with giant cells, lymphocytes, plasma cells, and eosinophils in greatly varying numbers.
- Langerhans cells are typically large cells with eosinophilic, granular cytoplasm and a distinct folded nucleus (Fig. 56.6).
- The Langerhans histiocytes are immunoreactive for S100 protein, CD1a, and Langerin (CD207) [49, 50].
- By electron microscopy, the cells show Birbeck granules.
- The diagnosis of Langerhans cell histiocytosis may be difficult, depending on the stage of the disease process. In late stages of the disease, fibrotic lesions with minimal inflammatory infiltrates are not uncommon.

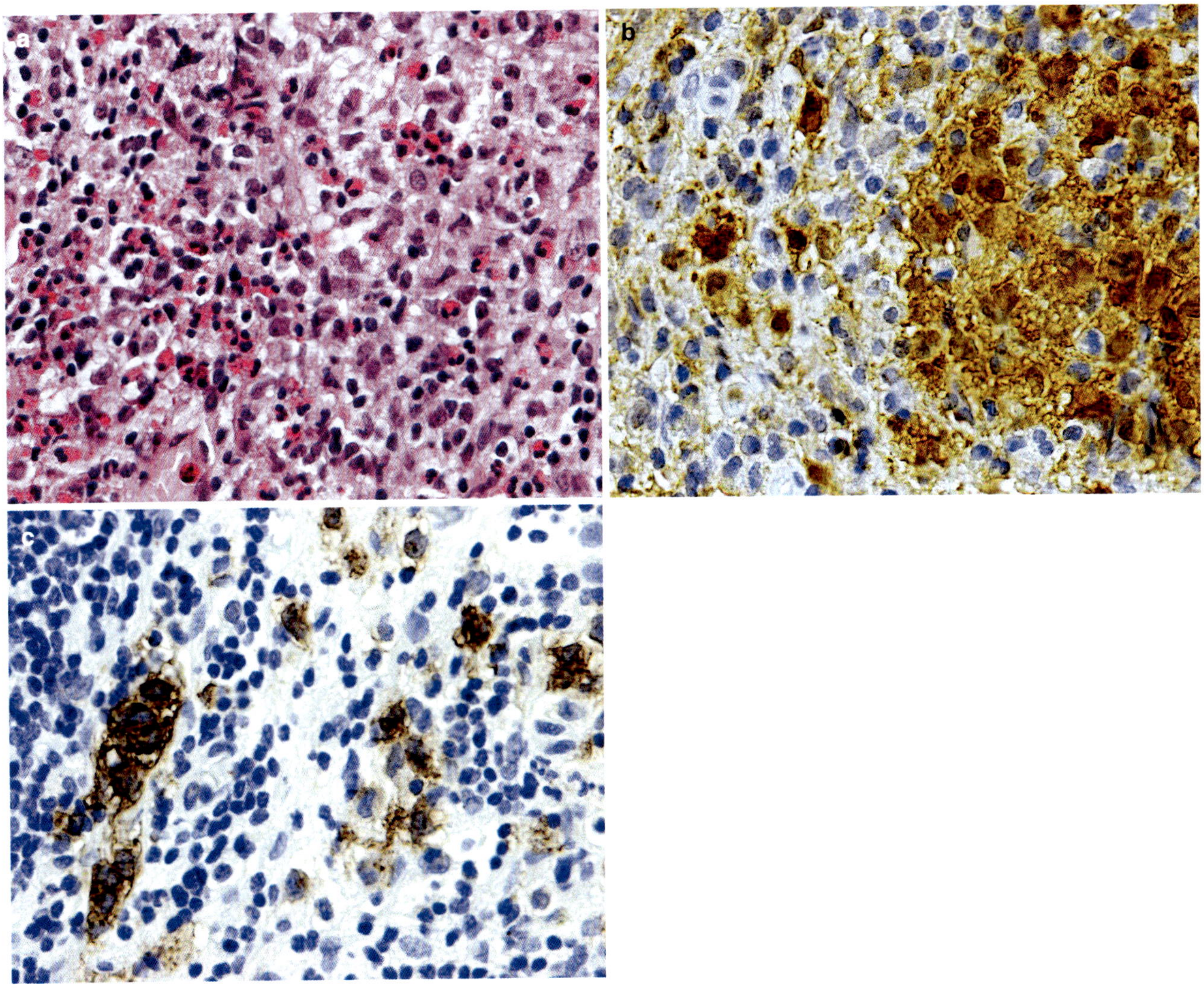

Fig. 56.6 Langerhans cell histiocytosis is characterized by a proliferation of Langerhans histiocytes admixed with giant cells, lymphocytes, plasma cells, and eosinophils in greatly varying numbers (**a**). Langerhans histiocytes are distinguished by large, folded nuclei and are immunoreactive for Langerin, S100 protein (**b**), and CD1a (**c**)

56.3.4 Clinical and Surgical Management

- Conservative management may be justified in many cases, as the disease is often self-limited and spontaneous resolution has been reported [51].
- Some LCH patients developing a suprasellar mass will already have skull or other bony lesions, obviating the need for a biopsy of the mass in the suprasellar region [38].
- If the diagnosis has already been established, serial imaging can often be performed to monitor the lesion.
- A biopsy for tissue diagnosis (in addition to CSF markers obtained via lumbar puncture) may be required, especially to differentiate between LCH and germinoma.
- Transsphenoidal resection of sellar and suprasellar LCH granulomas has been reported [52]; open craniotomies have also been used for biopsy and microsurgical resection [53].
- When necessary, adjunctive treatment often includes chemotherapy, low-dose radiation, and steroids, although many of these regimens remain controversial [54].
- Stereotactic radiosurgery has been successfully used to treat suprasellar LCH [55].
- Diabetes insipidus has been reported to improve in some patients following surgical resection [52, 53].
- Anterior hypopituitarism typically does not improve after treatment, and long-standing neuropsychological changes may be seen in many patients [40, 56].
- Endocrine replacement—particularly of the GH axis—may be required [43].

References

1. Carpinteri R, Patelli I, Casanueva FF, Giustina A. Pituitary tumours: inflammatory and granulomatous expansive lesions of the pituitary. Best Pract Res Clin Endocrinol Metab. 2009;23:639–50.
2. Hansen I, Petrossians P, Thiry A, Flandroy P, Gaillard RC, Kovacs K, et al. Extensive inflammatory pseudotumor of the pituitary. J Clin Endocrinol Metab. 2001;86:4603–10.
3. Dutta P, Hayatbhat M, Bhansali A, Bambery P, Kakar N. Wegener's granulomatosis presenting as diabetes insipidus. Exp Clin Endocrinol Diabetes. 2006;114:533–6.
4. Roberts GA, Eren E, Sinclair H, Pelling M, Burns A, Bradford R, et al. Two cases of Wegener's granulomatosis involving the pituitary. Clin Endocrinol (Oxf). 1995;42:323–8.
5. Bhansali A, Velayutham P, Radotra BD, Pathak A. Idiopathic granulomatous hypophysitis presenting as non-functioning pituitary adenoma: description of six cases and review of literature. Br J Neurosurg. 2004;18:489–94.
6. Mehndiratta MM, Phul P, Singh AK, Garg S, Bali R. Granulomatous hypophysitis--an interesting and rare cause mimicking pituitary mass. J Assoc Physicians India. 2007;55:653–4.
7. Toth M, Szabo P, Racz K, Szende B, Balogh I, Czirjak S, et al. Granulomatous hypophysitis associated with Takayasu's disease. Clin Endocrinol (Oxf). 1996;45:499–503.
8. Kanatani M, Nakamura R, Kurokawa K, Taoda M, Nemoto Y, Kamakura K, et al. Hypopituitarism associated with Cogan's syndrome; high-dose glucocorticoid therapy reverses pituitary swelling. Jpn J Med. 1991;30:164–9.
9. de Bruin WI, van 't Verlaat JW, de Bruin TW. Sellar granulomatous mass in a pregnant woman with active Crohn's disease. Neth J Med. 1991;39:136–41.
10. Pillai P, Ray-Chaudhury A, Ammirati M, Chiocca EA. Solitary pituitary sarcoidosis with normal endocrine function: case report. J Neurosurg. 2008;108:591–4.
11. Chen RC, McLeod JG. Neurological complications of sarcoidosis. Clin Exp Neurol. 1989;26:99–112.
12. Hoitsma E, Faber CG, Drent M, Sharma OP. Neurosarcoidosis: a clinical dilemma. Lancet Neurol. 2004;3:397–407.
13. Bihan H, Christozova V, Dumas JL, Jomaa R, Valeyre D, Tazi A, et al. Sarcoidosis: clinical, hormonal, and magnetic resonance imaging (MRI) manifestations of hypothalamic-pituitary disease in 9 patients and review of the literature. Medicine (Baltimore). 2007;86:259–68.
14. Lara Capellan JI, Cuellar Olmedo L, Martinez Martin J, del Marin Mar M, Garcia Villanueva M, Marin Zarza F, de la Blasco Calle H. Intrasellar mass with hypopituitarism as a manifestation of sarcoidosis. Case report. J Neurosurg. 1990;73:283–6.
15. Chevrette E, Morissette L, Gould P. Neurosarcoidosis presenting as an intrasellar pseudotumoral mass: case report. Can Assoc Radiol J. 1999;50:407–12.
16. Bullmann C, Faust M, Hoffmann A, Heppner C, Jockenhovel F, Muller-Wieland D, Krone W. Five cases with central diabetes insipidus and hypogonadism as first presentation of neurosarcoidosis. Eur J Endocrinol. 2000;142:365–72.
17. Sato N, Sze G, Kim JH. Cystic pituitary mass in neurosarcoidosis. AJNR Am J Neuroradiol. 1997;18:1182–5.
18. Gazioglu N, Tuzgen S, Oz B, Kocer N, Kafadar A, Akar Z, Kuday C. Idiopathic granulomatous hypophysitis: are there reliable, constant radiological and clinical diagnostic criterias? Neuroradiology. 2000;42:890–4.
19. Vasile M, Marsot-Dupuch K, Kujas M, Brunereau L, Bouchard P, Comoy J, Tubiana JM. Idiopathic granulomatous hypophysitis: clinical and imaging features. Neuroradiology. 1997;39:7–11.

20. Tabuena RP, Nagai S, Handa T, Shigematsu M, Hamada K, Ito I, et al. Diabetes insipidus from neurosarcoidosis: long-term follow-up for more than eight years. Intern Med. 2004;43:960–6.
21. Katzman GL, Langford CA, Sneller MC, Koby M, Patronas NJ. Pituitary involvement by Wegener's granulomatosis: a report of two cases. AJNR Am J Neuroradiol. 1999;20:519–23.
22. Wilson JD, Jacobs M, Shuer L, Atlas S, Horoupian DS. Idiopathic giant-cell granulomatous hypophysitis. Report of a case with autopsy follow-up. Clin Neuropathol. 2000;19:300–4.
23. Nowak DA, Widenka DC. Neurosarcoidosis: a review of its intracranial manifestation. J Neurol. 2001;248:363–72.
24. Sharma OP, Anders A. Neurosarcoidosis. A report of ten patients illustrating some usual and unusual manifestations. Sarcoidosis. 1985;2:96–106.
25. Murialdo G, Tamagno G. Endocrine aspects of neurosarcoidosis. J Endocrinol Invest. 2002;25:650–62.
26. Sharma OP. Neurosarcoidosis: a personal perspective based on the study of 37 patients. Chest. 1997;112:220–8.
27. Lexa FJ, Grossman RI. MR of sarcoidosis in the head and spine: spectrum of manifestations and radiographic response to steroid therapy. AJNR Am J Neuroradiol. 1994;15:973–82.
28. Yong TY, Li JY, Amato L, Mahadevan K, Phillips PJ, Coates PS, Coates PT. Pituitary involvement in Wegener's granulomatosis. Pituitary. 2008;11:77–84.
29. Garovic VD, Clarke BL, Chilson TS, Specks U. Diabetes insipidus and anterior pituitary insufficiency as presenting features of Wegener's granulomatosis. Am J Kidney Dis. 2001;37(1):E5.
30. Tenorio Jimenez C, Montalvo Valdivieso A, López Gallardo G, Mcgowan B. Pituitary involvement in Wegener's granulomatosis: unusual biochemical findings and severe malnutrition. BMJ Case Rep. 2011;2011. doi: 10.1136/bcr.02.2011.3850.
31. Hermann M, Bobek-Billewicz B, Bullo B, Hermann A, Rutkowski B. Wegener's granulomatosis with unusual cavernous sinus and sella turcica extension. Eur Radiol. 1999;9:1859–61.
32. Barlas NB, Hassan HH, Al Badr FB, Bilal A. Structural and functional involvement of pituitary gland in Wegener's granulomatosis. Clin Neuroradiol. 2011;21:31–3.
33. Woywodt A, Knoblauch H, Kettritz R, Schneider W, Göbel U. Sudden death and Wegener's granulomatosis of the pituitary. Scand J Rheumatol. 2000;29:264–6.
34. Hughes J, Barkhoudarian G, Ciarlini P, Laws ER, Mody E, Inzucchi SE, Woodmansee WW. Refractory pituitary granulomatosis with polyangiitis (Wegener's) treated with rituximab. Endocr Pract. 2013;19(1):e1–7.
35. Cochrane LA, Prince M, Clarke K. Langerhans' cell histiocytosis in the paediatric population: presentation and treatment of head and neck manifestations. J Otolaryngol. 2003;32:33–7.
36. Kaltsas GA, Powles TB, Evanson J, Plowman PN, Drinkwater JE, Jenkins PJ, et al. Hypothalamo-pituitary abnormalities in adult patients with Langerhans cell histiocytosis: clinical, endocrinological, and radiological features and response to treatment. J Clin Endocrinol Metab. 2000;85:1370–6.
37. Modan-Moses D, Weintraub M, Meyerovitch J, Segal-Lieberman G, Bielora B. Hypopituitarism in Langerhans cell histiocytosis: seven cases and literature review. J Endocrinol Invest. 2001;24:612–7.
38. Davidson L, McComb JG, Bowen I, Krieger MD. Craniospinal Langerhans cell histiocytosis in children: 30 years' experience at a single institution. J Neurosurg Pediatr. 2008;1:187–95.
39. Saeger W, Ludecke DK, Buchfelder M, Fahlbusch R, Quabbe HJ, Petersenn S. Pathohistological classification of pituitary tumors: 10 years of experience with the German Pituitary Tumor Registry. Eur J Endocrinol. 2007;156:203–16.
40. Makras P, Alexandraki KI, Chrousos GP, Grossman AB, Kaltsas GA. Endocrine manifestations in Langerhans cell histiocytosis. Trends Endocrinol Metab. 2007;18:252–7.
41. D'Ambrosio N, Soohoo S, Warshall C, Johnson A, Karimi S. Craniofacial and intracranial manifestations of Langerhans cell histiocytosis: report of findings in 100 patients. AJR Am J Roentgenol. 2008;191:589–97.
42. Atchison JA, Hedlund GL, Berkow R. Diabetes insipidus and histiocytosis X: a case of isolated pituitary involvement. Endocr Pract. 1995;1:318–9.
43. Donadieu J, Rolon MA, Thomas C, Brugieres L, Plantaz D, Emile JF, et al. Endocrine involvement in pediatric-onset Langerhans' cell histiocytosis: a population-based study. J Pediatr. 2004;144:344–50.
44. Donadieu J, Rolon MA, Pion I, Thomas C, Doz F, Barkaoui M, et al. Incidence of growth hormone deficiency in pediatric-onset Langerhans cell histiocytosis: efficacy and safety of growth hormone treatment. J Clin Endocrinol Metab. 2004;89:604–9.
45. Varan A, Cila A, Akyuz C, Kale G, Kutluk T, Buyukpamukcu M. Radiological evaluation of patients with pituitary Langerhans cell histiocytosis at diagnosis and at follow-up. Pediatr Hematol Oncol. 2008;25:567–74.
46. Prayer D, Grois N, Prosch H, Gadner H, Barkovich AJ. MR imaging presentation of intracranial disease associated with Langerhans cell histiocytosis. AJNR Am J Neuroradiol. 2004;25:880–91.
47. Isoo A, Ueki K, Ishida T, Yoshikawa T, Fujimaki T, Suzuki I, et al. Langerhans cell histiocytosis limited to the pituitary-hypothalamic axis--two case reports. Neurol Med Chir (Tokyo). 2000;40:532–5.
48. Hamilton BE, Salzman KL, Osborn AG. Anatomic and pathologic spectrum of pituitary infundibulum lesions. AJR Am J Roentgenol. 2007;188:W223–32.
49. Hieronimus S, Hadjali Y, Fredenrich A, Paquis P, Chanalet S, Grimaud A, et al. Hypothalamic-pituitary Langerhans cell histiocytosis: a diagnostic challenge. Ann Endocrinol (Paris). 2000;61:512–6.
50. Valladeau J, Ravel O, Dezutter-Dambuyant C, Moore K, Kleijmeer M, Liu Y, et al. Langerin, a novel C-type lectin specific to Langerhans cells, is an endocytic receptor that induces the formation of Birbeck granules. Immunity. 2000;12:71–81.
51. Gunny R, Clifton A, Al-Memar A. Spontaneous regression of supratentorial intracerebral Langerhans' cell histiocytosis. Br J Radiol. 2004;77:685–7.
52. Nishio S, Mizuno J, Barrow DL, Takei Y, Tindall GT. Isolated histiocytosis X of the pituitary gland: case report. Neurosurgery. 1987;21:718–21.
53. d'Avella D, Giusa M, Blandino A, Angileri FF, La Rosa G, Tomasello F. Microsurgical excision of a primary isolated hypothalamic eosinophilic granuloma. Case report. J Neurosurg. 1997;87:768–72.
54. Asano T, Goto Y, Kida S, Ohno K, Hirakawa K. Isolated histiocytosis X of the pituitary stalk. J Neuroradiol. 1999;26:277–80.
55. Hong WC, Murovic JA, Gibbs I, Vogel H, Chang SD. Pituitary stalk Langerhans cell histiocytosis treated with CyberKnife radiosurgery. Clin Neurol Neurosurg. 2013;115:573–7.
56. Fahrner B, Prosch H, Minkov M, Krischmann M, Gadner H, Prayer D, Grois N. Long-term outcome of hypothalamic pituitary tumors in Langerhans cell histiocytosis. Pediatr Blood Cancer. 2012;58:606–10.

Inflammatory Hypophysitis

57

Gabriel Zada, M. Beatriz S. Lopes,
Srinivasan Mukundan Jr., and Edward Laws Jr.

57.1 Epidemiology and Clinical Presentation

- Inflammatory diseases of the pituitary gland are uncommon and may mimic sellar masses. The most clinically relevant of these disorders is autoimmune lymphocytic hypophysitis, which is characterized by focal or diffuse inflammatory infiltration and the ultimate destruction of the gland. Hypophysitis may involve the adenohypophysis, neurohypophysis, infundibulum, or combined sites.
- On rare occasions, the pituitary gland may be involved secondarily by systemic inflammatory processes involving an infectious agent (bacterial, viral, or fungal) or a systemic disease (i.e., secondary hypophysitis).

57.1.1 Primary Hypophysitis

- Primary hypophysitis may be classified into one of three main histological categories: lymphocytic, granulomatous, and xanthomatous [1]. (The histologies of these categories are discussed separately below.)
- All types of inflammatory hypophysitis frequently present with severe hypopituitarism (60–80 %), headache (60–75 %), and visual loss (20–40 %) [2, 3].
- Taken together, inflammatory hypophysitis comprises roughly 0.5 % of lesions treated in major transsphenoidal series, with lymphocytic hypophysitis being more than twice as common as granulomatous or xanthomatous hypophysitis [4].
- Inflammatory hypophysitis is initially misdiagnosed as pituitary adenoma in up to 40 % of patients.
- The onset and development of symptoms in hypophysitis, however, are usually more rapid than in patients who have pituitary adenomas.
- Hypocortisolemia and hypothyroidism have been reported to occur earlier in the disease course than in patients with pituitary macroadenomas [2].
- Diabetes insipidus has been reported in approximately 15–30 % of patients [2].
- Aseptic meningitis and occlusion of the internal carotid artery have been rarely reported in association with this disorder [3].
- Lymphocytic hypophysitis is typically idiopathic, but often it is associated with recent pregnancy. An association with other autoimmune or inflammatory conditions has been reported, including paraneoplastic disease, thyroiditis, systemic lupus erythematosus, and temporal arteritis [3, 5].
- Lymphocytic hypophysitis most commonly affects women, but this syndrome also has been reported in males [1, 3, 5, 6]. Patients may have symptoms of an expanding pituitary mass, evidence of partial hypopituitarism or panhypopituitarism, or both. Mild hyperprolactinemia may be seen, owing to stalk compression. Diabetes insipidus has been described in some patients, indicating that the inflammatory process also may involve the posterior pituitary gland and pituitary stalk [6]. In this instance, the name of *infundibuloneurohypophysitis* is recognized.

G. Zada, MD, MS (✉)
Department of Neurological Surgery,
Keck School of Medicine, University of Southern California,
1200 N State Street, #3300, Los Angeles, CA 90033, USA
e-mail: gzada@usc.edu

M.B.S. Lopes, MD, PhD
Department of Pathology (Neuropathology),
University of Virginia School of Medicine,
1215 Lee Street, Room 3060–HEP, Charlottesville,
VA 22908, USA
e-mail: msl2e@virginia.edu

S. Mukundan Jr., PhD, MD
Department of Radiology, Brigham and Women's Hospital,
75 Francis Street, Boston, MA 02115, USA
e-mail: smukundan@partners.org

E. Laws Jr., MD
Department of Neurosurgery, Brigham and Women's Hospital,
15 Francis Street, Boston, MA 02115, USA
e-mail: elaws@partners.org

G. Zada et al. (eds.), *Atlas of Sellar and Parasellar Lesions: Clinical, Radiologic, and Pathologic Correlations*,
DOI 10.1007/978-3-319-22855-6_57

- Unlike lymphocytic hypophysitis, granulomatous hypophysitis has no relation to pregnancy. It most often involves middle-aged or elderly women, but the gender predilection is less strong [3, 7]. The majority of patients present with signs and symptoms of hypopituitarism [7].
- Xanthomatous hypophysitis is the least frequent form of primary hypophysitis [5, 7–9]. Although most cases are described in women, no association with pregnancy or the postpartum state has been described. Patients tend to be younger than those with lymphocytic or granulomatous hypophysitis [7]. Clinical symptoms most often are due to mild anterior pituitary axis failure and less commonly are associated with posterior pituitary involvement [7].

57.1.2 Secondary Hypophysitis

- Secondary hypophysitis occurs in the setting of known infectious or systemic inflammatory conditions, such as Wegener's granulomatosis, sarcoidosis, tuberculosis, Crohn's disease, or Langerhans cell histiocytosis.
- IgG4-related hypophysitis is a relatively new entity that is systemic in nature and affects multiple organ systems [10].
- Recently, an autoimmune hypophysitis has been described as an adverse effect of the anti-melanoma drug ipilimumab, a monoclonal immunomodulatory antibody targeting cytotoxic T-lymphocyte antigen 4 (CTLA-4) [11].
- Hypophysitis can be associated with an underlying structural lesion such as a Rathke cleft cyst or pituitary adenoma. In cases of Rathke cleft cysts, it has been postulated that leakage of caustic contents from the cyst may cause inflammation in the pituitary gland [12–15].
- Hypophysitis may be the initial histopathological finding prior to the diagnosis of a neoplastic disease such as a germinoma or lymphoma [16–18].

57.2 Imaging Features

- Hypophysitis is characterized by a sellar mass with suprasellar extension in 80 % of patients [3].
- It often mimics a pituitary adenoma on neuroimaging studies [19, 20].
- On MRI, the inflammatory mass is typically isointense on T1-weighted imaging and heterogeneously hyperintense on T2 imaging [21].
- A homogeneous contrast enhancement pattern is often seen on MRI (Figs. 57.1 and 57.2).
- Enhancement of the infundibulum can be observed in up to 31 % of patients [2, 3] (Fig. 57.1).
- Loss of the posterior pituitary bright spot has been described frequently [20].
- Cystic components may be seen on MRI.
- Tongue-shaped extension of the lesion along the base of the hypothalamus has been described [22].
- Cavernous sinus invasion may occur in up to 18 % of patients, but is an atypical feature of this entity [2, 3, 23].

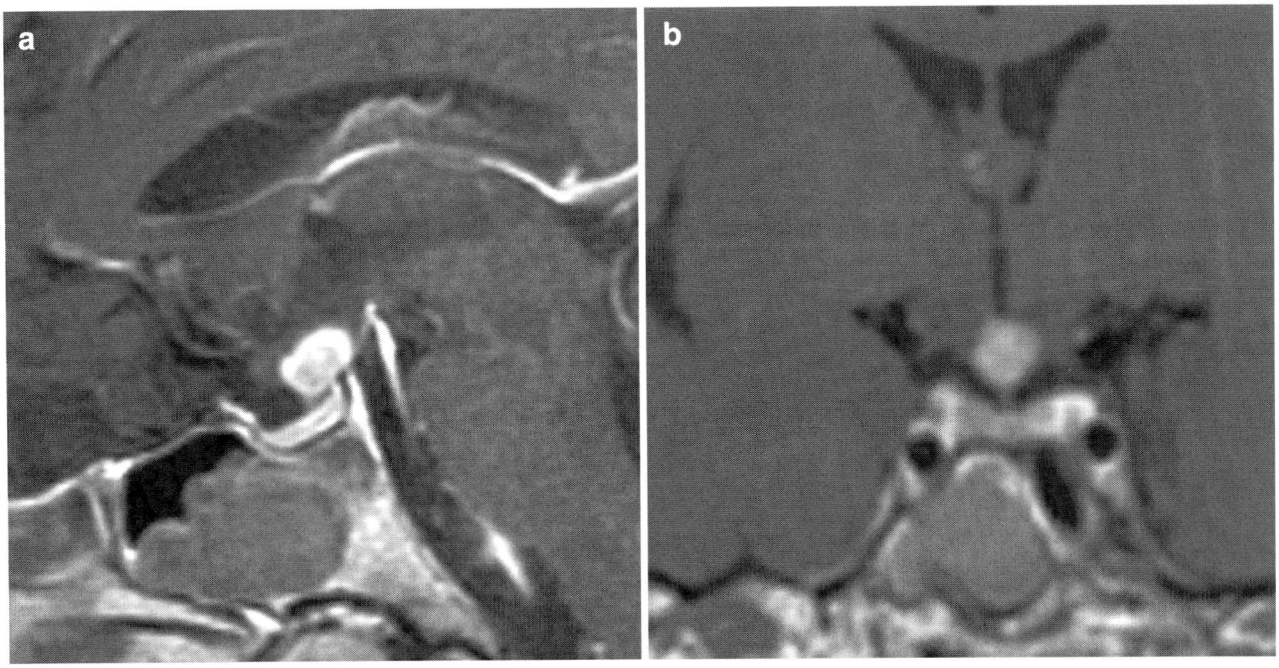

Fig. 57.1 Lymphocytic hypophysitis. (**a**) Sagittal T1-weighted gadolinium-enhanced MR image. (**b**) Coronal T1-weighted gadolinium-enhanced image. Nodular thickening involves the superior pituitary stalk. The pituitary gland appears normal in size

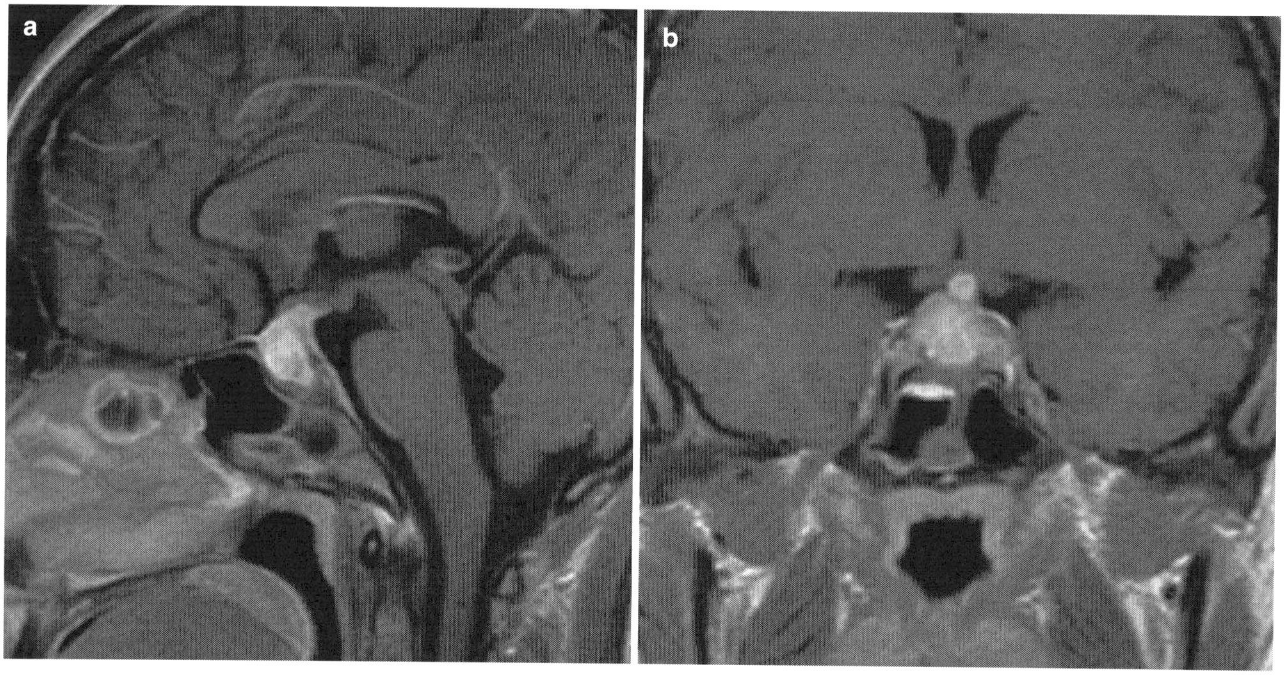

Fig. 57.2 Lymphocytic hypophysitis. (**a**) Sagittal T1-weighted gadolinium-enhanced MR image. (**b**) Coronal T1-weighted gadolinium-enhanced image. Nodular thickening involves the pituitary stalk and the pituitary gland, which is mildly enlarged. There is also mucosal thickening in the adjacent sphenoid sinuses

57.3 Histopathology

- Histologically, inflammatory hypophysitis may be classified into three main categories—lymphocytic, granulomatous, and xanthomatous (including xanthogranulomatous)—which frequently demonstrate overlapping features [7].

57.3.1 Lymphocytic Hypophysitis

- Histologically, lymphocytic hypophysitis is characterized by infiltration of the anterior pituitary gland by lymphocytes and plasma cells (Fig. 57.3). Germinal centers occasionally can be present.
- Later stages of the disease demonstrate atrophy of the gland parenchyma, a variable degree of fibrosis, and residual lymphocytic aggregates.
- The inflammatory infiltrate is rich in T cells with CD4+ and CD8+ immunoreactivity [24].

57.3.2 Granulomatous Hypophysitis

- Granulomatous hypophysitis is characterized by well-formed, noncaseating granulomas associated with variable lymphocytic infiltrates (Fig. 57.3e).
- Varying degrees of parenchymal fibrosis also may be present.
- Other granulomatous diseases (such as sarcoidosis and Langerhans cell histiocytosis) and infectious processes (such as tuberculosis) must be excluded before the final diagnosis.

57.3.3 Xanthomatous and Xanthogranulomatous Hypophysitis

- Xanthomatous hypophysitis is characterized by infiltration of foamy histiocytes with no granuloma formation.
- The cells are immunoreactive for CD68, but are negative for S100 protein and CD1a.
- Intact anterior pituitary acini and vasculature are present, with inflammatory infiltrates of foamy histiocytes, lymphocytes, and multinucleated giant cells [9, 25].
- Often granulation tissue and acellular debris can be seen [9].
- Positive immunoreactivity for CD68 (macrophage marker) has been reported [9].

57.3.4 IgG4 Hypophysitis

- IgG4 hypophysitis is characterized by dense, lymphoplasmacytic infiltration of the pituitary with sclerosis, phlebitis, and IgG4-positive plasma cells. Clinically, there may be high serum levels of IgG4 [10, 26].

57.4 Clinical and Surgical Management

- Medical management consists of high-dose corticosteroids and hormone replacement therapy.
- More recently, azathioprine has been utilized with favorable responses in some patients.
- Approximately half of patients will respond favorably to steroids, but those with visual loss on presentation or with

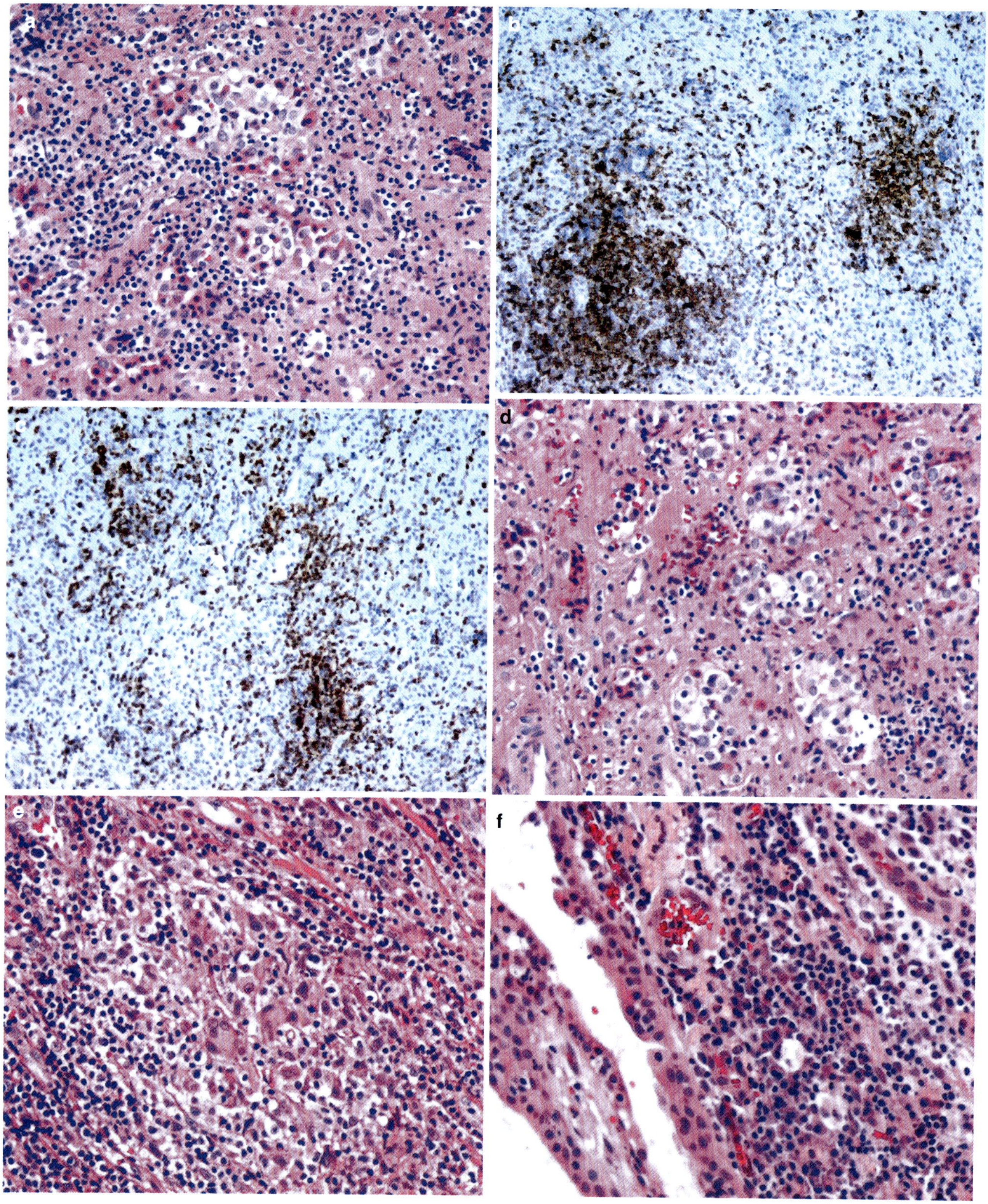

Fig. 57.3 Hypophysitis. Lymphocytic hypophysitis, the most common primary hypophysitis, is characterized by densely lymphoplasmacytic inflammatory cells that diffusely infiltrate the pituitary gland (**a**). The inflammatory infiltrate shows a mixed inflammatory population of CD3-positive T cells (**b**) and CD20-positive B cells (**c**). Extensive stromal fibrosis of the gland is seen in end-stage lymphocytic hypophysitis (**d**). Granulomatous hypophysitis displays dense, lymphoplasmacytic infiltrates and scattered granulomas with giant cells destroying and replacing the pituitary gland (**e**). Secondary hypophysitis is not uncommon in association with Rathke cleft cysts (**f**)

otherwise refractory or progressive disease may require surgical management. The role of surgical intervention is for biopsy, sellar decompression, and improvement of visual symptoms [3, 7].

- Transsphenoidal surgery is the mainstay procedure for biopsy, decompression, and partial resection of the mass.
- Intraoperatively, the pituitary gland is frequently noted to have a firm, indurated consistency.
- Most patients experience improvement in headaches and visual symptoms following surgical decompression [3].
- Hypopituitarism secondary to hypophysitis is less likely to improve after surgery, and a majority of patients require long-term hormone replacement.
- Medical therapy reduces the pituitary mass in 84 % of patients, improves anterior pituitary function in 45 %, and restores posterior pituitary function in 41 % [27].
- Recurrence occurs in up to 15 % of patients, mandating close hormonal monitoring for several years following initial remission [3, 28].
- It may be difficult to wean patients off high-dose corticosteroids, often mandating the use of other medical agents such as methotrexate, azathioprine, or rituximab [29, 30].
- Stereotactic radiotherapy and radiosurgery have been reported for refractory cases of invasive lymphocytic hypophysitis that do not respond to medical and surgical management [31, 32].

References

1. Cheung CC, Ezzat S, Smyth HS, Asa SL. The spectrum and significance of primary hypophysitis. J Clin Endocrinol Metab. 2001;86:1048–53.
2. Molitch ME, Gillam MP. Lymphocytic hypophysitis. Horm Res. 2007;68 Suppl 5:145–50.
3. Leung GK, Lopes MB, Thorner MO, Vance ML, Laws Jr ER. Primary hypophysitis: a single-center experience in 16 cases. J Neurosurg. 2004;101:262–71.
4. Saeger W, Ludecke DK, Buchfelder M, Fahlbusch R, Quabbe HJ, Petersenn S. Pathohistological classification of pituitary tumors: 10 years of experience with the German pituitary tumor registry. Eur J Endocrinol. 2007;156:203–16.
5. Tashiro T, Sano T, Xu B, Wakatsuki S, Kagawa N, Nishioka H, Yamada S, Kovacs K. Spectrum of different types of hypophysitis: a clinicopathologic study of hypophysitis in 31 cases. Endocr Pathol. 2002;13:183–95.
6. Carpinteri R, Patelli I, Casanueva FF, Giustina A. Pituitary tumours: inflammatory and granulomatous expansive lesions of the pituitary. Best Pract Res Clin Endocrinol Metab. 2009;23:639–50.
7. Gutenberg A, Hans V, Puchner MJ, Kreutzer J, Bruck W, Caturegli P, Buchfelder M. Primary hypophysitis: clinical-pathological correlations. Eur J Endocrinol. 2006;155:101–7.
8. Deodhare SS, Bilbao JM, Kovacs K, Horvath E, Nomikos P, Buchfelder M, et al. Xanthomatous hypophysitis: a novel entity of obscure etiology. Endocr Pathol. 1999;10:237–41.
9. Folkerth RD, Price Jr DL, Schwartz M, Black PM, De Girolami U. Xanthomatous hypophysitis. Am J Surg Pathol. 1998;22: 736–41.
10. Leporati P, Landek-Salgado MA, Lupi I, Chiovato L, Caturegli P. IgG4-related hypophysitis: a new addition to the hypophysitis spectrum. J Clin Endocrinol Metab. 2011;96:1971–80.
11. Juszczak A, Gupta A, Karavitaki N, Middleton MR, Grossman AB. Ipilimumab: a novel immunomodulating therapy causing autoimmune hypophysitis: a case report and review. Eur J Endocrinol. 2012;167:1–5.
12. Nishikawa T, Takahashi JA, Shimatsu A, Hashimoto N. Hypophysitis caused by Rathke's cleft cyst. Case report. Neurol Med Chir (Tokyo). 2007;47:136–9.
13. Moskowitz SI, Hamrahian A, Prayson RA, Pineyro M, Lorenz RR, Weil RJ. Concurrent lymphocytic hypophysitis and pituitary adenoma. Case report and review of the literature. J Neurosurg. 2006;105:309–14.
14. Murakami M, Nishioka H, Izawa H, Ikeda Y, Haraoka J. Granulomatous hypophysitis associated with Rathke's cleft cyst: a case report. Minim Invasive Neurosurg. 2008;51:169–72.
15. Zada G. Rathke cleft cysts: a review of clinical and surgical management. Neurosurg Focus. 2011;31(1):E1.
16. Bettendorf M, Fehn M, Grulich-Henn J, Selle B, Darge K, Ludecke DK, et al. Lymphocytic hypophysitis with central diabetes insipidus and consequent panhypopituitarism preceding a multifocal, intracranial germinoma in a prepubertal girl. Eur J Pediatr. 1999;158: 288–92.
17. Fehn M, Bettendorf M, Ludecke DK, Sommer C, Saeger W. Lymphocytic hypophysitis masking a suprasellar germinoma in a 12-year-old girl--a case report. Pituitary. 1999;1:303–7.
18. Huang YY, Lin SF, Dunn P, Wai YY, Hsueh C, Tsai JS. Primary pituitary lymphoma presenting as hypophysitis. Endocr J. 2005;52: 543–9.
19. Aste L, Bellinzona M, Meleddu V, Farci G, Manieli C, Godano U. Xanthomatous hypophysitis mimicking a pituitary adenoma: case report and review of the literature. J Oncol. 2010;2010:195323. doi:10.1155/2010/195323.

20. Bhansali A, Velayutham P, Radotra BD, Pathak A. Idiopathic granulomatous hypophysitis presenting as non-functioning pituitary adenoma: description of six cases and review of literature. Br J Neurosurg. 2004;18:489–94.
21. Gazioglu N, Tuzgen S, Oz B, Kocer N, Kafadar A, Akar Z, Kuday C. Idiopathic granulomatous hypophysitis: are there reliable, constant radiological and clinical diagnostic criterias? Neuroradiology. 2000;42:890–4.
22. Honegger J, Fahlbusch R, Bornemann A, Hensen J, Buchfelder M, Muller M, Nomikos P. Lymphocytic and granulomatous hypophysitis: experience with nine cases. Neurosurgery. 1997;40:713–22; discussion 722–3.
23. Kartal I, Yarman S, Tanakol R, Bilgic B. Lymphocytic panhypophysitis in a young man with involvement of the cavernous sinus and clivus. Pituitary. 2007;10:75–80.
24. Gutenberg A, Buslei R, Fahlbusch R, Buchfelder M, Bruck W. Immunopathology of primary hypophysitis: implications for pathogenesis. Am J Surg Pathol. 2005;29:329–38.
25. Burt MG, Morey AL, Turner JJ, Pell M, Sheehy JP, Ho KK. Xanthomatous pituitary lesions: a report of two cases and review of the literature. Pituitary. 2003;6:161–8.
26. Hsing MT, Hsu HT, Cheng CY, Chen CM. IgG4-related hypophysitis presenting as a pituitary adenoma with systemic disease. Asian J Surg. 2013;36:93–7.
27. Lupi I, Manetti L, Raffaelli V, Lombardi M, Cosottini M, Iannelli A, et al. Diagnosis and treatment of autoimmune hypophysitis: a short review. J Endocrinol Invest. 2011;34:e245–52.
28. Tsagarakis S, Vassiliadi D, Malagari K, Kontogeorgos G, Thalassinos N. Lymphocytic hypophysitis: late recurrence following successful transsphenoidal surgery. Endocrine. 2004;25: 85–90.
29. Curto L, Torre ML, Cotta OR, Losa M, Terreni MR, Santarpia L, et al. Lymphocytic hypophysitis: differential diagnosis and effects of high-dose pulse steroids, followed by azathioprine, on the pituitary mass and endocrine abnormalities--report of a case and literature review. Scientific World J. 2010;10:126–34. doi:10.1100/tsw.2010.24.
30. Schreckinger M, Francis T, Rajah G, Jagannathan J, Guthikonda M, Mittal S. Novel strategy to treat a case of recurrent lymphocytic hypophysitis using rituximab. J Neurosurg. 2012;116:1318–23.
31. Ray DK, Yen CP, Vance ML, Laws ER, Lopes B, Sheehan JP. Gamma knife surgery for lymphocytic hypophysitis. J Neurosurg. 2010;112:118–21.
32. Selch MT, DeSalles AA, Kelly DF, Frighetto L, Vinters HV, Cabatan-Awang C, et al. Stereotactic radiotherapy for the treatment of lymphocytic hypophysitis. Report of two cases. J Neurosurg. 2003;99:591–6.

Demyelinating Diseases: Multiple Sclerosis and Neuromyelitis Optica

58

Gabriel Zada, M. Beatriz S. Lopes, Srinivasan Mukundan Jr., and Edward Laws Jr.

58.1 Epidemiology and Clinical Presentation

- Multiple sclerosis (MS) is a demyelinating disease that more commonly affects women; its occurrence is partially determined by ancestral background.
- In patients with classic MS, hyperactivity of the hypothalamic-pituitary-adrenal axis and a chronically activated corticotropin-releasing hormone (CRH) system have been shown [1–3].
- Neuromyelitis optica (NMO) spectrum disorder, also known as Devic's disease, is a group of related demyelinating conditions with common manifestations in the suprasellar region and spinal cord. The optic chiasm, nerves, hypothalamus, and infundibulum are frequently affected. The spectrum of disease includes classic NMO, optic neuritis, Asian opticospinal MS, NMO with endocrinopathies, and other subtypes [4].
- NMO is part of a spectrum of diseases in which the body forms antibodies to aquaporin-4 [5].
- The mean age at diagnosis is 39 years [4].
- NMO often presents with severe visual loss, myelitis, and prodromal symptoms. Visual loss in NMO is often bilateral and simultaneous.
- Hypothalamic syndromes, including narcolepsy/sleepiness, hyperphagia, hypothermia, and obesity have been reported in association with NMO [6–9].
- In a recently described subset, NMO with endocrinopathies, patients have hypothalamic-pituitary axis deficiencies. Almost all affected patients are women, who present with amenorrhea and galactorrhea [10–12].
- Hyperprolactinemia is the most common endocrine finding in patients with NMO, and prolactin levels are noted to be significantly higher than in patients with classic MS [13].

G. Zada, MD, MS (✉)
Department of Neurological Surgery,
Keck School of Medicine, University of Southern California,
1200 N State Street, #3300, Los Angeles, CA 90033, USA
e-mail: gzada@usc.edu

M.B.S. Lopes, MD, PhD
Department of Pathology (Neuropathology),
University of Virginia School of Medicine,
1215 Lee Street, Room 3060–HEP,
Charlottesville, VA 22908, USA
e-mail: msl2e@virginia.edu

S. Mukundan Jr., PhD, MD
Department of Radiology, Brigham and Women's Hospital,
75 Francis Street, Boston, MA 02115, USA
e-mail: smukundan@partners.org

E. Laws Jr., MD
Department of Neurosurgery, Brigham and Women's Hospital,
15 Francis Street, Boston, MA 02115, USA
e-mail: elaws@partners.org

G. Zada et al. (eds.), *Atlas of Sellar and Parasellar Lesions: Clinical, Radiologic, and Pathologic Correlations*,
DOI 10.1007/978-3-319-22855-6_58

58.2 Imaging Features

- Demyelinating regions in the hypothalamus can be seen in 13 % of patients with MS; these regions are typically hyperintense on T2-weighted imaging and hypointense on T1-weighted imaging, without contrast enhancement [8, 14–16].
- In patients with NMO, MRI findings are more common in the upper cervical spinal cord. Longitudinal cord lesions are common findings in NMO and opticospinal MS (Figs. 58.1 and 58.2). In the brain, periventricular ovoid regions are seen and closely resemble those in classic MS [17].
- MRI in some patients with NMO is normal.
- Optical coherence tomography (OCT) may be used to measure the thickness of the retinal nerve fiber layer in MS and NMO.

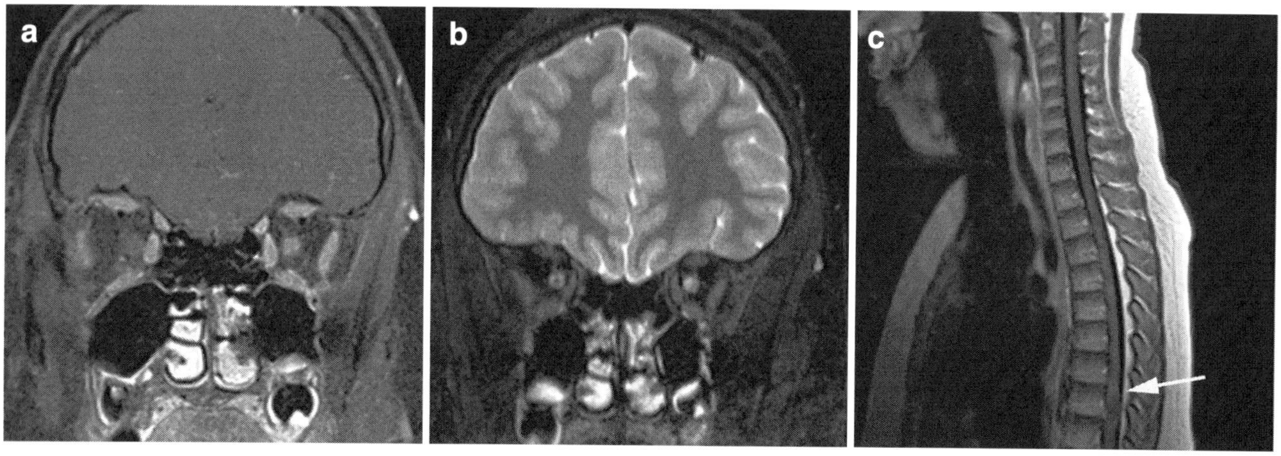

Fig. 58.1 Neuromyelitis optica (NMO). (**a**) Coronal fat-saturated T1-weighted gadolinium-enhanced MR image. (**b**) Coronal inversion recovery image. (**c**) Sagittal T1-weighted gadolinium-enhanced image. The left optic nerve demonstrates edema (**b**) and enhancement (**a**) consistent with neuritis. There is also focal enhancement of the lower thoracic cord (**c**) (*arrow*)

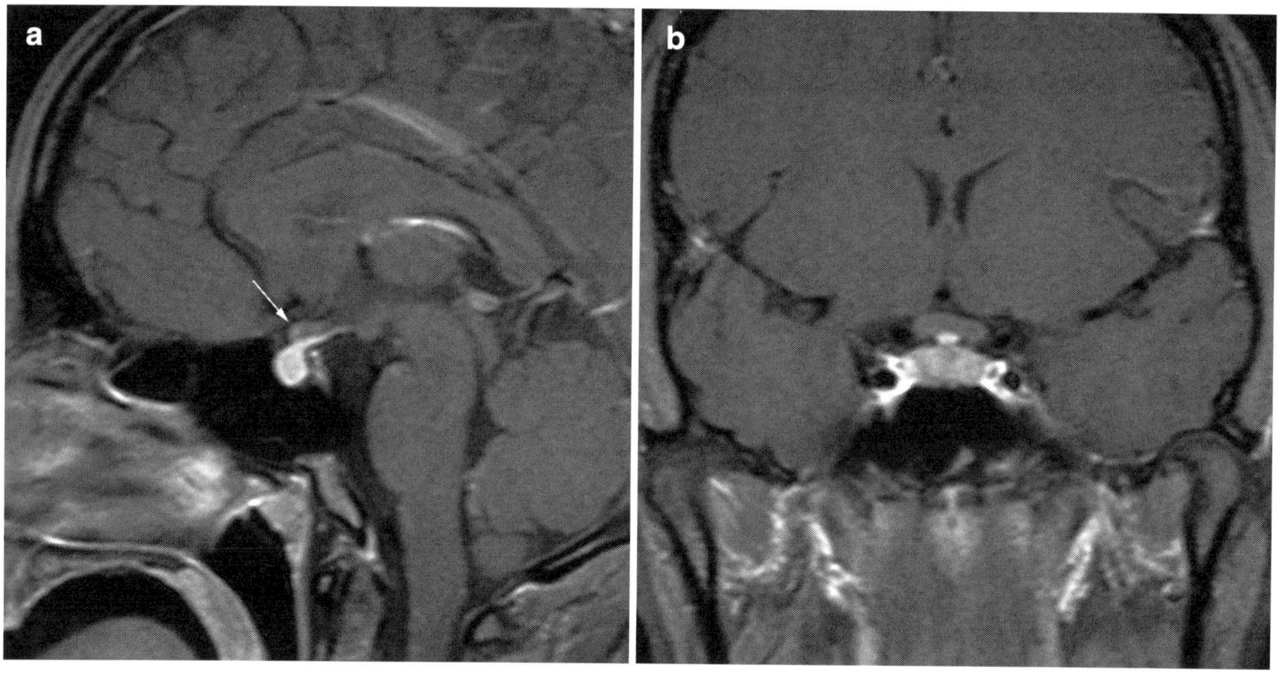

Fig. 58.2 NMO. (**a**) Sagittal T1-weighted gadolinium-enhanced MR image. (**b**) Coronal T1-weighted gadolinium-enhanced image. This young woman with vision loss and hypopituitarism was found to have NMO. There is slight enhancement of the optic chiasm (*arrow*) and infundibulum

58.3 Histopathology

- White matter plaques with demyelination and extensive perivenous infiltration of lymphocytes, macrophages, and plasma cells are commonly seen.
- Axonal tracts are typically preserved.
- Astrogliosis is often seen.
- In severe cases, necrotizing inflammation of the white matter can be seen.
- IgG and IgM antibodies are often positive in affected tissue.

58.4 Clinical Management

- Although not all patients with NMO are seroconverted, serum evidence of aquaporin-4 antibodies confirm the diagnosis (NMO-IgG antibody). This test has a sensitivity of 75 % in diagnosing NMO [18].
- Diagnostic criteria for NMO currently require optic neuritis, acute myelitis, and two of the following three characteristics [19]:
  - MRI that is nondiagnostic for MS
  - A longitudinal spinal cord lesion extending over three vertebral segments
  - NMO-IgG seropositive status
- Treatment for acute NMO includes high-dose corticosteroids and plasmapheresis.
- Long-term treatment may involve drugs such as azathioprine, mofetil mycophenolate, and rituximab [20].
- A frequent relapsing course is observed in over 80 % of patients with NMO [19].

References

1. Ysrraelit MC, Gaitán MI, Lopez AS, Correale J. Impaired hypothalamic-pituitary-adrenal axis activity in patients with multiple sclerosis. Neurology. 2008;71:1948–54.
2. Fassbender K, Schmidt R, Mössner R, Kischka U, Kühnen J, Schwartz A, Hennerici M. Mood disorders and dysfunction of the hypothalamic-pituitary-adrenal axis in multiple sclerosis: association with cerebral inflammation. Arch Neurol. 1998;55:66–72.
3. Huitinga I, Erkut ZA, van Beurden D, Swaab DF. Impaired hypothalamus-pituitary-adrenal axis activity and more severe multiple sclerosis with hypothalamic lesions. Ann Neurol. 2004;55: 37–45.
4. Storoni M, Davagnanam I, Radon M, Siddiqui A, Plant GT. Distinguishing optic neuritis in neuromyelitis optica spectrum disease from multiple sclerosis: a novel magnetic resonance imaging scoring system. J Neuroophthalmol. 2013;33:123–7.
5. Downer JJ, Leite MI, Carter R, Palace J, Küker W, Quaghebeur G. Diagnosis of neuromyelitis optica (NMO) spectrum disorders: is MRI obsolete? Neuroradiology. 2012;54:279–85.
6. Whitham RH, Brey RL. Neuromyelitis optica: two new cases and review of the literature. J Clin Neuroophthalmol. 1985;5:263–9.
7. Baba T, Nakashima I, Kanbayashi T, Konno M, Takahashi T, Fujihara K, et al. Narcolepsy as an initial manifestation of neuromyelitis optica with anti-aquaporin-4 antibody. J Neurol. 2009; 256:287–8.
8. Zhang Y, Dong R, Fan H, Li S, Geng D. Hypothalamus syndrome in opticospinal multiple sclerosis. AJNR Am J Neuroradiol. 2011;32:E153–5.
9. Suzuki K, Nakamura T, Hashimoto K, Miyamoto M, Komagamine T, Nagashima T, et al. Hypothermia, hypotension, hypersomnia, and obesity associated with hypothalamic lesions in a patient positive for the anti-aquaporin 4 antibody: a case report and literature review. Arch Neurol. 2012;69:1355–9.
10. Petravić D, Habek M, Supe S, Brinar VV. Recurrent optic neuromyelitis with endocrinopathies: a new syndrome or just a coincidence? Mult Scler. 2006;12:670–3.
11. Vernant JC, Cabre P, Smadja D, Merle H, Caubarrère I, Mikol J, Poser CM. Recurrent optic neuromyelitis with endocrinopathies: a new syndrome. Neurology. 1997;48:58–64.
12. Hui AC, Wong RS, Ma R, Kay R. Recurrent optic neuromyelitis with multiple endocrinopathies and autoimmune disorders. J Neurol. 2002;249:784–5.
13. Yamasaki K, Horiuchi I, Minohara M, Osoegawa M, Kawano Y, Ohyagi Y, et al. Hyperprolactinemia in optico-spinal multiple sclerosis. Intern Med. 2000;39:296–9.
14. Wang F, Liu Y, Duan Y, Li K. Brain MRI abnormalities in neuromyelitis optica. Eur J Radiol. 2011;80:445–9.
15. Qiu W, Raven S, Wu JS, Bundell C, Hollingsworth P, Carroll WM, et al. Hypothalamic lesions in multiple sclerosis. J Neurol Neurosurg Psychiatry. 2011;82:819–22.
16. Poppe AY, Lapierre Y, Melançon D, Lowden D, Wardell L, Fullerton LM, Bar-Or A. Neuromyelitis optica with hypothalamic involvement. Mult Scler. 2005;11:617–21.
17. O'Riordan JI, Gallagher HL, Thompson AJ, Howard RS, Kingsley DP, Thompson EJ, et al. Clinical, CSF, and MRI findings in Devic's neuromyelitis optica. J Neurol Neurosurg Psychiatry. 1996;60: 382–7.
18. Lennon VA, Wingerchuk DM, Kryzer TJ, Pittock SJ, Lucchinetti CF, Fujihara K, et al. A serum autoantibody marker of neuromyelitis optica: distinction from multiple sclerosis. Lancet. 2004;364: 2106–12.
19. Wingerchuk DM. Diagnosis and treatment of neuromyelitis optica. Neurologist. 2007;13:2–11.
20. Sato D, Callegaro D, Lana-Peixoto MA, Fujihara K, Brazilian Committee for Treatment and Research in Multiple Sclerosis. Treatment of neuromyelitis optica: an evidence based review. Arq Neuropsiquiatr. 2012;70:59–66.

Part VIII

Vascular Disorders of the Anterior Skull Base, Sellar, and Parasellar Region

Cerebral Aneurysms with Intrasellar Extension

59

Gabriel Zada, M. Beatriz S. Lopes, Srinivasan Mukundan Jr., and Edward Laws Jr.

59.1 Epidemiology and Clinical Presentation

- Sellar region aneurysms comprise a diverse group of cerebral aneurysms and may mimic the presentation of a cystic pituitary mass (cystic adenoma, craniopharyngioma, Rathke cleft cyst) [1–3].
- The repercussions of failure to diagnose an intrasellar aneurysm may be catastrophic. Fortunately, the advent of MRI and noninvasive vascular imaging (CT and MR angiography) has improved the ability to detect these lesions prior to any surgical intervention.
- Most patients presenting with intrasellar aneurysms will have unruptured aneurysms that present secondary to mass effect on surrounding structures [4].
- The most common signs and symptoms are headache, visual loss, endocrinopathy, hyponatremia, and cranial nerve paresis. Hyperprolactinemia and hypogonadism are the most common endocrinopathies associated with these lesions [4, 5].
- Some intrasellar aneurysms (approximately 20 %) are detected in the presence of a pituitary adenoma. Growth hormone (GH) adenomas are the adenomas most commonly associated with intrasellar aneurysms [6].
- Aneurysms with intrasellar extension fall into two major groups [4]:
  - *Infradiaphragmatic aneurysms*, which typically arise from the internal carotid artery (ICA) at the level of the cavernous sinuses and extend medially into the sella (Fig. 59.1). These aneurysms are more likely to present with endocrinopathy.
  - *Supradiaphragmatic aneurysms*, which arise from the ophthalmic segment of the ICA at the origin of the superior hypophysial artery, or anterior communicating artery aneurysms that point inferiorly into the sella (Fig. 59.2). These typically tend to be larger aneurysms (mean diameter 21 mm), and they are more likely to present with visual loss.
- Cranial nerve paresis is noted in 18 % of patients with intrasellar aneurysms [4].
- Rarely, bilateral ICA aneurysms may impinge on the pituitary gland and cause various endocrinopathies [7, 8].

G. Zada, MD, MS (✉)
Department of Neurological Surgery, Keck School of Medicine, University of Southern California, 1200 N State Street, #3300, Los Angeles, CA 90033, USA
e-mail: gzada@usc.edu

M.B.S. Lopes, MD, PhD
Department of Pathology (Neuropathology), University of Virginia School of Medicine, 1215 Lee Street, Room 3060–HEP, Charlottesville, VA 22908, USA
e-mail: msl2e@virginia.edu

S. Mukundan Jr., PhD, MD
Department of Radiology, Brigham and Women's Hospital, 75 Francis Street, Boston, MA 02115, USA
e-mail: smukundan@partners.org

E. Laws Jr., MD
Department of Neurosurgery, Brigham and Women's Hospital, 15 Francis Street, Boston, MA 02115, USA
e-mail: elaws@partners.org

G. Zada et al. (eds.), *Atlas of Sellar and Parasellar Lesions: Clinical, Radiologic, and Pathologic Correlations*, DOI 10.1007/978-3-319-22855-6_59

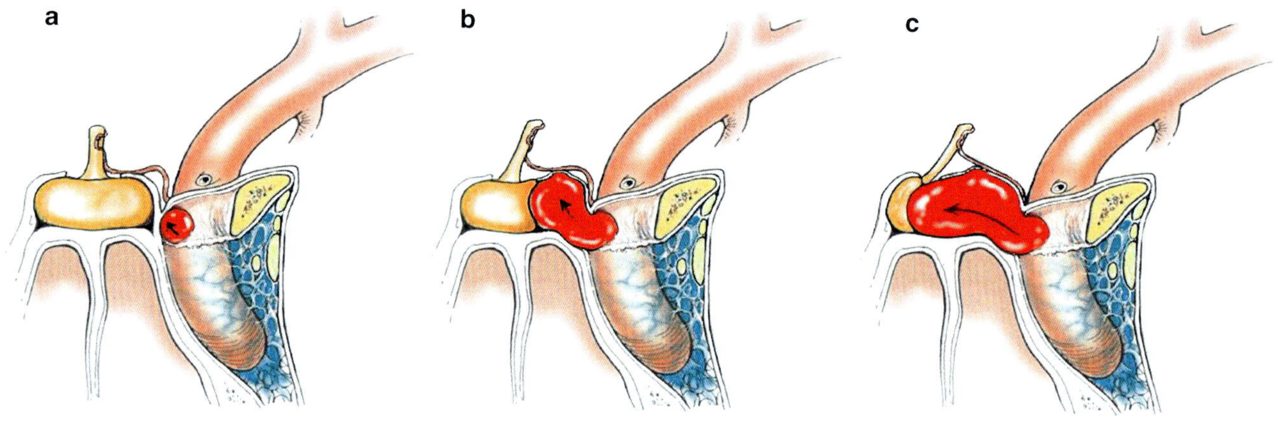

Fig. 59.1 The progressive growth pattern of cavernous and clinoid segment internal carotid artery (ICA) (infradiaphragmatic) aneurysms (**a**–**c**) medially into the sella, causing compression of the pituitary gland (Courtesy of Dr. Arthur L. Day)

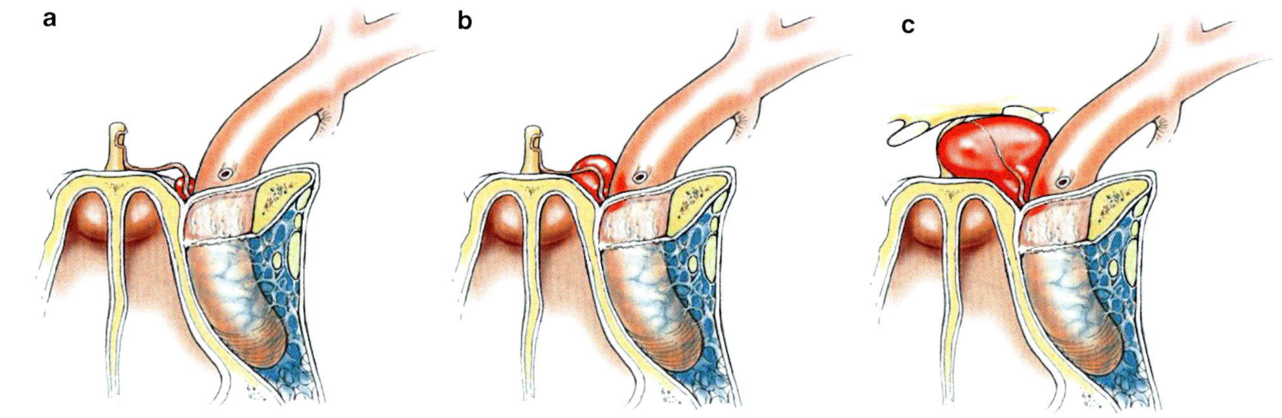

Fig. 59.2 The progressive growth pattern of superior hypophysial/ophthalmic ICA aneurysms (**a**–**c**)medially and intradurally above the diaphragma sellae, from where they may extend down into the sella turcica (Courtesy of Dr. Arthur L. Day)

59.2 Imaging Features

- Diagnosis of a sellar region aneurysm can be made with CT angiography, MR angiography, or conventional digital subtraction angiography (Figs. 59.3, 59.4, 59.5, 59.6, and 59.7).
- On CT scans, sellar aneurysms are more likely to be associated with a widened superior orbital fissure, nonfilling of the cavernous sinus, unilateral sellar erosion, calcification, and eccentric circular attenuation following contrast administration. On the other hand, pituitary adenomas are more likely to be associated with complete erosion of the pituitary fossa, soft tissue opacity in the sphenoid sinus, bilateral displacement of the cavernous sinuses, and general enlargement of the sella [9].
- On MRI, cerebral aneurysms with intrasellar extension often appear as round or ovoid masses, often with a "marbled" appearance and pulsation artifact.
- MR angiography or CT angiography can be used to make the diagnosis. The most common aneurysms presenting with intrasellar extension are cavernous and clinoidal ICA aneurysms, ophthalmic ICA aneurysms (especially superior hypophysial artery aneurysms), and inferiorly pointing anterior communicating aneurysms.
- Conventional angiography is the gold standard diagnostic modality.

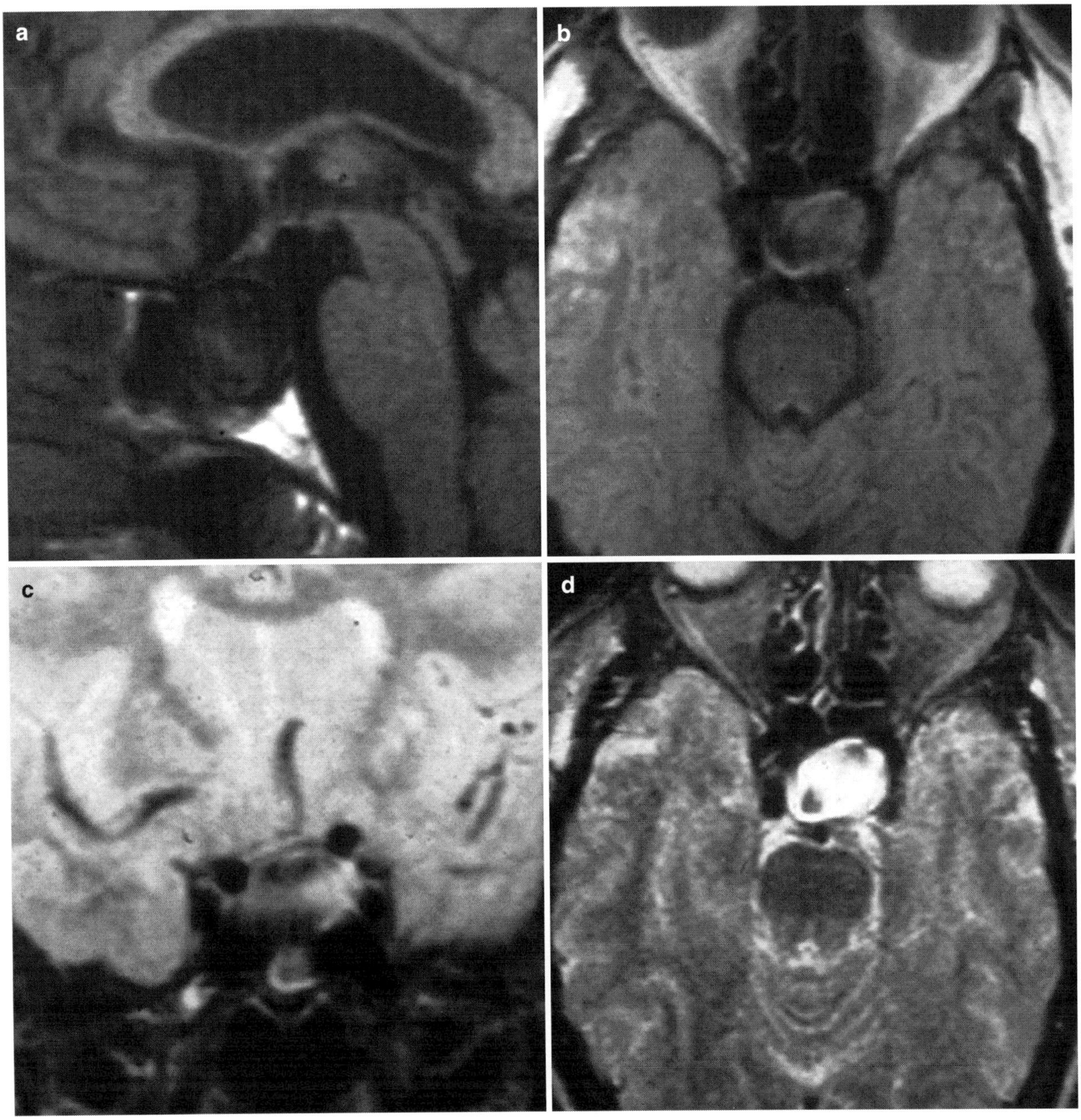

Fig. 59.3 Infradiaphragmatic sellar aneurysm. Sagittal T1-weighted (**a**), axial T1-weighted (**b**), coronal T2-weighted (**c**), and axial T2-weighted (**d**) MR images obtained in a patient with a left cavernous segment infradiaphragmatic aneurysm extending into the sella turcica (Reproduced with permission from Hanak et al. [4])

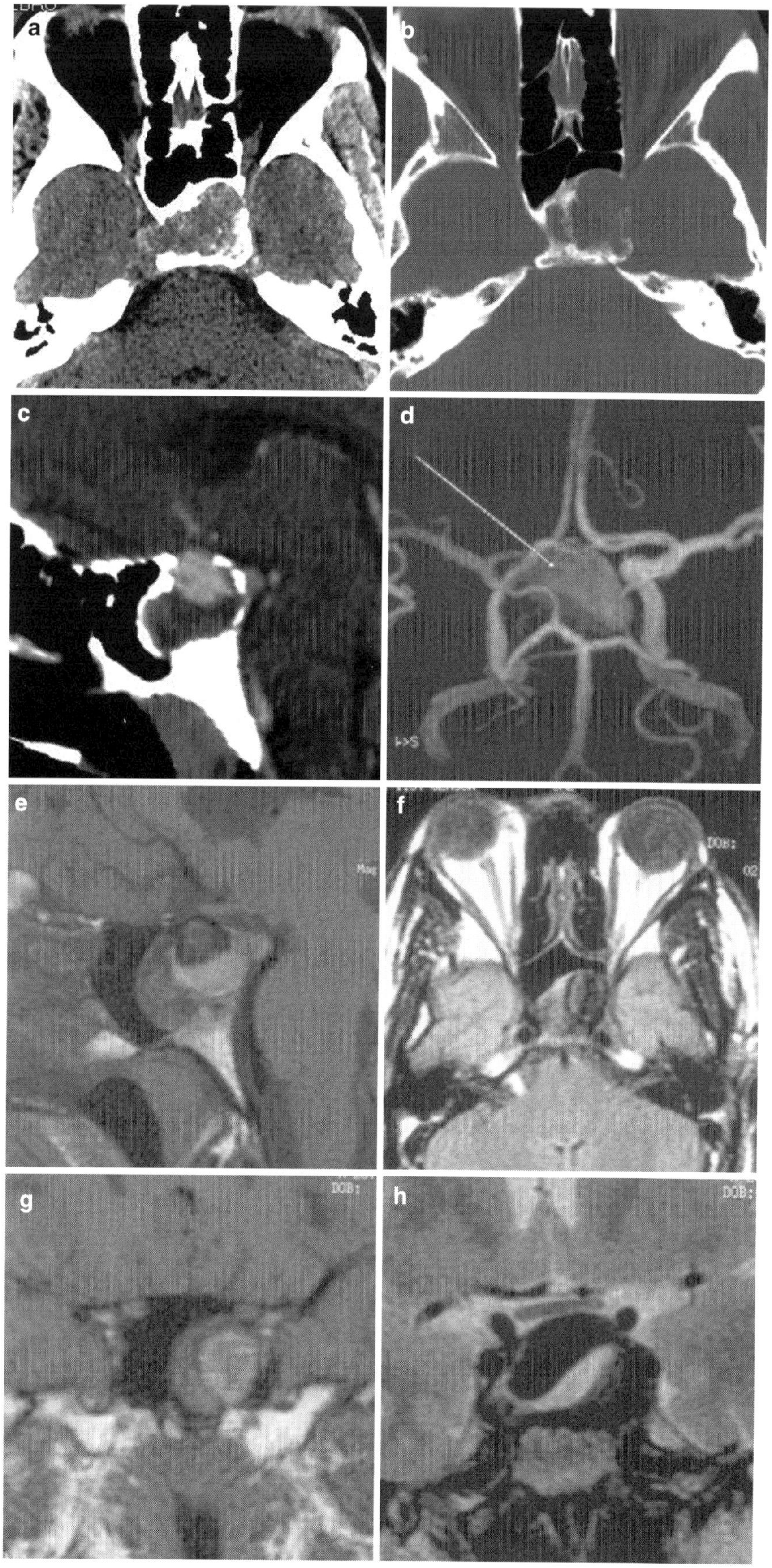

Fig. 59.4 Infradiaphragmatic sellar aneurysm. (**a**, **b**) Axial CT brain and bone windows obtained in a patient with a large, partially calcified cavernous ICA infradiaphragmatic aneurysm extending into the sella and sphenoid sinus. (**c**, **d**) Sagittal and 3D reconstructed CT angiograms demonstrating that the aneurysm is partially thrombosed. (**e**, **f**) Sagittal and axial T1-weighted postcontrast MR images also demonstrating partial thrombosis of this aneurysm. (**g**, **h**) Coronal T1-weighted postcontrast and T2-weighted MR images demonstrating extension into the sphenoid sinus and a marble-like appearance caused by the partial thrombosis (Reproduced with permission from Hanak et al. [4])

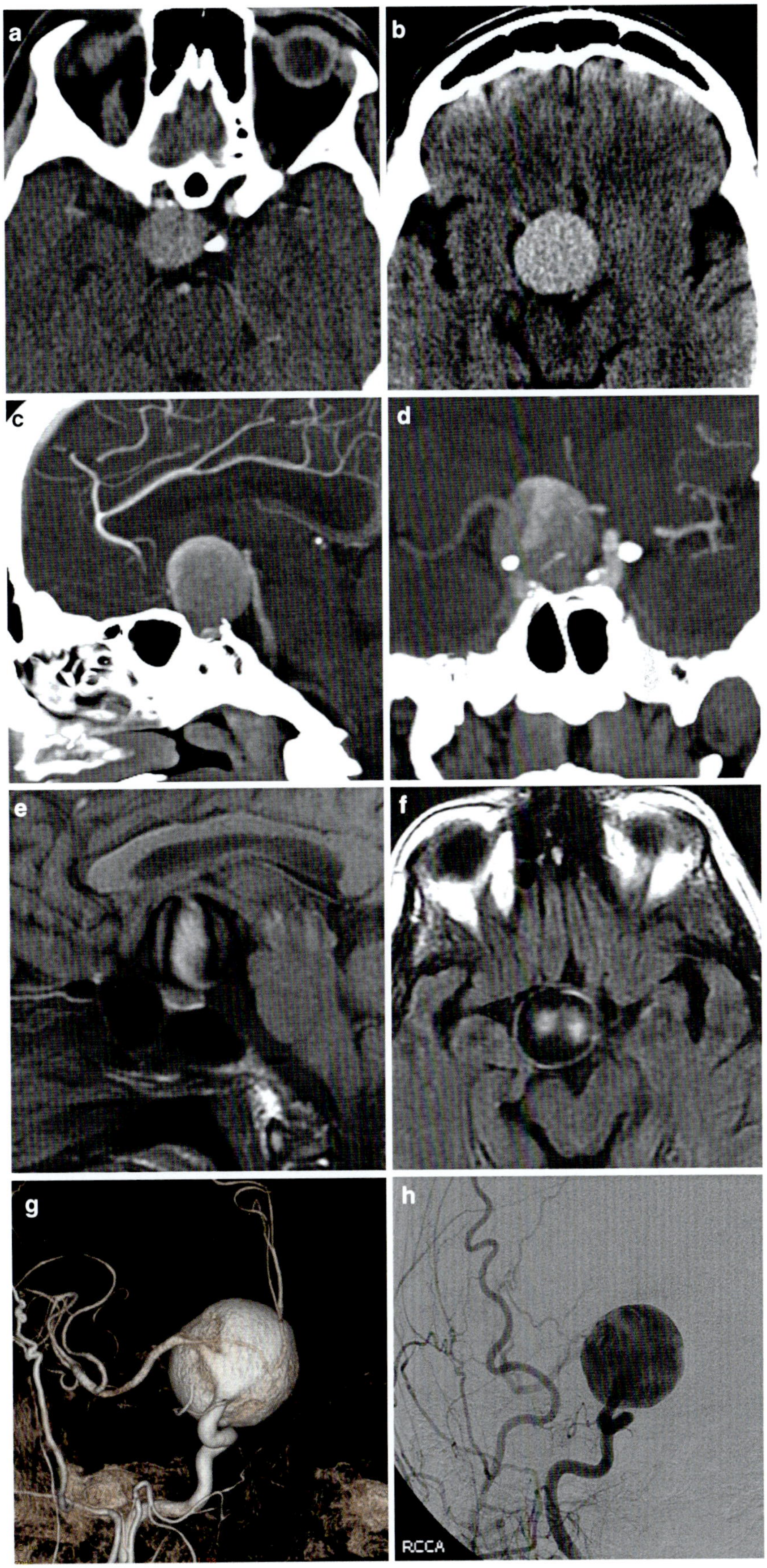

Fig. 59.5 Sellar aneurysm. (**a**, **b**) Axial CT scans obtained in a patient with a large superior hypophysial artery aneurysm projecting inferiorly into the sella. (**c**, **d**) Sagittal and coronal CT angiograms demonstrating suprasellar and infrasellar extension. (**e**, **f**) Sagittal and axial MR images demonstrating the marble-like appearance and location above the diaphragma sellae. (**g**, **h**) Reconstructed CT and digital subtraction angiograms of the aneurysm (Reproduced with permission from Hanak et al. [4])

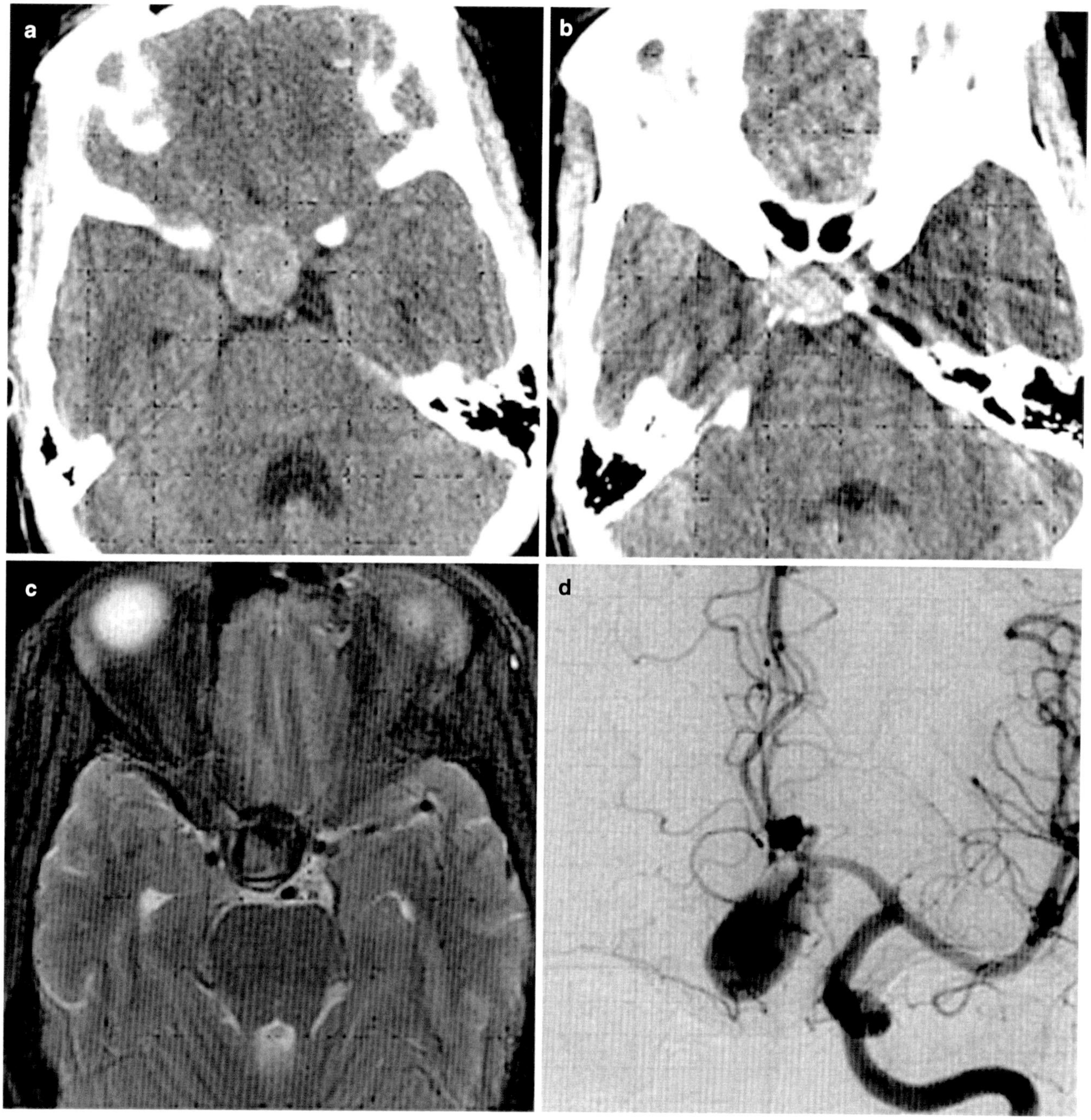

Fig. 59.6 Sellar aneurysm. (**a**, **b**) Axial CT scans obtained in a patient with a large sellar mass. (**c**, **d**) Axial T2-weighted MR image and digital subtraction angiogram (anteroposterior view) demonstrating a large left anterior communicating artery (ACoA) aneurysm projecting inferiorly into the sella (Reproduced with permission from Hanak et al. [4])

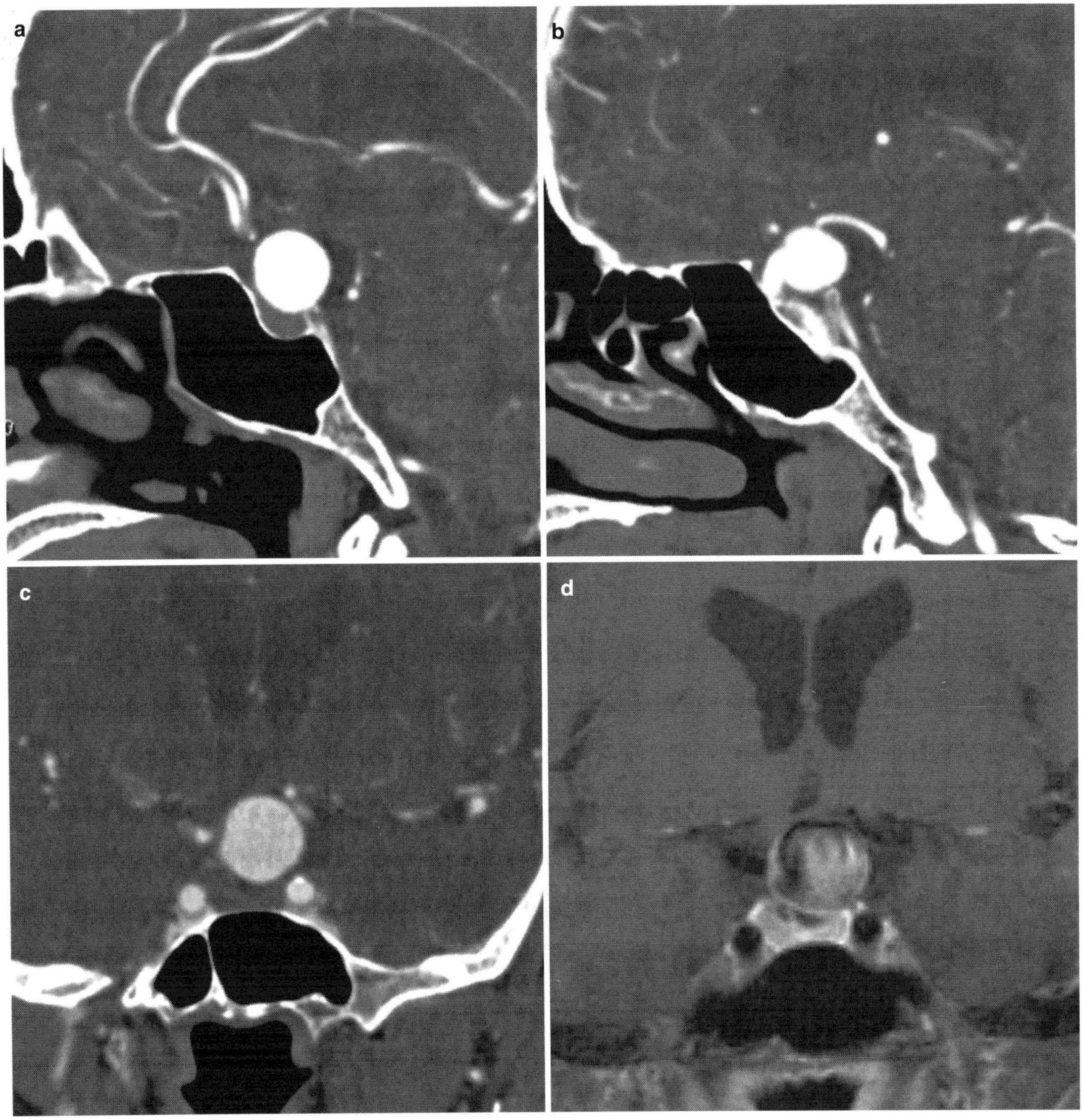

Fig. 59.7 Suprasellar aneurysm. (**a**) Sagittal CT image with contrast enhancement. (**b**) Sagittal CT image with contrast enhancement. (**c**) Coronal CT image with contrast enhancement. (**d**) Coronal T1-weighted gadolinium-enhanced image. (**a–c**) A round, homogeneously enhancing structure is seen in the suprasellar region. The degree of enhancement is similar to that of adjacent intracranial arteries. (**d**) Pulsation artifact in the horizontal orientation indicates that the lesion is vascular

59.3 Clinical and Surgical Management

- Clinical management of sellar region aneurysms is diverse. It depends on multiple factors that include the clinical status of the patient and the aneurysm's location, morphology, and rupture status.
- If there is a possibility of an intrasellar aneurysm during transsphenoidal surgery (with or without a pituitary adenoma), microvascular Doppler ultrasonography may be utilized to check for arterial flow. Another option is insertion of a long, 25-gauge spinal needle into the mass prior to opening the dura.
- Infradiaphragmatic aneurysms (typically cavernous or clinoidal segment ICA aneurysms) are more likely to be treated with endovascular coiling procedures, flow diversion, or with surgical bypass and trapping [4].
- Supradiaphragmatic aneurysms are often treated with either direct surgical clipping (with or without aneurysmal dome perforation), flow diversion, or with endovascular coiling [4].

References

1. Arseni C, Ghitescu M, Cristescu A, Mihăilă G. Intrasellar aneurysms simulating hypophyseal tumors. Eur Neurol. 1970;3:321–9.
2. White JC, Ballantine Jr HT. Intrasellar aneurysms simulating hypophyseal tumours. J Neurosurg. 1961;18:34–50.
3. Kayath MJ, Lengyel AM, Nogueira R, Tella Júnior O, Czepielewski MA. Giant aneurysms of the sellar region simulating pituitary adenomas: a diagnosis to be considered. J Endocrinol Invest. 1991;14:975–9.
4. Hanak BW, Zada G, Nayar VV, Thiex R, Du R, Day AL, Laws ER. Cerebral aneurysms with intrasellar extension: a systematic review of clinical, anatomical, and treatment characteristics. J Neurosurg. 2012;116:164–78.
5. Heshmati HM, Fatourechi V, Dagam SA, Piepgras DG. Hypopituitarism caused by intrasellar aneurysms. Mayo Clin Proc. 2001;76:789–93.
6. Weir B. Pituitary tumors and aneurysms: case report and review of the literature. Neurosurgery. 1992;30:585–91.
7. Friedman TC, Shahinian H. Bilateral cerebral aneurysms impinging on the pituitary. Pituitary. 2004;7:193–4.
8. Mindel JS, Sachdev VP, Kline LB, Sivak MA, Bergman DA, Yang WC, et al. Bilateral intracavernous carotid aneurysms mimicking a prolactin-secreting pituitary tumor. Surg Neurol. 1983;19:163–7.
9. Macpherson P, Anderson DE. Radiological differentiation of intrasellar aneurysms from pituitary tumours. Neuroradiology. 1981;21:177–83.

Arteriovenous Malformations

60

Gabriel Zada, M. Beatriz S. Lopes, Srinivasan Mukundan Jr., and Edward Laws Jr.

60.1 Epidemiology and Clinical Presentation

- Primary intrasellar arteriovenous malformations (AVMs) are exceedingly rare, being confined primarily to case reports [1].
- Dural AVMs of the cavernous sinus (AV fistulas) are a distinct entity, which is discussed in chapter 62.
- In the sellar and suprasellar region, true AVMs occur most commonly in the suprasellar region near the optic chiasm.
- Sellar and suprasellar region AVMs may be associated with the Bonnet–Dechaume–Blanc syndrome, also known as Wyburn–Mason syndrome or retinoencephalofacial angiomatosis [2–4]. This rare congenital syndrome is characterized by multiple AVMs that affect the optic structures, retina, midbrain, and face.
- The most commonly affected structures are the optic nerve, retina, optic chiasm, hypothalamus, thalamus, basal ganglia, and midbrain [5].
- The Bonnet–Dechaume–Blanc syndrome typically presents with visual loss, cranial nerve paresis, strokes, intracranial hemorrhage, epistaxis, and/or hydrocephalus.
- Optic nerve or chiasm apoplexy and AVM rupture have both been reported in conjunction with suprasellar AVMs [6, 7].
- In rare cases, abnormal venous varices or dilatations may become symptomatic by causing mass effect on the optic apparatus [8, 9].
- Cavernous malformations (angiomas), discussed in the next chapter, are also true vascular malformations that may be located anywhere in the brain.

G. Zada, MD, MS (✉)
Department of Neurological Surgery,
Keck School of Medicine, University of Southern California,
1200 N State Street, #3300, Los Angeles, CA 90033, USA
e-mail: gzada@usc.edu

M.B.S. Lopes, MD, PhD
Department of Pathology (Neuropathology),
University of Virginia School of Medicine,
1215 Lee Street, Room 3060–HEP,
Charlottesville, VA 22908, USA
e-mail: msl2e@virginia.edu

S. Mukundan Jr., PhD, MD
Department of Radiology, Brigham and Women's Hospital,
75 Francis Street, Boston, MA 02115, USA
e-mail: smukundan@partners.org

E. Laws Jr., MD
Department of Neurosurgery, Brigham and Women's Hospital,
15 Francis Street, Boston, MA 02115, USA
e-mail: elaws@partners.org

G. Zada et al. (eds.), *Atlas of Sellar and Parasellar Lesions: Clinical, Radiologic, and Pathologic Correlations*,
DOI 10.1007/978-3-319-22855-6_60

60.2 Imaging Features

- CT imaging often shows a hyperdense suprasellar mass. Subarachnoid hemorrhage may be seen in patients with ruptured suprasellar AVMs.
- MRI often shows distinct flow voids within the AVM nidus. T2-weighted imaging is extremely useful and may show a tangle of serpiginous, low-intensity bands (Fig. 60.1) [6].
- Noninvasive vascular imaging—CT angiography (CTA) or MR angiography (MRA)—can be used to confirm the diagnosis and is mandatory in planning for stereotactic radiosurgery.
- The gold standard diagnostic technique for diagnosis and surgical treatment planning is cerebral angiography.

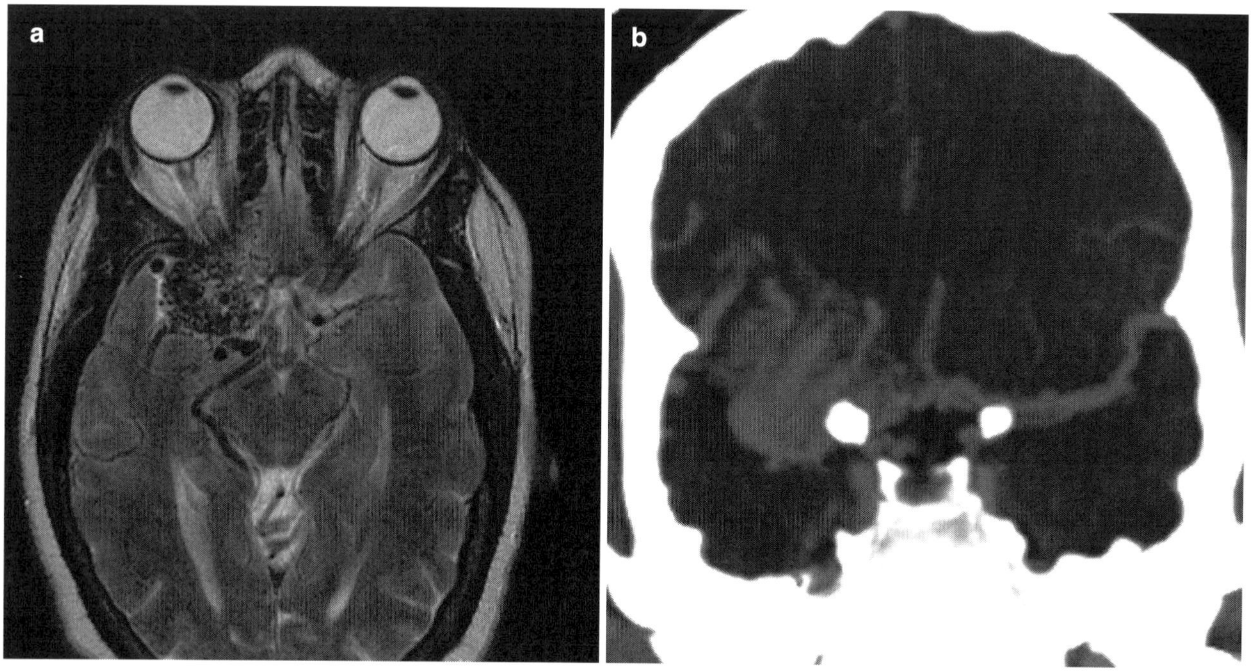

Fig. 60.1 Arteriovenous malformation (AVM) of the parasellar region. (**a**) Axial T2-weighted MR image. (**b**) Coronal contrast-enhanced CT image. Multiple tangles of the arteries and veins are present in the right parasellar region, indicating feeding arteries and draining veins of an AVM. The CT image (*cuc*) shows engorgement of the right cavernous ICA into the sella

60.3 Clinical and Surgical Management

- The individualized treatment of AVMs in the sellar region depends heavily on the location and architecture of the particular malformation.
- Emergent surgical intervention may be required for ruptured AVMs. Medical goals include blood pressure control.
- AVMs may be managed with multimodality treatment including endovascular embolization, surgical resection, and/or stereotactic radiosurgery [2, 3].

References

1. Gould TJ, Johnson LN, Colapinto EV, Spollen LE, Rodriguez FJ. Intrasellar vascular malformation mimicking a pituitary macroadenoma. J Neuroophthalmol. 1996;16:199–203.
2. Gibo H, Watanabe N, Kobayashi S, Sugita K. Removal of an arteriovenous malformation in the optic chiasm. A case of Bonnet-Dechaume-Blanc syndrome without retinal involvement. Surg Neurol. 1989;31:142–8.
3. Morgan MK, Johnston IH, de Silva M. Treatment of ophthalmofacial-hypothalamic arteriovenous malformation (Bonnet-Dechaume-Blanc syndrome). Case report. J Neurosurg. 1985;63:794–6.
4. Hopen G, Smith JL, Hoff JT, Quencer R. The Wyburn-Mason syndrome. Concomitant chiasmal and fundus vascular malformations. J Clin Neuroophthalmol. 1983;3:53–62.
5. Luo CB, Lasjaunias P, Bhattacharya J. Craniofacial vascular malformations in Wyburn-Mason syndrome. J Chin Med Assoc. 2006;69:575–80.
6. Muragaki Y, Ujiie H, Ohno M, Kubo O, Hori T. Optic nerve arteriovenous malformation causing optic apoplexy: case report. Neurosurgery. 2002;51:1075–8. discussion 1078.
7. Sasagawa Y, Akai T, Sasaki T, Iizuka H. Chiasmal and/or optic nerve apoplexy due to rupture of vascular malformation – case report. Neurol Med Chir (Tokyo). 2008;48:460–5.
8. Wolansky LJ, Shaderowfsky PD, Sander R, Frohman LP, Kalnin AJ, Lee HJ. Optic chiasmal compression by venous aneurysm: magnetic resonance imaging diagnosis. J Neuroimaging. 1997;7:46–7.
9. Mirabel S, Lindblom B, Halbach VV, Hoyt WF. Giant suprasellar varix: an unusual cause of chiasmal compression. J Clin Neuroophthalmol. 1991;11:268–72.

Cavernous Malformations (Angiomas) of the Sellar and Suprasellar Region

61

Gabriel Zada, M. Beatriz S. Lopes,
Srinivasan Mukundan Jr., and Edward Laws Jr.

61.1 Epidemiology and Clinical Presentation

- Cavernous malformations, also known as cavernous angiomas or cavernomas, are true vascular malformations that may be located anywhere in the brain. This section focuses on cavernous malformations of the sellar and suprasellar region.
- Cavernous malformations (angiomas) are distinct from cavernous sinus cavernous hemangiomas (CSCHs) (*see* Chap. 33) [1]. CSCHs are benign vascular tumors, not true vascular malformations.
- Cavernous malformations are congenital lesions that occur rarely in the sellar and suprasellar region, often within or adjacent to the optic nerves, chiasm, and hypothalamus [2]. They are typically intraparenchymal lesions, but they may also arise extra-axially in the optic cisterns [3–5].
- As a result, they may cause visual loss or chiasmal syndromes, often developing with a sudden onset [6–12].
- In some cases, ruptured cavernous malformations of the suprasellar region may result in subarachnoid hemorrhage or optic apoplexy [3, 10].

G. Zada, MD, MS (✉)
Department of Neurological Surgery, Keck School of Medicine, University of Southern California, 1200 N State Street, #3300, Los Angeles, CA 90033, USA
e-mail: gzada@usc.edu

M.B.S. Lopes, MD, PhD
Department of Pathology (Neuropathology), University of Virginia School of Medicine, 1215 Lee Street, Room 3060–HEP, Charlottesville, VA 22908, USA
e-mail: msl2e@virginia.edu

S. Mukundan Jr., PhD, MD
Department of Radiology, Brigham and Women's Hospital, 75 Francis Street, Boston, MA 02115, USA
e-mail: smukundan@partners.org

E. Laws Jr., MD
Department of Neurosurgery, Brigham and Women's Hospital, 15 Francis Street, Boston, MA 02115, USA
e-mail: elaws@partners.org

G. Zada et al. (eds.), *Atlas of Sellar and Parasellar Lesions: Clinical, Radiologic, and Pathologic Correlations*,
DOI 10.1007/978-3-319-22855-6_61

61.2 Imaging Features

- CT imaging usually shows a hyperdense suprasellar mass. Calcifications are evident in 56 % of patients [12].
- On MRI, cavernous malformations typically show mixed signal intensities and heterogeneous contents, with no contrast enhancement (Fig. 61.1). The mixed "popcorn"-like signal intensities are thought to represent blood products of various ages from intranidal hemorrhage (Fig. 61.2) [4, 12].
- Angiography is typically negative in patients with cavernous malformations.
- Developmental venous anomalies (DVAs) may be seen in conjunction with cavernous malformations.

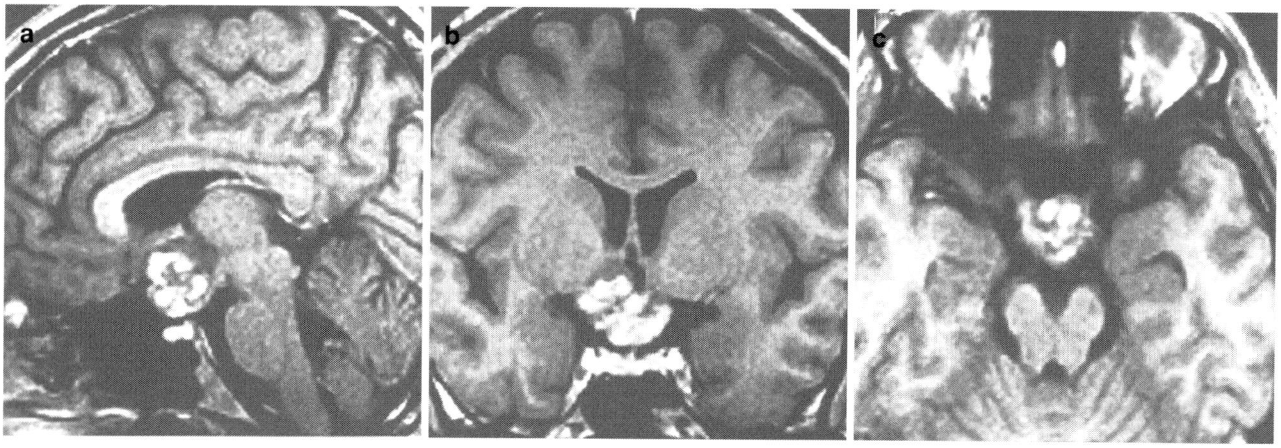

Fig. 61.1 Cavernous malformation (angioma). (**a**) Sagittal T1-weighted gadolinium-enhanced MR image showing a multilocular lesion with high signal intensity surrounded by a rim with low signal intensity, continuing anteriorly along both optic nerves. (**b**, **c**) Coronal and axial views of gadolinium-enhanced images show mild enhancement of the mass (From Shibuya et al. [5]; with permission)

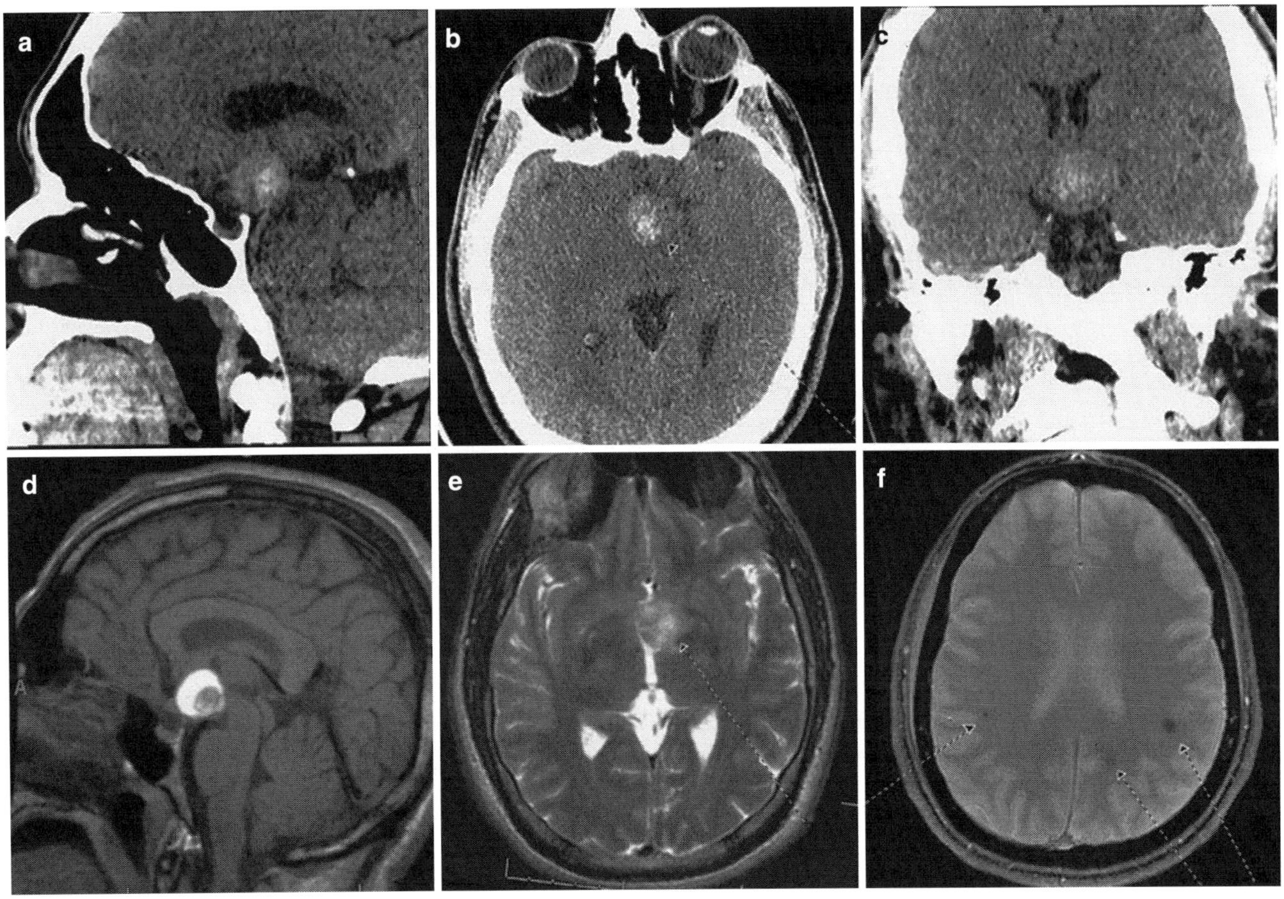

Fig. 61.2 Cavernous malformation (angioma). Sagittal (**a**), axial (**b**), and coronal (**c**) non-enhanced CT scans show a hyperdense mass in the suprasellar region. A sagittal T1-weighted non-enhanced MR image (**d**) demonstrates a predominantly T1-hyperintense mass in the suprasellar region at the level of the hypothalamus and tuber cinereum, abutting the distal basilar artery tip. Predominant signal characteristics are compatible with subacute methemoglobin. An internal nodular component demonstrates regional and circumferential low signals, which bloomed on gradient echo images compatible with hemosiderin at the site of the preexisting exophytic, hypothalamic cavernoma. An axial T2-weighted image (**e**) demonstrates a predominantly hyperintense signal compatible with extracellular methemoglobin within the 2-cm mass centered at the left paramedian, anteroinferior floor of the third ventricle. T2-weighted gradient echo images (**f**) demonstrate secondary areas of blooming signal void compatible with chronic hemosiderin deposition at sites of smaller cavernomas in the subcortical frontoparietal white matter and cervicomedullary junction (Adapted with permission from Rheinboldt and Blase [2])

61.3 Histopathology

- On gross examination, cavernous malformations are often well circumscribed, lobulated, and red/purple "mulberry"-like lesions.
- Cavernous angiomas (malformations) are congenital intraparenchymal lesions with thin-lined capillaries that are lined by a single-layer endothelium, separated by collagenous stroma with no intervening brain parenchyma, and contain sinusoidal spaces. Intranidal hemorrhage and thrombosis are commonly seen.

61.4 Clinical and Surgical Management

- Surgical treatment via craniotomy is recommended for most cases of symptomatic suprasellar cavernous malformations. Gross total resection is associated with improved visual outcomes [12].
- A pterional or subfrontal cranial approach is typically utilized for surgical resection [13].
- Emergent surgery is recommended for patients presenting with acute visual loss caused by chiasmal hemorrhage and/or apoplexy in the presence of a cavernous malformation [12, 14].
- Indocyanine green has been used to help identify and confirm the resection of optic cavernous malformations, because the lesion typically will not be visualized following administration of indocyanine green, whereas the brain, optic chiasm/nerves, and small vessels are visualized [11].
- The use of stereotactic radiosurgery for cavernous malformations is debated [15]. Radiosurgery has been reported to reduce the risk of rupture associated with cavernous malformations. In treating perioptic lesions in the suprasellar region, fractionated radiosurgery is typically required [16].

References

1. Gonzalez LF, Lekovic GP, Eschbacher J, Coons S, Porter RW, Spetzler RF. Are cavernous sinus hemangiomas and cavernous malformations different entities? Neurosurg Focus. 2006;21(1):e6.
2. Rheinboldt M, Blase J. Exophytic hypothalamic cavernous malformation mimicking an extra-axial suprasellar mass. Emerg Radiol. 2011;18:363–7.
3. Escott EJ, Rubinstein D, Cajade-Law AG, Sze CI. Suprasellar cavernous malformation presenting with extensive subarachnoid hemorrhage. Neuroradiology. 2001;43:313–6.
4. Loesch DV, Gilman S, Del Dotto J, Rosenblum ML. Cavernous malformation of the mammillary bodies: neuropsychological implications. Case report. J Neurosurg. 1995;83:354–8.
5. Shibuya M, Baskaya MK, Saito K, Suzuki Y, Ooka K, Hara M. Cavernous malformations of the optic chiasma. Acta Neurochir (Wien). 1995;136:29–36.
6. Stephenson G, Afshar F. Suprasellar cavernous angioma causing pituitary and hypothalamic dysfunction. Br J Neurosurg. 1994;8:225–7.
7. Udayakumaran S, Paraskevopoulos D, Cagnano E, Roth J, Constantini S. Spontaneous bleeding into a suprasellar cavernous angioma of a neonate: case report and literature review. Childs Nerv Syst. 2011;27:303–11.
8. Hassler W, Zentner J, Wilhelm H. Cavernous angiomas of the anterior visual pathways. J Clin Neuroophthalmol. 1989;9:160–4.
9. Muta D, Nishi T, Koga K, Yamashiro S, Fujioka S, Kuratsu J. Cavernous malformation of the optic chiasm: case report. Br J Neurosurg. 2006;20:312–5.
10. Ferreira NP, Ferreira MP. Optic nerve apoplexy caused by a cavernous angioma: case report. Neurosurgery. 1992;30:262–4.
11. Murai Y, Adachi K, Koketsu K, Teramoto A. Indocyanine green videoangiography of optic cavernous angioma – case report. Neurol Med Chir (Tokyo). 2011;51:296–8.
12. Liu JK, Lu Y, Raslan AM, Gultekin SH, Delashaw Jr JB. Cavernous malformations of the optic pathway and hypothalamus: analysis of 65 cases in the literature. Neurosurg Focus. 2010;29(3):E17.
13. Sun XY, Yu F. Microsurgical resection of a cavernous angioma that involves the optic pathway using a pterional approach: a case report and literature review. Br J Neurosurg. 2012;26:882–5.
14. Newman H, Nevo M, Constantini S, Maimon S, Kesler A. Chiasmal cavernoma: a rare cause of acute visual loss improved by prompt surgery. Pediatr Neurosurg. 2008;44:414–7.
15. Steiner L, Karlsson B, Yen CP, Torner JC, Lindquist C, Schlesinger D. Radiosurgery in cavernous malformations: anatomy of a controversy. J Neurosurg. 2010;113:16–21; discussion 21–2.
16. Niranjan A, Lunsford LD. Stereotactic radiosurgery guidelines for the management of patients with intracranial cavernous malformations. Prog Neurol Surg. 2013;27:166–75.

Vascular Fistulas of the Sellar and Parasellar Region

62

Gabriel Zada, M. Beatriz S. Lopes, Srinivasan Mukundan Jr., and Edward Laws Jr.

62.1 Epidemiology and Clinical Presentation

- Primary arteriovenous malformations (AVMs) of the pituitary gland and sellar region are exceedingly rare [1].
- More commonly, vascular malformations in surrounding structures (such as the cavernous sinus) have a secondary effect on the pituitary gland and its physiology.
- The most common of these conditions are cavernous-carotid fistulas (CCFs) and dural arteriovenous malformations (AVMs) of the cavernous sinus.
- The Barrow classification system is often used to categorize these lesions [2]. Classic, direct CCFs are Type A, and Types B through D are collectively called "indirect fistulas" or "dural AVMs."
  - Type A fistulas are direct, high-flow CCFs between the ICA and cavernous sinus.
  - Type B fistulas are caused by communication between smaller ICA branches and the cavernous sinus.
  - Type C fistulas are caused by dural branches of the external carotid artery (ECA).
  - Type D fistulas are those caused by a combination of ICA and ECA branches.

62.1.1 Cavernous-Carotid Fistulas

- Type A CCFs can be traumatic (80 %) or spontaneous, or they can develop as a result of a ruptured cavernous segment ICA aneurysm [3].
- The most common clinical presentation of Type A CCFs includes visual loss, headache, diplopia, and orbital pain. Common clinical signs include an orbital bruit, elevated intraocular pressure, exophthalmos, and cranial nerve paresis. Abducens nerve palsies are most commonly associated with CCF [3].
- CCFs may also rarely have secondary effects on the pituitary gland, including hypopituitarism [4, 5].

G. Zada, MD, MS (✉)
Department of Neurological Surgery, Keck School of Medicine, University of Southern California, 1200 N State Street, #3300, Los Angeles, CA 90033, USA
e-mail: gzada@usc.edu

M.B.S. Lopes, MD, PhD
Department of Pathology (Neuropathology), University of Virginia School of Medicine, 1215 Lee Street, Room 3060–HEP, Charlottesville, VA 22908, USA
e-mail: msl2e@virginia.edu

S. Mukundan Jr., PhD, MD
Department of Radiology, Brigham and Women's Hospital, 75 Francis Street, Boston, MA 02115, USA
e-mail: smukundan@partners.org

E. Laws Jr., MD
Department of Neurosurgery, Brigham and Women's Hospital, 15 Francis Street, Boston, MA 02115, USA
e-mail: elaws@partners.org

G. Zada et al. (eds.), *Atlas of Sellar and Parasellar Lesions: Clinical, Radiologic, and Pathologic Correlations*, DOI 10.1007/978-3-319-22855-6_62

62.1.2 Cavernous Sinus Dural AVMs

- Indirect cavernous sinus dural AVMs (Types B–D) are most commonly caused by communications with the meningohypophyseal trunk and the artery of the inferior cavernous sinus [2].
- About 70 % occur in women over the age of 50. The mean age is 60 years [6].
- Symptoms in patients with cavernous sinus dural AVMs are similar to those in patients with CCFs, albeit to a lesser degree. Misdiagnosis is common [3].
- Venous congestion caused by cavernous sinus dural AVMs may infrequently result in congestion of the pituitary gland [7] or even remote hemorrhages in the brainstem [8, 9].

62.2 Imaging Features

- Standard CT imaging may show widening of the cavernous sinus in conjunction with a CCF or high-flow cavernous dural AVM. The superior ophthalmic vein and extraocular muscles may be larger because of venous congestion.
- Orbital ultrasonography may confirm superior ophthalmic venous congestion and show reversal of flow through the vein [3].
- In patients with CCFs, MRI may show abnormal flow voids, signal changes, and widening of the cavernous sinus (Fig. 62.1).
- MRI often shows an enlarged (congested) pituitary gland in patients with cavernous sinus dural AVMs [10].
- Time-of-flight MR angiography is highly sensitive in detecting flow-related enhancement at the fistula connection extending to the cavernous sinuses immediately adjacent to the fistula (Fig. 62.1b).
- Dynamic MRI has been shown to demonstrate asymmetric filling in patients with cavernous sinus AVMs. The side with the dural AVM typically shows reduced enhancement, and the pituitary gland on the whole enhances more slowly than in control subjects [10].
- Angiography is the gold standard modality for visualization (and often treatment) of parasellar vascular malformations (Fig. 62.2).

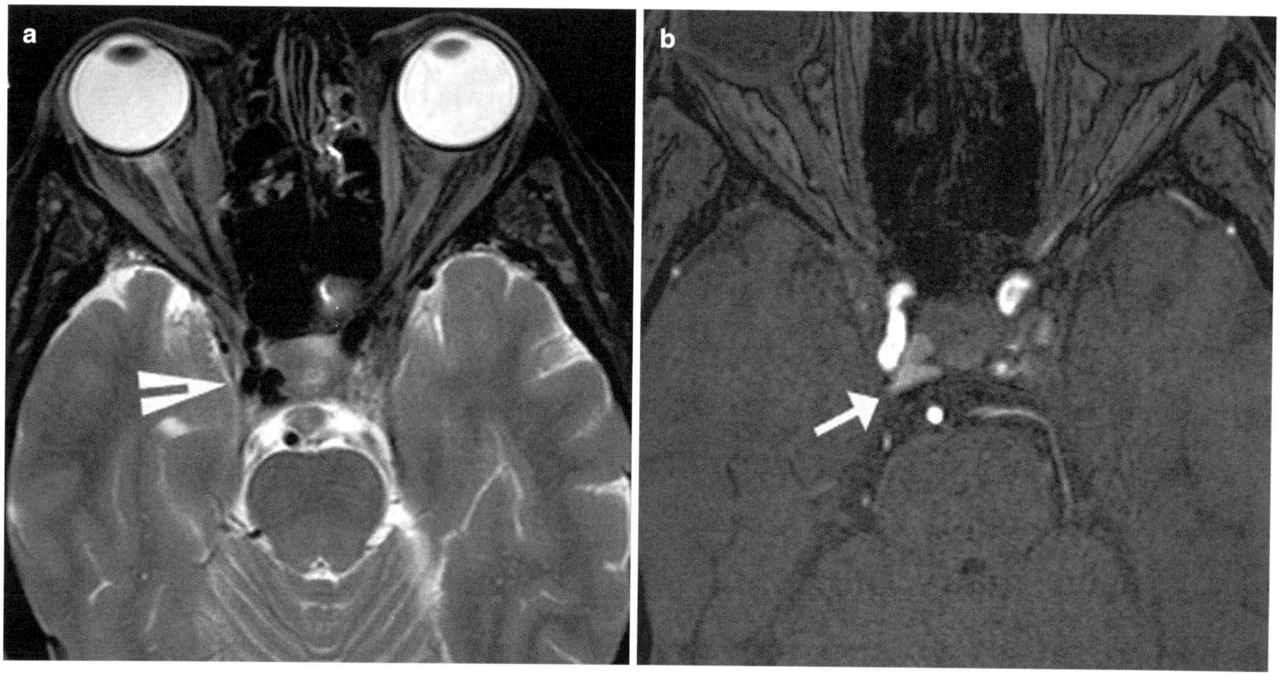

Fig. 62.1 Cavernous-carotid fistula. (**a**) Axial T2-weighted MR image. (**b**) Time-of-flight intracranial MR angiography image. Arterial flow void is observed in the right cavernous sinus (**a**, *arrowhead*). The right globe is mildly proptotic, with mild enlargement of the extraocular muscles. Flow-related enhancement is seen in the right cavernous sinus (**b**, *arrow*), indicating arterialization of the right cavernous sinus

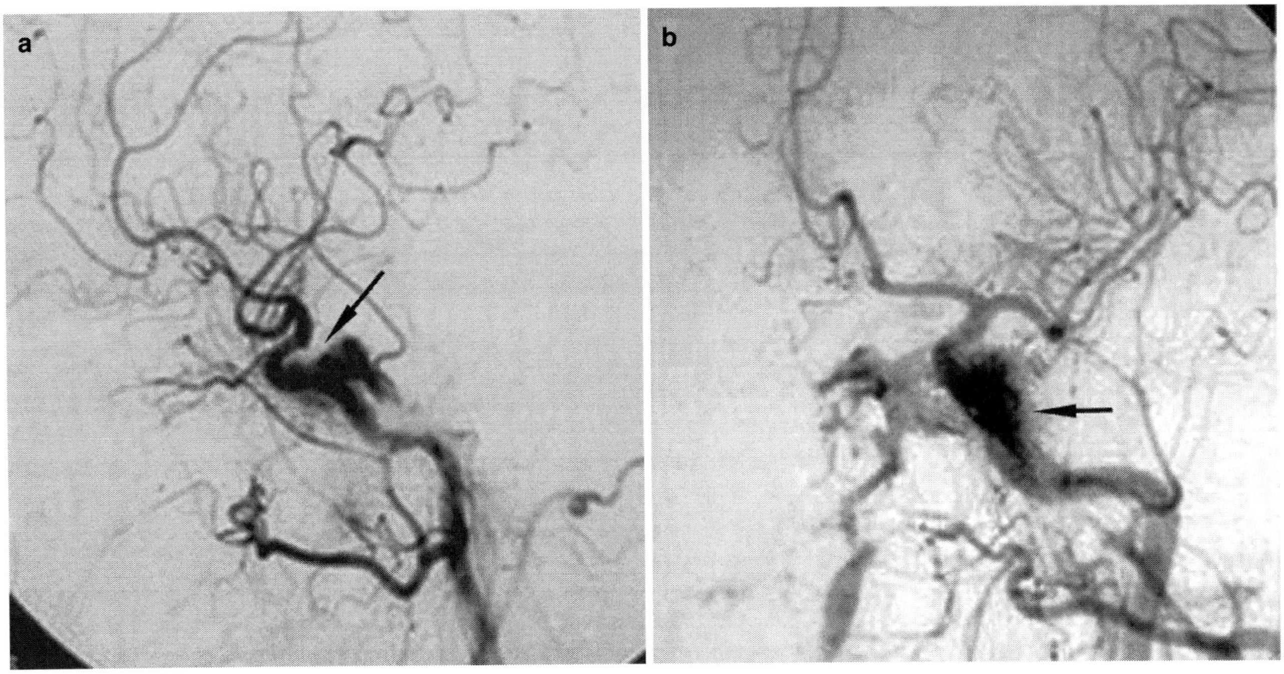

Fig. 62.2 Cavernous sinus dural arteriovenous fistula (DAVF) seen on lateral (**a**) and anteroposterior (**b**) digital subtraction angiography (DSA) (Adapted with permission from Kashiwazaki et al. [13])

62.3 Clinical and Surgical Management

- Some patients with low-flow cavernous sinus dural AVMs will have spontaneous thrombosis and resolution of the fistula.
- In patients with high-flow CCFs and dural AVMs that require intervention, management strategies vary. They typically involve endovascular techniques with embolization of the fistula. The available techniques include coil embolization, balloon embolization, and stent placement. The approach may be done transarterially or transvenously. Every attempt is made to obliterate the fistula while preserving ICA flow.
- Successful superselective coil embolization of cavernous sinus dural AVMs has been reported. A majority of patients have excellent outcomes and can be treated in one setting [11, 12]. Cranial nerve paresis may occur in the setting of endovascular treatment for parasellar AVFs and CCFs [13].
- Successful long-term embolization of direct (Type A) CCFs is possible in up to 95 % of patients [14].
- Five years following treatment, over 80 % of patients with indirect fistulas (Types B–D) are typically cured [6, 14, 15].
- Improvement in pituitary gland congestion size has been shown following embolization of cavernous sinus AVMs [7, 10].
- Recanalization or recurrence occurs in about 9 % of patients after successful initial embolization [15].
- Stereotactic surgery has been successfully used to treat patients with refractory low-flow fistulas. According to one study, 90 % of patients had resolution of the fistula at 7 months following the procedure [16].

References

1. Gould TJ, Johnson LN, Colapinto EV, Spollen LE, Rodriguez FJ. Intrasellar vascular malformation mimicking a pituitary macroadenoma. J Neuroophthalmol. 1996;16:199–203.
2. Barrow DL, Spector RH, Braun IF, Landman JA, Tindall SC, Tindall GT. Classification and treatment of spontaneous carotid-cavernous sinus fistulas. J Neurosurg. 1985;62:248–56.
3. Feiner L, Bennett J, Volpe NJ. Cavernous sinus fistulas: carotid cavernous fistulas and dural arteriovenous malformations. Curr Neurol Neurosci Rep. 2003;3:415–20.
4. Yarandi SS, Khoshnoodi MA, Chandra P. Hypopituitarism caused by carotid cavernous fistula. Intern Med. 2011;50:1105–8.
5. Goto A, Takahashi Y, Kishimoto M, Tanabe A, Kajio H, Hasuo K, Noda M. Hypopituitarism caused by bilateral internal carotid artery aneurysms with a carotid-cavernous fistula. Intern Med. 2008; 47:815–6.
6. Meyers PM, Halbach VV, Dowd CF, Lempert TE, Malek AM, Phatouros CC, et al. Dural carotid cavernous fistula: definitive endovascular management and long-term follow-up. Am J Ophthalmol. 2002;134:85–92.
7. Sato N, Putman CM, Chaloupka JC, Glenn BJ, Vinuela F, Sze G. Pituitary gland enlargement secondary to dural arteriovenous fistula in the cavernous sinus: appearance at MR imaging. Radiology. 1997;203:263–7.
8. Miyagishima T, Hara T, Inoue M, Terano N, Ohno H, Okamoto K, Hasuo K. Pontine venous congestion due to dural arteriovenous fistula of the cavernous sinus: case report and review of the literature. Surg Neurol Int. 2012;3:53.
9. Furuya K, Segawa H, Shiokawa Y, Ide K, Sano K. Brain stem haemorrhage during transsphenoidal surgery. Possible risk of the manoeuvre of increasing the endexpiratory pressure in a case of pituitary adenoma associated with dural arteriovenous malformation. Case report. Acta Neurochir (Wien). 1993;125:188–91.
10. Shigematsu Y, Korogi Y, Kitajima M, Ishii A, Liang L, Yamura M, et al. Abnormal perfusion of the pituitary gland secondary to dural arteriovenous fistulas in the cavernous sinus: dynamic MR findings. AJNR Am J Neuroradiol. 2003;24:930–6.
11. Satow T, Murao K, Matsushige T, Fukuda K, Miyamoto S, Iihara K. Superselective shunt occlusion for the treatment of cavernous sinus dural arteriovenous fistulae. Neurosurgery. 2013;73:ons100–5.
12. Kupersmith MJ, Berenstein A, Choi IS, Warren F, Flamm E. Management of nontraumatic vascular shunts involving the cavernous sinus. Ophthalmology. 1988;95:121–30.
13. Kashiwazaki D, Kuwayama N, Akioka N, Kuroda S. Delayed abducens nerve palsy after transvenous coil embolization for cavernous sinus dural arteriovenous fistulae. Acta Neurochir (Wien). 2014;156:97–101.
14. Ducruet AF, Albuquerque FC, Crowley RW, McDougall CG. The evolution of endovascular treatment of carotid cavernous fistulas: a single-center experience. World Neurosurg. 2013;80:538–48.
15. Yoshida K, Melake M, Oishi H, Yamamoto M, Arai H. Transvenous embolization of dural carotid cavernous fistulas: a series of 44 consecutive patients. AJNR Am J Neuroradiol. 2010;31:651–5.
16. Barcia-Salorio JL, Soler F, Barcia JA, Hernández G. Stereotactic radiosurgery for the treatment of low-flow carotid-cavernous fistulae: results in a series of 25 cases. Stereotact Funct Neurosurg. 1994;63:266–70.

Carotid Artery Dolichoectasia and Kissing Internal Carotid Arteries

63

Gabriel Zada, M. Beatriz S. Lopes,
Srinivasan Mukundan Jr., and Edward Laws Jr.

63.1 Epidemiology and Clinical Presentation

- Various vascular anomalies of the internal carotid arteries (ICAs) may occasionally arise in the sellar and parasellar region and warrant attention from treating physicians.
- Dolichoectasia is a term used to describe dilatation, elongation, and tortuosity of cerebral arteries. It most commonly affects the vertebrobasilar system, but it may also occur in unilateral or bilateral ICAs [1].
- Dolichoectasia is commonly associated with hypertension and may be associated with polycystic kidney disease.
- In rare cases, ectasia of the ICA may result in compression of the optic nerve, chiasm, or both, with corresponding visual loss. The median age of patients with this condition is 72 years [2, 3].
- ICA ectasia and calcification may be associated with low-tension glaucoma [4–6].
- "Kissing carotid arteries" is a term used when bilateral ICA tortuosity causes them to come into close contact with one another. In rare cases, this entity may cause hypopituitarism or visual loss. It becomes especially important when planning surgical approaches, as it may be an absolute contraindication to a selected surgical approach [7–9].
- The caliber and tortuosity of the ICA may be abnormal in conjunction with various diseases. In patients with acromegaly, the caliber and tortuosity of the ICA are greater, and special attention to these structures on preoperative imaging studies is imperative prior to performing transsphenoidal surgery [10, 11].

G. Zada, MD, MS (✉)
Department of Neurological Surgery, Keck School of Medicine,
University of Southern California, 1200 N State Street, #3300,
Los Angeles, CA 90033, USA
e-mail: gzada@usc.edu

M.B.S. Lopes, MD, PhD
Department of Pathology (Neuropathology),
University of Virginia School of Medicine,
1215 Lee Street, Room 3060–HEP, Charlottesville,
VA 22908, USA
e-mail: msl2e@virginia.edu

S. Mukundan Jr., PhD, MD
Department of Radiology, Brigham and Women's Hospital,
75 Francis Street, Boston, MA 02115, USA
e-mail: smukundan@partners.org

E. Laws Jr., MD
Department of Neurosurgery, Brigham and Women's Hospital,
15 Francis Street, Boston, MA 02115, USA
e-mail: elaws@partners.org

G. Zada et al. (eds.), *Atlas of Sellar and Parasellar Lesions: Clinical, Radiologic, and Pathologic Correlations*,
DOI 10.1007/978-3-319-22855-6_63

63.2 Imaging Features

- Noninvasive vascular imaging includes CT and MR angiography (Fig. 63.1). These studies allow visualization of the relationship of the vasculature to surrounding neural structures, such as the optic nerves and chiasm.
- On MRI, asymptomatic unilateral ectasia of the ICA, in which the ICA comes in direct contact with the optic nerve but no visual loss occurs, has been reported in up to 70 % of patients. Bilateral optic nerve compression by the ICAs was seen in 12 % of patients. The diameter of the ICA was correlated with optic nerve compression [12].
- Kissing carotid arteries can be assessed on noninvasive imaging including CT angiogram and MR angiograms (Fig. 63.2).

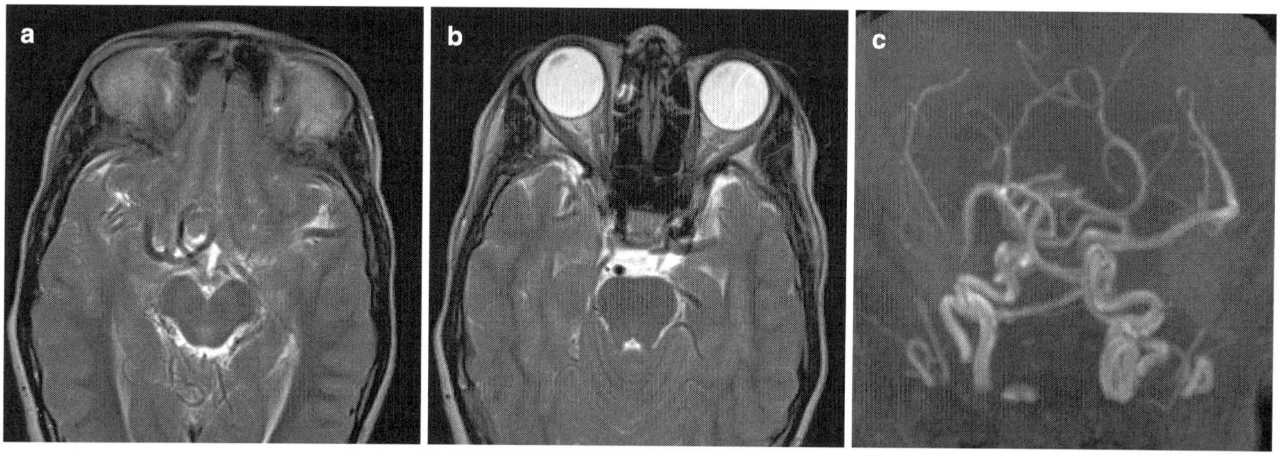

Fig. 63.1 Dolichoectasia. (**a**, **b**) Axial T2-weighted MR images. (**c**) Maximum-intensity-projection (MIP) time-of-flight MR angiography. The intracranial internal carotid arteries appear ectatic, with marked tortuosity, in a 10-year-old boy with a diagnosis of Ehlers-Danlos syndrome

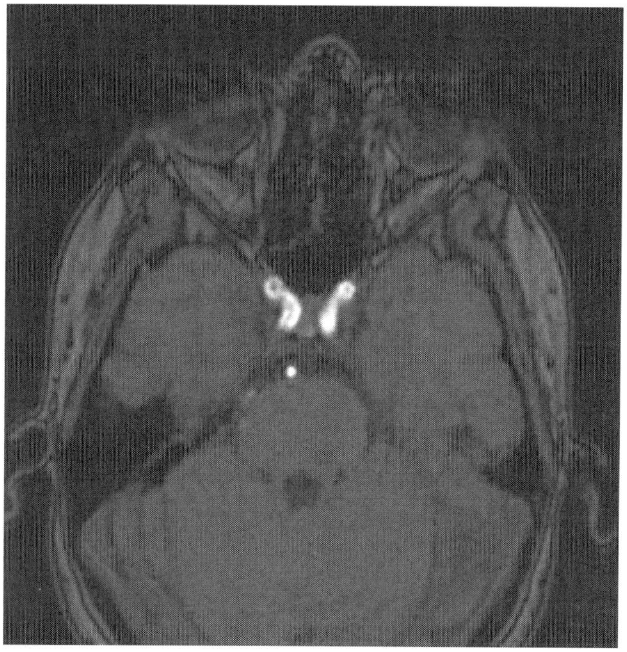

Fig. 63.2 Kissing internal carotid arteries. Axial MRI through the sellar region, showing significant bilateral dolichoectasia of the ICAs, also known as "kissing" ICAs (Adapted with permission from Sahin et al. [8])

63.3 Clinical and Surgical Management

- Anomalies in the course and caliber of the ICA—especially kissing ICAs (Fig. 63.2)—can be a contraindication to various surgical approaches. Surgeons planning any operations in the sellar and suprasellar region must routinely and habitually study the anatomy and course of the ICA prior to any operation.
- Patients with acromegaly require additional attention in surgical planning, as they are known to have fusiform dilatation and increased tortuosity of the ICAs [11, 13].
- In rare cases, visual loss from ICA ectasia may be treated surgically via craniotomy to decompress the optic structures. Visual outcomes are excellent following these procedures [2, 14].

References

1. Takeuchi S, Takasato Y, Masaoka H, Hayakawa T, Otani N, Yoshino Y, et al. Dolichoectasia involving the vertebrobasilar and carotid artery systems. J Clin Neurosci. 2009;16:1344–6.
2. Fargen KM, Blackburn S. Surgical decompression for optic neuropathy from carotid artery ectasia: case report with technical considerations. World Neurosurg. 2014;82:239. e9–12.
3. Jacobson DM. Symptomatic compression of the optic nerve by the carotid artery: clinical profile of 18 patients with 24 affected eyes identified by magnetic resonance imaging. Ophthalmology. 1999; 106:1994–2004.
4. Ellis MF, Scott M, Erwin G. Carotid artery ectasia coexistent with primary open angle glaucoma. Clin Experiment Ophthalmol. 2001; 29:44–6.
5. Ogata N, Imaizumi M, Kurokawa H, Arichi M, Matsumura M. Optic nerve compression by normal carotid artery in patients with normal tension glaucoma. Br J Ophthalmol. 2005;89:174–9.
6. Gutman I, Melamed S, Ashkenazi I, Blumenthal M. Optic nerve compression by carotid arteries in low-tension glaucoma. Graefes Arch Clin Exp Ophthalmol. 1993;231:711–7.
7. Pereira Filho Ade A, Gobbato PL, Pereira Filho Gde A, Silva SB, Kraemer JL. Intracranial intrasellar kissing carotid arteries: case report. Arq Neuropsiquiatr. 2007;65:355–7.
8. Sahin M, Dilli A, Karbek B, Unsal IO, Gungunes A, Colak N, et al. Unusual cause of primary amenorrhea due to kissing internal carotid arteries. Pituitary. 2012;15:258–9.
9. Slavin ML. Bitemporal hemianopia associated with dolichoectasia of the intracranial carotid arteries. J Clin Neuroophthalmol. 1990; 10:80–1.
10. Sacher M, Som PM, Shugar JM, Leeds NE. Kissing intrasellar carotid arteries in acromegaly: CT demonstration. J Comput Assist Tomogr. 1986;10:1033–5.
11. Zada G, Cavallo LM, Esposito F, Fernandez-Jimenez JC, Tasiou A, De Angelis M, et al. Transsphenoidal surgery in patients with acromegaly: operative strategies for overcoming technically challenging anatomical variations. Neurosurg Focus. 2010;29(4):E8.
12. Jacobson DM, Warner JJ, Broste SK. Optic nerve contact and compression by the carotid artery in asymptomatic patients. Am J Ophthalmol. 1997;123:677–83.
13. Sivakumar W, Chamoun RB, Riva-Cambrin J, Salzman KL, Couldwell WT. Fusiform dilatation of the cavernous carotid artery in acromegalic patients. Acta Neurochir (Wien). 2013;155:1077–83; discussion 1083.
14. Colapinto EV, Cabeen MA, Johnson LN. Optic nerve compression by a dolichoectatic internal carotid artery: case report. Neurosurgery. 1996;39:604–6.

Sheehan's Pituitary Infarction

64

Gabriel Zada, M. Beatriz S. Lopes,
Srinivasan Mukundan Jr., and Edward Laws Jr.

64.1 Epidemiology and Clinical Presentation

- Sheehan's syndrome is the eponymous name for pituitary insufficiency caused by ischemia. It is classically associated with hypovolemia and hypotension following severe postpartum hemorrhage.
- The incidence of Sheehan's syndrome has dramatically decreased over the course of the past century and is currently very low in developed nations [1].
- The pathophysiology of Sheehan's syndrome is likely multifactorial; the disease has been associated with larger pituitary gland size, smaller sella turcica size, blood clotting disorders, and blood loss.
- Pituitary infarction resembling Sheehan's syndrome (Simmond's disease) has been shown to develop following severe trauma, snakebites from the Russell's viper [2], coronary artery bypass surgery [3], gastrointestinal hemorrhage [4], severe burns [5], and cocaine abuse [6].
- Sheehan's syndrome often develops in a delayed fashion, with a delay in diagnosis of 9 years or more following the inciting event [7]. The mean age at the time of diagnosis is 46 years [8].
- Aside from primary ischemia and infarction as a mechanism for the development of Sheehan's syndrome, it has been shown that the slower time course of the disease may also be mediated by pituitary autoimmunity and antipituitary antibodies caused by the release of tissue factor antigens associated with primary injury [9].
- Sheehan's syndrome is characterized by anterior hypopituitarism in most cases. It often presents clinically with fatigue, headache, lactation failure (agalactia), loss of axillary and pubic hair, and amenorrhea [7]. Other classic symptoms and signs include decreased muscle strength, dryness and wrinkling of the skin, premature aging, hypotension, cold intolerance, constipation, pallor, anemia, bradycardia, hypoglycemia, insulin hypersensitivity, infertility, breast atrophy, decreased vaginal secretions, mental slowing, apathy, and psychiatric disturbances [10].
- On laboratory studies, deficient prolactin and growth hormone axes are most commonly seen. Hyponatremia is another common manifestation [11].
- Posterior pituitary function is also commonly affected in patients with Sheehan's syndrome, with up to 30 % meeting criteria for diabetes insipidus [12].

G. Zada, MD, MS (✉)
Department of Neurological Surgery, Keck School of Medicine, University of Southern California, 1200 N State Street, #3300, Los Angeles, CA 90033, USA
e-mail: gzada@usc.edu

M.B.S. Lopes, MD, PhD
Department of Pathology (Neuropathology), University of Virginia School of Medicine, 1215 Lee Street, Room 3060–HEP, Charlottesville, VA 22908, USA
e-mail: msl2e@virginia.edu

S. Mukundan Jr., PhD, MD
Department of Radiology, Brigham and Women's Hospital, 75 Francis Street, Boston, MA 02115, USA
e-mail: smukundan@partners.org

E. Laws Jr., MD
Department of Neurosurgery, Brigham and Women's Hospital, 15 Francis Street, Boston, MA 02115, USA
e-mail: elaws@partners.org

G. Zada et al. (eds.), *Atlas of Sellar and Parasellar Lesions: Clinical, Radiologic, and Pathologic Correlations*, DOI 10.1007/978-3-319-22855-6_64

64.2 Imaging Features

- An empty sella is often seen on CT or MRI in patients with Sheehan's syndrome [13–15].
- A completely empty sella is seen in two thirds of patients, and a partially empty sella in one third (Fig. 64.1) [16].
- In some cases, prolapse of the optic chiasm into an empty sella may be seen [17].
- In acute stage, the pituitary gland demonstrates diffuse central hypoenhancement on MRI, indicating infarction.

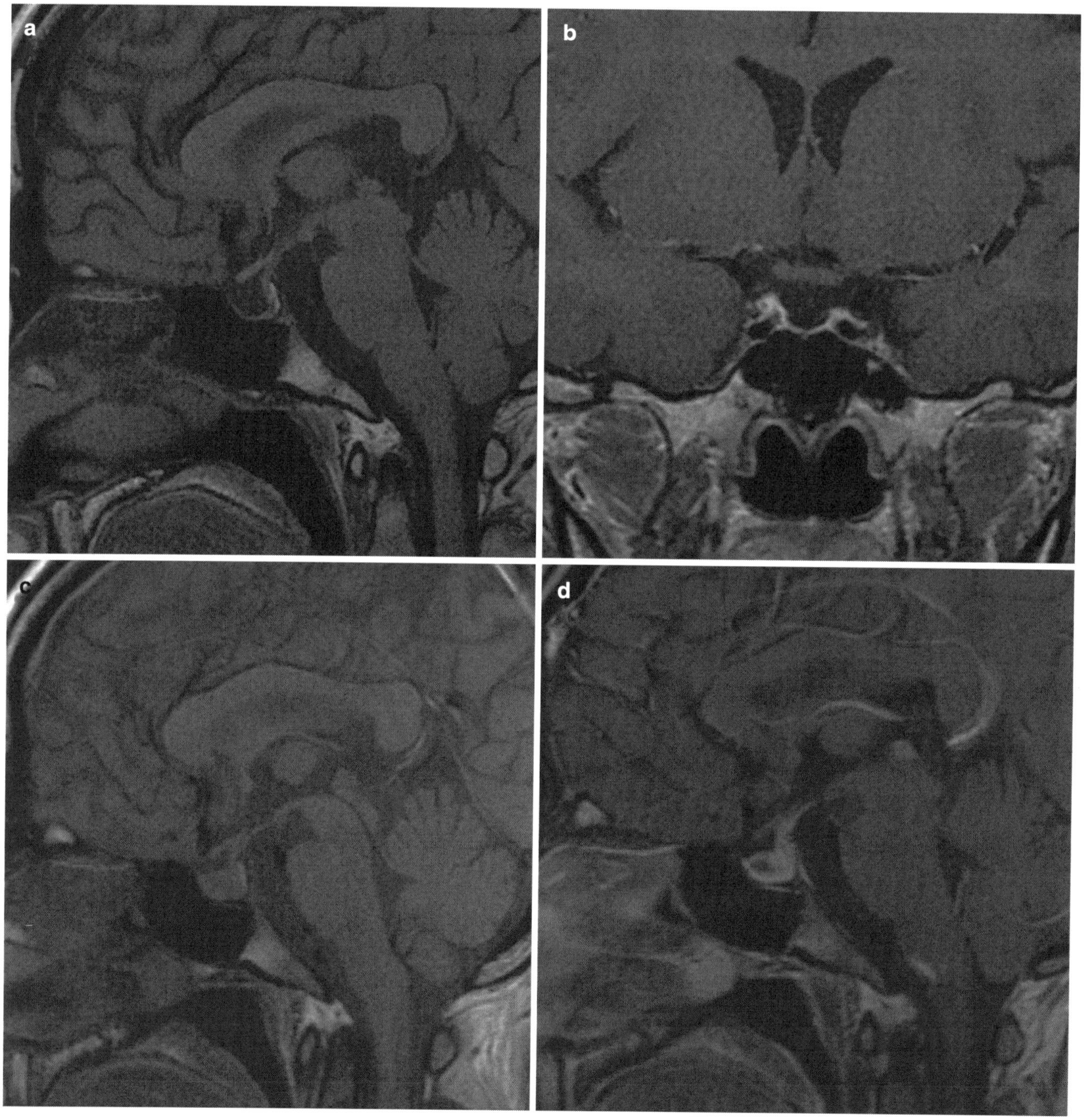

Fig. 64.1 Sheehan's infarction. (**a**) Sagittal T1-weighted precontrast MR image. (**b**) Coronal T1-weighted gadolinium-enhanced image. (**c**) Sagittal T1-weighted precontrast image. (**d**) Sagittal T1-weighted gadolinium-enhanced image. The pituitary gland is markedly thinned (**a**, **b**) compared with 1 year earlier, when the patient presented with acute endocrinopathy and necrosis within the normal-size pituitary gland (**d**)

64.3 Histopathology

- Sheehan's syndrome is characterized microscopically by extensive necrosis of the pituitary gland and fibrous scar formation.
- Atrophy of the pituitary gland is often seen on autopsy studies.
- Normal adenohypophyseal cells may be replaced with scar formation, ghost cells, necrotic debris, an inflammatory infiltrate, collagen scar formation, and chronic blood products [10].

64.4 Clinical Management

- Clinical management in patients with suspected pituitary infarction relies on timely diagnosis and hormonal replacement.
- Acute and severe hypocortisolemia is an uncommon but life-threatening aspect of this condition; rapid replacement of the cortisol axis is imperative.
- Many patients will require hormonal replacement for multiple anterior pituitary hormonal axes and potentially desmopressin acetate (DDAVP) to treat diabetes insipidus.
- Growth hormone replacement may be beneficial in patients with Sheehan's syndrome [18].

References

1. Kelestimur F. Sheehan's syndrome. Pituitary. 2003;6:181–8.
2. Tun-Pe, Phillips RE, Warrell DA, Moore RA, Tin-Nu-Swe, Myint-Lwin, Burke CW. Acute and chronic pituitary failure resembling Sheehan's syndrome following bites by Russell's viper in Burma. Lancet. 1987;2(8562):763–7.
3. Zayour DH, Azar ST. Silent pituitary infarction after coronary artery bypass grafting procedure: case report and review of literature. Endocr Pract. 2006;12:59–62.
4. Jones NS, Finer N. Pituitary infarction and development of the empty sella syndrome after gastrointestinal haemorrhage. Br Med J (Clin Res Ed). 1984;289:661–2.
5. Liu J, Zhang Q, Zheng JX, Liu Y, Niu YW, Tang JJ, Gomez M. Management of a patient with extensive burns and Sheehan's syndrome. Burns. 2013;39:e17–9.
6. Insel JR, Dhanjal N. Pituitary infarction resulting from intranasal cocaine abuse. Endocr Pract. 2004;10:478–82.
7. Ramiandrasoa C, Castinetti F, Raingeard I, Fenichel P, Chabre O, Brue T, Courbière B. Delayed diagnosis of Sheehan's syndrome in a developed country. A retrospective cohort study. Eur J Endocrinol. 2013;169:431–8.
8. Kelestimur F, Jonsson P, Molvalilar S, Gomez JM, Auernhammer CJ, Colak R, et al. Sheehan's syndrome: baseline characteristics and effect of 2 years of growth hormone replacement therapy in 91 patients in KIMS – Pfizer International Metabolic Database. Eur J Endocrinol. 2005;152:581–7.
9. Goswami R, Kochupillai N, Crock PA, Jaleel A, Gupta N. Pituitary autoimmunity in patients with Sheehan's syndrome. J Clin Endocrinol Metab. 2002;87:4137–41.
10. Kovacs K. Sheehan syndrome. Lancet. 2003;361:520–2.
11. Kilicli F, Dokmetas HS, Acibucu F. Sheehan's syndrome. Gynecol Endocrinol. 2013;29:292–5.
12. Atmaca H, Tanriverdi F, Gokce C, Unluhizarci K, Kelestimur F. Posterior pituitary function in Sheehan's syndrome. Eur J Endocrinol. 2007;156:563–7.
13. Barkan AL. Pituitary atrophy in patients with Sheehan's syndrome. Am J Med Sci. 1989;298:38–40.
14. Laway BA, Mir SA, Gojwari T, Shah TR, Zargar AH. Selective preservation of anterior pituitary functions in patients with Sheehan's syndrome. Indian J Endocrinol Metab. 2011;15 Suppl 3:S238–41.
15. Otsuka F, Kageyama J, Ogura T, Hattori T, Makino H. Sheehan's syndrome of more than 30 years' duration: an endocrine and MRI study of 6 cases. Endocr J. 1998;45:451–8.
16. Sanyal D, Raychaudhuri M. Varied presentations of Sheehan's syndrome at diagnosis: a review of 18 patients. Indian J Endocrinol Metab. 2012;16 Suppl 2:S300–1.
17. Scheller TF, Nader S. Magnetic resonance imaging in Sheehan's syndrome: case report and literature review of imaging studies. Endocr Pract. 1997;3:82–4.
18. Tanriverdi F, Unluhizarci K, Kula M, Guven M, Bayram F, Kelestimur F. Effects of 18-month of growth hormone (GH) replacement therapy in patients with Sheehan's syndrome. Growth Horm IGF Res. 2005;15:231–7.

Persistent Trigeminal Artery of the Sellar Region

65

Gabriel Zada, M. Beatriz S. Lopes, Srinivasan Mukundan Jr., and Edward Laws Jr.

65.1 Epidemiology and Clinical Presentation

- A persistent trigeminal artery (PTA) is a remnant structure from the fetal vasculature that may fail to regress during development.
- PTA is the most common and most cephalad of the persistent communications between the carotid and vertebrobasilar systems [1].
- The incidence of PTA ranges from 0.1 to 0.76 % in the general population [1].
- Although PTAs are almost always asymptomatic and are usually incidental findings, the existence of a PTA may have major implications for selection of a surgical approach for any coexistent lesions in the sellar region.
- PTAs have been reported to coexist with pituitary adenomas [2–4], craniopharyngiomas, cerebral aneurysms [5, 6], or cavernous fistulas [1, 7].
- Rarely, PTAs can present clinically with trigeminal neuralgia or hyperprolactinemia caused by pituitary stalk effect [8].

65.2 Imaging Features

- On standard MR sequences, a flow void may be seen coursing through the sella or lateral to it.
- Confirmation of a PTA can be made using CT or MR angiography or with standard cerebral angiography as needed (Fig. 65.1).
- PTAs arise from the intracavernous ICA and run caudally, either passing beneath the dorsum sellae (lateral type) or passing directly through the sella and dorsum sellae (medial type), to communicate with the basilar artery. The types occur with equal frequency [9, 10].
- The Saltzman classification of PTA has also been widely used to classify these anomalies. In the Saltzman type 1 PTA, the posterior communicating (PCOM) artery is absent. In the Saltzman type 2 PTA, the ipsilateral posterior cerebral artery (PCA) arises directly from the ICA, and the P1 segment is absent, indicating a fetal origin of the PCA. A hypoplastic basilar artery proximal to the anastomotic point is usually seen with both types [10, 11].
- PTAs occur on the left side in 62.5 % of cases [12].

G. Zada, MD, MS (✉)
Department of Neurological Surgery, Keck School of Medicine, University of Southern California, 1200 N State Street, #3300, Los Angeles, CA 90033, USA
e-mail: gzada@usc.edu

M.B.S. Lopes, MD, PhD
Department of Pathology (Neuropathology), University of Virginia School of Medicine, 1215 Lee Street, Room 3060–HEP, Charlottesville, VA 22908, USA
e-mail: msl2e@virginia.edu

S. Mukundan Jr., PhD, MD
Department of Radiology, Brigham and Women's Hospital, 75 Francis Street, Boston, MA 02115, USA
e-mail: smukundan@partners.org

E. Laws Jr., MD
Department of Neurosurgery, Brigham and Women's Hospital, 15 Francis Street, Boston, MA 02115, USA
e-mail: elaws@partners.org

G. Zada et al. (eds.), *Atlas of Sellar and Parasellar Lesions: Clinical, Radiologic, and Pathologic Correlations*, DOI 10.1007/978-3-319-22855-6_65

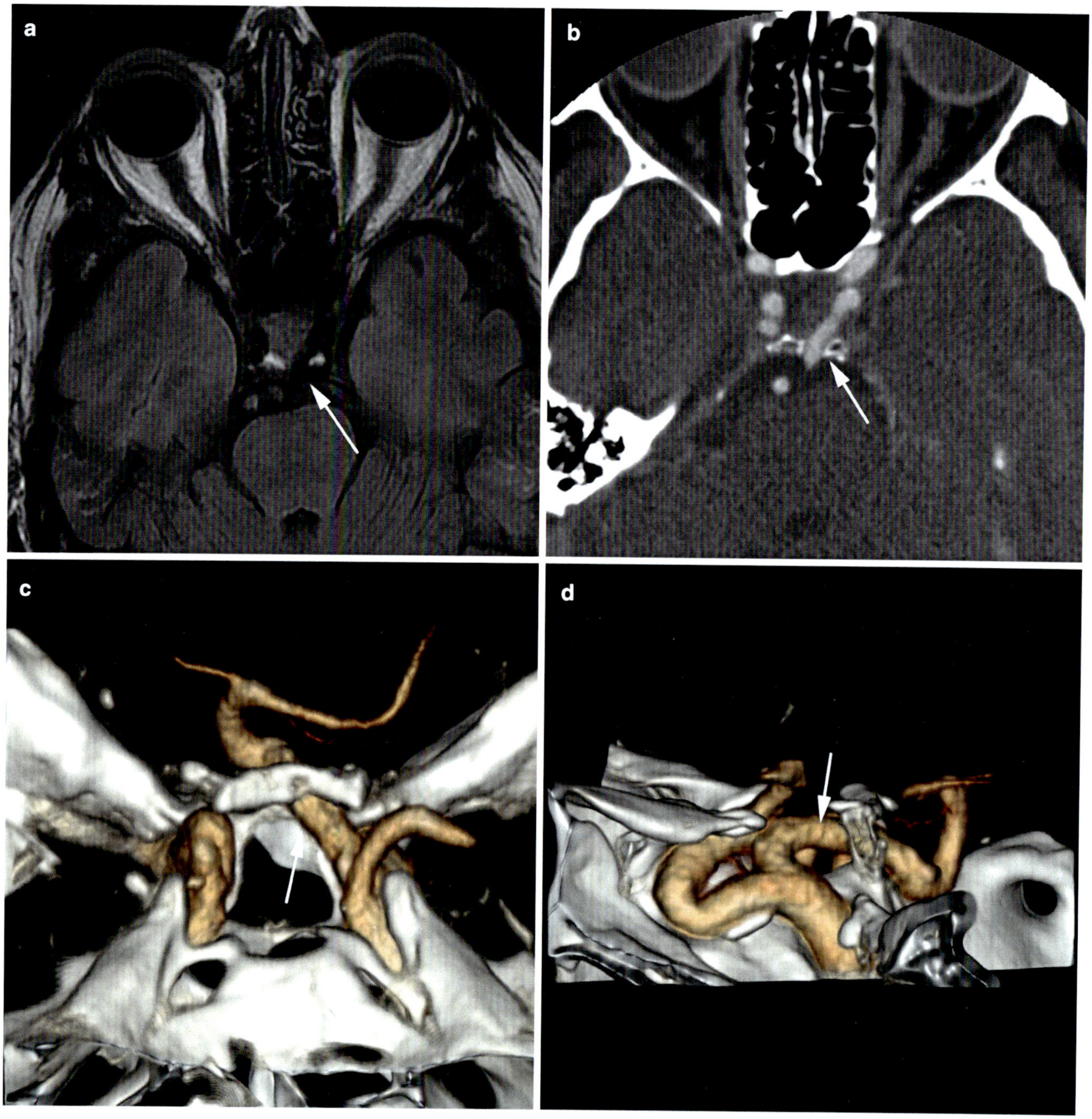

Fig. 65.1 Persistent trigeminal artery (PTA) extending through the sella turcica and pituitary gland. (**a**) Axial noncontrast MRI showing a flow void through the dorsum sellae (*arrow*) arising from the left ICA. (**b**) Axial CT angiogram showing the PTA arising from the left ICA (*arrow*) and communicating with the basilar artery system after passing through the dorsum sellae. (**c**) Three-dimensional reconstruction (anteroposterior view) showing PTA arising from the left ICA and communicating with the basilar artery (*arrow*). (**d**) Three-dimensional reconstruction (lateral view) showing PTA arising from the left ICA and communicating with the basilar artery (*arrow*)

65.3 Clinical and Surgical Management

- No clinical management is required. The importance of a sellar PTA is that it may affect surgical planning for other lesions of the sellar and parasellar region [13].
- Successful transsphenoidal surgery for a pituitary adenoma has been performed in a patient with an intrasellar PTA [3].
- In rare cases, microvascular decompression or coil embolization may be warranted in patients with PTA causing trigeminal neuralgia [1, 14].

References

1. Meckel S, Spittau B, McAuliffe W. The persistent trigeminal artery: development, imaging anatomy, variants, and associated vascular pathologies. Neuroradiology. 2013;55:5–16.
2. Abe T, Fujita S, Ozawa H, Kawamura N, Shimazu M, Ikeda H, et al. Haemorrhagic nonsecreting pituitary adenoma associated with persistent primitive trigeminal artery. Acta Neurochir (Wien). 2000;142:1423–4.
3. Lee KS, Kelly Jr DL. Intrasellar persistent trigeminal artery associated with a pituitary adenoma. Case report. J Neurosurg. 1989; 70:271–3.
4. Salcman M. Persistent trigeminal artery and pituitary adenoma. J Neurosurg. 1989;71:301–2.
5. Bai M, Guo Q, Sun Y. Rare saccular aneurysm in a medial type persistent trigeminal artery trunk and literature review. Surg Radiol Anat. 2014;36:299–302.
6. Li MH, Li WB, Pan YP, Fang C, Wang W. Persistent primitive trigeminal artery associated with aneurysm: report of two cases and review of the literature. Acta Radiol. 2004;45:664–8.
7. Tokunaga K, Sugiu K, Kameda M, Sakai K, Terasaka K, Higashi T, Date I. Persistent primitive trigeminal artery-cavernous sinus fistula with intracerebral hemorrhage: endovascular treatment using detachable coils in a transarterial double-catheter technique. Case report and review of the literature. J Neurosurg. 2004;101:697–9.
8. Ekinci G, Baltacioğlu F, Kiliç T, Cimşit C, Akpinar I, Pamir N, Erzen C. A rare cause of hyperprolactinemia: persistent trigeminal artery with stalk-section effect. Eur Radiol. 2001;11:648–50.
9. Richardson DN, Elster AD, Ball MR. Intrasellar trigeminal artery. AJNR Am J Neuroradiol. 1989;10:205.
10. Uchino A, Sawada A, Takase Y, Kudo S. MR angiography of anomalous branches of the internal carotid artery. AJR Am J Roentgenol. 2003;181:1409–14.
11. Saltzman GF. Patent primitive trigeminal artery studied by cerebral angiography. Acta Radiol. 1959;51:329–36.
12. Weon YC, Choi SH, Hwang JC, Shin SH, Kwon WJ, Kang BS. Classification of persistent primitive trigeminal artery (PPTA): a reconsideration based on MRA. Acta Radiol. 2011;52:1043–51.
13. Warnke JP, Tschabitscher M, Thalwitzer J, Galzio R. Endoscopic anatomy for transnasal transsphenoidal pituitary surgery in the presence of a persistent trigeminal artery. Cent Eur Neurosurg. 2009;70:207–10.
14. Ladner TR, Ehtesham M, Davis BJ, Khan IS, Ghiassi M, Ghiassi M, Singer RJ. Resolution of trigeminal neuralgia by coil embolization of a persistent primitive trigeminal artery aneurysm. J Neurointerv Surg. 2014;6(3), e22.

Part IX

Congenital and Developmental Anomalies of the Anterior Skull Base and Sellar Region

Meningoceles and Encephaloceles

66

Gabriel Zada, M. Beatriz S. Lopes, Srinivasan Mukundan Jr., and Edward Laws Jr.

66.1 Epidemiology and Clinical Presentation

- Skull base meningoceles and encephaloceles are developmental or acquired defects that result in outward protrusion or herniation of the dura and arachnoid (meningocele), sometimes with involvement of the brain parenchyma (encephalocele).
- Meningoceles and encephaloceles may develop following cranial trauma or surgery and are often located in the region of the cribriform plate and fovea ethmoidalis [1].
- Isolated sphenoid encephaloceles are rare findings, but may develop in the region of Sternberg's canal (lateral craniopharyngeal canal), a fusion point between the greater wing of the sphenoid and basisphenoid. Herniation of the temporal lobe into the lateral sphenoid recess may occur in this region.
- Patients with symptomatic meningoencephaloceles may present with CSF rhinorrhea, meningitis, seizures, visual loss, or a combination of these. Tension pneumocephalus has also been reported as a rare development of meningoencephaloceles [2, 3].
- In patients with spontaneous CSF rhinorrhea, a skull base defect and meningoencephalocele should be ruled out with dedicated imaging studies. Similarly, a consideration of intracranial hypertension should be considered. (See the Sect. on 73.1.1 in Chap. 73.)
- Sphenoidal encephaloceles may present with optic nerve dysfunction, vision loss, and the "morning glory syndrome" (coloboma of the optic nerve). This finding arises from a congenitally undeveloped optic nerve and disk. On funduscopic examination, it appears as a funnel-shaped excavation of the posterior fundus incorporating the optic nerve, surrounded by an elevated annulus of chorioretinal pigment, which resembles a morning glory flower [4, 5].
- Midline transsellar sphenoid encephaloceles are even rarer; they are typically larger defects associated with congenital syndromes and craniofacial anomalies. Hypothalamic and pituitary dysfunction can be seen in these patients [6–10].

G. Zada, MD, MS (✉)
Department of Neurological Surgery, Keck School of Medicine, University of Southern California, 1200 N State Street, #3300, Los Angeles, CA 90033, USA
e-mail: gzada@usc.edu

M.B.S. Lopes, MD, PhD
Department of Pathology (Neuropathology), University of Virginia School of Medicine, 1215 Lee Street, Room 3060–HEP, Charlottesville, VA 22908, USA
e-mail: msl2e@virginia.edu

S. Mukundan Jr., PhD, MD
Department of Radiology, Brigham and Women's Hospital, 75 Francis Street, Boston, MA 02115, USA
e-mail: smukundan@partners.org

E. Laws Jr., MD
Department of Neurosurgery, Brigham and Women's Hospital, 15 Francis Street, Boston, MA 02115, USA
e-mail: elaws@partners.org

G. Zada et al. (eds.), *Atlas of Sellar and Parasellar Lesions: Clinical, Radiologic, and Pathologic Correlations*,
DOI 10.1007/978-3-319-22855-6_66

66.2 Imaging Features

- Thin-cut CT imaging with coronal and sagittal reconstruction is the preferred modality for assessment of the bony skull base defect.
- MRI is the preferred modality for diagnosis of an encephalocele (Figs. 66.1, 66.2, 66.3, 66.4, and 66.5) [11, 12]. On MRI, encephaloceles are often associated with T2 hyperintensity in the affected lobe. Depending on the size of the encephalocele, widening of the surrounding cerebral fissures (such as the Sylvian fissure) may be noted, with elongated vessels caused by herniation of the affected lobe [13].

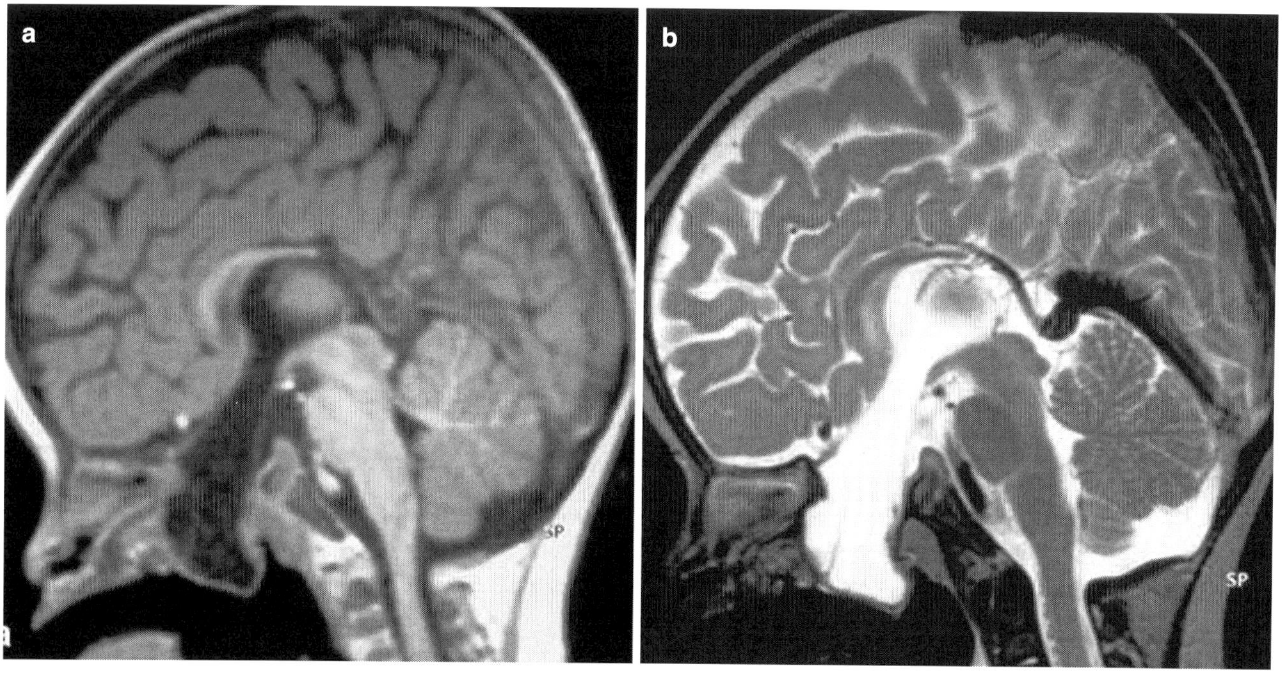

Fig. 66.1 Encephalocele. Sagittal T1-weighted MR image (**a**) and sagittal T2-weighted MR image (**b**) showing a basal encephalocele extending into the nasopharynx (*From* Chen et al. [10]; *with permission*)

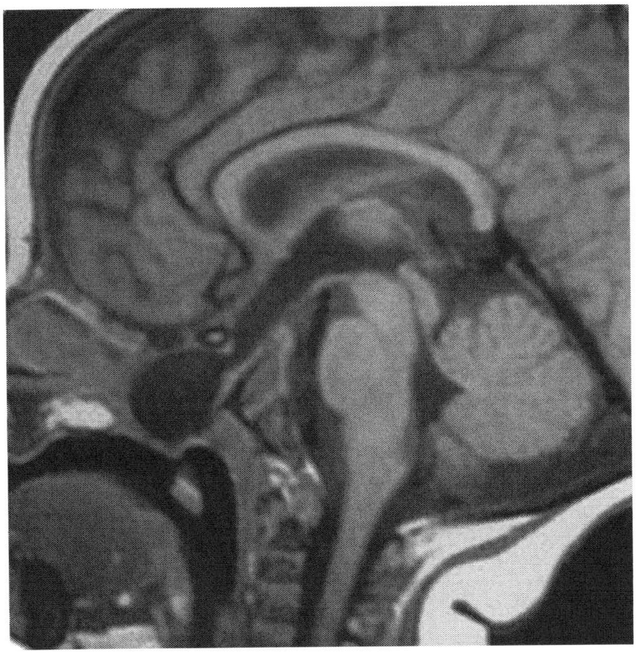

Fig. 66.2 Meningocele. Sagittal T1-weighted MRI showing a transsphenoidal meningocele extending to the posterior portion of the palate (From Franco et al. [11]; with permission)

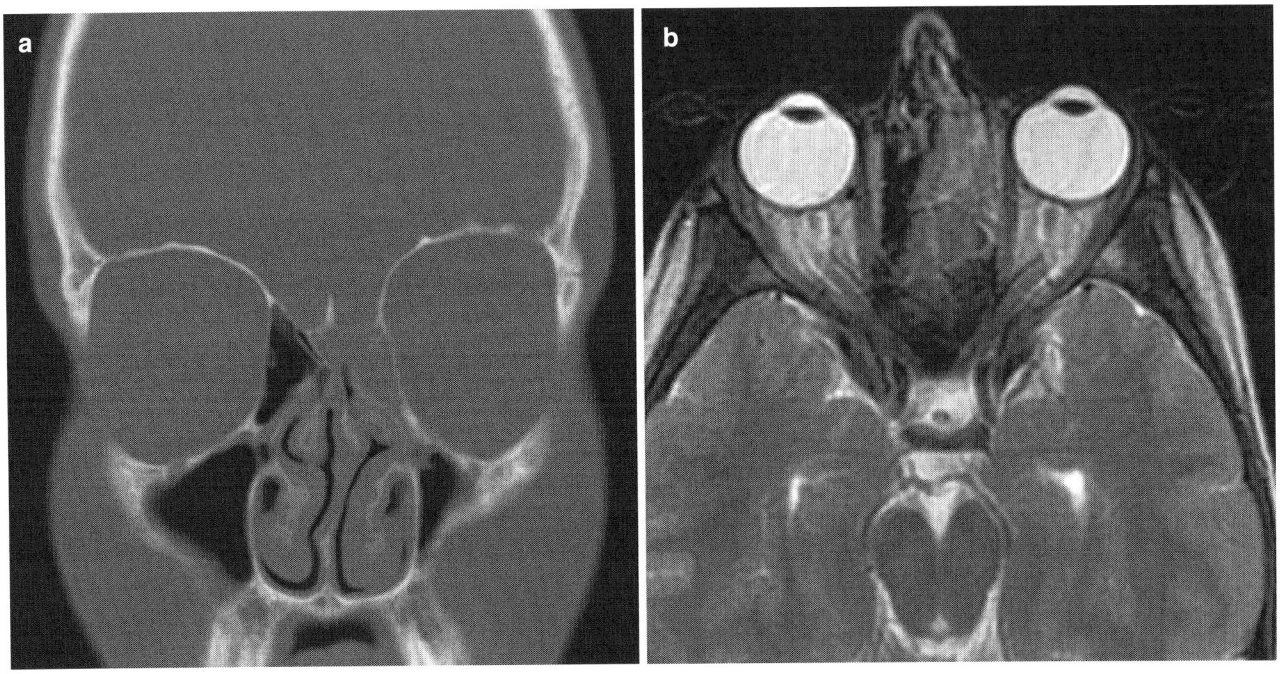

Fig. 66.3 Encephalocele. (**a**) Coronal CT image. (**b**) Axial T2-weighted MR image. Soft tissue is present in the left ethmoid (**b**) and there is a defect in the roof of the left ethmoid (**a**), consistent with an ethmoid encephalocele

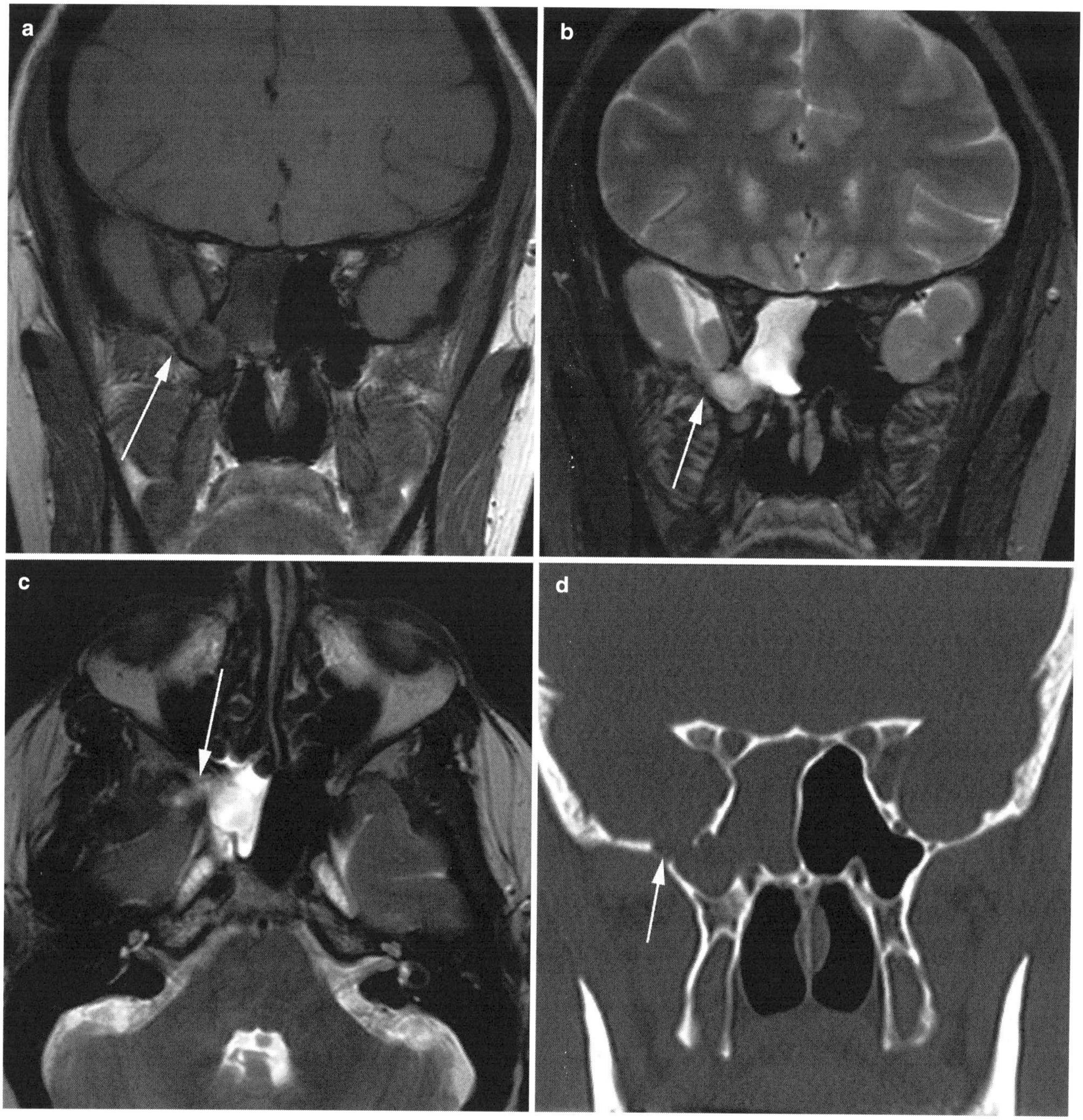

Fig. 66.4 Meningoencephalocele. Coronal T1-weighted MRI (**a**), T2-weighted MRI (**b**), and axial T2-weighted MRI (**c**) showing a large right middle fossa meningoencephalocele (*arrow*) with extension into the sphenoid sinus. A coronal CT scan (**d**) shows the bony defect in the floor of the right middle fossa (*arrow*)

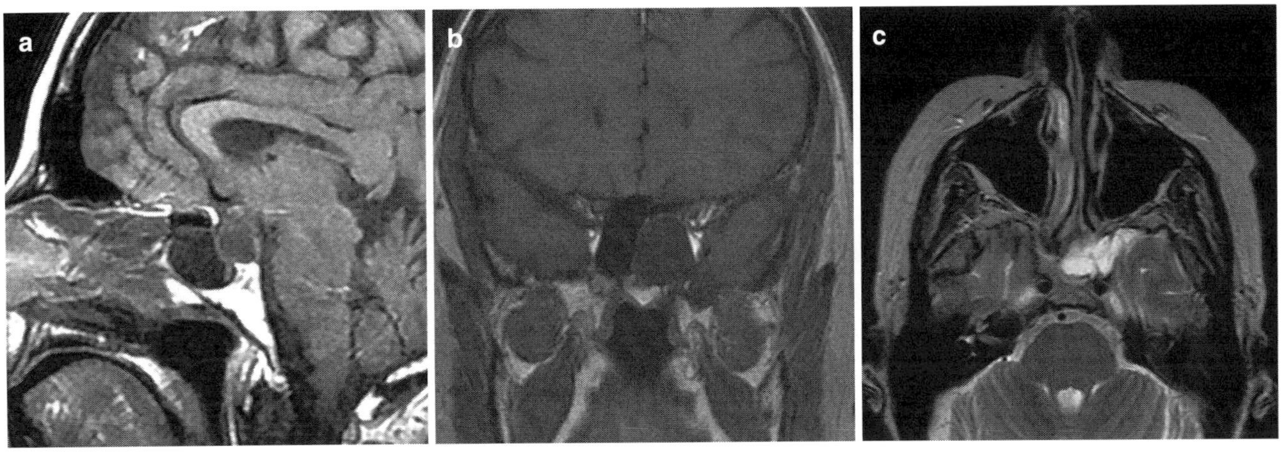

Fig. 66.5 Meningoencephalocele. Sagittal (**a**) and coronal (**b**) T1-weighted MR images in a patient with a middle fossa meningoencephalocele extending into the sphenoid sinus. An axial T2-weighted MR image (**c**) shows a hyperintense CSF collection arising from the left temporal region and extending into the sphenoid sinus

66.3 Histopathology

- Marked gliosis of the brain is often noted in an encephalocele. Evidence of lymphocytic infiltrate and dural thickening may be present in cases of infection.

66.4 Clinical and Surgical Management

- Both open cranial and endoscopic endonasal approaches have been widely utilized for the surgical repair of symptomatic meningoencephaloceles. Rates of successful repair appear similar for both approaches, but complication rates may be lower in patients treated with endoscopic surgery [14].
- In recent years, extended endonasal endoscopic approaches have been used to repair the skull base defects. These cases often involve endonasal transmaxillary and/or transpterygoid approaches; the use of a pedicled nasoseptal flap and possibly a lumbar drain is recommended for larger defects. In many cases, the encephalocele brain is nonfunctional (or even a seizure focus) and should be resected [3, 15].
- Outcomes following repair of sphenoid meningoencephaloceles are excellent, with high success rates (>90 %) and rare recurrences [3, 16–18].
- In rare cases of midline transsellar encephaloceles, thorough screening for hypopituitarism should be performed, with hormone replacement.

References

1. Lee TJ, Chang PH, Huang CC, Chuang CC. Endoscopic treatment of traumatic basal encephaloceles: a report of 8 cases. J Neurosurg. 2008;108:729–35.
2. Ohkawa T, Nakao N, Uematsu Y, Itakura T. Temporal lobe encephalocele in the lateral recess of the sphenoid sinus presenting with intraventricular tension pneumocephalus. Skull Base. 2010;20:481–6.
3. Tabaee A, Anand VK, Cappabianca P, Stamm A, Esposito F, Schwartz TH. Endoscopic management of spontaneous meningoencephalocele of the lateral sphenoid sinus. J Neurosurg. 2010;112:1070–7.
4. Itakura T, Miyamoto K, Uematsu Y, Hayashi S, Komai N. Bilateral morning glory syndrome associated with sphenoid encephalocele. Case report. J Neurosurg. 1992;77:949–51.
5. Storms M, Dralands L, Leys A, Vanderschueren D, Bouillon R. Morning glory syndrome and basal encephalocele mimicking a pituitary adenoma. Bull Soc Belge Ophtalmol. 1987;225:97–103.
6. Booth JD, Josse RG, Singer W. Pituitary and hypothalamic dysfunction in a patient with a basal encephalocele. J Endocrinol Invest. 1983;6:473–8.
7. Ellyin F, Khatir AH, Singh SP. Hypothalamic-pituitary functions in patients with transsphenoidal encephalocele and midfacial anomalies. J Clin Endocrinol Metab. 1980;51:854–6.
8. Lieblich JM, Rosen SE, Guyda H, Reardan J, Schaaf M. The syndrome of basal encephalocele and hypothalamic-pituitary dysfunction. Ann Intern Med. 1978;89:910–6.
9. Raman Sharma R, Mahapatra AK, Pawar SJ, Thomas C, Al-Ismaily M. Trans-sellar trans-sphenoidal encephaloceles: report of two cases. J Clin Neurosci. 2002;9:89–92.
10. Chen CS, David D, Hanieh A. Morning glory syndrome and basal encephalocele. Childs Nerv Syst. 2004;20:87–90.
11. Franco D, Alonso N, Ruas R, da Silva Freitas R, Franco T. Transsphenoidal meningoencephalocele associated with cleft lip and palate: challenges for diagnosis and surgical treatment. Childs Nerv Syst. 2009;25:1455–8.
12. Tanimoto K, Onda S, Sawaki H, Hiraiwa T, Sano H, Ohnishi M, et al. Hypopituitarism in a patient with transsphenoidal cephalocele: longitudinal changes in endocrinological abnormalities. Endocr J. 2011;58:193–8.
13. Schuknecht B, Simmen D, Briner HR, Holzmann D. Nontraumatic skull base defects with spontaneous CSF rhinorrhea and arachnoid herniation: imaging findings and correlation with endoscopic sinus surgery in 27 patients. AJNR Am J Neuroradiol. 2008;29:542–9.
14. Komotar RJ, Starke RM, Raper DM, Anand VK, Schwartz TH. Endoscopic endonasal versus open repair of anterior skull base CSF leak, meningocele, and encephalocele: a systematic review of outcomes. J Neurol Surg A Cent Eur Neurosurg. 2013;74:239–50.
15. Schmidt RF, Choudhry OJ, Raviv J, Baredes S, Casiano RR, Eloy JA, Liu JK. Surgical nuances for the endoscopic endonasal transpterygoid approach to lateral sphenoid sinus encephaloceles. Neurosurg Focus. 2012;32(6), E5.
16. Lai SY, Kennedy DW, Bolger WE. Sphenoid encephaloceles: disease management and identification of lesions within the lateral recess of the sphenoid sinus. Laryngoscope. 2002;112:1800–5.
17. Pasquini E, Sciarretta V, Farneti G, Mazzatenta D, Modugno GC, Frank G. Endoscopic treatment of encephaloceles of the lateral wall of the sphenoid sinus. Minim Invasive Neurosurg. 2004;47:209–13.
18. Tomazic PV, Stammberger H. Spontaneous CSF-leaks and meningoencephaloceles in sphenoid sinus by persisting Sternberg's canal. Rhinology. 2009;47:369–74.

Empty Sella Syndrome

67

Gabriel Zada, M. Beatriz S. Lopes, Srinivasan Mukundan Jr., and Edward Laws Jr.

67.1 Epidemiology and Clinical Presentation

- An empty sella refers to a condition in which an arachnoid diverticulum extends into the sella, often causing reshaping and flattening of the pituitary gland and stalk.
- This entity is frequently characterized as either a primary or secondary empty sella syndrome, depending on the etiology and associated conditions.
  - Suggested causes of primary empty sella (PES) include numerous congenital and developmental syndromes, congenital defects in the diaphragma sella, and chronic elevations in intracranial pressure (such as idiopathic intracranial hypertension) [1–3]. Defects of the diaphragma sella appear to be necessary—but not sufficient—in causing arachnoidal diverticula and PES [4].
  - Secondary empty sella syndrome occurs in association with or following treatment for other conditions, including pituitary adenomas, apoplexy, infections, autoimmune disease, trauma, prior surgery, and prior radiation.
- An empty sella is diagnosed more frequently in women than in men (over 4:1 sex ratio). It occurs more commonly in multiparous and obese women [5].
- The mean age at diagnosis is 43–52 years [6, 7]. In rare symptomatic cases, the mean duration of symptoms prior to diagnosis is over 5 years [7].
- An empty sella is frequently an incidental finding, but it can be associated with various hormonal, visual, and/or neurological symptoms and signs. The most common findings associated with PES syndrome are headache (33 %), endocrinopathy (31 %), and visual loss (9 %) [5].
- Spontaneous CSF rhinorrhea is associated with the empty sella syndrome, which also is associated with intracranial hypertension, another occasional cause of CSF rhinorrhea. Elevated intracranial pressures have been reported in 65–77 % of patients with PES [2, 3]. Papilledema has been noted in 25 % of patients with PES and headache [7].
- Visual disturbances consist mainly of disturbances in visual acuity. These changes may be caused by tension on the optic complex due to prolapse or compression, by microvascular compromise of the optic apparatus, or both [6, 7].
- Endocrine dysfunction has been reported upon initial diagnosis in 19–31 % of patients with empty sella syndrome. The most common endocrinopathy in patients with PES is GH axis deficiency (mainly subclinical). The most frequent symptomatic endocrine abnormality is hyperprolactinemia, which often results in oligomenorrhea in women and sexual dysfunction in men [5, 6, 8, 9].
- Panhypopituitarism in association with PES is rare, occurring in about 2 % of cases [6].

G. Zada, MD, MS (✉)
Department of Neurological Surgery, Keck School of Medicine, University of Southern California, 1200 N State Street, #3300, Los Angeles, CA 90033, USA
e-mail: gzada@usc.edu

M.B.S. Lopes, MD, PhD
Department of Pathology (Neuropathology), University of Virginia School of Medicine, 1215 Lee Street, Room 3060–HEP, Charlottesville, VA 22908, USA
e-mail: msl2e@virginia.edu

S. Mukundan Jr., PhD, MD
Department of Radiology, Brigham and Women's Hospital, 75 Francis Street, Boston, MA 02115, USA
e-mail: smukundan@partners.org

E. Laws Jr., MD
Department of Neurosurgery, Brigham and Women's Hospital, 15 Francis Street, Boston, MA 02115, USA
e-mail: elaws@partners.org

G. Zada et al. (eds.), *Atlas of Sellar and Parasellar Lesions: Clinical, Radiologic, and Pathologic Correlations*, DOI 10.1007/978-3-319-22855-6_67

67.2 Imaging Features

- An arachnoid diverticulum extending from the intracranial subarachnoid space into the sella is frequently noted. This is a different entity from an arachnoid cyst.
- T2-weighted MR imaging demonstrates isointensity to CSF.
- The pituitary gland and stalk are often compressed inferiorly and posteriorly by the arachnoid diverticulum (Figs. 67.1, 67.2, and 67.3).
- Optic chiasm prolapse may be noted in some cases, especially in secondary empty sella syndrome following the resection of large sellar tumors.
- Empty sella syndrome may be characterized as partial (65 % of patients) or complete (35 % of patients) [6].
- The degree of empty sella has not been correlated to the severity of clinical symptoms [11].

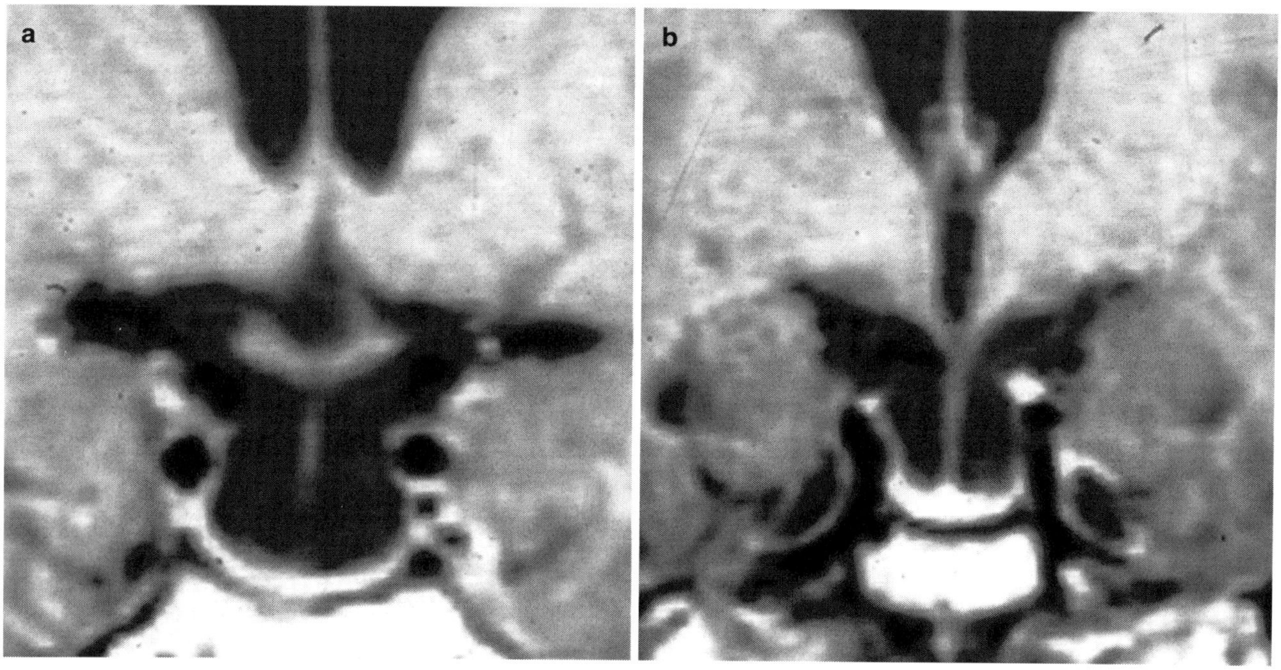

Fig. 67.1 Empty sella syndrome. (**a**, **b**) Coronal T1-weighted gadolinium-enhanced MR images. The pituitary gland appears flattened, with increased cerebrospinal fluid (CSF) space above the gland. The optic chiasm is slightly prolapsed

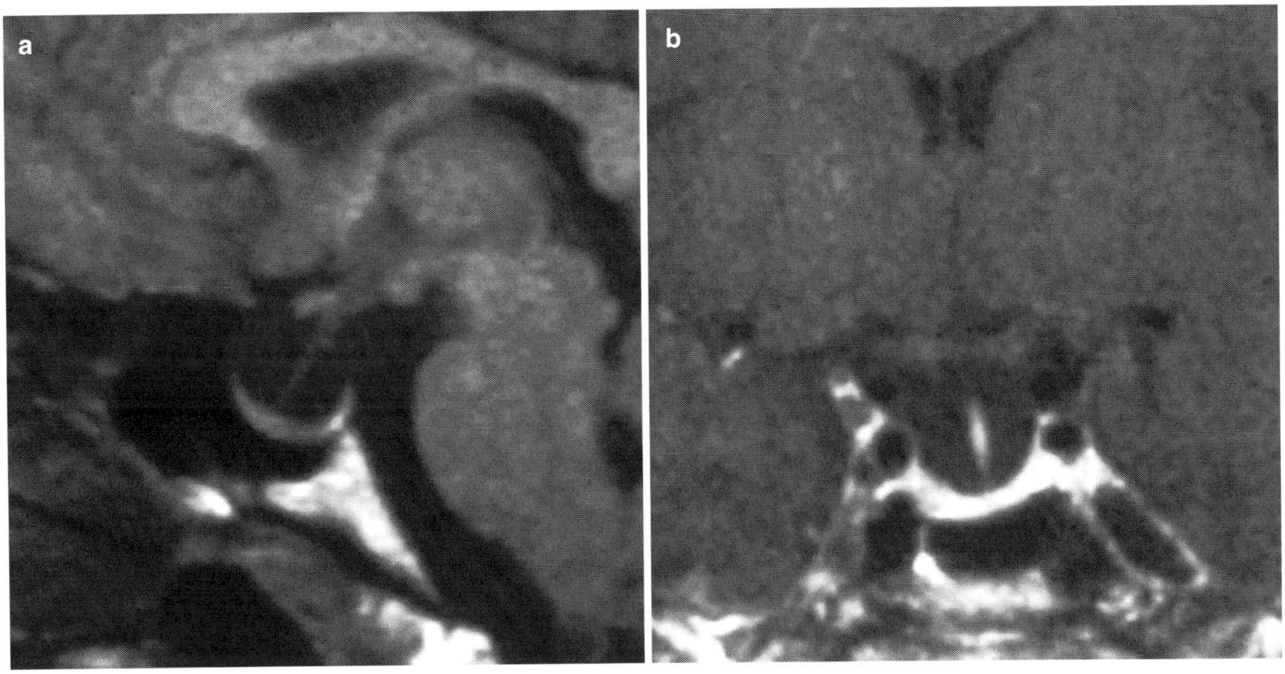

Fig. 67.2 Empty sella syndrome. (**a**) Sagittal T1-weighted precontrast MR image. (**b**) Coronal T1-weighted gadolinium-enhanced image. The pituitary gland appears flattened, with increased CSF space above the gland

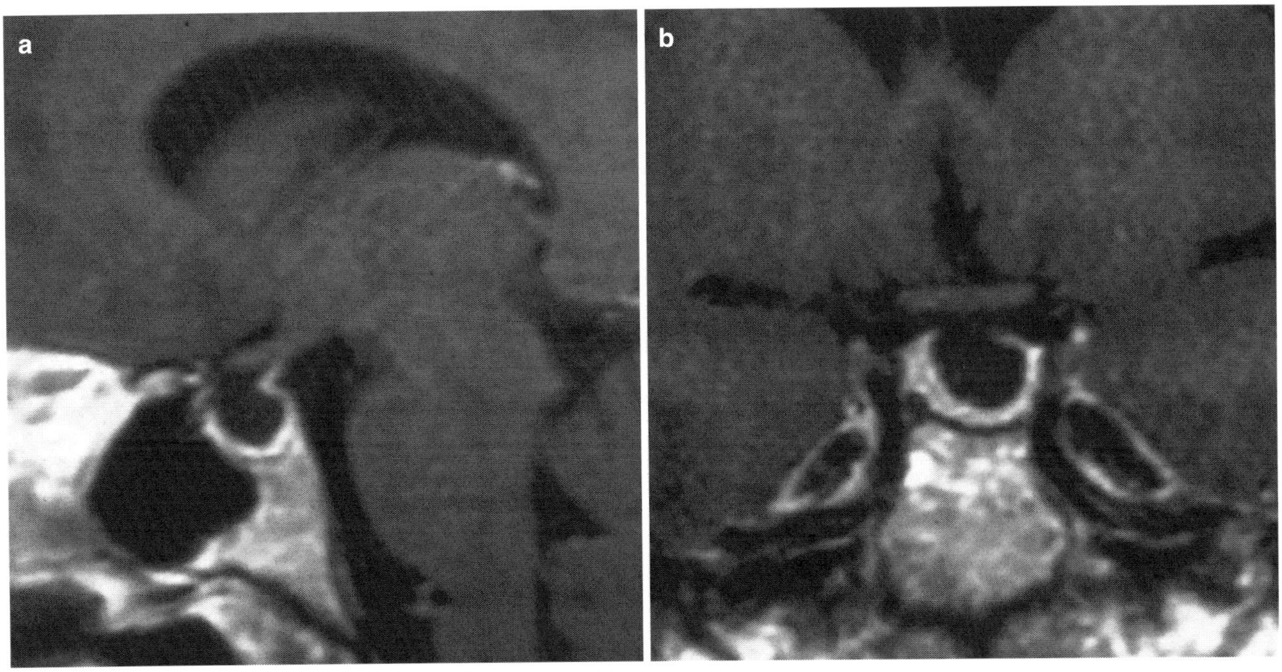

Fig. 67.3 Empty sella syndrome. (**a**) Sagittal T1-weighted gadolinium-enhanced MR image. (**b**) Coronal T1-weighted gadolinium-enhanced image. The pituitary gland appears flattened, with increased CSF space above the gland. The pituitary stalk is mildly displaced posteriorly (**a**)

67.3 Clinical and Surgical Management

- The optimal management of empty sella syndrome has been controversial.
- Few patients require surgical management, as an empty sella is often an incidental finding and most patients are asymptomatic at the time of diagnosis.
- Conservative management is usually indicated, unless signs of intracranial hypertension, hypopituitarism, visual loss, or CSF rhinorrhea are noted.
- A thorough endocrine evaluation should be performed on all symptomatic patients with empty sella syndrome.
- Symptomatic patients with PES should be screened for symptoms and signs of intracranial hypertension (papilledema, headache, visual symptoms). Medical management may be indicated, including weight loss and possible carbonic anhydrase inhibitors.
- Patients with suspected or documented intracranial hypertension and those with CSF rhinorrhea may require insertion of a CSF-diverting shunt, transsphenoidal repair of a sellar floor defect, or both.
- Patients with optic nerve prolapse and visual symptoms may benefit from optic chiasmopexy, in which an abdominal fat graft is used to elevate and buttress the chiasm [10].

References

1. Ommaya AK, Di Chiro G, Baldwin M, Pennybacker JB. Nontraumatic cerebrospinal fluid rhinorrhoea. J Neurol Neurosurg Psychiatry. 1968;31:214–25.
2. Foley KM, Posner JB. Does pseudotumor cerebri cause the empty sella syndrome? Neurology. 1975;25:565–9.
3. Brismar K, Bergstrand G. CSF circulation in subjects with the empty sella syndrome. Neuroradiology. 1981;21:167–75.
4. Hubbard JL, McDonald TJ, Pearson BW, Laws Jr ER. Spontaneous cerebrospinal fluid rhinorrhea: evolving concepts in diagnosis and surgical management based on the Mayo Clinic experience from 1970 through 1981. Neurosurgery. 1985;16:314–21.
5. Guitelman M, Garcia Basavilbaso N, Vitale M, Chervin A, Katz D, Miragaya K, et al. Primary empty sella (PES): a review of 175 cases. Pituitary. 2013;16:270–4.
6. De Marinis L, Bonadonna S, Bianchi A, Maira G, Giustina A. Primary empty sella. J Clin Endocrinol Metab. 2005;90:5471–7.
7. Maira G, Anile C, Mangiola A. Primary empty sella syndrome in a series of 142 patients. J Neurosurg. 2005;103:831–6.
8. Brismar K, Efendic S. Pituitary function in the empty sella syndrome. Neuroendocrinology. 1981;32:70–7.
9. Durodoye OM, Mendlovic DB, Brenner RS, Morrow JS. Endocrine disturbances in empty sella syndrome: case reports and review of literature. Endocr Pract. 2005;11:120–4.
10. Hamlyn PJ, Baer R, Afshar F. Transsphenoidal chiasmopexy for long standing visual failure in the secondary empty sella syndrome. Br J Neurosurg. 1988;2:277–9.
11. Gallardo E, Schächter D, Cáceres E, Becker P, Colin E, Martínez C, Henríquez C. The empty sella: results of treatment in 76 successive cases and high frequency of endocrine and neurological disturbances. Clin Endocrinol (Oxf). 1992;37:529–33.

Pituitary Hypoplasia and Other Midline Developmental Anomalies

68

Gabriel Zada, M. Beatriz S. Lopes, Srinivasan Mukundan Jr., and Edward Laws Jr.

68.1 Epidemiology and Clinical Presentation

- Hypoplasia of the pituitary gland, infundibulum, septum pellucidum, corpus callosum, and optic nerve(s) may be seen in an isolated fashion or in combination with one another. These related midline developmental anomalies are thought to represent a spectrum of congenital and developmental conditions with varying degrees of penetrance, including holoprosencephaly and/or septo-optic dysplasia (SOD) [1].
- Pituitary hypoplasia may occur as an isolated entity (IPH) or in association with various (often overlapping) syndromes [2]:
  - Septo-optic dysplasia (SOD, de Morsier's syndrome)
  - Kallmann syndrome
  - Holoprosencephaly
  - Coffin-Siris syndrome [3]
  - Worster-Drought syndrome (congenital bilateral perisylvian syndrome) [4]
  - Hall-Pallister syndrome [5]
- Although usually sporadic conditions, pituitary hypoplasia and related midline anomaly spectrum disorders have been associated with mutations in a number of genes:
  - *Pit-1* [6, 7]
  - *Sonic Hedgehog* (*SHH*)
  - Growth hormone-releasing hormone (*GHRH*) receptor [8, 9]
  - *HESX1* [10]
  - *SOX2* and *SOX3*
  - Additional genes on the long arm of chromosome 14 [11]
- Isolated pituitary hypoplasia most commonly affects the growth hormone (GH), thyroid, and prolactin axes. Most patients with pituitary hypoplasia present with short stature. Clinically, these syndromes are known as isolated GH deficiency or combined pituitary hormone deficiency [12–14].
- Pituitary hypoplasia may be accompanied by adrenal cortical hypoplasia [15].
- Optic nerve hypoplasia is a leading cause of congenital blindness and is typically diagnosed on funduscopic examination. Additional midline anomalies are often identified with neuroimaging studies [16].
- Septo-optic dysplasia (SOD) and septo-optic-pituitary dysplasia are developmental disorders that involve hypoplasia of one or more midline structures. These conditions have been associated with maternal drug and alcohol use and in rare cases can be congenital.
  - The incidence of SOD is 1 in 10,000 newborns.
  - Affected expression of hypothalamic *Sonic Hedgehog* (*SHH*) has been shown to cause classic SOD [17].
  - The most common finding is optic nerve hypoplasia. Pituitary hypoplasia, agenesis of the septum pellucidum, and cortical developmental malformations can all be seen in combination or as isolated entities. Concurrent pituitary hypoplasia is seen in 64 % of

G. Zada, MD, MS (✉)
Department of Neurological Surgery, Keck School of Medicine, University of Southern California, 1200 N State Street, #3300, Los Angeles, CA 90033, USA
e-mail: gzada@usc.edu

M.B.S. Lopes, MD, PhD
Department of Pathology (Neuropathology), University of Virginia School of Medicine, 1215 Lee Street, Room 3060–HEP, Charlottesville, VA 22908, USA
e-mail: msl2e@virginia.edu

S. Mukundan Jr., PhD, MD
Department of Radiology, Brigham and Women's Hospital, 75 Francis Street, Boston, MA 02115, USA
e-mail: smukundan@partners.org

E. Laws Jr., MD
Department of Neurosurgery, Brigham and Women's Hospital, 15 Francis Street, Boston, MA 02115, USA
e-mail: elaws@partners.org

G. Zada et al. (eds.), *Atlas of Sellar and Parasellar Lesions: Clinical, Radiologic, and Pathologic Correlations*, DOI 10.1007/978-3-319-22855-6_68

patients with optic nerve hypoplasia, and agenesis of the septum pellucidum is seen in 50 % [12, 18].
   - Patients with SOD often present with developmental delay, communication difficulties, visual loss, nystagmus, and hypopituitarism.
   - The presence and degree of endocrinopathy correlate with the absence of multiple midline structures. Patients with absence of the septum pellucidum and hypothalamic-pituitary axis on MRI have the highest degree of endocrinopathy [19].
- Rarely, isolated pituitary stalk hypoplasia, also known as the pituitary stalk interruption syndrome (PSIS), can be seen [20]. This discrete entity has been associated with genes involved in holoprosencephaly (*SHH*, *TGIF*, *SIX3*).

68.2 Imaging Features

- Hypoplasia of the pituitary gland, infundibulum, septum pellucidum, corpus callosum, and/or optic nerve(s) can be seen on MRI (Fig. 68.1) [18, 20].
- The height of a hypoplastic pituitary gland, when present, is typically less than 3 mm; the normal height is more than 5 mm [8].
- An ectopic pituitary gland may be visualized [21].
- In patients with congenital GH deficiency, the triad of an ectopic posterior pituitary (EPP), pituitary aplasia/hypoplasia, and stalk defects is correlated with the presence of other endocrine abnormalities (Fig. 68.2) [22].
- The presence of diabetes insipidus has been shown to correlate with loss of the posterior pituitary bright spot [23, 24].
- Pituitary hypoplasia or ectopia can be associated with agenesis of an internal carotid artery [25, 26].
- On MRI, the cross-sectional area of the optic nerve can be used to support the diagnosis of optic nerve hypoplasia [27].

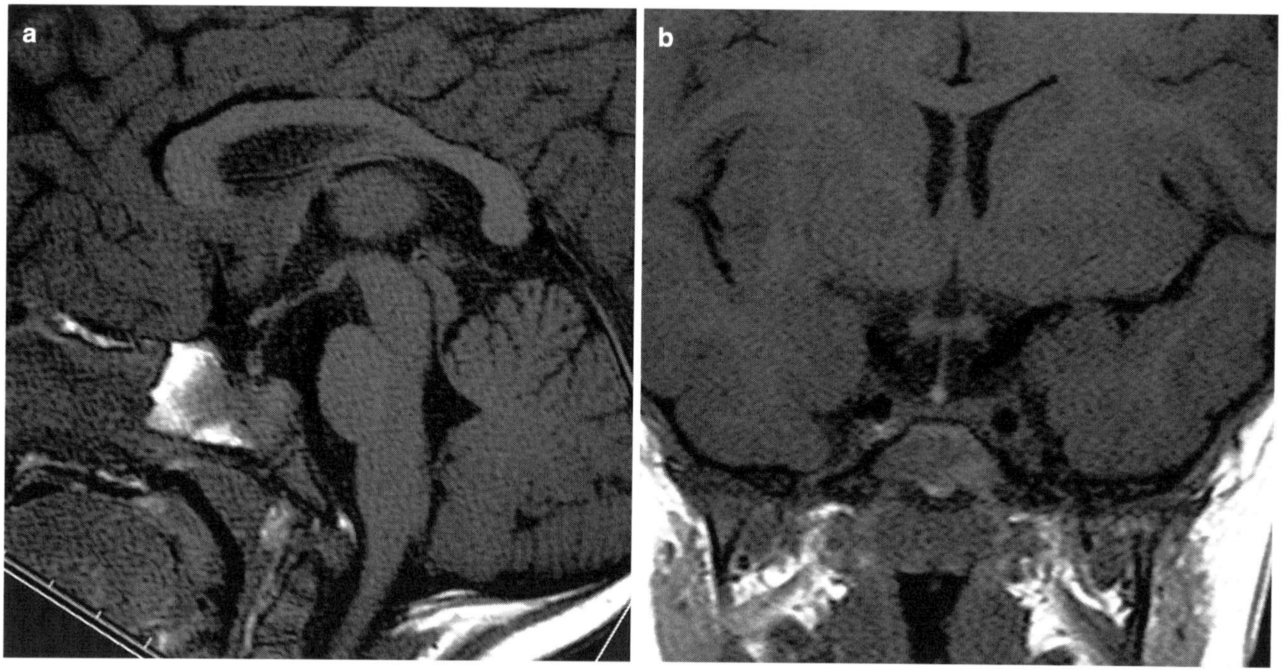

Fig. 68.1 Pituitary hypoplasia. (**a**) Sagittal T1-weighted precontrast MR image. (**b**) Coronal T1-weighted precontrast image. The anterior pituitary gland is hypoplastic and the posterior pituitary T1 shortening is visible in the center of the sella. The stalk is present

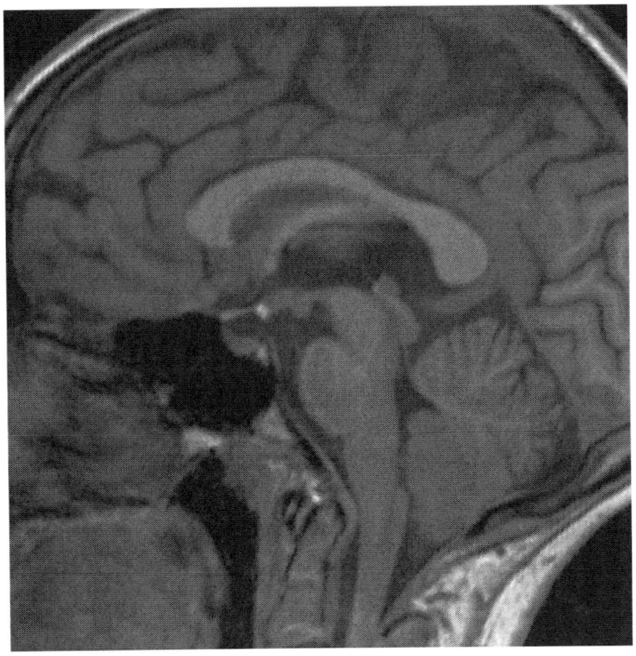

Fig. 68.2 Pituitary hypoplasia. Sagittal T1-weighted precontrast MR image. There is a T1-hyperintense spot in the infundibular recess, indicating ectopic neurohypophysis, and the pituitary stalk is not seen. The anterior pituitary gland is present in the sella

68.3 Clinical Management

- Clinical management is centered on prompt diagnosis and hormone replacement.
- Favorable responses to GH replacement have been shown in many patients [28].
- Multidisciplinary management is recommended for patients with any midline developmental disorders. Among the clinicians required may be endocrinologists, ophthalmologists, psychiatrists, neurologists, neurosurgeons, genetic counselors, and visual and occupational therapists.

References

1. Tatsi C, Sertedaki A, Voutetakis A, Valavani E, Magiakou MA, Kanaka-Gantenbein C, et al. Pituitary stalk interruption syndrome and isolated pituitary hypoplasia may be caused by mutations in holoprosencephaly-related genes. J Clin Endocrinol Metab. 2013; 98:E779–84.
2. Raivio T, Avbelj M, McCabe MJ, Romero CJ, Dwyer AA, Tommiska J, et al. Genetic overlap in Kallmann syndrome, combined pituitary hormone deficiency, and septo-optic dysplasia. J Clin Endocrinol Metab. 2012;97:E694–9.
3. Baban A, Moresco L, Divizia MT, Rossi A, Ravazzolo R, Lerone M, De Toni T. Pituitary hypoplasia and growth hormone deficiency in Coffin-Siris syndrome. Am J Med Genet A. 2008;146A:384–8.
4. Baş F, Darendeliler F, Yapici Z, Gökalp S, Bundak R, Saka N, Günöz H. Worster-Drought syndrome (congenital bilateral perisylvian syndrome) with posterior pituitary ectopia, pituitary hypoplasia, empty sella and panhypopituitarism: a patient report. J Pediatr Endocrinol Metab. 2006;19:535–40.
5. Cianfarani S, Vitale S, Stanhope R, Boscherini B. Imperforate anus, bilateral hydronephrosis, bilateral undescended testes and pituitary hypoplasia: a variant of Hall-Pallister syndrome or a new syndrome. Acta Paediatr. 1995;84:1322–4.
6. Frisch H, Kim C, Häusler G, Pfäffle R. Combined pituitary hormone deficiency and pituitary hypoplasia due to a mutation of the Pit-1 gene. Clin Endocrinol (Oxf). 2000;52:661–5.
7. Pfäffle RW, DiMattia GE, Parks JS, Brown MR, Wit JM, Jansen M, et al. Mutation of the POU-specific domain of Pit-1 and hypopituitarism without pituitary hypoplasia. Science. 1992;257:1118–21.
8. Murray RA, Maheshwari HG, Russell EJ, Baumann G. Pituitary hypoplasia in patients with a mutation in the growth hormone-releasing hormone receptor gene. AJNR Am J Neuroradiol. 2000;21:685–9.
9. Shohreh R, Sherafat-Kazemzadeh R, Jee YH, Blitz A, Salvatori R. A novel frame shift mutation in the GHRH receptor gene in familial isolated GH deficiency: early occurrence of anterior pituitary hypoplasia. J Clin Endocrinol Metab. 2011;96:2982–6.
10. Thomas PQ, Dattani MT, Brickman JM, McNay D, Warne G, Zacharin M, et al. Heterozygous *HESX1* mutations associated with isolated congenital pituitary hypoplasia and septo-optic dysplasia. Hum Mol Genet. 2001;10:39–45.
11. Nolen LD, Amor D, Haywood A, St Heaps L, Willcock C, Mihelec M, et al. Deletion at 14q22–23 indicates a contiguous gene syndrome comprising anophthalmia, pituitary hypoplasia, and ear anomalies. Am J Med Genet A. 2006;140:1711–8.
12. Margalith D, Tze WJ, Jan JE. Congenital optic nerve hypoplasia with hypothalamic-pituitary dysplasia. A review of 16 cases. Am J Dis Child. 1985;139:361–6.
13. Costin G, Murphree AL. Hypothalamic-pituitary function in children with optic nerve hypoplasia. Am J Dis Child. 1985;139:249–54.
14. Lettau M, Laible M. Kallmann's syndrome with pituitary hypoplasia. Rofo. 2011;183:576–8.
15. Mosier HD. Hypoplasia of the pituitary and adrenal cortex; report of occurrence in twin siblings and autopsy findings. J Pediatr. 1956;48:633–9.
16. Garcia-Filion P, Borchert M. Optic nerve hypoplasia syndrome: a review of the epidemiology and clinical associations. Curr Treat Options Neurol. 2013;15:78–89.
17. Zhao L, Zevallos SE, Rizzoti K, Jeong Y, Lovell-Badge R, Epstein DJ. Disruption of SoxB1-dependent Sonic hedgehog expression in the hypothalamus causes septo-optic dysplasia. Dev Cell. 2012; 22:585–96.
18. Acers TE. Optic nerve hypoplasia: septo-optic-pituitary dysplasia syndrome. Trans Am Ophthalmol Soc. 1981;79:425–57.
19. Birkebaek NH, Patel L, Wright NB, Grigg JR, Sinha S, Hall CM, et al. Endocrine status in patients with optic nerve hypoplasia: relationship to midline central nervous system abnormalities and appearance of the hypothalamic-pituitary axis on magnetic resonance imaging. J Clin Endocrinol Metab. 2003;88:5281–6.
20. Kaufman LM, Miller MT, Mafee MF. Magnetic resonance imaging of pituitary stalk hypoplasia. A discrete midline anomaly associated with endocrine abnormalities in septo-optic dysplasia. Arch Ophthalmol. 1989;107:1485–9.
21. Tajima T, Hattori T, Nakajima T, Okuhara K, Tsubaki J, Fujieda K. A novel missense mutation (P366T) of the LHX4 gene causes severe combined pituitary hormone deficiency with pituitary hypoplasia, ectopic posterior lobe and a poorly developed sella turcica. Endocr J. 2007;54:637–41.
22. Deal C, Hasselmann C, Pfäffle RW, Zimmermann AG, Quigley CA, Child CJ, et al. Associations between pituitary imaging abnormalities and clinical and biochemical phenotypes in children with congenital growth hormone deficiency: data from an international observational study. Horm Res Paediatr. 2013;79:283–92.
23. Mark AS, Kolsky M. Optic nerve hypoplasia: absence of posterior pituitary bright signal on magnetic resonance imaging correlates with diabetes insipidus. Am J Ophthalmol. 1997;123(5):715.
24. Sorkin JA, Davis PC, Meacham LR, Parks JS, Drack AV, Lambert SR. Optic nerve hypoplasia: absence of posterior pituitary bright signal on magnetic resonance imaging correlates with diabetes insipidus. Am J Ophthalmol. 1996;122:717–23.
25. Shulman DI, Martinez CR. Association of ectopic posterior pituitary and anterior pituitary hypoplasia with absence of the left internal carotid. J Pediatr Endocrinol Metab. 1996;9:539–42.
26. Inamo Y, Harada K. Agenesis of the internal carotid artery and congenital pituitary hypoplasia: proposal of a cause of congenital hypopituitarism. Eur J Pediatr. 2003;162:610–2.
27. Birkebaek NH, Patel L, Wright NB, Grigg JR, Sinha S, Hall CM, et al. Optic nerve size evaluated by magnetic resonance imaging in children with optic nerve hypoplasia, multiple pituitary hormone deficiency, isolated growth hormone deficiency, and idiopathic short stature. J Pediatr. 2004;145:536–41.
28. Dattani M, Preece M. Growth hormone deficiency and related disorders: insights into causation, diagnosis, and treatment. Lancet. 2004;363:1977–87.

Duplication of the Pituitary Gland

69

Gabriel Zada, M. Beatriz S. Lopes, Srinivasan Mukundan Jr., and Edward Laws Jr.

69.1 Epidemiology and Clinical Presentation

- Duplication of the pituitary gland, stalk, or both may occur either in an isolated fashion or in association with other developmental and congenital disorders. The pathogenesis is thought to relate to defective blastogenesis and incomplete twinning [1].
- Pituitary gland duplication has been described in patients with median cleft facial/palate syndromes and nasal or oral teratomas [1–5].
- It has also been reported in conjunction with dermoid tumors and hypothalamic hamartomas [6–9].
- Other less common findings related to blastogenesis include duplication of the tongue, basilar artery, and odontoid process. Duplication of the pituitary gland can also be seen with clival encephalocele, hypertelorism, and callosal agenesis [10, 11].
- The pathophysiology is thought to be related to duplication of the prechordal plate and anterior notochord [12].
- Mutations in chromosome 14 and the thyroid transcription factor-1 (TTF-1) gene have been reported in association with this finding [13].
- In rare cases, duplication of the pituitary can cause precocious puberty [14–16].

G. Zada, MD, MS (✉)
Department of Neurological Surgery, Keck School of Medicine, University of Southern California, 1200 N State Street, #3300, Los Angeles, CA 90033, USA
e-mail: gzada@usc.edu

M.B.S. Lopes, MD, PhD
Department of Pathology (Neuropathology), University of Virginia School of Medicine, 1215 Lee Street, Room 3060–HEP, Charlottesville, VA 22908, USA
e-mail: msl2e@virginia.edu

S. Mukundan Jr., PhD, MD
Department of Radiology, Brigham and Women's Hospital, 75 Francis Street, Boston, MA 02115, USA
e-mail: smukundan@partners.org

E. Laws Jr., MD
Department of Neurosurgery, Brigham and Women's Hospital, 15 Francis Street, Boston, MA 02115, USA
e-mail: elaws@partners.org

G. Zada et al. (eds.), *Atlas of Sellar and Parasellar Lesions: Clinical, Radiologic, and Pathologic Correlations*,
DOI 10.1007/978-3-319-22855-6_69

69.2 Imaging Features

- On MRI, duplication of the pituitary gland, the infundibulum, or both may be seen (Fig. 69.1). This finding is often associated with hypothalamic hamartomas and midline basisphenoid clefts [8, 12].
- Nasopharyngeal and oral teratomas, hamartomas, and dermoid tumors may be seen.
- Other rare findings include duplication or fenestration of the basilar artery, odontoid process, and tongue.

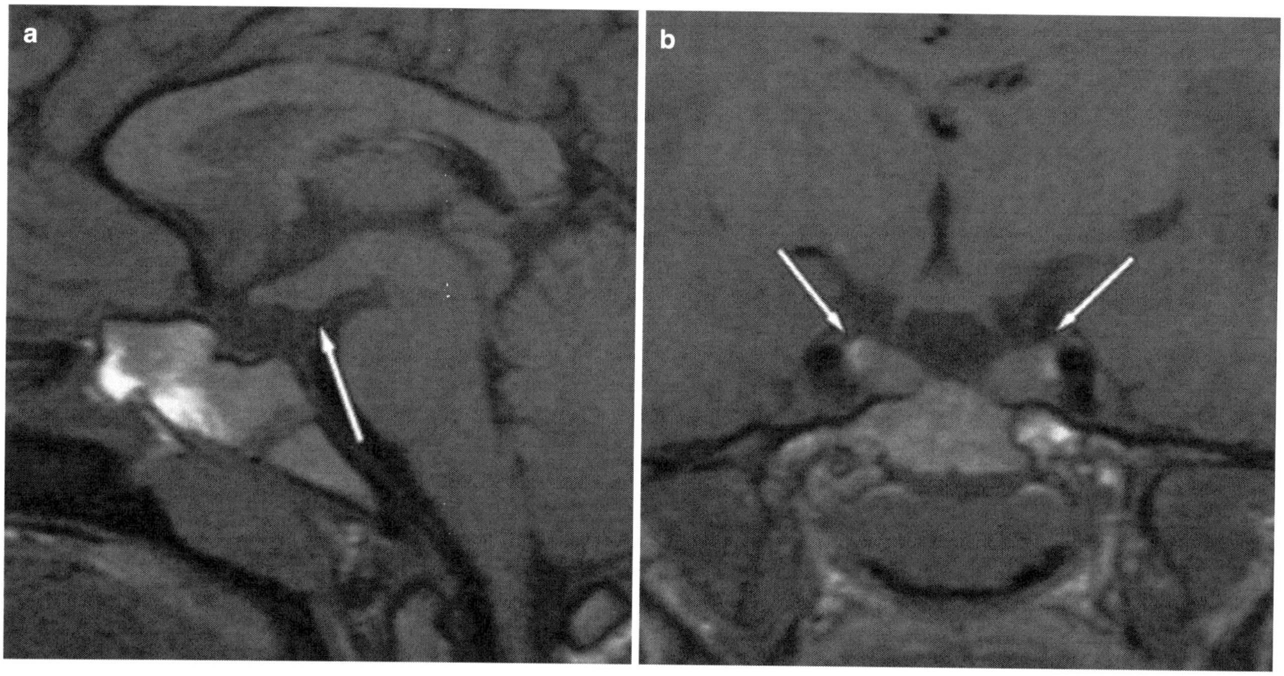

Fig. 69.1 Duplication of the pituitary gland. (**a**) Sagittal T1-weighted MR scan shows hypothalamic thickening (*arrow*). (**b**) Coronal T1-weighted MR scan shows two separate anterior and posterior pituitary glands with two separate pituitary stalks (*arrows*) (Adapted with permission from Akin et al. [14])

69.3 Clinical Management

- Treatment in patients with duplicated pituitary glands is highly individualized. Treatment may not be necessary. When it is needed, treatment includes screening for and management of precocious puberty and treatment of any associated tumors.

References

1. Slavotinek A, Parisi M, Heike C, Hing A, Huang E. Craniofacial defects of blastogenesis: duplication of pituitary with cleft palate and orophgaryngeal tumors. Am J Med Genet A. 2005;135:13–20.
2. Hamon-Kérautret M, Ares GS, Demondion X, Rouland V, Francke JP, Pruvo JP. Duplication of the pituitary gland in a newborn with median cleft face syndrome and nasal teratoma. Pediatr Radiol. 1998;28:290–2.
3. Chariker M, Ford R, Morrison C, Theile A, Moeller K, Moriarty T. Pituitary duplication with nasopharyngeal teratoma and cleft palate. J Craniofac Surg. 2011;22:755–8.
4. Huisman TA, Fischer U, Boltshauser E, Straube T, Gysin C. Pituitary duplication and nasopharyngeal teratoma in a newborn: CT, MRI, US and correlative histopathological findings. Neuroradiology. 2005;47:558–61.
5. Maeda Y, Suenaga H, Sugiyama M, Saijo H, Hoshi K, Mori Y, Takato T. Clinical presentation of epignathus teratoma with cleft palate; and duplication of cranial base, tongue, mandible, and pituitary gland. J Craniofac Surg. 2013;24:1486–91.
6. Madhusudhan KS, Kandpal H. Pituitary stalk duplication with intrasellar dermoid and herniation of the third ventricle. Pediatr Radiol. 2009;39:1013.
7. Mutlu H, Paker B, Gunes N, Emektar A, Keceli M, Kantarci M. Pituitary duplication associated with oral dermoid and corpus callosum hypogenesis. Neuroradiology. 2004;46:1036–8.
8. Ryals BD, Brown DC, Levin SW. Duplication of the pituitary gland as shown by MR. AJNR Am J Neuroradiol. 1993;14:137–9.
9. Shah S, Pereira JK, Becker CJ, Roubal SE. Duplication of pituitary gland. J Comput Assist Tomogr. 1997;21:459–61.
10. Manjila S, Miller EA, Vadera S, Goel RK, Khan FR, Crowe C, Geertman RT. Duplication of the pituitary gland associated with multiple blastogenesis defects: duplication of the pituitary gland (DPG)-plus syndrome. Case report and review of literature. Surg Neurol Int. 2012;3:23.
11. Shroff M, Blaser S, Jay V, Chitayat D, Armstrong D. Basilar artery duplication associated with pituitary duplication: a new finding. AJNR Am J Neuroradiol. 2003;24:956–61.
12. Kollias SS, Ball WS, Prenger EC. Review of the embryologic development of the pituitary gland and report of a case of hypophyseal duplication detected by MRI. Neuroradiology. 1995;37:3–12.
13. Accornero S, Danesino C, Bastianello S, D'Errico I, Guala A, Chiovato L. Duplication of the pituitary stalk in a patient with a heterozygous deletion of chromosome 14 harboring the thyroid transcription factor-1 gene. J Clin Endocrinol Metab. 2010;95:3595–6.
14. Akin L, Kendirci M, Doğanay S, Kurtoğlu S, Tucer B, Coskun A. Pituitary duplication: a rare cause of precocious puberty. Childs Nerv Syst. 2011;27:1157–60.
15. de Penna GC, Pimenta MP, Drummond JB, Sarquis M, Martins JC, de Campos RC, Dias EP. Duplication of the hypophysis associated with precocious puberty: presentation of two cases and review of pituitary embryogenesis. Arq Bras Endocrinol Metabol. 2005;49:323–7.
16. Vieira TC, Chinen RN, Ribeiro MR, Nogueira RG, Abucham J. Central precocious puberty associated with pituitary duplication and midline defects. J Pediatr Endocrinol Metab. 2007;20:1141–4.

Fibrous Dysplasia

70

Gabriel Zada, M. Beatriz S. Lopes, Srinivasan Mukundan Jr., and Edward Laws Jr.

70.1 Epidemiology and Clinical Presentation

- Fibrous dysplasia (FD) is a developmental disorder that may result in expansion and distortion of mature bone and replacement with weaker, immature bone.
- The disease is often sporadic. It may occur as part of the McCune-Albright syndrome (polyostotic fibrous dysplasia, endocrine hypersecretion disorders, café au lait spots, and precocious puberty) [1].
- FD may also occur in association with pituitary adenomas that secrete both GH and prolactin [1–5].
- FD comprises approximately 0.1 % of patients undergoing transsphenoidal operations [6].
- The disease often presents during the first three decades of life, with a mean age of 24 years [7].
- FD can be monostotic (70–80 %) or polyostotic (20–30 %) [8, 9].
- Bony involvement can occur anywhere in the craniofacial region or along the skull base, including the paranasal sinuses. The ethmoid, frontal, and sphenoid bones are the most commonly affected craniofacial bones [9, 10].
- Dysplastic bony overgrowth may result in visual loss, exophthalmos, cranial nerve impingement, cosmetic deformity, sinus disease, headache, or a combination of these [11–14].
- Cystic degeneration of the mass has also been associated with progressive visual loss [14, 15].
- In rare cases, FD involves the clivus, where it may cause headache and lower cranial nerve paresis [8, 16, 17].

G. Zada, MD, MS (✉)
Department of Neurological Surgery, Keck School of Medicine, University of Southern California, 1200 N State Street, #3300, Los Angeles, CA 90033, USA
e-mail: gzada@usc.edu

M.B.S. Lopes, MD, PhD
Department of Pathology (Neuropathology), University of Virginia School of Medicine, 1215 Lee Street, Room 3060–HEP, Charlottesville, VA 22908, USA
e-mail: msl2e@virginia.edu

S. Mukundan Jr., PhD, MD
Department of Radiology, Brigham and Women's Hospital, 75 Francis Street, Boston, MA 02115, USA
e-mail: smukundan@partners.org

E. Laws Jr., MD
Department of Neurosurgery, Brigham and Women's Hospital, 15 Francis Street, Boston, MA 02115, USA
e-mail: elaws@partners.org

G. Zada et al. (eds.), *Atlas of Sellar and Parasellar Lesions: Clinical, Radiologic, and Pathologic Correlations*,
DOI 10.1007/978-3-319-22855-6_70

70.2 Imaging Features

- CT scans typically demonstrate ground-glass opacification, widening of diploic spaces, and expansion of the bone (Fig. 70.2). Stenosis of skull base foramina may be seen on CT. FD is characterized by lesions with 70–130 Hounsfield units (HU), compared with 20–40 HU for other benign entities [18].
- MRI typically demonstrates low T1 signal and low or isointense T2 signal with nonenhancing bony expansion (Fig. 70.1) [16, 19–21].

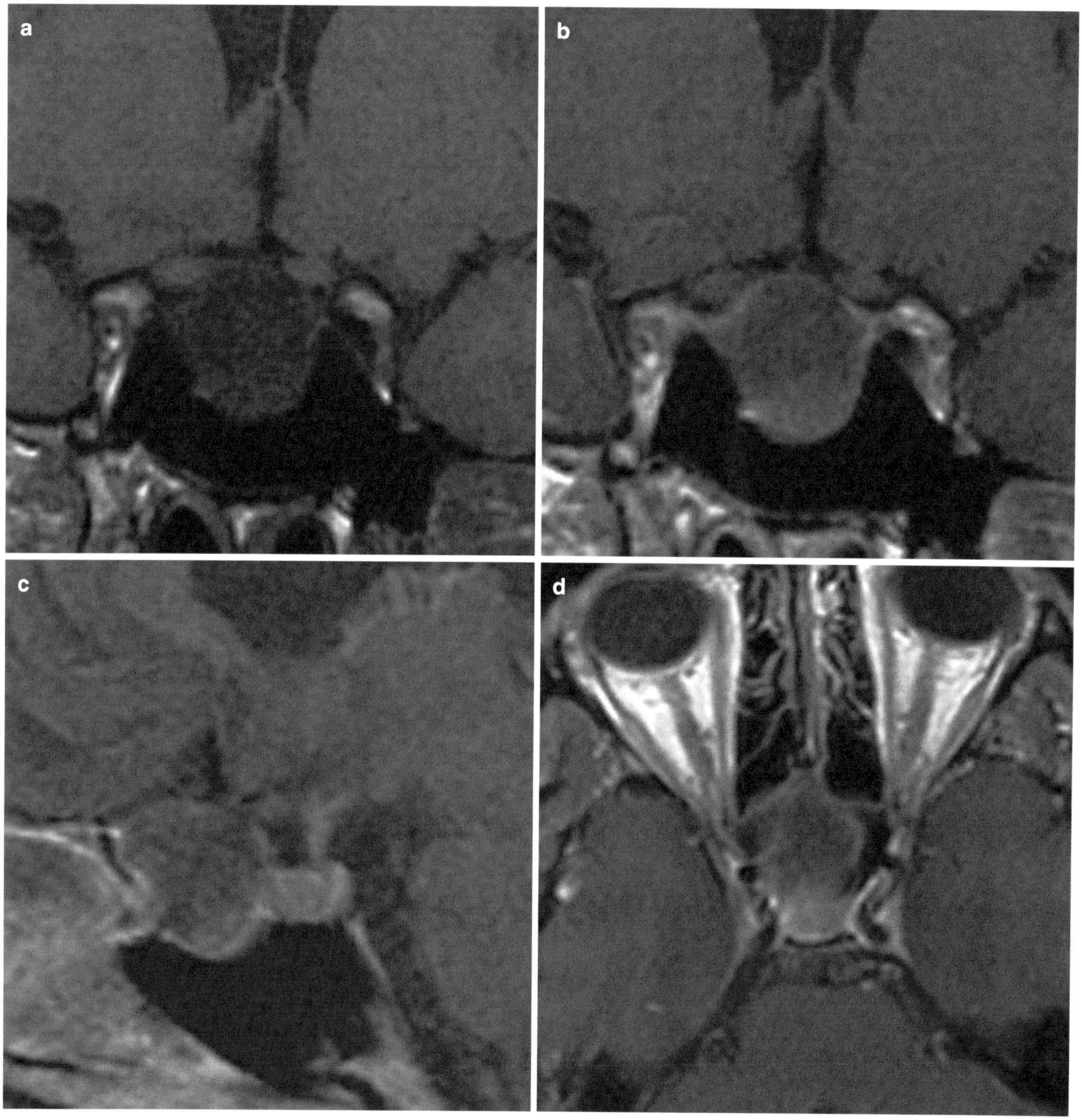

Fig. 70.1 Fibrous dysplasia. (**a**) Coronal T1-weighted precontrast MR image. (**b**) Coronal T1-weighted gadolinium-enhanced image. (**c**) Sagittal T1-weighted gadolinium-enhanced image. (**d**) Axial T1-weighted gadolinium-enhanced image. An expansile lesion is centered in the body of the sphenoid, demonstrating heterogeneous signal intensity and faint contrast enhancement. The pituitary gland is posterior to the lesion

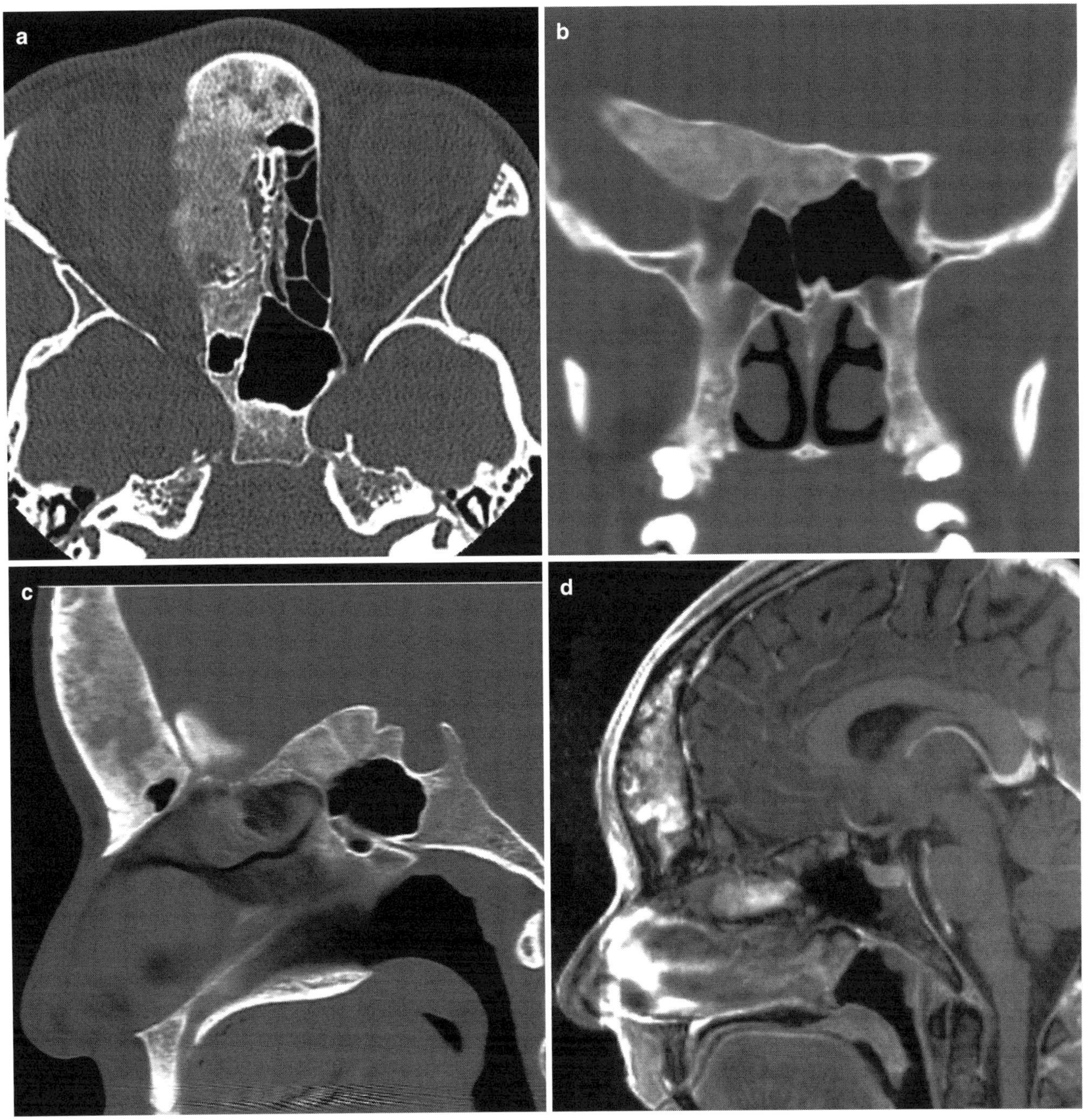

Fig. 70.2 Fibrous dysplasia. (**a**) Axial CT image in bone algorithm. (**b**) Coronal CT image in bone window. (**c**) Sagittal CT image in bone algorithm. (**d**) Sagittal T1-weighted gadolinium-enhanced MR image. Bony expansion with ground-glass attenuation is observed in the right frontal bone, right ethmoid bone, and right sphenoid wing. The lesion involves the medial right orbital wall and displaces the orbital contents. MRI shows heterogeneous enhancement within the lesion

70.3 Histopathology

- FD is characterized by abnormal fibroblast maturation and proliferation resulting in replacement of normal bone with weaker, immature woven bone.
- FD rarely undergoes malignant transformation to osteosarcoma, fibrosarcoma, or chondrosarcoma [22].
- FD has also been noted to coexist with aneurysmal bone cysts [23, 24].

70.4 Clinical and Surgical Management

- Conservative management is recommended in most cases, as the disease is often benign and self-limited.
- Bisphosphonate therapy may benefit some patients with pain and neurological symptoms [25, 26].
- Corticosteroids may benefit some patients with progressive visual changes [27].
- A biopsy may be necessary if the imaging features are atypical or questionable, especially in a monostotic lesion where the diagnosis has not yet been established.
- Surgical decompression (especially optic nerve decompression) may be warranted in a minority of cases with cranial nerve compression or craniocervical joint involvement [10, 16].
- A transsphenoidal approach may be used to obtain a biopsy specimen or achieve surgical decompression for appropriate skull base lesions [4, 28].
- In recent years, extended endoscopic approaches have been used to treat symptomatic FD lesions [4, 29].
- In cases of McCune-Albright syndrome, primary management of the endocrinopathy and hypersecretion syndromes using surgery, medications, and/or radiation may be needed to achieve endocrinological remission.

References

1. Lipson A, Hsu TH. The Albright syndrome associated with acromegaly: report of a case and review of the literature. Johns Hopkins Med J. 1981;149:10–4.
2. Garcia MB, Koppeschaar HP, Lips CJ, Thijssen JH, Krenning EP. Acromegaly and hyperprolactinemia in a patient with polyostotic fibrous dysplasia: dynamic endocrine studies and treatment with the somatostatin analogue octreotide. J Endocrinol Invest. 1994;17:59–65.
3. O'Laughlin RL, Selinger SE, Moriarty PE. Pituitary adenoma in McCune-Albright syndrome: MR demonstration. J Comput Assist Tomogr. 1989;13:685–8.
4. Singh N, Abou-Zeid A, King A, du Plessis D, Gnanalingham K. Endoscopic transsphenoidal surgery for isolated fibrous dysplasia of the clivus. Minim Invasive Neurosurg. 2009;52:190–2.
5. Christoforidis A, Maniadaki I, Stanhope R. McCune-Albright syndrome: growth hormone and prolactin hypersecretion. J Pediatr Endocrinol Metab. 2006;19:623–5.
6. Saeger W, Lüdecke DK, Buchfelder M, Fahlbusch R, Quabbe HJ, Petersenn S. Pathohistological classification of pituitary tumors: 10 years of experience with the German Pituitary Tumor Registry. Eur J Endocrinol. 2007;156:203–16.
7. MacDonald-Jankowski D. Fibrous dysplasia: a systematic review. Dentomaxillofac Radiol. 2009;38:196–215.
8. Levy ML, Chen TC, Weiss MH. Monostotic fibrous dysplasia of the clivus. Case report. J Neurosurg. 1991;75:800–3.
9. Srinivas N, DeLong SR, Amilineni VK. Monostotic fibrous dysplasia of the sphenoid sinus: a serendipitous finding on a bone scan. Clin Nucl Med. 2000;25:477–9.
10. Lustig LR, Holliday MJ, McCarthy EF, Nager GT. Fibrous dysplasia involving the skull base and temporal bone. Arch Otolaryngol Head Neck Surg. 2001;127:1239–47.
11. Weisman JS, Hepler RS, Vinters HV. Reversible visual loss caused by fibrous dysplasia. Am J Ophthalmol. 1990;110:244–9.
12. Amit M, Fliss DM, Gil Z. Fibrous dysplasia of the sphenoid and skull base. Otolaryngol Clin North Am. 2011;44:891–902.
13. Bollen E, Vielvoye J, Van Dijk JG, Roos RA. Trigeminal neuralgia-like pain in an aged woman with fibrous dysplasia of the skull base. Headache. 1990;30:277–9.
14. Dumont AS, Boulos PT, Jane Jr JA, Ellegala DB, Newman SA, Jane Sr JA. Cranioorbital fibrous dysplasia: with emphasis on visual impairment and current surgical management. Neurosurg Focus. 2001;10(5):E6.
15. Michael CB, Lee AG, Patrinely JR, Stal S, Blacklock JB. Visual loss associated with fibrous dysplasia of the anterior skull base. Case report and review of the literature. J Neurosurg. 2000;92:350–4.
16. Adada B, Al-Mefty O. Fibrous dysplasia of the clivus. Neurosurgery. 2003;52:318–22; discussion 323.
17. Sato K, Kubota T, Kaneko M, Kawano H, Kobayashi H. Fibrous dysplasia of the clivus. Surg Neurol. 1993;40:522–5.
18. Khalil HS, Toynton S, Steventon N, Adams W, Gibson J. Radiological difficulties in the diagnosis of fibrous dysplasia of the sphenoid sinus and the cranial base. Rhinology. 2001;39:49–51.
19. Maeda M, Kimura H, Tsuchida C, Ishii Y, Kubota T. MR imaging of monostotic fibrous dysplasia of the clivus. A case report. Acta Radiol. 1993;34:527–8.
20. Jee WH, Choi KH, Choe BY, Park JM, Shinn KS. Fibrous dysplasia: MR imaging characteristics with radiopathologic correlation. AJR Am J Roentgenol. 1996;167:1523–7.
21. Sirvanci M, Karaman K, Onat L, Duran C, Ulusoy OL. Monostotic fibrous dysplasia of the clivus: MRI and CT findings. Neuroradiology. 2002;44:847–50.
22. Yabut Jr SM, Kenan S, Sissons HA, Lewis MM. Malignant transformation of fibrous dysplasia. A case report and review of the literature. Clin Orthop Relat Res. 1988;228:281–9.
23. Haddad GF, Hambali F, Mufarrij A, Nassar A, Haddad FS. Concomitant fibrous dysplasia and aneurysmal bone cyst of the skull base. Case report and review of the literature. Pediatr Neurosurg. 1998;28:147–53.
24. Itshayek E, Spector S, Gomori M, Segal R. Fibrous dysplasia in combination with aneurysmal bone cyst of the occipital bone and the clivus: case report and review of the literature. Neurosurgery. 2002;51:815–7; discussion 817–8.
25. DiCaprio MR, Enneking WF. Fibrous dysplasia. Pathophysiology, evaluation, and treatment. J Bone Joint Surg Am. 2005;87:1848–64.
26. DiMeglio LA. Bisphosphonate therapy for fibrous dysplasia. Pediatr Endocrinol Rev. 2007;4:440–5.
27. Arroyo JG, Lessell S, Montgomery WW. Steroid-induced visual recovery in fibrous dysplasia. J Clin Neuroophthalmol. 1991;11:259–61.
28. Contratti F, Menniti A, Fraioli MF, Fraioli B. Fibrous dysplasia of the clivus with a second T8 bone lesion: case report. Surg Neurol. 2006;65:202–5; discussion 205–6.
29. Salmasi V, Blitz AM, Ishii M, Gallia GL. Expanded endonasal endoscopic approach for resection of a large skull base aneurysmal bone cyst in a pediatric patient with extensive cranial fibrous dysplasia. Childs Nerv Syst. 2011;27:649–56.

Basilar Impression and Invagination

71

Gabriel Zada, M. Beatriz S. Lopes, Srinivasan Mukundan Jr., and Edward Laws Jr.

71.1 Epidemiology and Clinical Presentation

- Basilar impression (secondary/acquired) and invagination (primary) develop when the odontoid process of C2 migrates into the foramen magnum, causing compression of the brainstem and upper cervical spine. The terms are often used interchangeably because the symptoms and treatment are similar. For the purposes of this chapter, both basilar impression and invagination will be referred to as BI.
- Basilar invagination is more commonly associated with congenital anomalies such as the Klippel-Feil syndrome and hindbrain herniation.
- Basilar impression is more commonly associated with conditions causing softening of the bone and secondary settling, including Paget disease, rheumatoid arthritis, hyperparathyroidism, Hajdu-Cheney syndrome, and osteogenesis imperfecta.
- The mean age of patients requiring surgical decompression is 43 years for basilar impression and 22 years for basilar invagination [1, 2].
- Clinical signs and symptoms may include weakness, neck pain, myelopathy/spasticity, ataxia, swallowing difficulty, and other lower cranial nerve deficits.
- Craniocervical instability may be present and requires a thorough assessment, as discussed below.

G. Zada, MD, MS (✉)
Department of Neurological Surgery, Keck School of Medicine, University of Southern California, 1200 N State Street, #3300, Los Angeles, CA 90033, USA
e-mail: gzada@usc.edu

M.B.S. Lopes, MD, PhD
Department of Pathology (Neuropathology), University of Virginia School of Medicine, 1215 Lee Street, Room 3060–HEP, Charlottesville, VA 22908, USA
e-mail: msl2e@virginia.edu

S. Mukundan Jr., PhD, MD
Department of Radiology, Brigham and Women's Hospital, 75 Francis Street, Boston, MA 02115, USA
e-mail: smukundan@partners.org

E. Laws Jr., MD
Department of Neurosurgery, Brigham and Women's Hospital, 15 Francis Street, Boston, MA 02115, USA
e-mail: elaws@partners.org

G. Zada et al. (eds.), *Atlas of Sellar and Parasellar Lesions: Clinical, Radiologic, and Pathologic Correlations*,
DOI 10.1007/978-3-319-22855-6_71

71.2 Imaging Features

- In patients with BI, upward migration of the odontoid process through the foramen magnum can be seen, often with compression of the ventral brainstem or upper cervical spinal cord.
- An assessment of craniocervical instability should be made. Methods available to help make this determination include Chamberlain's line, McGregor's line, and McRae's line.
- On CT scans, the mean position of the odontoid process is 1.4 mm below Chamberlain's line, 0.8 mm below McGregor's line, and 5 mm below McRae's line [3].
- On MRI, the mean position of the odontoid peg was 1.2 mm below Chamberlain's line, 0.9 mm below McGregor's line, and 4.6 mm below McRae's line [4].
- Chiari I malformation, syringomyelia, and loss of height and volume of the posterior fossa may be seen may be seen in conjunction with BI (Fig. 71.1).
- Platybasia refers to flattening of the angulation of the clivus with respect to the cervical spine. It may be an incidental finding, or it may play a role in the development of BI.

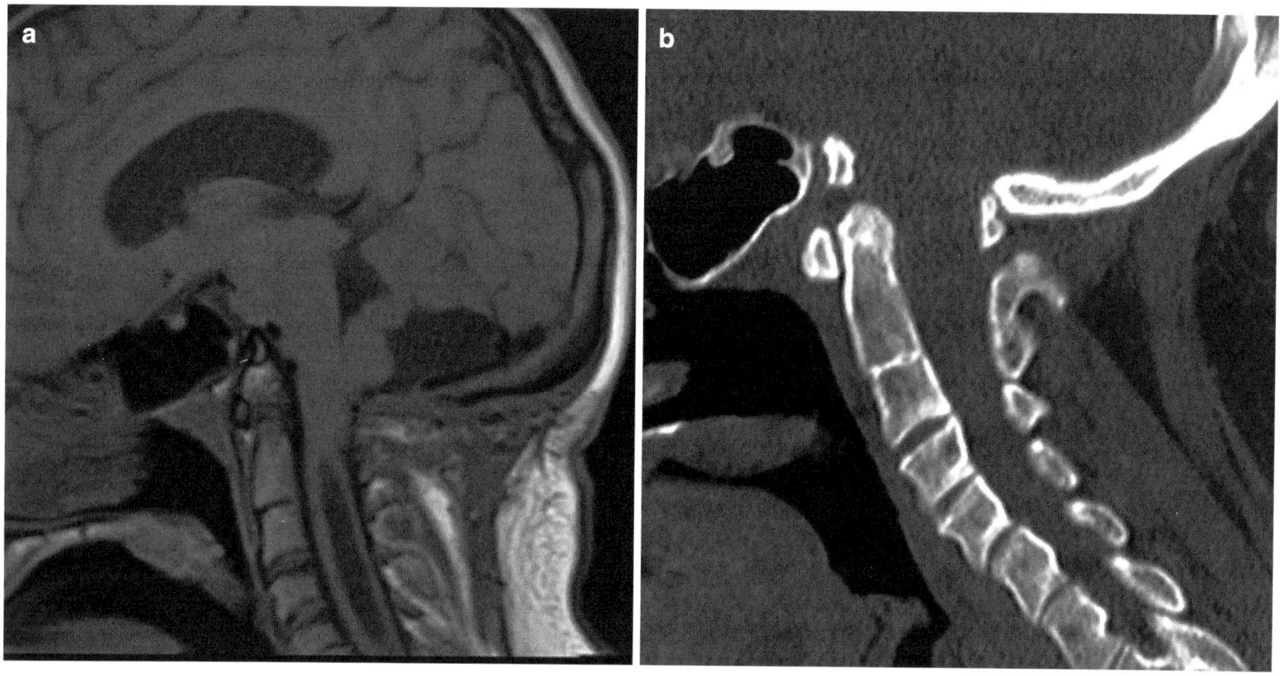

Fig. 71.1 Basilar impression/invagination. (**a**) Sagittal T1-weighted precontrast MR image. (**b**) Sagittal CT image. The clivus is hypoplastic, and there is incomplete segmentation of C2 and C3. The odontoid process of C2 is high riding and the foramen magnum is narrowed. A posterior fossa arachnoid cyst is displacing the cerebellar tonsils anteriorly. (**a**) A cervical cord syrinx is present

71.3 Clinical and Surgical Management

- The management of BI should be individualized. It is often based on the patient's signs and symptoms, degree of anterior (brainstem) compression, presence of a Chiari malformation, presence of craniocervical instability, and the patient's age and comorbidities [5].
- In some patients, especially younger ones with primary basilar invagination, cervical traction and fixation can be used successfully to achieve decompression and stabilization [2, 6, 7].
- In the presence of a Chiari I malformation and reduction of posterior fossa volume, posterior decompression (with or without fixation) is a preferred approach for many patients [8].
- Classically, a transoral approach has been used in treating anterior craniocervical pathology with direct brainstem compression, often followed by posterior fixation and fusion. These approaches offer good exposure of the affected region, and many patients improve with regard to compression symptoms, but complication rates are relatively high [9, 10].
- In recent years, extended endoscopic endonasal and transcervical approaches to the odontoid region and clivus have expanded the ability to treat these disorders [1, 11].
- The sublabial approach has been used frequently to treat patients with basilar impression [12, 13].
- Endonasal surgery may be a more feasible option in patients with platybasia, which is associated with an increased height of the odontoid process relative to the palatine line.

References

1. Dasenbrock HH, Clarke MJ, Bydon A, Sciubba DM, Witham TF, Gokaslan ZL, Wolinsky JP. Endoscopic image-guided transcervical odontoidectomy: outcomes of 15 patients with basilar invagination. Neurosurgery. 2012;70:351–9; discussion 359–60.
2. Peng X, Chen L, Wan Y, Zou X. Treatment of primary basilar invagination by cervical traction and posterior instrumented reduction together with occipitocervical fusion. Spine (Phila Pa 1976). 2011;36:1528–31.
3. Cronin CG, Lohan DG, Mhuircheartigh JN, Meehan CP, Murphy J, Roche C. CT evaluation of Chamberlain's, McGregor's, and McRae's skull-base lines. Clin Radiol. 2009;64:64–9.
4. Cronin CG, Lohan DG, Mhuircheartigh JN, Meehan CP, Murphy JM, Roche C. MRI evaluation and measurement of the normal odontoid peg position. Clin Radiol. 2007;62:897–903.
5. Goel A. Basilar invagination, Chiari malformation, syringomyelia: a review. Neurol India. 2009;57:235–46.
6. Goel A. Treatment of basilar invagination by atlantoaxial joint distraction and direct lateral mass fixation. J Neurosurg Spine. 2004;1:281–6.
7. Goel A, Shah A. Atlantoaxial joint distraction as a treatment for basilar invagination: a report of an experience with 11 cases. Neurol India. 2008;56:144–50.
8. Goel A, Bhatjiwale M, Desai K. Basilar invagination: a study based on 190 surgically treated patients. J Neurosurg. 1998;88:962–8.
9. Ibrahim AG, Crockard HA. Basilar impression and osteogenesis imperfecta: a 21-year retrospective review of outcomes in 20 patients. J Neurosurg Spine. 2007;7:594–600.
10. Perrini P, Benedetto N, Guidi E, Di Lorenzo N. Transoral approach and its superior extensions to the craniovertebral junction malformations: surgical strategies and results. Neurosurgery. 2009;64:331–42; discussion 342.
11. Rawal RB, Shah RN, Zanation AM. Endonasal odontoidectomy for basilar impression and brainstem compression due to radiation fibrosis. Laryngoscope. 2013;123:584–7.
12. Asadi-Moghaddam K, Otto BA, Carrau RL, Prevedello DM. Sublabial approach for symptomatic basilar impression. Neurosurgery. 2012;70:E1054–5.
13. Bettegowda C, Shajari M, Suk I, Simmons OP, Gokaslan ZL, Wolinsky JP. Sublabial approach for the treatment of symptomatic basilar impression in a patient with Klippel-Feil syndrome. Neurosurgery. 2011;69(1 Suppl Operative):ons77–82; discussion ons82.

Part X

Acquired Anomalies of the Sellar Region

Traumatic Injury of the Sellar Region, Pituitary Stalk Disruption, and Posttraumatic Anosmia

72

Gabriel Zada, M. Beatriz S. Lopes, Srinivasan Mukundan Jr., and Edward Laws Jr.

72.1 Epidemiology and Clinical Presentation

- Under certain circumstances, traumatic brain injury (TBI) may result in fractures of the anterior and middle skull base.
- The pituitary gland and stalk are at particular risk of injury in high-speed acceleration-deceleration shear-type injuries, because the stalk is surrounded anatomically by the rigid diaphragma sella and the gland is encased within the rigid bony sella. Furthermore, the pituitary stalk is composed of axonal tracts arising from hypothalamic neurons, in addition to a portal venous system, rendering it susceptible to traumatic injury.
- The incidence of sella turcica fractures among TBI patients is 3.6 % according to major series; these fractures are more common in children. In about half of cases, these fractures are associated with CSF leaks [1].
- Risk factors for developing hypopituitarism following TBI include diffuse axonal injury, basal skull fractures, and older age [2].
- It has been shown recently that the development of hypopituitarism following TBI may be mediated by autoimmune mechanisms, namely, the circulation of antipituitary antibodies [3].
- Sellar region trauma may result in a variety of clinical problems, including CSF leaks, meningitis, meningoceles and encephaloceles, pneumocephalus, panhypopituitarism, diabetes insipidus, visual loss, cranial nerve paresis, pseudoaneurysms, and cavernous-carotid and cavernous dural fistulas [4–8].
- The incidence of acute posttraumatic hypopituitarism of any anterior pituitary hormonal axis is 50–76 % [9–11]. The incidence of posterior pituitary dysfunction (diabetes insipidus) in the acute state following moderate or severe TBI is 21.6 %; permanent diabetes insipidus develops in 6.9 % of patients [12].

G. Zada, MD, MS (✉)
Department of Neurological Surgery, Keck School of Medicine, University of Southern California, 1200 N State Street, #3300, Los Angeles, CA 90033, USA
e-mail: gzada@usc.edu

M.B.S. Lopes, MD, PhD
Department of Pathology (Neuropathology), University of Virginia School of Medicine, 1215 Lee Street, Room 3060–HEP, Charlottesville, VA 22908, USA
e-mail: msl2e@virginia.edu

S. Mukundan Jr., PhD, MD
Department of Radiology, Brigham and Women's Hospital, 75 Francis Street, Boston, MA 02115, USA
e-mail: smukundan@partners.org

E. Laws Jr., MD
Department of Neurosurgery, Brigham and Women's Hospital, 15 Francis Street, Boston, MA 02115, USA
e-mail: elaws@partners.org

G. Zada et al. (eds.), *Atlas of Sellar and Parasellar Lesions: Clinical, Radiologic, and Pathologic Correlations*, DOI 10.1007/978-3-319-22855-6_72

- The hormonal axis most often chronically affected in patients with traumatic hypopituitarism is the growth hormone axis. In the acute phase following TBI, the hormonal axes most often affected are the gonadotropin axis (41.6 %), the growth hormone axis (20.4 %), the ACTH axis (9.8 %), and the thyroid axis (5.8 %). One year following the injury, the most prevalent hormonal axis deficiencies involved the growth hormone axis (37.7 %), the ACTH axis (19.2 %), the gonadotropin axis (7.7 %), and the thyroid axis (5.8 %). Hormonal dysfunction tends to at least partially improve in up to 60 % of patients following a traumatic injury [9, 13].
- The incidence of anosmia caused by shear stress to olfactory nerves in the cribriform plate is as high as 56 % following a TBI, but many of these patients are not aware of the anosmia [14].
- A spectrum of clinical symptoms related to anosmia may be present, including hyposmia, dysosmia (distortion of smell), hypogeusia (reduced taste sensation), and dysgeusia (distortion of taste) [15].
- The finding of anosmia following TBI has been associated with more prominent neuropsychiatric dysfunction, especially as it pertains to frontal lobe function [16].

72.2 Imaging Features

- CT imaging, often using thin cuts and multiplanar reconstruction, is the most sensitive method for detecting fractures of the sellar region (Fig. 72.1) [1].
- On MRI, enlargement of the pituitary gland may be seen. Specific changes within the pituitary gland, such as hemorrhage or infarction, are seen in 30 % of cases following TBI [17].
- MRI may show pituitary stalk disruption with loss of the normal posterior pituitary bright spot; this loss has been reported to correlate clinically with the development of diabetes insipidus (Fig. 72.2) [7, 18, 19].
- In up to 80 % of long-term survivors of TBI with clinical hypopituitarism, MRI may show an empty sella, perfusion deficits, and loss of the posterior pituitary bright spot [20].
- In patients with posttraumatic anosmia, MR imaging is often negative, or it may show diffuse white matter changes consistent with prior TBI. The orbitofrontal cortex is most likely to show evidence of injury in patients with anosmia.
- SPECT imaging has been used to measure perfusion, which may be altered in the frontal lobes in patients with posttraumatic anosmia [21].

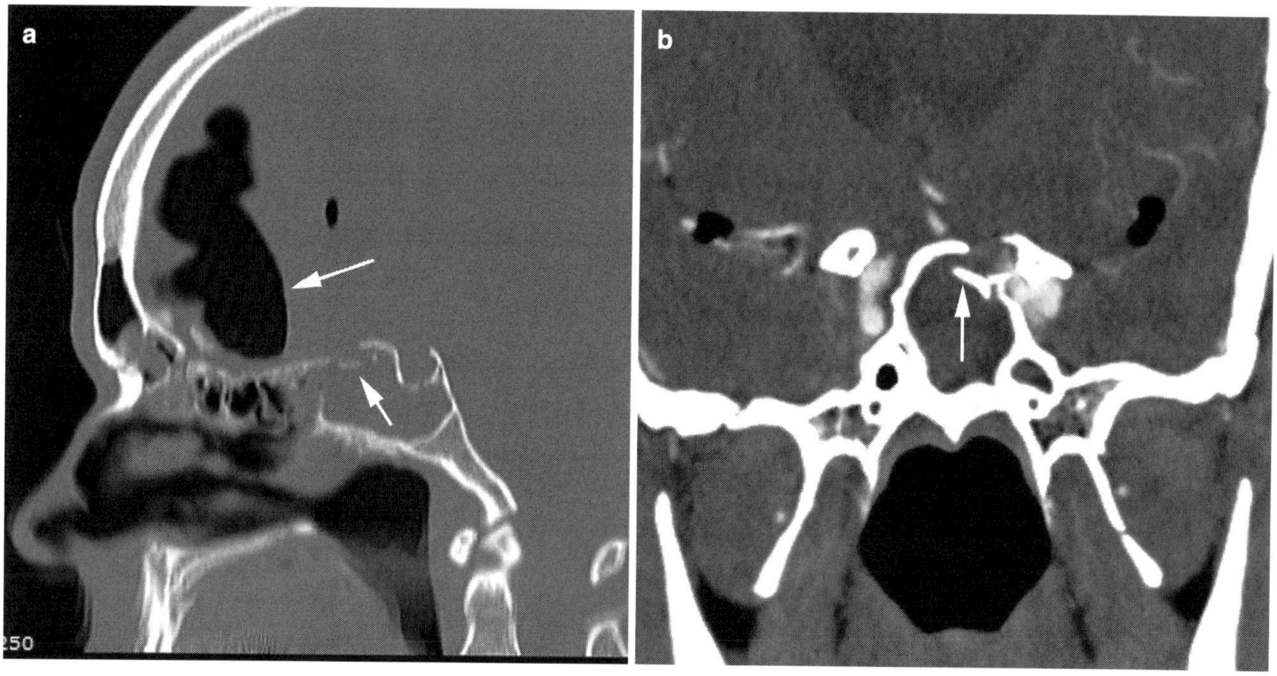

Fig. 72.1 Traumatic injury to anterior skull base fracture. (**a**) Sagittal CT image reconstructed in bone algorithm. (**b**) Coronal CT image with intravenous contrast enhancement. Comminuted fractures of the planum sphenoidale are seen on both images (*arrows*), with complete opacification of the sphenoid sinuses and pneumocephalus (**a**, *upper arrow*)

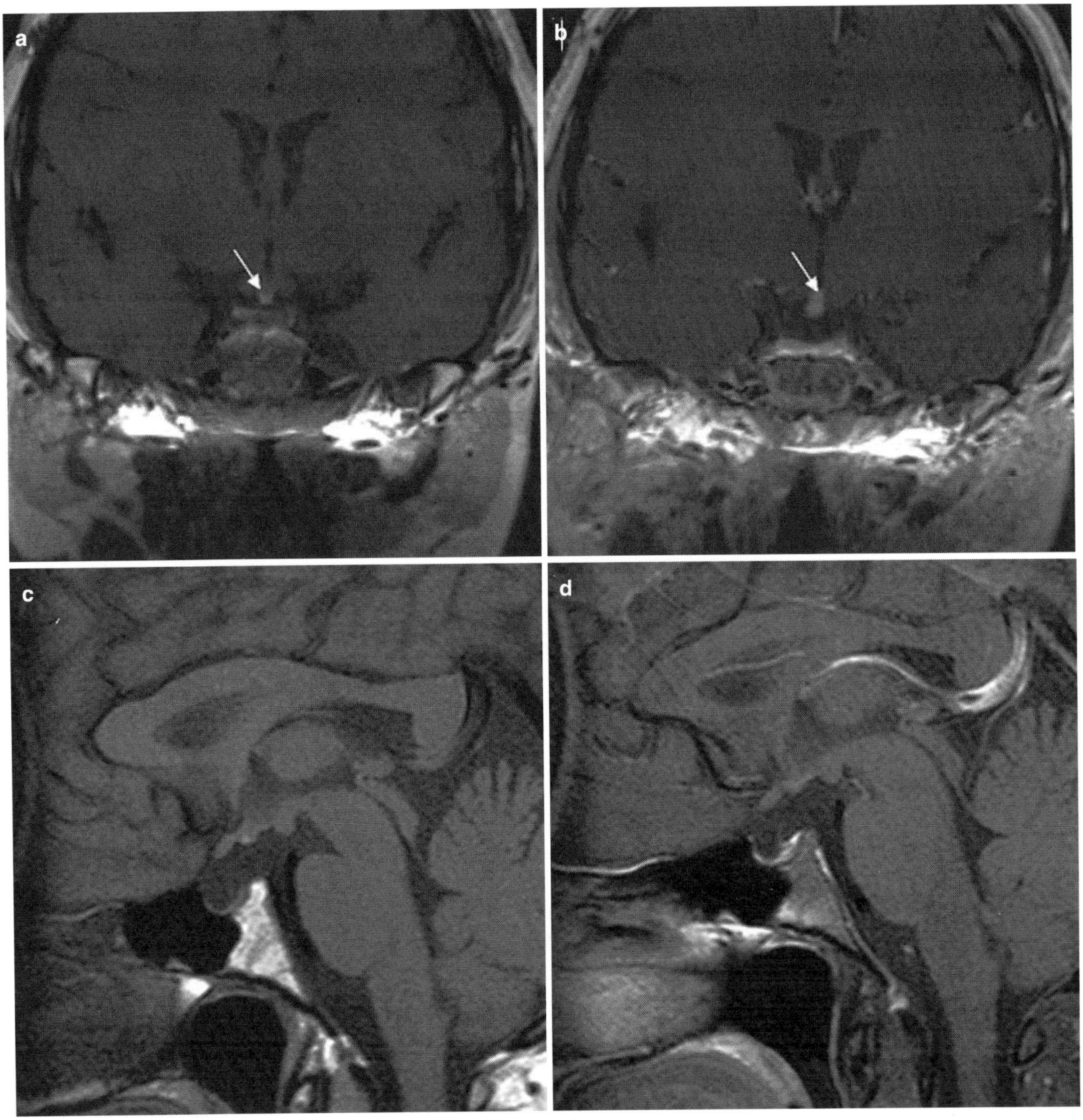

Fig. 72.2 Pituitary stalk transection. (**a**, **b**) Coronal pituitary MR images before and after contrast administration in a patient with pituitary stalk transection. Residual pituitary (*arrows*) is seen at the floor of the third ventricle. The figure also illustrates the small anterior pituitary gland and absent infundibulum. (**c**, **d**) Sagittal pituitary MR images before and after contrast administration (*Adapted with permission from* Ioachimescu et al. [19])

72.3 Histopathology

- Microscopic histological analysis of the pituitary gland following severe TBI shows a pattern of infarction and widespread necrosis of the anterior pituitary gland [22].
- In patients with traumatic anosmia, microscopic degeneration of the olfactory vesicles and loss of cilia are seen. A common finding is bald olfactory vesicles with basal bodies. In severe cases, atrophy or complete loss of the olfactory epithelium may be seen [23, 24].

72.4 Clinical and Surgical Management

- Standard neurocritical management in patients with TBI includes monitoring and treatment of intracranial pressure, supportive care, seizure control, and evacuation of any compressive lesions.
- Management of traumatic CSF leaks should be performed in a timely fashion (in stable TBI patients) to prevent pneumocephalus or meningitis.
- Screening for hypopituitarism is recommended for patients with severe TBI, especially children, older adults, and patients with evidence of basilar skull fractures. Some patients will require additional stress doses of hormones that they are unable to produce in a posttraumatic state, and growth hormone deficiency has more profound effects on children than on adults.
- In some patients with visual loss following TBI, decompression of the optic nerve or chiasm is recommended. This can be done via a craniotomy or endoscopic endonasal approach. Approximately one third to one half of patients will have improvement in vision following surgical decompression of the optic nerve. Steroids do not appear to provide an additional clinical benefit [8, 25, 26].
- In patients with posttraumatic anosmia, the key aspects of clinical management involve recognizing the anosmia and treating any associated conditions, including CSF leaks, infections, and neuropsychiatric dysfunction.
- Patients with craniofacial trauma and anosmia are more likely to have psychosocial and vocational dysfunction for years following an injury; these patients may need multidisciplinary treatment involving therapists, psychiatrists, and others.
- Recovery of olfactory function has been reported in 10 % of patients, occurring between 8 weeks and 2 years after the injury [27].
- The management of CSF leaks is discussed in the next chapter. See also the discussions of encephaloceles (Chap. 66) and traumatic vascular conditions such as cavernous-carotid fistulas (Chap. 62).

References

1. Ceviker N, Baykaner K, Keskil S, Işik S, Tokyay M, Kaymaz M, Aykol S. Sella turcica fractures in a trauma series and their clinical significance. Surg Neurol. 1995;44:28–30.
2. Schneider M, Schneider HJ, Yassouridis A, Saller B, von Rosen F, Stalla GK. Predictors of anterior pituitary insufficiency after traumatic brain injury. Clin Endocrinol (Oxf). 2008;68: 206–12.
3. Tanriverdi F, De Bellis A, Bizzarro A, Sinisi AA, Bellastella G, Pane E, et al. Antipituitary antibodies after traumatic brain injury: is head trauma-induced pituitary dysfunction associated with autoimmunity? Eur J Endocrinol. 2008;159:7–13.
4. Alkhani A, Willinsky R, TerBrugge K. Spontaneous resolution of bilateral traumatic carotid cavernous fistulas and development of trans-sellar intercarotid vascular communication: case report. Surg Neurol. 1999;52:627–9.
5. Kanade A, Ruiz AE, Tornyos K, Wakabayashi I, Kastin AJ. Panhypopituitarism and anemia secondary to traumatic fracture of the sella turcica. J Endocrinol Invest. 1978;1:263–8.
6. Resneck JD, Lederman IR. Traumatic chiasmal syndrome associated with pneumocephalus and sellar fracture. Am J Ophthalmol. 1981;92:233–7.
7. Halimi P, Sigal R, Doyon D, Delivet S, Bouchard P, Pigeau I. Posttraumatic diabetes insipidus: MR demonstration of pituitary stalk rupture. J Comput Assist Tomogr. 1988;12:135–7.
8. Kojima T, Waga S, Furuno M. Fracture of the sella turcica. Neurosurgery. 1985;16:225–9.
9. Tanriverdi F, Senyurek H, Unluhizarci K, Selcuklu A, Casanueva FF, Kelestimur F. High risk of hypopituitarism after traumatic brain injury: a prospective investigation of anterior pituitary function in the acute phase and 12 months after trauma. J Clin Endocrinol Metab. 2006;91:2105–11.
10. Niederland T, Makovi H, Gál V, Andréka B, Abrahám CS, Kovács J. Abnormalities of pituitary function after traumatic brain injury in children. J Neurotrauma. 2007;24:119–27.
11. Klose M, Juul A, Struck J, Morgenthaler NG, Kosteljanetz M, Feldt-Rasmussen U. Acute and long-term pituitary insufficiency in traumatic brain injury: a prospective single-centre study. Clin Endocrinol (Oxf). 2007;67:598–606.
12. Agha A, Thornton E, O'Kelly P, Tormey W, Phillips J, Thompson CJ. Posterior pituitary dysfunction after traumatic brain injury. J Clin Endocrinol Metab. 2004;89:5987–92.
13. Tanriverdi F, De Bellis A, Ulutabanca H, Bizzarro A, Sinisi AA, Bellastella G, et al. A five year prospective investigation of anterior pituitary function after traumatic brain injury: is hypopituitarism long-term after head trauma associated with autoimmunity? J Neurotrauma. 2013;30:1426–33.
14. Callahan CD, Hinkebein JH. Assessment of anosmia after traumatic brain injury: performance characteristics of the University of Pennsylvania Smell Identification Test. J Head Trauma Rehabil. 2002;17:251–6.
15. Schechter PJ, Henkin RI. Abnormalities of taste and smell after head trauma. J Neurol Neurosurg Psychiatry. 1974;37: 802–10.
16. Callahan CD, Hinkebein J. Neuropsychological significance of anosmia following traumatic brain injury. J Head Trauma Rehabil. 1999;14:581–7.
17. Maiya B, Newcombe V, Nortje J, Bradley P, Bernard F, Chatfield D, et al. Magnetic resonance imaging changes in the pituitary gland following acute traumatic brain injury. Intensive Care Med. 2008;34:468–75.

18. Massol J, Humbert P, Cattin F, Bonneville JF. Post-traumatic diabetes insipidus and amenorrhea-galactorrhea syndrome after pituitary stalk rupture. Neuroradiology. 1987;29:299–300.
19. Ioachimescu AG, Hamrahian AH, Stevens M, Zimmerman RS. The pituitary stalk transection syndrome: multifaceted presentation in adulthood. Pituitary. 2012;15:405–11.
20. Schneider HJ, Sämann PG, Schneider M, Croce CG, Corneli G, Sievers C, et al. Pituitary imaging abnormalities in patients with and without hypopituitarism after traumatic brain injury. J Endocrinol Invest. 2007;30:RC9–12.
21. Mann NM, Vento JA. A study comparing SPECT and MRI in patients with anosmia after traumatic brain injury. Clin Nucl Med. 2006;31:458–62.
22. Salehi F, Kovacs K, Scheithauer BW, Pfeifer EA, Cusimano M. Histologic study of the human pituitary gland in acute traumatic brain injury. Brain Inj. 2007;21:651–6.
23. Hasegawa S, Yamagishi M, Nakano Y. Microscopic studies of human olfactory epithelia following traumatic anosmia. Arch Otorhinolaryngol. 1986;243:112–6.
24. Jafek BW, Eller PM, Esses BA, Moran DT. Post-traumatic anosmia. Ultrastructural correlates. Arch Neurol. 1989;46:300–4.
25. Ropposch T, Steger B, Meço C, Emesz M, Reitsamer H, Rasp G, Moser G. The effect of steroids in combination with optic nerve decompression surgery in traumatic optic neuropathy. Laryngoscope. 2013;123:1082–6.
26. Li H, Zhou B, Shi J, Cheng L, Wen W, Xu G. Treatment of traumatic optic neuropathy: our experience of endoscopic optic nerve decompression. J Laryngol Otol. 2008;122:1325–9.
27. Jimenez DF, Sundrani S, Barone CM. Posttraumatic anosmia in craniofacial trauma. J Craniomaxillofac Trauma. 1997;3:8–15.

Spontaneous, Traumatic, and Postoperative CSF Rhinorrhea

73

Gabriel Zada, M. Beatriz S. Lopes, Srinivasan Mukundan Jr., and Edward Laws Jr.

73.1 Epidemiology and Clinical Presentation

- Cerebrospinal fluid (CSF) rhinorrhea may occur when a communication (fistula) develops between the nasal cavity and subarachnoid space. For this to occur, the bone, dura, and arachnoid membrane must all be breached by the offending process. CSF rhinorrhea may develop spontaneously or as a result of a variety of inciting factors, including craniofacial trauma, surgery, radiation, or medical treatment.
- If left untreated, CSF rhinorrhea may result in meningitis, pneumocephalus, and intracranial hypotension.

73.1.1 Spontaneous CSF Rhinorrhea

- Spontaneous CSF rhinorrhea classically develops in obese patients with idiopathic intracranial hypertension, also known as pseudotumor cerebri. The condition is more common in middle-aged women, especially those with obesity and/or multiparity [1–3].
- The mean age of patients with spontaneous CSF rhinorrhea is 50–53 years [3, 4].
- Concomitant findings often associated with spontaneous CSF rhinorrhea include elevated intracranial pressure, meningoencephaloceles, visual loss, an empty sella, and skull base erosion [5].
- The most common locations of CSF fistulas causing rhinorrhea are the lateral lamina of the ethmoid and the fovea ethmoidalis [6].
- Spontaneous CSF rhinorrhea may also develop in the setting of a pituitary adenoma or other skull base tumor, most commonly following successful medical treatment of large, invasive prolactinomas. CSF leaks following radiation and radiosurgery have also been reported [7, 8].

73.1.2 Traumatic CSF Rhinorrhea

- The incidence of CSF rhinorrhea following traumatic brain injury is 4.6 % [9].

G. Zada, MD, MS (✉)
Department of Neurological Surgery, Keck School of Medicine, University of Southern California, 1200 N State Street, #3300, Los Angeles, CA 90033, USA
e-mail: gzada@usc.edu

M.B.S. Lopes, MD, PhD
Department of Pathology (Neuropathology), University of Virginia School of Medicine, 1215 Lee Street, Room 3060–HEP, Charlottesville, VA 22908, USA
e-mail: msl2e@virginia.edu

S. Mukundan Jr., PhD, MD
Department of Radiology, Brigham and Women's Hospital, 75 Francis Street, Boston, MA 02115, USA
e-mail: smukundan@partners.org

E. Laws Jr., MD
Department of Neurosurgery, Brigham and Women's Hospital, 15 Francis Street, Boston, MA 02115, USA
e-mail: elaws@partners.org

G. Zada et al. (eds.), *Atlas of Sellar and Parasellar Lesions: Clinical, Radiologic, and Pathologic Correlations*, DOI 10.1007/978-3-319-22855-6_73

- CSF rhinorrhea following traumatic brain injury may be associated with skull base fractures, visual loss, anosmia, hypopituitarism, vascular injuries, and meningoencephaloceles. (*See* the previous section on Traumatic Injury of the Sellar Region.)

73.1.3 Postoperative CSF Rhinorrhea

- Following standard transsphenoidal operations for pituitary tumors, the incidence of CSF rhinorrhea is as high as 10 %. In recent series, however, the usual incidence is 1–4 % [10].
- In extended endonasal endoscopic surgeries, the incidence of postoperative CSF rhinorrhea was initially as high as 58 %. The more frequent use of lumbar drainage and pedicled nasoseptal flaps, however, has greatly reduced this incidence to approximately 5 % [11, 12].

73.2 Imaging Features

- Plain axial CT imaging will often show pneumocephalus but is not highly sensitive in identifying the fistula site (Fig. 73.3).
- Thin-slice CT imaging with sagittal and coronal reconstruction will often show the site of the bony defect (>90 % sensitivity) and sometimes an encephalocele (Fig. 73.2) [13].
- CT cisternography is a highly effective modality for identifying the site of CSF fistula (Fig. 73.1). It often shows contrast extravasation through a bony defect and pooling in a paranasal sinus. The technique is accurate in over 90 % of patients, but only 30–40 % in the absence of an active CSF leak [14, 15].
- MR cisternography is also a highly effective test for identifying a specific CSF leak site, with a sensitivity of 92 % and specificity of 100 %. It often shows a T2-hyperintense column of CSF communicating between the subarachnoid space and sinuses (Fig. 73.4). An encephalocele may be seen, often with corresponding encephalomalacia, edema, and downward traction of the lobe of origin [14–17].
- Radionuclide cisternography can be used to confirm the presence of a skull base CSF leak and to aid in its localization [18].

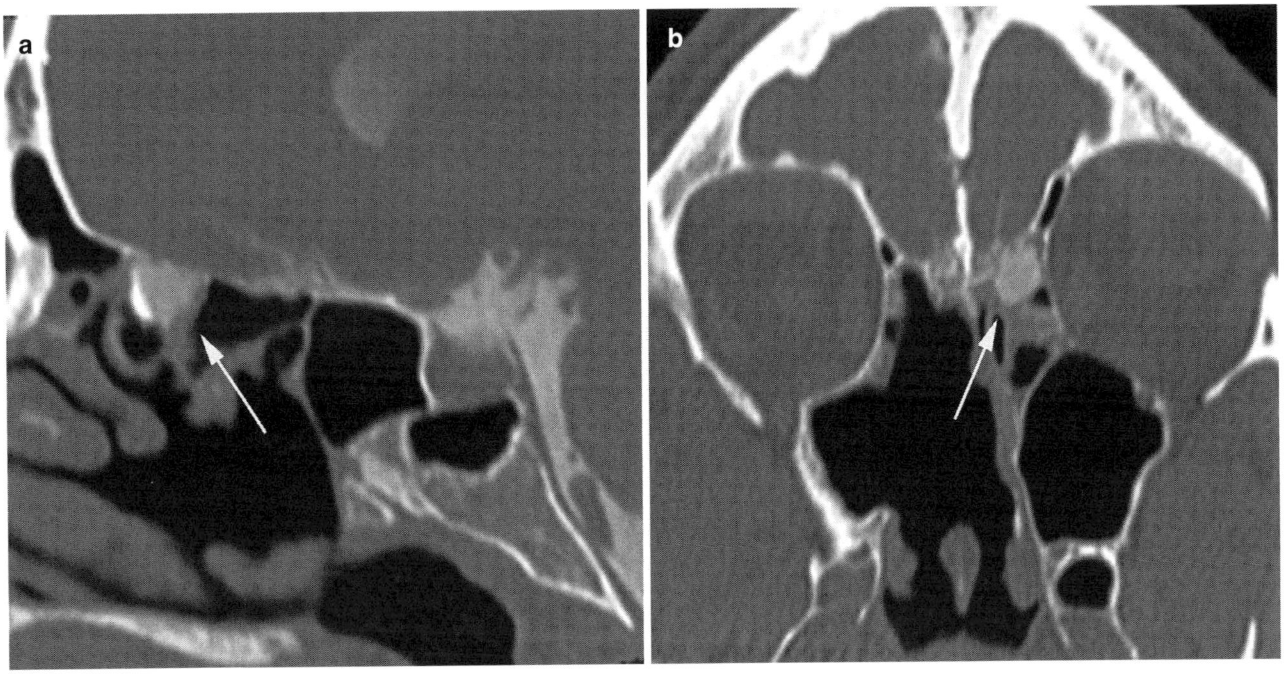

Fig. 73.1 CSF leak. (**a**) Sagittal CT cisternogram image. (**b**) Coronal CT cisternogram image. Postoperative changes from prior right ethmoid resection and medial maxillary antrostomy are present. In both images, contrast pooling is detected in one of the ethmoid air cells on the left, immediately below the roof (*arrows*), consistent with leakage of CSF. A bony defect is not directly visualized

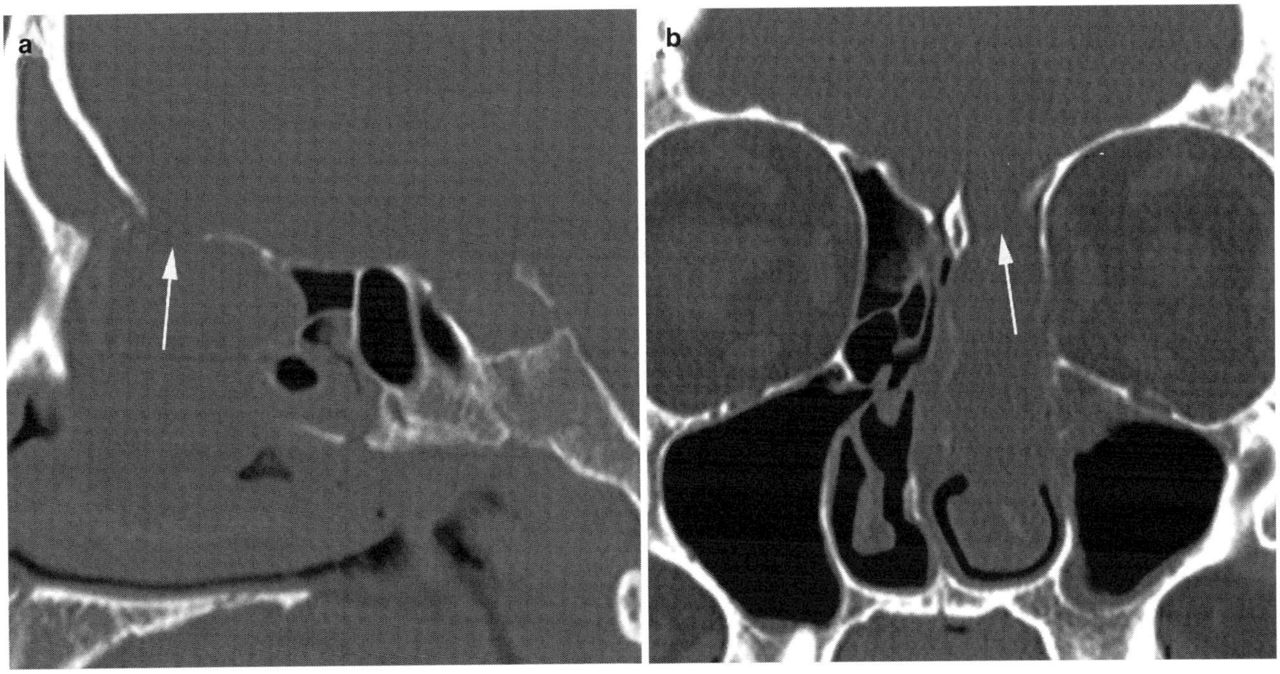

Fig. 73.2 CSF leak. (**a**) Sagittal CT image without contrast. (**b**) Coronal CT image without contrast. In both images, a bony defect is seen in the roof of the left ethmoid (*arrows*), with complete opacification of the left ethmoid air cells and part of the left nasal cavity

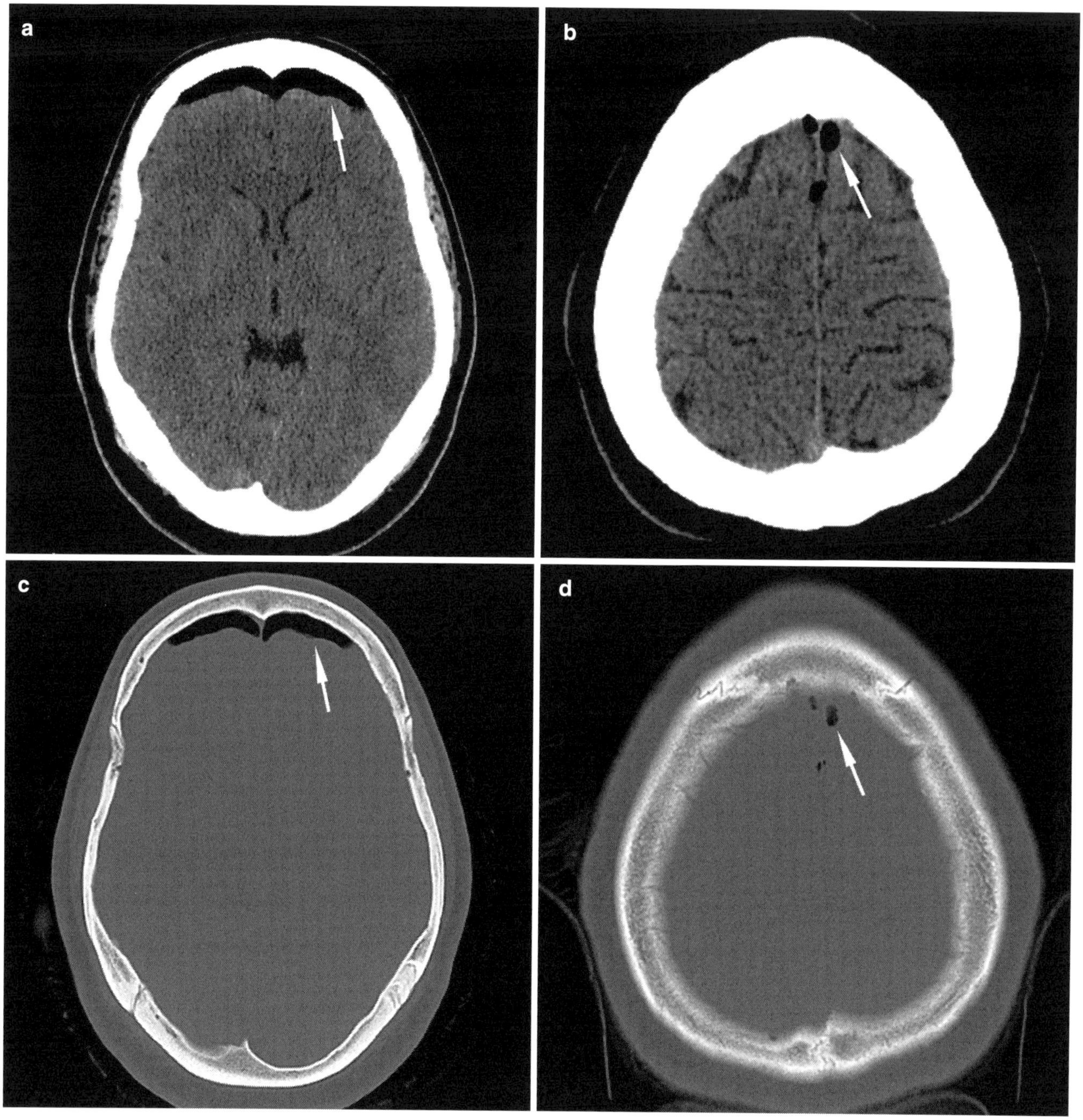

Fig. 73.3 CSF leak. Noncontrast axial CT images in a patient with a postoperative CSF leak following pituitary surgery. Images (**a**, **b**) are windowed for brain soft tissue, and images (**c**, **d**) are windowed for bone imaging. Pneumocephalus (*arrows*) can be seen in the frontal region in (**a**, **c**) and near the superior sagittal sinus, along the convexity, in (**b**, **d**)

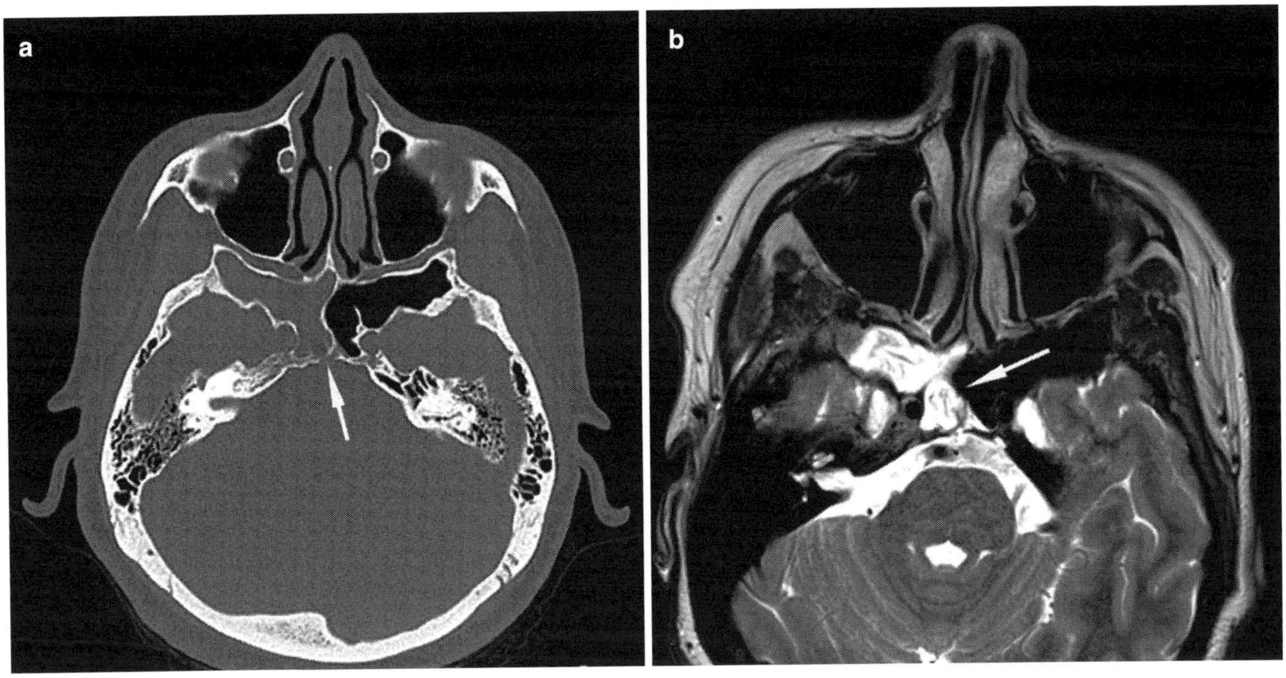

Fig. 73.4 CSF leak. Axial noncontrast CT image (**a**) and noncontrast T2-weighted MR image (**b**) in a patient with a CSF leak arising from the clivus and presenting with right-sided rhinorrhea. CT imaging shows the area of bony dehiscence (*arrow*) and opacification of the right sphenoid sinus (**a**). MR imaging shows T2-hyperintense CSF pooling (*arrow*) in the right sphenoid sinus (**b**)

73.3 Clinical and Surgical Management

73.3.1 Diagnosis of CSF Leaks

- In most patients, the diagnosis of CSF rhinorrhea is clinical. The rhinorrhea may be dependent on exertion or on position, worsening when the patient leans forward ("tilt test"). CSF leaks often appear as clear or blood-tinged fluid that looks like a drip from a faucet as a patient tilts forward. Also associated with CSF leaks is the "halo" sign, in which a yellowish ring forms on paper or gauze when CSF is present.
- Confirmation of CSF may be done via laboratory analysis for beta-2-transferrin, which is highly specific in differentiating CSF from other clear fluids such as nasal secretions or tears.
- A CT scan of the head may show pneumocephalus, which is highly suggestive of a CSF fistula.
- In some patients with CSF rhinorrhea, the exact fistula point cannot be identified with standard imaging. In these patients, tests such as CT cisternography or radionuclide cisternography studies can be performed to help identify the site of leakage [18].
- Intraoperatively, during a transsphenoidal operation, a Valsalva maneuver should be performed to assess for a CSF leak. Many postoperative CSF leaks develop because the leak was not identified during surgery, rather than representing a failed sellar repair [19].
- In other patients, the intraoperative use of intrathecal fluorescein can help to identify and confirm the fistula site [19, 20].

73.3.2 Management of CSF Rhinorrhea

- CSF leaks resolve spontaneously in some patients, depending on the etiology.
- Medical management with acetazolamide, which reduces the production of CSF and therefore reduces intracranial pressure, can be used as a temporizing measure. It may cause severe nausea and vomiting, however, which can exacerbate the CSF leak, so acetazolamide should be used only after weighing the risks and benefits.
- Lumbar punctures and temporary lumbar drains are often successful treatments for CSF leaks causing rhinorrhea. These maneuvers usually work for smaller leaks and those where there is sufficient tissue in place to form a permanent scar, or seal, at the fistula point.
- Many surgical options are available for repair of skull base CSF leaks, including autologous fat and fascia, dural substitutes, collagen sponge, fibrin glue, and dural sealants. Multilayer closures tend to offer the best chance of achieving a permanent repair.
- For larger leaks with wide bony deficits, the use of a rigid buttress may be beneficial. This can be crafted from bone (the vomer or turbinate), cartilage, titanium, or an absorbable synthetic plate.
- The use of pedicled nasal or temporalis flaps can be highly successful in closing larger skull base defects, greatly adding to the armamentarium of endoscopic skull base surgeons. The most commonly used flap is the pedicled nasoseptal flap [21–23].
- Patients with refractory CSF leaks despite multiple attempts at surgical repair often have underlying intracranial hypertension, and the definitive management option may be insertion of a CSF-diverting shunt, such as a permanent ventriculoperitoneal or lumbar-peritoneal shunt.
- Intracranial pressure may increase following successful repair of a CSF leak, causing new symptoms or leaks in other locations [4].
- Outcomes following CSF leak repair are generally excellent, with the leak being repaired on the first attempt in over 90 % of patients [4, 24].

References

1. Badia L, Loughran S, Lund V. Primary spontaneous cerebrospinal fluid rhinorrhea and obesity. Am J Rhinol. 2001;15:117–9.
2. Rosenfeld E, Dotan G, Kimchi TJ, Kesler A. Spontaneous cerebrospinal fluid otorrhea and rhinorrhea in idiopathic intracranial hypertension patients. J Neuroophthalmol. 2013;33:113–6.
3. Yang Z, Wang B, Wang C, Liu P. Primary spontaneous cerebrospinal fluid rhinorrhea: a symptom of idiopathic intracranial hypertension? J Neurosurg. 2011;115:165–70.
4. Chaaban MR, Illing E, Riley KO, Woodworth BA. Spontaneous cerebrospinal fluid leak repair: a five-year prospective evaluation. Laryngoscope. 2014;124:70–5.
5. Dempsey PK, Harbaugh RE. Encephalomeningocele presenting with spontaneous cerebrospinal fluid rhinorrhea in an elderly man: case report. Neurosurgery. 1988;23:637–40.
6. Tóth M, Selivanova O, Schaefer S, Mann W. Spontaneous cerebrospinal fluid rhinorrhea: a clinical and anatomical study. Laryngoscope. 2010;120:1724–9.
7. Hu Z, Godoy BL, Zadeh G. Spontaneous cerebrospinal fluid rhinorrhea secondary to anterior fossa osteoradionecrosis. J Clin Neurosci. 2013;20:1314–5.
8. Lam G, Mehta V, Zada G. Spontaneous and medically induced cerebrospinal fluid leakage in the setting of pituitary adenomas: review of the literature. Neurosurg Focus. 2012;32(6):E2.
9. Bell RB, Dierks EJ, Homer L, Potter BE. Management of cerebrospinal fluid leak associated with craniomaxillofacial trauma. J Oral Maxillofac Surg. 2004;62:676–84.
10. Ciric I, Ragin A, Baumgartner C, Pierce D. Complications of transsphenoidal surgery: results of a national survey, review of the literature, and personal experience. Neurosurgery. 1997;40:225–36; discussion 236–7.
11. Gardner PA, Kassam AB, Snyderman CH, Carrau RL, Mintz AH, Grahovac S, Stefko S. Outcomes following endoscopic, expanded endonasal resection of suprasellar craniopharyngiomas: a case series. J Neurosurg. 2008;109:6–16.
12. Gardner PA, Kassam AB, Thomas A, Snyderman CH, Carrau RL, Mintz AH, Prevedello DM. Endoscopic endonasal resection of

anterior cranial base meningiomas. Neurosurgery. 2008;63:36–52; discussion 52–4.
13. La Fata V, McLean N, Wise SK, DelGaudio JM, Hudgins PA. CSF leaks: correlation of high-resolution CT and multiplanar reformations with intraoperative endoscopic findings. AJNR Am J Neuroradiol. 2008;29:536–41.
14. Choong CC, Venkatesh SK, Phadke RV. Spontaneous cerebrospinal fluid rhinorrhoea: computed tomography and magnetic resonance imaging findings. Singapore Med J. 2013;54:176–80; quiz 181.
15. Shetty PG, Shroff MM, Sahani DV, Kirtane MV. Evaluation of high-resolution CT and MR cisternography in the diagnosis of cerebrospinal fluid fistula. AJNR Am J Neuroradiol. 1998;19: 633–9.
16. Schuknecht B, Simmen D, Briner HR, Holzmann D. Nontraumatic skull base defects with spontaneous CSF rhinorrhea and arachnoid herniation: imaging findings and correlation with endoscopic sinus surgery in 27 patients. AJNR Am J Neuroradiol. 2008;29:542–9.
17. Eljamel MS, Pidgeon CN, Toland J, Phillips JB, O'Dwyer AA. MRI cisternography, and the localization of CSF fistulae. Br J Neurosurg. 1994;8:433–7.
18. Kraft O, Safarcik K, Bartos V. Detection of spontaneous cerebrospinal fluid rhinorrhea. Hell J Nucl Med. 2004;7:56–7.
19. Jakimovski D, Bonci G, Attia M, Shao H, Hofstetter C, Tsiouris AJ, et al. Incidence and significance of intraoperative cerebrospinal fluid leak in endoscopic pituitary surgery using intrathecal fluorescein. World Neurosurg. 2014;82:e513–23.
20. Seth R, Rajasekaran K, Benninger MS, Batra PS. The utility of intrathecal fluorescein in cerebrospinal fluid leak repair. Otolaryngol Head Neck Surg. 2010;143:626–32.
21. Kassam AB, Thomas A, Carrau RL, Snyderman CH, Vescan A, Prevedello D, et al. Endoscopic reconstruction of the cranial base using a pedicled nasoseptal flap. Neurosurgery. 2008;63:ONS44–52; discussion ONS52–3.
22. Hadad G, Bassagasteguy L, Carrau RL, Mataza JC, Kassam A, Snyderman CH, Mintz A. A novel reconstructive technique after endoscopic expanded endonasal approaches: vascular pedicle nasoseptal flap. Laryngoscope. 2006;116:1882–6.
23. Patel MR, Taylor RJ, Hackman TG, Germanwala AV, Sasaki-Adams D, Ewend MG, Zanation AM. Beyond the nasoseptal flap: outcomes and pearls with secondary flaps in endoscopic endonasal skull base reconstruction. Laryngoscope. 2014;124:846–52.
24. Daele JJ, Goffart Y, Machiels S. Traumatic, iatrogenic, and spontaneous cerebrospinal fluid (CSF) leak: endoscopic repair. B-ENT. 2011;7:47–60.

Pseudoaneurysms of the Internal Carotid Artery in the Sellar Region

74

Gabriel Zada, M. Beatriz S. Lopes, Srinivasan Mukundan Jr., and Edward Laws Jr.

74.1 Epidemiology and Clinical Presentation

- A pseudoaneurysm (false aneurysm) develops when all three walls of an artery (intima, media, and adventitia) are violated. In the sellar region, pseudoaneurysms of the internal carotid artery (ICA) usually occur iatrogenically as a result of surgical injury.
- ICA pseudoaneurysms may also develop as a result of blunt or penetrating traumatic injuries [1].
- The incidence of ICA injury during transsphenoidal pituitary surgery is typically less than 1 % [2–4].
- In extended endoscopic endonasal operations for more complex skull base pathology, the incidence may be as high as 5 %.
- Intraoperative ICA injury is characterized by profuse arterial bleeding that is often accompanied by a rapid drop in systemic blood pressure.
- In some cases, no intraoperative ICA injury is seen, but a traumatic pseudoaneurysm is diagnosed in a delayed fashion.
- Delayed rupture of an ICA pseudoaneurysm may present with severe—sometimes fatal—epistaxis [5, 6].

G. Zada, MD, MS (✉)
Department of Neurological Surgery, Keck School of Medicine, University of Southern California, 1200 N State Street, #3300, Los Angeles, CA 90033, USA
e-mail: gzada@usc.edu

M.B.S. Lopes, MD, PhD
Department of Pathology (Neuropathology), University of Virginia School of Medicine, 1215 Lee Street, Room 3060–HEP, Charlottesville, VA 22908, USA
e-mail: msl2e@virginia.edu

S. Mukundan Jr., PhD, MD
Department of Radiology, Brigham and Women's Hospital, 75 Francis Street, Boston, MA 02115, USA
e-mail: smukundan@partners.org

E. Laws Jr., MD
Department of Neurosurgery, Brigham and Women's Hospital, 15 Francis Street, Boston, MA 02115, USA
e-mail: elaws@partners.org

G. Zada et al. (eds.), *Atlas of Sellar and Parasellar Lesions: Clinical, Radiologic, and Pathologic Correlations*, DOI 10.1007/978-3-319-22855-6_74

74.2 Imaging Features

- Digital subtraction angiography (DSA) is the gold standard modality for evaluation of the ICA following an acute injury. Findings shown may include a pseudoaneurysm, dissection, occlusion, contrast extravasation, or vessel wall irregularities (Figs. 74.1 and 74.2) [7].
- Noninvasive vascular imaging, such as CT angiography (CTA) and MR angiography (MRA), may be used as follow-up measures when angiography is not required [8].
- Any region of the ICA is susceptible to injury, including the paraclival ICA, cavernous ICA, and suprasellar ICA.

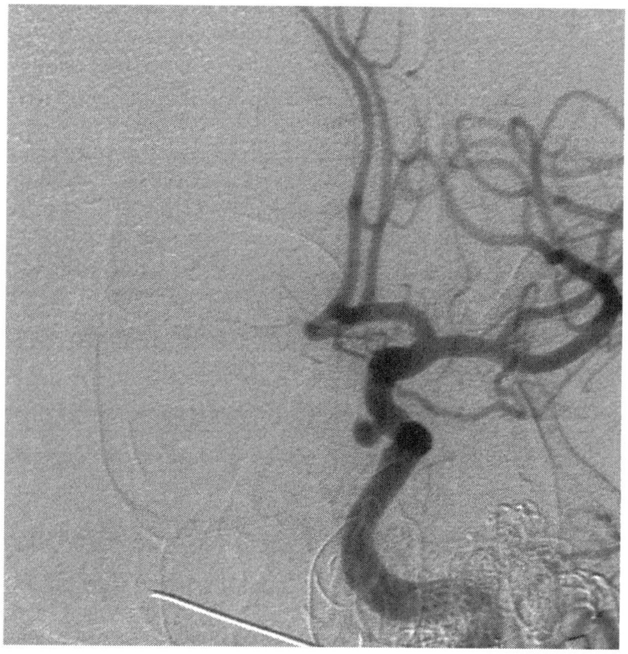

Fig. 74.1 Digital subtraction angiography (DSA) image of pseudoaneurysm. This anterior-posterior projection following left internal carotid artery (ICA) injection shows a small, medially projecting aneurysm arising from the cavernous segment of the ICA

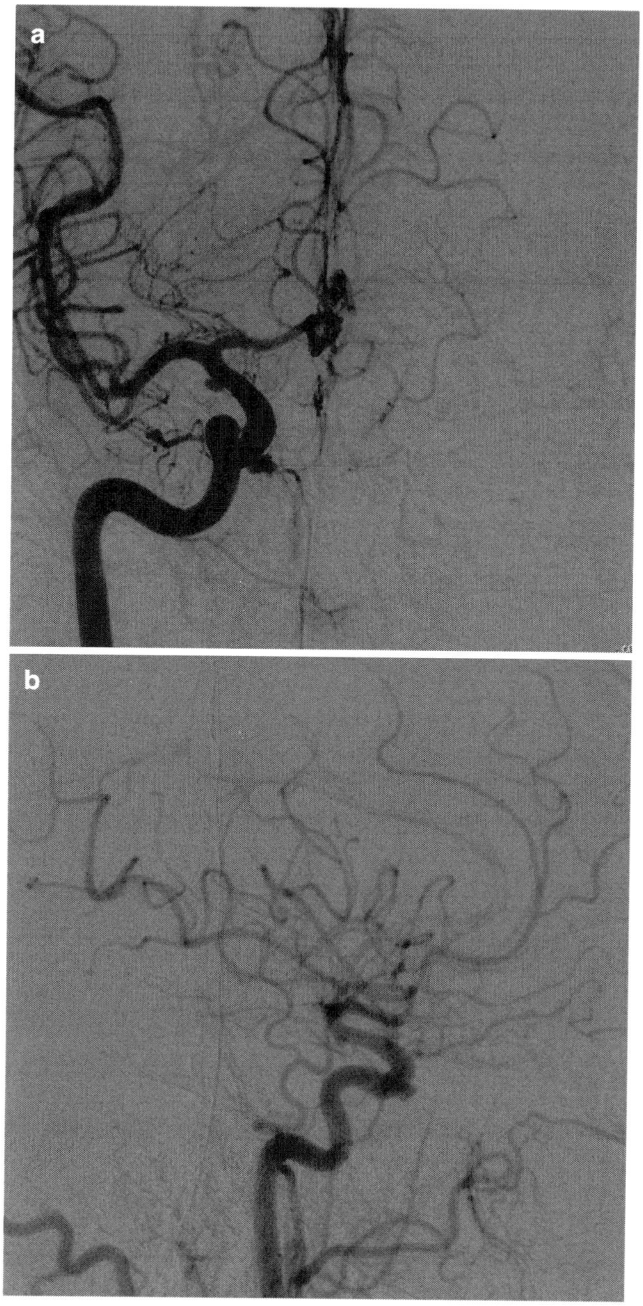

Fig. 74.2 DSA images of pseudoaneurysm. (**a**) Anterior-posterior projection. (**b**) Lateral projection following right common carotid artery (CCA) injection. An irregularly shaped, anteriorly/medially projecting aneurysm is seen arising from the cavernous segment of the ICA. An additional small, right supraclinoid aneurysm is also present, likely an incidental posterior communicating artery (PCOM) aneurysm

74.3 Clinical and Surgical Management

- Prevention of an ICA injury is of paramount importance for any endoscopic skull base operation. Several key steps can be used to minimize the risk of ICA injury, including optimal patient positioning, microDoppler ultrasonography, neuronavigation, and avoidance of sharp instruments in the region of the ICA [9].
- In the event of an intraoperative ICA injury, rapid packing of the site of bleeding is recommended. This often requires the use of optimal suctioning techniques and positioning of the endoscope, in order to identify the site and selectively pack it off. Possible packing materials include gelatin sponge, cottonoids, gauze sponges, or autologous muscle, fat, or fascia. Autologous muscle grafting is the prefered packing/repair material.
- It is critical to avoid overpacking the site of an acute arterial bleed, as overpacking may result in worsened avulsion or complete occlusion of the parent vessel.
- Close communication with the anesthesia team is mandatory in the event of an ICA injury. When possible, enough time should be given to allow them to catch up and stabilize the patient from a physiological standpoint, with fluids, pressors, blood, and so forth.
- Once the patient and the site of arterial injury have been stabilized, the patient is usually transported to the angiography suite for angiography and possible embolization of the pseudoaneurysm, which can be done using various techniques, including the use of coils, balloons, particles, or glue.
- In some cases, a patient's pseudoaneurysm will be temporarily embolized, and a definitive procedure (stent insertion or flow diversion with or without coiling) may be performed later, as such procedures often require concomitant anticoagulation [10].
- If the pseudoaneurysm cannot be successfully coiled, a number of endovascular and open surgical alternatives exist. A balloon test occlusion of the ICA may be performed, and the parent artery sacrificed if the patient passes the occlusion test. If occlusion of the ICA is not possible, some form of ECA-ICA bypass may be necessary to provide alternate means of perfusion prior to sacrificing the parent vessel.
- Frequent follow-up angiography is recommended to rule out recurrence of the pseudoaneurysm and to evaluate the patency of the parent vessel.
- Patients are often prescribed antiplatelet agents (e.g., aspirin) for a year or more following the injury and repair.

References

1. Magge D, Farber A, Vladimir F, Woodson J, Collins K, Shaw P, Gibbons G. Diagnosis and management of traumatic pseudoaneurysm of the carotid artery: case report and review of the literature. Vascular. 2008;16:350–5.
2. Gardner PA, Tormenti MJ, Pant H, Fernandez-Miranda JC, Snyderman CH, Horowitz MB. Carotid artery injury during endoscopic endonasal skull base surgery: incidence and outcomes. Neurosurgery. 2013;73:ons261–9; discussion ons269–70.
3. Laws Jr ER. Vascular complications of transsphenoidal surgery. Pituitary. 1999;2:163–70.
4. Ciric I, Ragin A, Baumgartner C, Pierce D. Complications of transsphenoidal surgery: results of a national survey, review of the literature, and personal experience. Neurosurgery. 1997;40:225–36; discussion 236–7.
5. Adeel M, Ikram M. Post-traumatic pseudoaneurysm of internal carotid artery: a cause of intractable epistaxis. BMJ Case Rep. 2012;2012. pii: bcr0220125927.
6. Chen D, Concus AP, Halbach VV, Cheung SW. Epistaxis originating from traumatic pseudoaneurysm of the internal carotid artery: diagnosis and endovascular therapy. Laryngoscope. 1998;108:326–31.
7. Cinar C, Bozkaya H, Parildar M, Oran I. Endovascular management of vascular injury during transsphenoidal surgery. Interv Neuroradiol. 2013;19:102–9.
8. Buerke B, Tombach B, Stoll W, Heindel W, Niederstadt T. Magnetic resonance angiography follow-up examinations to detect iatrogenic pseudoaneurysms following otorhinolaryngological surgery. J Laryngol Otol. 2007;121:698–701.
9. Dusick JR, Esposito F, Malkasian D, Kelly DF. Avoidance of carotid artery injuries in transsphenoidal surgery with the Doppler probe and micro-hook blades. Neurosurgery. 2007;60:322–8; discussion 328–9.
10. Amenta PS, Starke RM, Jabbour PM, Tjoumakaris SI, Gonzalez LF, Rosenwasser RH, et al. Successful treatment of a traumatic carotid pseudoaneurysm with the Pipeline stent: case report and review of the literature. Surg Neurol Int. 2012;3:160.

Iatrogenic Pituitary Abscess

75

Gabriel Zada, M. Beatriz S. Lopes, Srinivasan Mukundan Jr., and Edward Laws Jr.

75.1 Epidemiology and Clinical Presentation

- Spontaneous pituitary abscesses are rarely encountered; they represent less than 0.6 % of patients with sellar lesions undergoing surgical resection [1–3]. (*See* Chap. 51.)
- Acquired or iatrogenic pituitary abscesses are also uncommon. They develop rarely following cerebral trauma or transsphenoidal surgery, especially in the presence of a CSF leak. Iatrogenic abscesses are usually bacterial [4–6]. Risk factors for postoperative pituitary abscess include paranasal sinus disease and sphenoid sinusitis or a spontaneous or traumatic CSF leak. Sepsis is also known to be another inciting factor [2, 7–10].
- Pituitary abscesses may present clinically with headache, fever, hypopituitarism (85 %), meningitis, diabetes insipidus, visual loss, cranial nerve paresis, altered mental status, and/or toxemia [2, 10].
- Diabetes insipidus is relatively commonly in patients with sellar abscess, being present in up to 70 % at the time of diagnosis [10].
- The most common offending bacterial organisms are staphylococcus, streptococcus, and pneumococcus species [3, 6, 10].
- Only one third of patients have an increased peripheral white blood cell count [6].

G. Zada, MD, MS (✉)
Department of Neurological Surgery, Keck School of Medicine, University of Southern California, 1200 N State Street, #3300, Los Angeles, CA 90033, USA
e-mail: gzada@usc.edu

M.B.S. Lopes, MD, PhD
Department of Pathology (Neuropathology), University of Virginia School of Medicine, 1215 Lee Street, Room 3060–HEP, Charlottesville, VA 22908, USA
e-mail: msl2e@virginia.edu

S. Mukundan Jr., PhD, MD
Department of Radiology, Brigham and Women's Hospital, 75 Francis Street, Boston, MA 02115, USA
e-mail: smukundan@partners.org

E. Laws Jr., MD
Department of Neurosurgery, Brigham and Women's Hospital, 15 Francis Street, Boston, MA 02115, USA
e-mail: elaws@partners.org

G. Zada et al. (eds.), *Atlas of Sellar and Parasellar Lesions: Clinical, Radiologic, and Pathologic Correlations*, DOI 10.1007/978-3-319-22855-6_75

75.2 Imaging Features

- CT scan generally shows a homogenous, low-density mass with rim enhancement following contrast administration.
- MRI typically demonstrates a cystic mass with homogenous, low-intensity, or isointense signal on T1-weighted imaging and high-intensity signals on T2-weighted images, with rim enhancement following gadolinium administration (Fig. 75.1) [11, 12].
- Sellar abscess may seldom resemble a cystic or hemorrhagic pituitary adenoma, Rathke cleft cyst, or cystic craniopharyngioma [11].
- Restricted diffusion-weighted imaging (DWI) often supports the presence of a sellar abscess, but its usefulness is somewhat limited along the skull base and paranasal sinuses [13, 14].
- A thickened, enhancing infundibulum may be associated with sellar abscess on MRI with contrast [15, 16].

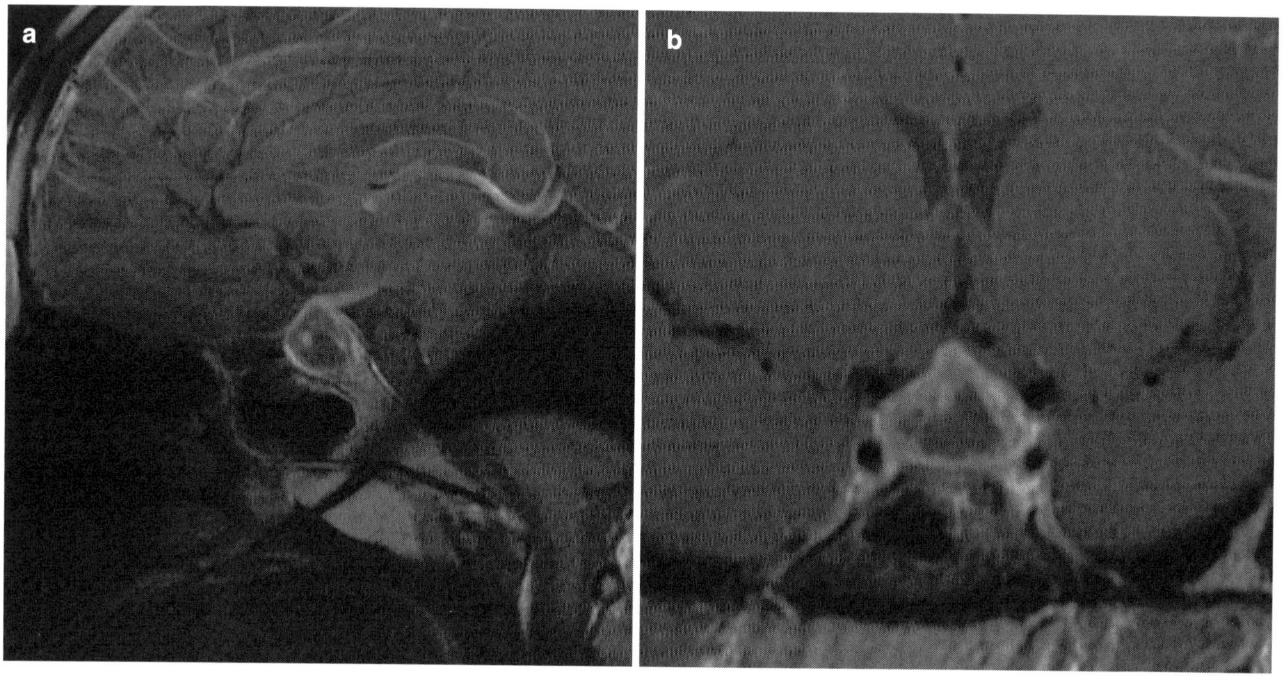

Fig. 75.1 Postoperative pituitary abscess. (**a**) Sagittal T1-weighted gadolinium-enhanced MR image. (**b**) Coronal T1-weighted gadolinium-enhanced image. A peripherally enhancing lesion in the sella displaces the pituitary stalk superiorly. The wall of the lesion is thick and irregular

75.3 Histopathology

- A wide variety of bacterial and fungal organisms have been implicated in the formation of sellar abscesses.
- Histopathology may demonstrate necrosis and abscess wall, with infiltration by polymorphonuclear leukocytes or macrophages [2].
- In over 80 % of cases, organisms are not isolated on cultures [10].
- PCR (polymerase chain reaction) testing may be useful in establishing a definitive diagnosis.

75.4 Clinical and Surgical Management

- The diagnosis of sellar abscess is often missed prior to surgery, but it should be considered for postoperative patients [10].
- The standard management includes transsphenoidal surgical drainage and marsupialization of the abscess wall [10, 17].
- In some cases, conservative management with antibiotics may be attempted, but there is little evidence to support this management strategy [18].
- Intraoperative cultures for aerobic, anaerobic, fungal, and acid-fast bacilli should be used.
- Sellar floor reconstruction is not recommended unless a CSF leak is present.
- For bacterial abscesses, intravenous antibiotics are typically required for at least 6 weeks after drainage.
- Tubercular or fungal abscesses should be treated with the appropriate antibiotic regimens.
- Symptoms from mass effect generally improve following drainage, whereas hypopituitarism typically fails to do so [6, 19].
- Recurrence rates have been reported to range from 0 to 18 % following surgical and antibiotic management of sellar abscess [6, 10].

References

1. Saeger W, Lüdecke DK, Buchfelder M, Fahlbusch R, Quabbe HJ, Petersenn S. Pathohistological classification of pituitary tumors: 10 years of experience with the German Pituitary Tumor Registry. Eur J Endocrinol. 2007;156:203–16.
2. Dutta P, Bhansali A, Singh P, Kotwal N, Pathak A, Kumar Y. Pituitary abscess: report of four cases and review of literature. Pituitary. 2006;9:267–73.
3. Jain KC, Varma A, Mahapatra AK. Pituitary abscess: a series of six cases. Br J Neurosurg. 1997;11:139–43.
4. Henegar MM, Koby MB, Silbergeld DL, Rich KM, Moran CJ. Intrasellar abscess following transsphenoidal surgery. Surg Neurol. 1996;45:183–8.
5. Sudhakar N, Ray A, Vafidis JA. Complications after transsphenoidal surgery: our experience and a review of the literature. Br J Neurosurg. 2004;18:507–12.
6. Vates GE, Berger MS, Wilson CB. Diagnosis and management of pituitary abscess: a review of twenty-four cases. J Neurosurg. 2001;95:233–41.
7. Verdalle P, Roquet E, Hor F, Raynal M, Courtois A, Bauduceau B, et al. Pituitary abscess. A rare complication of sinusitis. Rev Laryngol Otol Rhinol (Bord). 1997;118:327–9.
8. Somali MH, Anastasiou AL, Goulis DG, Polyzoides C, Avramides A. Pituitary abscess presenting with cranial nerve paresis. Case report and review of literature. J Endocrinol Invest. 2001;24:45–50.
9. Shono T, Nishio S, Muratani H, Yasuda T, Fukui M, Moutai K. Pituitary abscess secondary to isolated sphenoid sinusitis. Minim Invasive Neurosurg. 1999;42:204–6.
10. Zhang X, Sun J, Shen M, Shou X, Qiu H, Qiao N, et al. Diagnosis and minimally invasive surgery for the pituitary abscess: a review of twenty nine cases. Clin Neurol Neurosurg. 2012;114:957–61.
11. Wolansky LJ, Gallagher JD, Heary RF, Malantic GP, Dasmahapatra A, Shaderowfsky PD, Budhwani N. MRI of pituitary abscess: two cases and review of the literature. Neuroradiology. 1997;39: 499–503.
12. Sabbah P, Bonardel G, Herve R, Marjou F, Hor F, Pharaboz C, Bauduceau B. CT and MRI findings in primitive pituitary abscess: a case report and review of literature. J Neuroradiol. 1999;26:196–9.
13. Takayasu T, Yamasaki F, Tominaga A, Hidaka T, Arita K, Kurisu K. A pituitary abscess showing high signal intensity on diffusion-weighted imaging. Neurosurg Rev. 2006;29:246–8.
14. Taguchi Y, Yoshida K, Takashima S, Tanaka K. Diffusion-weighted MRI findings in a patient with pituitary abscess. Intern Med. 2012;51:683.
15. Sinha S, Singh AK, Tatke M, Singh D. Hypophyseal tuberculoma: direct radiosurgery is contraindicated for a lesion with a thickened pituitary stalk: case report. Neurosurgery. 2000;46:735–8; discussion 738–9.
16. Patankar T, Patkar D, Bunting T, Castillo M, Mukherji SK. Imaging in pituitary tuberculosis. Clin Imaging. 2000;24:89–92.
17. Ciappetta P, Calace A, D'Urso PI, De Candia N. Endoscopic treatment of pituitary abscess: two case reports and literature review. Neurosurg Rev. 2008;31:237–46; discussion 246.
18. Uchida Y, Tsuchimochi N, Oku M, Fujihara N, Shimono N, Okada K, Harada M. Successful treatment of pituitary abscess with oral administration of sparfloxacin. Intern Med. 2008;47: 1147–51.
19. Hernández I, Garcia L, Guinto G, Cabrera L, Mercado M. Bacterial pituitary abscess: an unusual cause of panhypopituitarism. Endocr Pract. 2002;8:424–8.

Index

G. Zada et al. (eds.), *Atlas of Sellar and Parasellar Lesions: Clinical, Radiologic, and Pathologic Correlations*,
DOI 10.1007/978-3-319-22855-6

D

S